3RD EDITION

T0195332

DRUG DISCOVERY AND DEVELOPMENT

TECHNOLOGY IN TRANSITION

Raymond G Hill, BPharm, PhD, DSc (hc), FMedSci, HonFBPhS
President Emeritus, British Pharmacological Society
Honorary Professor of Pharmacology
Imperial College
London

Duncan B Richards, MA, DM, FRCP, FFPM
Professor
Clinical Therapeutics
University of Oxford
United Kingdom

ELSEVIER

ELSEVIER

Copyright © 2022 by Elsevier Limited. All rights reserved.
Previous editions copyrighted 2005, and 2012.

No part of this publication may be reproduced or transmitted in any form or by any means, electronic or mechanical, including photocopying, recording, or any information storage and retrieval system, without permission in writing from the publisher. Details on how to seek permission, further information about the Publisher's permissions policies and our arrangements with organizations such as the Copyright Clearance Center and the Copyright Licensing Agency, can be found at our website: www.elsevier.com/permissions

This book and the individual contributions contained in it are protected under copyright by the Publisher (other than as may be noted herein).

Notices

Practitioners and researchers must always rely on their own experience and knowledge in evaluating and using any information, methods, compounds or experiments described herein. Because of rapid advances in the medical sciences, in particular, independent verification of diagnoses and drug dosages should be made. To the fullest extent of the law, no responsibility is assumed by Elsevier, authors, editors or contributors for any injury and/or damage to persons or property as a matter of products liability, negligence or otherwise, or from any use or operation of any methods, products, instructions, or ideas contained in the material herein.

ISBN: 978-0-7020-7804-0

Content Strategist: Alexandra Mortimer
Content Development Specialist: Andrae Akeh
Publishing Services Manager: Deepthi Unni
Project Manager: Haritha Dharmarajan
Design: Margaret Reid

Printed in India

Last digit is the print number: 9 8 7 6 5 4

Working together to grow libraries in developing countries

ELSEVIER · Book Aid International

www.elsevier.com · www.bookaid.org

Preface to 3rd edition

As the third edition goes into production, the globe is in the grip of the coronavirus disease 2019 (COVID-19) pandemic caused by severe acute respiratory syndrome coronavirus 2 (SARS-CoV-2). This has challenged world health systems on an unprecedented scale and disrupted the global economy in a profound way. Never has there been a greater need for rapid development of effective therapies, and the crisis has put the role of therapeutics and the pharmaceutical industry into sharp relief. Our current commercially based model for the discovery and development of novel therapeutics is based on healthy competition, expecting this will stimulate innovation and drive rapid progress. By contrast, a key feature of the response to COVID-19 has been an unprecedented degree of cooperation between regulators, payers, academics and industry to facilitate evaluation of novel and repurposed treatments. It is too early to say whether this cooperative model proves to be more efficient than the usual model, but many have shown a willingness to work together for public benefit in a way that has not been seen before.

The range of therapeutic modalities available to prosecute putative targets has never been wider and is expanding rapidly. Such is the pace of change that it is beyond the scope of any textbook to provide a definitive contemporary view of all the options. We have included sections on some of the most important novel modalities such as cell-based therapy and nucleotide-based treatments. Vaccination has long been the cornerstone of our fight against infectious disease, but the immunological principles have wider utility. In a new chapter on vaccines we review the current state of the art and look forward to opportunities for the future.

The traditional schema for development of a small-molecule drug is being disrupted by new technologies for drug discovery, safety assessment and approaches to clinical development. The updated chapters on these topics reflect the changing nature of discovery and development in a world where biological molecules are a substantial proportion of new medicines.

We have again tried to invite authors from the key constituencies of drug discovery and development so that large and small companies, contract research organisations and scientists and clinicians working in academic groups all have their voice.

We speculated on how the future might look in the preface to the second edition, and if we have learned anything in the intervening time it is that life becomes more rather than less unpredictable. Many new therapeutic agents and approaches have been introduced in the last 10 years and some long-term projects (such as oligonucleotide drugs) have at last reached the stage of becoming marketed products. The reduction in investment in pharmaceuticals research has been reversed and the industry looks in a healthy state as we again look forward to the future of our fascinating subject.

We hope that this new edition continues to fill the niche occupied by its predecessors and provides a primer for those studying drug discovery and development in the academic sphere, an introduction to the topic for those contemplating careers in the industry and a guide of where to look next for those already engaged with drug discovery but needing their knowledge refreshed.

DB Richards
RG Hill

Preface to 2nd Edition

The intention that we set out with when starting the task of editing this new edition was to bring the book fully up to date but to try to keep the style and ethos of the original. All of the chapters have been updated and many have been extensively revised or completely rewritten by new authors. There are two completely novel topics given chapters of their own (Protein Scaffolds as Antibody Replacements; Imaging in Clinical Drug Development) as these topics were judged to be of increasing importance for the future. There are a greater number of authors contributing to this new edition and an attempt has been made to recruit some of our new authors from the traditional stronghold of our subject in the large pharmaceutical companies but also to have contributions from individuals who work in biotechnology companies, academic institutions and CROs. These segments of the industry are of increasing importance in sustaining the flow of new drugs yet have a different culture and different needs to those of the bigger companies. We are living in turbulent times and the traditional models of drug discovery and development are being questioned. Rather than the leadership position in research being automatically held by traditional large pharmaceutical companies we now have the creative mixture of a small number of very large companies (often with a focus on outsourcing a large part of their research activities), a vigorous and growing biotechnology/small specialty pharmaceutical company sector and a significant number of academic institutions engaged in drug discovery. It is interesting to speculate on how the face of drug discovery may look 5 years from now but it will certainly be different with movement of significant research investment to growth economies such as China and a reduction in such investment being made in the US and Western Europe. We hope that this new edition continues to fill the need for a general guide and primer to drug discovery and development and has moved with the times to reflect the changing face of our industry.

RG Hill
HP Rang

Preface to 1st edition

A large pharmaceutical company is an exceptionally complex organization. Several features stand out. First, like any company, it must make a profit, and handle its finances efficiently in order to survive. Modern pharmaceutical companies are so large that they are financially comparable to a small nation, and the average cost of bringing a new drug to market – about $800m – is a sum that any government would think twice about committing.

Second, there is an underlying altruism in the mission of a pharmaceutical company, in the sense that its aim is to provide therapies that meet a significant medical need, and thereby relieve human suffering. Though cynics will point to examples where the profit motive seems to have prevailed over ethical and altruistic concerns, the fact remains that the modern pharmacopeia has enormous power to alleviate disease, and owes its existence almost entirely to the work of the pharmaceutical industry.

Third, the industry is research-based to an unusual extent. Biomedical science has arguably advanced more rapidly than any other domain of science in the last few decades, and new discoveries naturally create expectations that they will lead on improved therapies. Though discoveries in other fields may have profound implications for our understanding of the natural world, their relevance for improving the human condition is generally much less direct. For this reason, the pharmaceutical industry has to stay abreast of leading-edge scientific progress to a greater extent than most industries.

Finally, the products of the pharmaceutical industry have considerable social impact, producing benefits in terms of life expectancy and relief of disability, risks of adverse effects, changes in lifestyle – for example, the contraceptive pill – and financial pressures which affect healthcare policy on a national and international scale. In consequence, an elaborate, and constantly changing, regulatory system exists to control the approval of new drugs, and companies need to devote considerable resources to negotiating this tricky interface.

This book provides an introduction to the way a pharmaceutical company goes about its business of discovering and developing new drugs. The first part gives a brief historical account of the evolution of the industry from its origins in the mediaeval apothecaries' trade, and discusses the changing understanding of what we mean by disease, and what therapy aims to achieve, as well as summarizing case histories of the discovery and development of some important drugs.

The second part focuses on the science and technology involved in the discovery process, that is the stages by which a promising new chemical entity is identified, from the starting point of a medical need and an idea for addressing it. A chapter on biopharmaceuticals, whose discovery and development tend to follow routes somewhat different from synthetic compounds, is included here, as well as accounts of patent issues that arise in the discovery phase, and a chapter on research management in this environment. Managing drug discovery scientists can be likened in some ways to managing a team of huskies on a polar journey. Huskies provide the essential driving force, but are somewhat wayward and unpredictable creatures, prone to fighting each other, occasionally running off on their own, and inclined to bite the expedition leader. Success in husky terms means gaining the respect of other huskies, not of humans. (We must not, of course, push the analogy too far. Scientists, unlike huskies, do care about reaching the goal, and the project management plan – in my experience at least – does not involve killing them to feed their colleagues.)

The third section of the book deals with drug development, that is the work that has to be undertaken to turn the drug candidate that emerges from the discovery process into a product on the market, and a final chapter presents some facts and figures about the way the whole process operates in practice.

No small group on its own can produce a drug, and throughout the book there is strong emphasis on the need for interdisciplinary team-work. The main reason for writing it was to help individual specialists to understand better the work of colleagues who address different aspects of the problem. The incentive came from my own experience when, after a career in academic pharmacology, I joined Sandoz as a research director in 1985, motivated by a wish to see whether my knowledge of pharmacology could be put to use in developing useful new medicines. It was a world startlingly different from what I was used to, full of people – mostly very friendly and forthcoming – whose work I really did not understand. Even the research laboratories worked in a different way. Enjoyable though it was to explore this new territory, and to come to understand the language and preoccupations of colleagues in other disciplines, it would have been a lot quicker and more painless had I been able to read a book about it first! No such book existed, nor has any appeared since. Hence this book, which is aimed not only at scientists who want to understand better the broad range of activities involved in producing a new drug, but also non-scientists who want to understand the realities of drug discovery research. Inevitably, in covering such a broad range, the treatment has to be superficial, concentrating on general principles rather than technical details, but further reading is suggested for those seeking more detail. I am much indebted to my many friends and colleagues, especially to those who have taken the time to write chapters, but also to those with whom I have worked over the years and who taught me many valuable lessons.

It is hoped that those seeking a general guide to pharmaceutical R & D will find the book helpful.

H P Rang

Contributors

Paul Beswick, BSc, PhD
Director
UK Chemistry and IP
Bicycle Therapeutics
Cambridge, United Kingdom

Britta Bonn, MSc, PhD
Associate Director DMPK Design Leads and Biotransformation
Early Research and Development Respiratory and Inflammation,
Biopharmaceuticals R&D, AstraZeneca
Sweden

Federica Cappuccini, PhD
Senior Post-Doctoral Research Scientist
University of Oxford
United Kingdom

Helen Carnaghan, MB BChir (Cantab), BSc, MRCS, PhD
Clinical Trials Physician
GlaxoSmithKline, United Kingdom

Nicola Colclough, PhD
Principal Scientist, DMPK
Early Research and Development Oncology DMPK,
Oncology R&D, AstraZeneca
United Kingdom

Brian Cordery, MA (Oxon)
Partner
Bristows LLP
London
United Kingdom

David Cronk, CBiol. MRSB
Domainex Ltd
Great Chesterford
United Kingdom

Steven Grant, PhD
Scientific Leader
Biopharm Discovery
Medicine Design,
Medicinal Science & Technology (MST)
United Kingdom

Jeremy Griggs, PhD
Business Development
GlaxoSmithKline
Stevenage, United Kingdom

Stephanie Harlfinger, PhD
Principal Scientist
AstraZeneca, Oncology R&D, DMPK
United Kingdom

Constanze Hilgendorf, FCP, PhD
Associate Director ADME
DMPK Project Leader
Early Research and Development Cardiovascular Renal
and Metabolism, Biopharmaceuticals R&D, AstraZeneca
Sweden

Raymond G Hill, BPharm, PhD, DSc (hc), FMedSci, HonFBPhS
President Emeritus, British Pharmacological Society
Honorary Professor of Pharmacology
Imperial College
London, United Kingdom

Jakub Kopycinski, MSc, PhD
Senior Post-Doctoral Scientist
Nuffield Department of Medicine
University of Oxford
Oxford, United Kingdom

Vincent M Lawton, BSc, MSc, PhD CBE
Chairman
Addex Therapeutics
Switzerland

Bo Lindmark, MSc
DMPK Project Leader
Early Research and Development Cardiovascular Renal
and Metabolism, Biopharmaceuticals R&D, AstraZeneca
Sweden

Contributors

Antonio Llinas, MSc, PhD
Principal Scientist, Senior DMPK Design Lead
Early Research and Development Respiratory and Inflammation,
Biopharmaceuticals R&D, AstraZeneca
Sweden

Ricardo Macarrón, MSE, PhD
Vice-president of Applied Technology
Incyte
Wilmington, Delaware, USA

Paul M Matthews, MD, DPhil, FRCP, FMedSci
Edmond and Lily Safra Professor of Translational Neuroscience
and Therapeutics
Director, UK Dementia Research Centre at Imperial
Head of Department, Department of Brain Sciences
Imperial College London
London
United Kingdom

Philip Stephen Murphy, PhD
GlaxoSmithKline
United Kingdom

Chris Parkinson BSc, PhD, FTOPRA
Director, Therapeutic Groups
Global Regulatory Affairs
GlaxoSmithKline Research & Development Ltd
United Kingdom

Claire Phipps-Jones, MSc, GDL, LPP, PGDip
Senior Associate
Bristows LLP
Stevenage
United Kingdom

Kendall G Pitt, FRPharmS, AFIChemE, PhD
Senior Technical Director
Manufacturing, Science & Technology
Pharma Supply Chain, GSK
United Kingdom

Humphrey P Rang, MB, BS, MA, DPhil, FMedSci, FRS
Emeritus Professor of Pharmacology
University College London
London, United Kingdom

Duncan B Richards, MA, DM, FRCP, FFPM
Professor
Clinical Therapeutics
University of Oxford
Oxford, United Kingdom

Jim M Ritter, MA, DPhil, FRCP, FMedSci, HonFBPhS
Emeritus Professor
Clinical Pharmacology at King's College
London, United Kingdom

Lea Sarov-Blat, PhD
Senior Director
Human Genetics
GlaxoSmithKline
Philadelphia, USA

Joanne Shearer, PhD
Charles River Laboratories
Great Chesterford
United Kingdom

Rachel Tanner, DPhil (Oxon)
Post-Doctoral Research Scientist
The Jenner Institute, Nuffield Department of Medicine
University of Oxford
United Kingdom

Beth Williamson, BSc, PhD
DMPK Project Representative
Early Research and Development Oncology DMPK,
Oncology R&D, AstraZeneca
United Kingdom

Contents

Preface to 3rd Edition...iii
Preface to 2nd Edition.. iv
Preface to 1st Edition v
Contributors vii

Section 1: Introduction and background

1. The development of the pharmaceutical industry 1
Humphrey P Rang, Jim M Ritter

2. The nature of disease and the purpose of therapy 19
Duncan B Richards, Raymond G Hill

3. Therapeutic modalities...................................33
Duncan B Richards

Section 2: Drug discovery

4. Target selection 43
Ricardo Macarrón, Duncan B Richards, Lea Sarov-Blat

5. From drug target to drug discovery.................56
Jeremy Griggs

6. High-throughput screening...........................65
David Cronk, Joanne Shearer

7. The role of medicinal chemistry in the drug discovery process 91
Paul Beswick

8. Therapeutic antibodies................................. 108
Steven D Grant

9. Emerging modalities: nucleotide-based therapies, cell-based therapies, gene therapy 123
Helen Carnaghan, Raymond G Hill, Duncan B Richards

10. Metabolism and pharmacokinetic optimization strategies in drug discovery.......................................134
Beth Williamson, Britta Bonn, Bo Lindmark, Nicola Colclough, Stephanie Harlfinger, Antonio Llinas, Constanze Hilgendorf

11. Pharmacology 159
Duncan B Richards

12. Nonclinical safety assessment......................174
Duncan B Richards

13. Therapeutic vaccines...................................186
Federica Cappuccini, Jakub Kopycinski, Rachel Tanner

Section 3: Drug development

14. An introduction to drug development 217
Duncan B Richards, Raymond G Hill

15. Clinical assessment of safety.........................225
Duncan B Richards

16. Pharmaceutical development 234
Kendall G Pitt

17. Clinical development 245
Duncan B Richards

18. Clinical imaging in drug development 259
Philip Stephen Murphy, Paul M Matthews

19. Intellectual property in drug discovery and development..281
Brian Cordery, Claire Phipps-Jones

20. Regulatory affairs 290
Chris Parkinson

21. The role of pharmaceutical marketing 311
Vincent M Lawton

Section 4: Facts and figures

22. Drug discovery and development: the future? 332
Raymond G Hill, Duncan B Richards

Index 349

ix

Chapter | 1 |

The development of the pharmaceutical industry

Humphrey P Rang, Jim M Ritter

Antecedents and origins

Our task in this book is to give an account of the principles underlying drug discovery as it happens today, and to provide pointers to the future. The present situation, of course, represents merely the current frame of a long-running movie. To understand the significance of the different elements that appear in the frame, and to predict what is likely to change in the next few frames, we need to know something about what has gone before. In this chapter, we give a brief and selective account of some of the events and trends that have shaped the pharmaceutical industry. Most of the action in our metaphorical movie happened in the last 150 years, despite the film having started at the birth of civilization, some 10,000 years ago. The next decade or two will probably see at least as much change as the past century.

Many excellent and extensive histories of medicine and the pharmaceutical and biotechnology industries have been published, to which readers seeking more detailed information are referred (Bud, 1993; Caruthers, 1985; Mann, 1984; Porter, 1997; Sneader, 1985; Weatherall, 1990; see also Drews, 2000, 2003).

Plagues of infectious diseases arrived as soon as humans began to congregate in settlements about 5000 years ago. Early writings on papyrus and clay tablets describe many kinds of disease and list a wide variety of herbal and other remedies used to treat them. The earliest such surviving document, the famous Ebers papyrus, dating from around 1550 BCE, describes more than 800 such remedies. Disease was regarded as an affliction sent by the gods; consequently, the remedies were aimed partly at neutralizing or purging the affliction, and partly at appeasing the deities. Despite its essentially theistic basis, early medicine nevertheless discovered, through empiricism and common sense, many plant extracts whose pharmacological properties we recognize and still use today; their active principles include morphine, ephedrine, emetine, cannabis, senna and many others.[1]

In contrast to the ancient Egyptians, who would, one feels, have been completely unsympathetic to medical science had they been time-warped into the 21st century, the ancient Greeks might have felt much more at home in the present era. They sought to understand nature, work out its rules and apply them to alleviate disease, just as we aim to do today. The Hippocratic tradition had little time for theistic explanations. However, the Greeks were not experimenters, and so the basis of Greek medicine remained essentially theoretical. Their theories were philosophical constructs, whose perceived validity rested on their elegance and logical consistency; the idea of testing theory by experiment came much later, and this essential aspect of present-day science would have found no resonance in ancient Greece. The basic concept of four humours—black bile, yellow bile, blood and phlegm—proved, with the help of Greek reasoning, to be an extremely versatile framework for 'explaining' health and disease. Given the right starting point—cells, molecules and tissues instead of humours—they might quickly have come to terms with

---

[1] There were, it should be added, far more—such as extracts of asses' testicles, bats' eyes and crocodile dung—that have yet to find their way into modern medicine, although 'fecal transplantation' is currently attracting interest within conventional medicine (see, e.g., Kassam et al., 2013)—so never say never!

1

modern medicine. From a therapeutic perspective, Greek medicine placed rather little emphasis on herbal remedies, incorporating earlier teachings on the subject but making few advances of its own. The Greek traditions formed the basis of the CE 2nd century writings of Galen, whose influence dominated the practice of medicine in Europe well into the Renaissance. Other civilizations, notably Indian, Arabic and Chinese, developed their own medical traditions, which still flourish independently of Western medicine.

Despite growing scientific interest in herbal remedies from the 18th century onwards, it was only in the mid-19th century that chemistry and biology advanced sufficiently to give a scientific basis to drug therapy, and it was not until the beginning of the 20th century that this knowledge actually began to be applied to the discovery of new drugs. In the long interim, the apothecaries' trade flourished; closely controlled by guilds and apprenticeship schemes, it formed the supply route for various exotic preparations. Treatment failures were attributed to failure to use the right ingredients or to follow the recipe correctly, and elaborate systems to regulate the quality of ingredients and manufacture were developed by the professional bodies of apothecaries and physicians, long before requirements based on scientific evidence of safety or efficacy (Griffin, 2004). The early development of therapeutics—based mainly on superstition and on speculations that have been swept away by scientific advances—represents the prehistory of the pharmaceutical industry which retains few, if any, traces of it.[2]

Therapeutics in the 18th–19th centuries

Preventive medicine made spectacular early advances; for example, in controlling scurvy [Lind, 1763], vaccination [Jenner, 1798], curtailment of the London cholera epidemic of 1854 by disabling the Broad Street pump [Snow, 1854] and control of childbirth infection ('puerperal sepsis') and surgical infections using antiseptic techniques [Lister, 1867; Semmelweis, 1861]. In contrast, therapeutic medicine was virtually nonexistent until the end of the 19th century.

Oliver Wendell Holmes—a pillar of the medical establishment—wrote in 1860: 'I firmly believe that if

the whole materia medica, as now used, could be sunk to the bottom of the sea, it would be all the better for mankind—and the worse for the fishes' (see Porter, 1997). This may have been somewhat ungenerous, for some contemporary medicines—for example, digitalis, famously described by Withering in 1785, extract of willow bark (salicylic acid), and *Cinchona* extract (quinine)—had potentially beneficial pharmacological effects. But on balance, Holmes was right—medicines did more harm than good.

We can obtain an idea of the state of therapeutics in 1864 from the first edition of the *British Pharmacopoeia*, published in that year and which lists 311 preparations. Of these, 187 were plant-derived materials, only nine of which were purified substances. Many of the plant products—lemon juice, rose hips, yeast, etc.—are rich sources of vitamins and some—digitalis, castor oil, ergot, colchicum—are pharmacologically active sources of drugs as distinct from nutrients. Of the 311 preparations, 103 were 'chemicals', mainly inorganic—iodine, ferrous sulfate, sodium bicarbonate, and many toxic salts of bismuth, arsenic, lead and mercury—but also a few synthetic organic chemicals, such as diethyl ether and chloroform. The remainder comprised miscellaneous materials and a few animal products, such as lard, cantharidin and cochineal.

An industry begins to emerge

For the pharmaceutical industry, the transition from prehistory to actual history occurred late in the 19th century (3Q19C, as managers of today might like to call it), when three essential strands came together. These were: the evolving sciences of biomedicine (especially pharmacology, pathology and bacteriology); the emergence of synthetic organic chemistry and the development of a chemical industry in Europe, coupled with a medical supplies trade—the result of buoyant entrepreneurship, mainly in America.

Developments in biomedicine

Science began to be applied wholeheartedly to medicine—as to almost every other aspect of life—in the 19th century. Among the most important milestones from the point of view of drug discovery was the elaboration in 1858 of cell theory, by the German pathologist Rudolf Virchow. Virchow was a remarkable man: preeminent as a pathologist, he also designed the Berlin sewage system and instituted hygiene inspections in schools, and later became an active member of the Reichstag. The tremendous reductionist leap of the cell theory gave biology—and the pharmaceutical industry—the scientific foundation it needed. It is only

---

[2]Plenty of traces remain outside the pharmaceutical industry, in the form of a wide variety of 'alternative' and 'complementary' therapeutic procedures, such as herbalism, moxibustion, reflexology and acupuncture, whose underlying principles originated in the prescientific era and remain largely beyond the boundaries of science. It may not be long, given the growing appeal of such approaches in the public's eye, before the mainstream pharmaceutical industry decides that it must follow this trend. That will indeed be a challenge for drug discovery research.

by thinking of living systems in terms of the function of their cells that one can begin to understand how molecules affect them.

A second milestone was the birth of pharmacology as a scientific discipline when the world's first pharmacological institute was set up in 1847 at Dorpat by Rudolf Buchheim—literally by Buchheim himself, as the institute was in his own house and funded by him personally. It gained such recognition that the university built him a new one 13 years later. Buchheim foresaw that pharmacology as a science was needed to exploit the great advances in integrative physiology being made, in particular, by Claude Bernard and link this to therapeutics. Since this was at a time when organic chemistry and physiology were both in their cradles, and therapeutics was ineffectual, Buchheim's vision seems bold, if not slightly crazy. Nevertheless, his institute was a spectacular success. Although he made no truly seminal discoveries, Buchheim imposed on himself and his staff extremely high standards of experimentation and argument, which eclipsed the empiricism of the old therapeutic principles and attracted some exceptionally gifted students. Among these was the legendary Oswald Schmiedeberg, who later moved to Strasbourg, where he set up an institute of pharmacology of unrivalled size and grandeur, which soon became the Mecca for would-be pharmacologists all over the world.

A third milestone came with Louis Pasteur's germ theory of disease, proposed in Paris in 1878. A chemist by training, Pasteur's initial interest was in the process of fermentation of wine and beer, and the souring of milk. He showed that these were caused by microorganisms, and demonstrated famously, the potential for airborne infection. Particular organisms, he argued, were pathogenic to humans and accounted for many forms of disease, including anthrax, cholera and rabies. Pasteur successfully introduced several specific immunization procedures to protect against infectious diseases. Robert Koch, Pasteur's rival and near-contemporary, clinched the infection theory by articulating rigorous criteria for demonstrating disease causation ('Koch's postulates') and applying these experimentally in laboratory and clinic.

The founder of chemotherapy—some would say the founder of molecular pharmacology—was Paul Ehrlich (see Drews, 2004 for a brief biography). Born in 1854 and trained in pathology, Ehrlich became interested in histological stains and tested a wide range of synthetic dyes. He invented 'vital staining'—staining by dyes injected into living animals—and described how the chemical properties of the dyes, particularly their acidity and lipid solubility, influenced the distribution of dye to particular tissues and cellular structures. Thence came the idea of binding of molecules to specific cellular components, which directed not only Ehrlich's study of chemotherapeutic agents, but much of pharmacological thinking ever since. 'Receptor' and

'magic bullets' are Ehrlich's terms. He envisaged receptors as targets for toxins and systematically sought agents that would be selectively toxic to invading pathogens while leaving host cells unscathed. Working in Koch's institute, Ehrlich developed diphtheria antitoxin for clinical use and put forwards a theory of antibody action based on specific chemical recognition of microbial macromolecules, work for which he won the 1908 Nobel Prize. Ehrlich became director of his own institute in Frankfurt, close to a large dye works, and returned to his idea of using the specific binding properties of synthetic dyes to develop selective antimicrobial drugs.

Meanwhile, Langley (professor of physiology in Cambridge, UK) independently evolved the concept of 'receptive substances' capable of combining with agonists such as nicotine or pilocarpine or competitive antagonists such as 'curari' or atropine, foreshadowing the 20th century discoveries of acetylcholine as the mammalian neuromuscular transmitter and of its nicotinic and muscarinic receptors.

At this point, we interrupt the biological theme at the end of the 19th century, with Ehrlich in full flood, on the verge of introducing the first designer drugs, and turn to the chemical and commercial developments that were going on simultaneously.

Developments in chemistry

The first synthetic chemicals to be used for medical purposes were not therapeutic agents of themselves, but anaesthetics—enablers of the extraordinary advances in surgery that have occurred in the past 150 years. Diethyl ether ('sweet oil of vitriol') had been first made and described in 1540. Early in the 19th century, it and nitrous oxide (prepared by Humphrey Davy in 1799 and found—by experiments on himself—to have disinhibiting as well as stupefying properties) were used to liven up parties and sideshows, their usefulness as surgical anaesthetics was demonstrated, amid much controversy, only in the 1840s,[3] by which time chloroform had also made a controversial appearance. Its use during labour became socially acceptable after it was adopted by Queen Victoria during the birth of her last two children. Synthetic chemistry at the time could deal only with very simple molecules, made by recipe rather than reason, as our understanding of molecular structure was still in its infancy. The first therapeutic drug to come from synthetic chemistry was amyl nitrite, prepared in 1859 by Guthrie and introduced, because of

---

[3]An event welcomed, in his inimitable prose style, by Oliver Wendell Holmes in 1847: 'The knife is searching for disease, the pulleys are dragging back dislocated limbs – Nature herself is working out the primal curse which doomed the tenderest of her creatures to the sharpest of her trials, but the fierce extremity of suffering has been steeped in the waters of forgetfulness, and the deepest furrow in the knotted brow of agony has been smoothed forever'.

its vasodilator activity, for treating angina by Brunton in 1864—the first example of a drug born in a recognizably 'modern' way, through the application of synthetic chemistry, physiology and clinical medicine. This was a landmark indeed, for it was nearly 40 years before synthetic chemistry made any further significant contribution to therapeutics, and not until well into the 20th century that physiological and pharmacological knowledge began to be applied to the invention of new drugs.

It was during the latter half of the 19th century that the foundations of synthetic organic chemistry were laid, the impetus coming from work on aniline, a copious by-product of the coal-tar industry. An English chemist, Perkin, prepared a vivid purple compound, *mauvein*, from aniline in 1856. This discovery was a chemical accident, as Perkin's aim had been to synthesize quinine. Nevertheless, the discovery gave birth to the synthetic dyestuffs industry, which played a major part in establishing the commercial potential of synthetic organic chemistry—a technology which later became a lynchpin of the evolving pharmaceutical industry. A systematic approach to organic synthesis went hand in hand with improved understanding of chemical structure. Crucial steps were the establishment of the rules of chemical equivalence (valency), and the elucidation of the structure of benzene by Von Kekulé in 1865. The first representation of a structural formula depicting the bonds between atoms in two dimensions, based on valency rules, also appeared in 1865.[4]

The reason why Perkin had sought to synthesize quinine was that the drug, prepared from *Cinchona* bark, was much in demand for the treatment of malaria, a protozoal infection associated with high fever. Quinine was (wrongly, as it turned out) designated as an antipyretic drug and used to treat fevers of all kinds. Because quinine itself could not be synthesized, fragments of the molecule were made instead; these included antipyrine, phenacetin and various others, which were introduced with great success in the 1880s and 1890s. These were the first drugs to be 'designed' on chemical principles.[5]

The apothecaries' trade

Despite the lack of efficacy of the pharmaceutical preparations available in the 19th century, the apothecaries' trade flourished. Then, as now, physicians issued prescriptions to satisfy the expectations of their patients for some token of remedial intent. Prescriptions comprised individualized mixtures prepared by local apothecaries, often including plant extracts of unknown chemical composition. Early in the 19th century, a few enterprising chemists set about isolating the active substances from these plant extracts. This was a bold and inspired leap, and one that attracted a good deal of ridicule. Although the old idea of 'signatures', which held that plants owed their medicinal properties to their physical appearance,[6] was falling into disrepute, few were willing to accept that individual chemical substances could be responsible for the effects these plants produced, such as emesis, narcosis, purgation or suppression of fever. The trend began with Friedrich Sertürner, a junior apothecary in Westphalia, who in 1805 isolated and purified morphine, barely surviving a test of its potency on himself. This was the first 'alkaloid': a pharmacologically active nitrogenous base of plant origin. This discovery led to the isolation of several more alkaloids, including emetine, strychnine, caffeine and quinine, mainly by two remarkably prolific chemists, Caventou and Pelletier, working in Paris in the period 1810–25. The recognition that medicinal plants owed their properties to their individual chemical constituents, rather than to some intangible property associated with their living nature, marks a critical point in the history of the pharmaceutical industry. It was the starting point of two of the three strands from which the industry grew—the 'industrialization' of the apothecary's trade and the emergence of the science of pharmacology. And by revealing the chemical nature of medicinal preparations, it hinted at the possibility of making medicines artificially by organic synthesis and provided the impetus that turned the chemical industry, at a very early stage in its history, to making drugs.

The first local apothecary business to move, in 1827, into large-scale production and marketing of pharmaceuticals was the old-established Darmstadt firm Merck, founded in 1668, closely followed by other German- and Swiss-based apothecary businesses, several of which later evolved into giant pharmaceutical companies, such as Schering and Boehringer. The American pharmaceutical industry emerged in the middle of the 19th century. Squibb began in 1858, with ether as its main product.

---

[4]Its author, the Edinburgh chemist Alexander Crum Brown, was also a pioneer of pharmacology and was the first person to use a chemical reaction—quaternization of amines—to modify naturally occurring substances, such as strychnine and morphine. With Thomas Fraser, in 1868, he found that this drastically altered their pharmacological properties, changing strychnine, for example, from a convulsant to a paralysing agent. Although they knew neither the structures of these molecules nor the mechanisms by which they acted, theirs was the first systematic study of structure-activity relationships.

[5]These drugs belong pharmacologically to the class of nonsteroidal antiinflammatory drugs (NSAIDs), the most famous of which is aspirin (acetylsalicylic acid). Ironically, aspirin itself had been synthesized many years earlier, in 1855, with no pharmacological purpose in mind. It was developed commercially in 1899, subsequently generating huge revenues for Bayer, first as an antiinflammatory (a property it shares with other NSAIDs), and then as an antiplatelet drug for the prevention of arterial thrombosis.

[6]*Pulmonaria officinalis* (lungwort) was used to treat respiratory disorders because its leaves resembled lungs, saffron to treat jaundice, and so on; Hepatica nobilis, whose leaves were thought to resemble the three lobes of the liver, was used to treat liver disease—unfortunately so, since it contains a potent hepatotoxin (Oakley, 2015).

Soon after came the manufacturing chemists Parke Davis (1866) and Eli Lilly (1876). In the 1890s, Parke Davis became the world's largest pharmaceutical company, one of whose early successes was to purify crystalline adrenaline from adrenal glands and sell it in ampoules for injection. The US scientific community contested the adoption of the word 'adrenaline' as a trade name, but industry won the day, and American scientists were forced to call the hormone 'epinephrine'. Nowadays epinephrine autoinjectors had sales exceeding $1.5 billion in 2015, being used mainly for anaphylaxis and other allergic emergencies.

Bayer, Hoechst, Agfa, Sandoz, Geigy and others, which had begun not as apothecaries but as dyestuffs manufacturers, followed the move into pharmaceuticals. Notwithstanding the recent introduction of mauvein (discovered in 1856, see earlier) and related aniline dyes, the dyestuffs industry at that time was also still based largely on plant products, which had to be refined, and were sold in relatively small quantities, so the commercial parallels with the pharmaceutical industry were plain. Dye factories were usually located close to large rivers, accounting for the present-day location of many of the large European pharmaceutical companies. As we shall see, the link with the dyestuffs industry later came to have profound implications for drug discovery.

From about 1870—following Kekulé's elucidation of the structure of benzene—the dyestuffs industry turned increasingly to synthetic chemistry as a source of new products. Synthetic aromatic compounds, based on the benzene ring structure, remain prominent among therapeutically useful drugs. Understanding the nature of aromaticity was critical. Many of these dyestuffs companies saw the potential of the medicines business and, from 1880 onwards, moved into the area hitherto occupied by the apothecaries. The result was the first wave of companies ready to apply chemical technology to the production of medicines. Many of these founder companies remained in business for years, several names disappearing only in the late 20th century because of mergers and takeovers.

Thus the beginnings of a recognizable pharmaceutical industry date from about 1860 to 1880, its origins being in the apothecaries and medical supplies trades on the one hand and the dyestuffs industry on the other. In those early days, however, they had rather few products to sell; these were mainly inorganic compounds of varying degrees of toxicity and others best described as concoctions. Holmes (see earlier) dismissed the pharmacopoeia of 1860 as worse than useless.

To turn this ambitious new industry into a source of human benefit, rather than just corporate profit, required two things. First, it had to embrace the principles of pathology and pharmacology, which provided a basis for understanding how disease and drugs, respectively, affect the function of living organisms. Second, it had to embrace the principles of chemistry, going beyond the descriptors of colour, crystallinity, taste, volatility, etc., towards an understanding of the structure and properties of molecules, and how to make them in the laboratory. Both fields had made tremendous progress towards the end of the 19th century, so at the start of the 20th century the time was right for the industry to seize its chance. Nevertheless, several decades passed before the inventions coming from the industry began to make a major positive impact on the treatment of disease.

The industry enters the 20th century

By the end of the 19th century, various synthetic drugs had been made and tested, including the 'antipyretics' and various central nervous system depressants (see earlier). Chemical developments based on chloroform had produced chloral hydrate, the first nonvolatile CNS depressant, which was in clinical use for many years as a hypnotic (i.e., sleep-inducing) drug and is still sometimes used for this purpose in children in the UK. Independently, various compounds based on urea were found to have similar effects, and von Mering followed this lead to produce the first barbiturate, *barbitone* (since renamed barbital), which was introduced in 1903 by Bayer and gained widespread clinical use as a hypnotic, tranquillizer and antiepileptic drug—an early blockbuster. Almost simultaneously, Einthorn in Munich synthesized *procaine*, the first synthetic local anaesthetic, which followed the naturally occurring alkaloid cocaine. The local anaesthetic action of cocaine on the eye was discovered by Sigmund Freud and his ophthalmologist colleague Koeller in the late 19th century, and its use was heralded as a major advance for ophthalmic surgery. After several chemists had tried, with limited success, to make synthetic compounds with the same actions, procaine was finally produced and introduced commercially in 1905 by Hoechst. Barbitone and procaine were triumphs of chemical ingenuity but owed little or nothing to physiology or pharmacology. Indeed, 70 years elapsed before the mechanisms of action of these agents were elucidated at the molecular level.

From this stage, where chemistry began to make an impact on drug discovery, up to the last quarter of the 20th century, when molecular biology began to emerge as a dominant technology, we can discern three main routes by which new drugs were discovered: chemistry-driven approaches, target-directed approaches and accidental clinical discoveries. In many of the most successful case histories, graphically described by Weatherall (1990), the three were closely interwoven. The remarkable family of diverse and important drugs that came from the original sulfonamide lead, described later, exemplifies this pattern very well.

Chemistry-driven drug discovery

Synthetic chemistry

The pattern of drug discovery driven by synthetic chemistry—with biology often struggling to keep up—emerged in the early part of the 20th century and prevailed for at least 50 years. The balance of research in the pharmaceutical industry up to the 1970s placed chemistry as the key discipline in drug discovery, the task of biologists being mainly to devise and perform assays capable of revealing possible useful therapeutic activity among the many anonymous white powders that arrived for testing. Research management in the industry was largely in the hands of chemists. This strategy produced many successes, including antiepileptic, antihypertensive, antidepressant and antipsychotic drugs. The surviving practice of classifying many drugs based on their chemical structure (e.g., phenothiazines, benzodiazepines, thiazides, etc.), rather than on the more logical basis of their site or mode of action, stems from this era. The development of antiepileptic drugs exemplifies this approach well. Following the success of barbital (see earlier), several related compounds were made, including the phenyl derivative *phenobarbital*, first made in 1911. This proved to be an effective hypnotic drug, helpful in allowing peaceful nights in a ward full of restive patients. By chance, it was found by Alfred Hauptmann also to reduce the frequency of seizures when tested in epileptic patients—an example of clinical serendipity (see later), possibly prompted by the known anticonvulsant effect of sedatives such as bromide (Yasiri & Shorvon, 2012)—and it became widely used as an anticonvulsant. Phenobarbital proved more effective for this indication than barbital itself. About 20 years later, Putnam, working in Boston, developed a model of epilepsy-like seizures in mice by electrical stimulation of the brain via extracranial electrodes. This simple model allowed hundreds of compounds to be tested for potential antiepileptic activity, *phenytoin* being an early success, followed by *carbamazepine*, *valproate* and others. Clinical serendipity subsequently led to repurposing of several such agents as mood stabilizers for bipolar disorder and as analgesics for neuropathic pain. None of this relied on an understanding of the mechanism of action of these compounds—which remains controversial; what was needed were green-fingered chemists, a robust bioassay that predicted efficacy in the clinic and astute clinicians aided by clinical registers.

Natural product chemistry

We have mentioned the early days of pharmacology, and purification of plant-derived drugs such as *morphine, atropine, tubocurarine, strychnine, digitalis* and *ergot alkaloids*, which predominated in the clinic until well into the 20th century. Despite the rise of synthetic chemistry, natural products remain a significant source of new drugs, particularly in the field of chemotherapy but also in other applications. Following the discovery of *penicillin* by Fleming in 1929—described by Mann (1984) as 'the most important medical discovery of all time'—and its development as an antibiotic for clinical use by Chain and Florey in 1938, an intense search was undertaken for antibacterial compounds produced by fungi and other microorganisms, much of it in academic/industry collaborations; for example, that between Merck, who developed the process for manufacturing penicillin at Rutgers University, and an academic group at Rutgers led by Selman Waksman. This approach yielded many useful antibiotics, including *chloramphenicol* (1947), *tetracyclines* (1948), *streptomycin* (1949) and *ivermectin* (1981), an antiparasitic drug which, after 20 years as the world's top-selling veterinary product, has raised hopes for the global eradication of major human diseases including river blindness (onchocerciasis) and filarial lymphedema (elephantiasis). The same bacterial source (*Actinomyces*) that yielded streptomycin also yielded *actinomycin D*, which was isolated by Waksman and Woodruff in 1940 and approved by the US Food and Drug Administration (FDA) in 1964, the first antibiotic with demonstrated anticancer activity. It binds DNA, blocking its transcription, and is now mainly used therapeutically to treat childhood cancers such as Wilms' tumour and Ewing's sarcoma. Plants have continued to yield useful drugs, including *vincristine* and *vinblastine* (1958) and *paclitaxel* (1971). *Artemisinin*, extracted from sweet wormwood in a Chinese programme originating in the 1960s in response to chloroquine-resistant malaria in Vietnam (Youyou, 2015), has saved millions of lives worldwide.

Outside the field of chemotherapy, successful drugs derived from natural products include *ciclosporin* (1972) and *tacrolimus* (1993), fungal-derived immunosuppressants, and *mevastatin* (1976), another fungal metabolite, which was the first of the 'statin' series of cholesterol-lowering drugs that act by inhibiting HMG CoA reductase.

The pharmaceutical industry continues to have something of a love–hate relationship with such plant- or microorganism-derived natural products. They often have weird and wonderful structures that cause hardened chemists to turn pale; they are often near-impossible to synthesize, troublesome to produce from natural sources and 'optimizing' such molecules to make them suitable for therapeutic use is akin to remodelling Westminster Abbey to improve its acoustics. But the fact remains that Nature unexpectedly provides some of our most useful drugs, evolved over millennia presumably during various interspecies 'arms races', with much untapped potential.

Animal-derived natural products have also featured in the pharmacopeia since the early 20th century and have exploded in importance with the introduction of recombinant proteins, monoclonal antibodies (Galfré & Milstein, 1981) and oligonucleotides (Caruthers, 1985). In addition to *adrenaline* and *insulin* (mentioned earlier), natural desiccated thyroid hormones from pig thyroid glands provided effective replacement therapy for hypothyroidism. *Thyroxine* was synthesized by Harington and Barger [1926], and synthetic L-thyroxine is now standard for replacement therapy. Banting and Best in collaboration with Macleod succeeded in extracting biologically active *insulin* in 1920, initially from dogs, and later from calves, and then adult bovines, and subsequent collaboration with Eli Lilly led to a commercially viable method; soon after (1923) Hagedorn founded the Nordisk Insulinlaboratorium in Denmark—forerunner of today's Novo Nordisk. Different formulations of animal insulins (pig and beef) remained standard until recombinant technology led to the introduction by Novo Nordisk of human insulin in 1988 and 'designer' variants such as *insulin lispro* [Lilly, 1996] and *glargine* [Sanofi-Aventis, 2000] modified to optimize their pharmacokinetic properties.

Target-directed drug discovery

Although chemistry was the preeminent discipline in drug discovery until the 1970s, the seeds of the biological revolution had long since been sown and began to bear fruit quite early within the chemistry-led culture of the pharmaceutical industry. This happened most notably in the field of chemotherapy, where Ehrlich played such an important role as the first 'modernist' who defined the principles of drug specificity in terms of a specific interaction between the drug molecule and a target molecule—the 'receptive substance'—in the organism, an idea summarized in his famous Latin catchphrase *Corpora non agunt nisi fixata*. Although we now take it for granted that the chemical nature of the target molecule, as well as that of the drug molecule, determines what effects a drug will produce, nobody before Ehrlich had envisaged drug action in this way. By linking chemistry and biology, Ehrlich effectively set the stage for drug discovery in the modern style. But despite Ehrlich's seminal role in the evolution of the pharmaceutical industry, discoveries in his favourite field of endeavour, chemotherapy, remain empirical as well as target directed, with important new therapeutic drugs such as the taxanes and artemisinin continuing to emerge through a combination of serendipity and sophisticated chemistry.

Indeed, Ehrlich's preoccupation with the binding of chemical dyes, as exemplified by biological stains, for specific constituents of cells and tissues, turned out to be misplaced, and not applicable to the problem of achieving selective toxicity. Although he soon came to realize that the dye-binding moieties of cells were not equivalent

to the hypothesized drug-binding moieties, neither he nor any of his contemporaries succeeded in identifying the latter and using them as defined targets for new compounds. The history of successes in the field of chemotherapy prior to the antibiotic era, some of which are listed in Table 1.1, represents a series of striking achievements in synthetic chemistry, coupled to the development of assay systems in animals, according to the chemistry-led model that we have already discussed. The use of bioassay was key to discovering the unexpected activities of chemical variants (e.g., diuretic and hypoglycaemic actions of sulfonamide derivatives, see later), as well as the in vivo antibacterial activity of prodrugs such as Prontosil—see later. This potential for serendipity remains an advantage of bioassay over the vastly more specific and precise physical assays, such as mass spectrometry. Bioassay enabled, for example, the discovery of prostacyclin during a search in vascular tissue for a mediator (thromboxane) with opposite pharmacological properties.

The popular image of 'magic bullets' designed to home in, like cruise missiles, on defined targets is actually a misleading one in the context of the early days of chemotherapy, but there is no doubt that Ehrlich's thinking prepared the ground for the steady advance of target-directed approaches to drug discovery, a trend that, from the 1950s onwards, steadily shifted the industry's focus from chemistry to biology (Lednicer, 1993; Maxwell & Eckhardt, 1990). A few selected case histories exemplify this general trend.

The sulfonamide story

Ehrlich's discovery in 1910 of *Salvarsan* ('Compound 606'), and its success over the next 40 years in treating syphilis, was triumphant proof of the concept of selective toxicity in antimicrobial therapy. However, other common bacterial infections, such as pneumonia and wound infections, proved unresponsive to drug treatment for many years, despite strenuous efforts of the pharmaceutical industry. In 1927, IG Farbenindustrie, which had a long-standing interest in discovering antimicrobial drugs, appointed Gerhard Domagk to direct their research. Among the various leads that he followed was a series of azo dyes, including some sulfonamide derivatives (a modification introduced earlier into dyestuffs to improve their affinity for certain fibres). These were much more effective in animals, and less toxic, than anything that had gone before, and *Prontosil*—a dark-red azo dye—was introduced in 1935. In the same year, it cured Domagk's daughter, who had developed septicaemia after a needle prick. It was soon discovered that the azo linkage in the Prontosil molecule was rapidly cleaved in the body, yielding the colourless compound *sulfanilamide*, which accounted for the antibacterial effect of Prontosil. If

Table 1.1 Examples of drugs from different sources: natural products, synthetic chemistry and biopharmaceuticals

Natural products (extracted from microorganisms, plants or animal tissue)	Synthetic chemistry	Biopharmaceuticals (synthesized either by recombinant technology or from hybridoma clones)
Antibiotics (penicillin, streptomycin, tetracyclines, cephalosporins, etc.) Anticancer drugs (doxorubicin, bleomycin, actinomycin, vincristine, vinblastine, paclitaxel (Taxol), etc.) Atropine, hyoscine Ciclosporin Cocaine Colchicine Digitalis (digoxin) Ephedrine Heparin	Early successes include: Antiepileptic drugs Antihypertensive drugs Antimetabolites Barbiturates Bronchodilators Diuretics Local anaesthetics Sulfonamides (*Since c.1950, more new drugs have been synthetic chemicals than natural products.*)	Human insulin (the first biotech product, registered 1982) Human growth hormone α-Interferon, γ-interferon Hepatitis B vaccine Tissue plasminogen activator (t-PA) Hirudin-derived antithrombin drugs Blood clotting factors Erythropoietin G-CSF, GM-CSF Infliximab (chimeric monoclonal TNF antagonist) Adalimumab (fully human monoclonal TNF antagonist marketed since 2002) (*Biopharmaceuticals accounted for approximately 25%–30% of new drug approvals from 2012 to 2018.*)
Opium alkaloids (morphine, papaverine) Physostigmine *Rauwolfia* alkaloids (reserpine) Statins Streptokinase Tubocurarine Vaccines		

G-CSF, Granulocyte colony-stimulating factor; *GM-CSF,* granulocyte macrophage colony-stimulating factor; *TNF,* tumour necrosis factor.

Prontosil had been screened only for in vitro activity against cultured bacteria, it would have appeared to be inactive.

With chemistry still firmly in the driving seat, and little concern about mechanisms or targets, many sulfonamides were made in the next few years. These dramatically improved the prognosis of patients suffering from acute bacterial infections including, notably, infection following childbirth—puerperal sepsis—previously a major cause of maternal mortality.

The mechanistic light began to dawn in 1940, when D. D. Woods, a microbiologist in Oxford, discovered that the antibacterial effect of sulfonamides was antagonized by *p*-aminobenzoic acid (PABA), a closely related compound and a precursor in the biosynthesis of folic acid (Fig. 1.1). Bacteria, unlike eukaryotic cells, must synthesize their own folic acid to support DNA synthesis. Woods deduced that sulfonamides compete with PABA for a target enzyme, now known to be dihydropteroate synthase, and thus prevent folic acid synthesis.

The discovery of sulfonamides and the elucidation of their mechanism of action had great repercussions, scientifically as well as clinically. In the drug discovery field, it set off two major lines of inquiry. First, the sulfonamide structure proved to be a rich source of molecules with many different, and useful, pharmacological properties—an exuberant vindication of the chemistry-led approach to drug discovery. Second, attacking the folic acid pathway proved to be a highly successful strategy for producing therapeutically useful drugs—a powerful boost for the 'targeteers'.

The chemical dynasty originating with sulfanilamide is shown in Fig. 1.2. An early spin-off came from the clinical observation that some sulfonamides produced an alkaline diuresis, associated with an increased excretion of sodium bicarbonate in the urine. Carbonic anhydrase, an enzyme which catalyses the interconversion of carbon

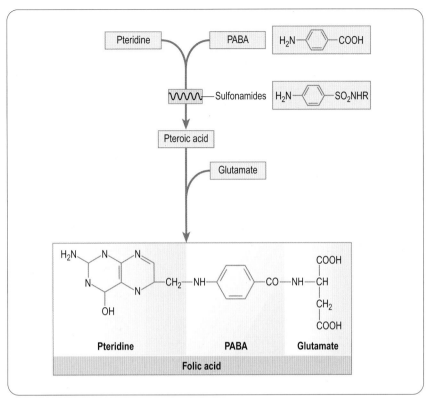

Fig. 1.1 Folic acid synthesis and *p*-aminobenzoic acid (PABA).

dioxide and carbonic acid, was described in 1940, and its role in renal bicarbonate excretion was discovered a few years later, presaging the finding that some, but not all, sulfonamides inhibit this enzyme. Modification of the sulfonamide structure led eventually to the introduction of *acetazolamide,* the first commercially available carbonic anhydrase inhibitor, as a diuretic in 1952. Carbonic anhydrase is involved in forming the aqueous humour in the eye and acetazolamide, or its derivative *dorzolamide,* which is administered topically as eye drops, is still used therapeutically to lower intraocular pressure in patients with glaucoma. Following the diuretic trail led in turn to *chlorothiazide* (1957), the first of the thiazide diuretics. These are much more effective than acetazolamide in increasing sodium excretion, acting as subsequently determined via inhibition of distal tubular Na^+/Cl^- cotransport rather than inhibition of carbonic anhydrase, and which remain mainstays in the treatment of arterial hypertension. Further modifications led to *furosemide* (1962), the first of the loop diuretics that work by inhibiting $Na^+/K^+/2Cl^-$ co-transport in the thick ascending limb of Henle's loop. These are more effective than thiazides in causing a diuresis and remain central in the treatment of heart failure and other disorders characterized by Na^+ overload. Other modifications of the thiazide structures led to the accidental but important discovery of hypotensive vasodilator drugs, such as *hydralazine* and *diazoxide*. In yet another development, *carbutamide,* one of the sulfonamides synthesized by Boehringer in 1954 as part of an antibacterial drug programme, was found accidentally to cause hypoglycaemia. This drug was the first of the sulfonylurea series, from which many further derivatives, such as *tolbutamide* and *glibenclamide,* were produced and used successfully to treat type 2 diabetes. Many of these products of the sulfonamide dynasty are widely used today. Their chemical relationship to sulfonamides is clear, though none of them has antibacterial activity. Their biochemical targets in smooth muscle, the kidney, the pancreas and elsewhere, are all different. Chemistry, not biology, was the guiding principle in their discovery and synthesis.

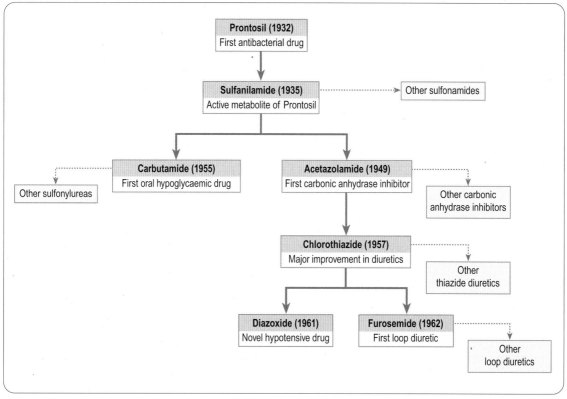

Fig. 1.2 Sulfonamide dynasty.

Target-directed approaches to drug design have played a much more significant role in areas other than antibacterial chemotherapy, the approaches being made possible by advances on two important fronts, separated, as it happens, by the Atlantic Ocean. In the United States, the antimetabolite principle, based on interfering with defined metabolic pathways, proved to be highly successful, due largely to the efforts of George Hitchings and Gertrude Elion at Burroughs Wellcome. In Europe, drug discovery took its lead more from physiology than biochemistry and sprung from advances in knowledge of chemical transmitters and their receptors. The names of Henry Dale and James Black deserve special mention here.

Hitchings and Elion and the antimetabolite principle

George Hitchings and Gertrude Elion came together in 1944 in the biochemistry department of Burroughs Wellcome in Tuckahoe, New York. Their biochemical interest lay in the synthesis of folic acid, based on the importance of this pathway for the action of sulfonamides, and they set about synthesizing potential 'antimetabolites' of purines and pyrimidines as chemotherapeutic agents. At the time, it was known that this pathway was important for DNA synthesis, but the role of DNA in cell function was uncertain. It turned out to be an inspired choice, and theirs was one of the first drug discovery programmes to focus on a biochemical pathway, rather than on a series of chemical compounds.

Starting from a series of purine and pyrimidine analogues, which had antibacterial activity, Hitchings and Elion identified a key enzyme in the folic acid pathway, namely dihydrofolate reductase, which was necessary for DNA synthesis and was inhibited by many of their antibacterial pyrimidine analogues. Because all cells, not just bacteria, use this reaction to make DNA, they wondered why the drugs showed selectivity in their ability to block cell division and found that the enzyme showed considerable species variation in its susceptibility to inhibitors. This led them to seek inhibitors that would selectively attack bacteria, protozoa and human neoplasms, which they achieved with great success. Drugs to emerge from this programme included the antimalarial drug *pyrimethamine*, the antibacterial *trimethoprim* and the anticancer drug *6-mercaptopurine*, as well as its prodrug *azathioprine*, an immunosuppressant widely used to prevent transplant rejection. Another spin-off from the work of Hitchings and Elion was *allopurinol*, an inhibitor of purine synthesis that is used in the prevention of gout. Subsequently, Elion—her enthusiasm for purines and pyrimidines undiminished—led the research group, which in 1977 discovered one of the first effective antiviral drugs, *aciclovir*, an inhibitor of DNA polymerase, and later the first antiretroviral drug, *zidovudine* (AZT), which inhibits reverse transcriptase. Hitchings and Elion, by focusing on the metabolic pathways involved in DNA synthesis, invented an extraordinary range of valuable therapeutic drugs, an achievement unsurpassed in the history of drug discovery.

James Black and receptor-targeted drugs

As already mentioned, the concept of 'receptors' as recognition sites for hormones and other physiological mediators came from J. N. Langley's analysis of the mechanisms of action of nicotine, 'curari' and other drugs that influence cholinergic neurotransmission. A. V. Hill, then a student working in Langley's laboratory, was the first to express the receptor idea quantitatively in terms of a bimolecular reaction obeying the law of mass action (Hill, 1909). Henry Dale's work on the distinct 'muscarinic' and 'nicotinic' actions of acetylcholine also pointed to the existence of two distinct types of cholinergic receptor, though Dale himself dismissed the receptor concept as an abstract and unhelpful cloak for ignorance.[7]

During the 1920s and 1930s, major discoveries highlighting the role of chemical mediators were made by physiologists, including the discovery of insulin, adrenal steroids and several neurotransmitters. The realization that chemical signalling is crucial for normal function focused attention on the receptor mechanisms needed to decode these signals. Pharmacologists, particularly A. J. Clark, J. H. Gaddum and H. O. Schild, applied the law of mass action to put ligand–receptor interactions on a quantitative basis. Schild's studies on drug antagonism allowed the binding affinity of competitive antagonists to receptors to be estimated from pharmacological experiments and were an important step forwards which provided the first—and still widely used—quantitative basis for receptor classification. R. P. Ahlquist in 1948 proposed the existence of two distinct classes of adrenoceptor, α and β, to account for the varied effects of adrenaline, noradrenaline, isoprenaline and related agonists on autonomic function.

This discovery inspired James Black, working in the research laboratories of Imperial Chemical Industries in the UK, to seek antagonists that would act selectively on β-adrenoceptors and thus block the effects of adrenaline on the heart. His chemical starting point was *dichloroisoprenaline*, a partial agonist which had been found by Slater in 1957 to block the relaxant effects of adrenaline on bronchial smooth muscle. The result of Black's efforts was the first β-adrenoceptor-blocking drug, *pronethalol* (1960), which had the desired pharmacological effects but was carcinogenic in the strain of mice tested. It was quickly followed by *propranolol* (registered in 1964[8])—which has found many important applications in cardiovascular medicine, including the treatment of dysrhythmias, of ischaemic heart disease, of heart failure and (most recently) of severe haemangiomas in children (Léauté-Labrèze et al., 2015). This was the first time that a receptor, identified pharmacologically, had been deliberately targeted in a drug discovery project.

Black, after moving to Smith Kline and French, went on from this success to look for novel histamine antagonists that would block the stimulatory effect of histamine on gastric acid secretion, this effect being resistant to the then-known antihistamine drugs. The result of this project, in which the chemistry effort proved much tougher than the β-adrenoceptor antagonist project, was the first H_2-receptor antagonist, *burimamide* (1972), a major conceptual advance, followed by *cimetidine* (1976), which transformed the treatment of peptic ulcers (the options for which had previously been surgery, antacids or prolonged bed rest). In 1988, Black, along with Hitchings and Elion, was awarded the Nobel Prize, the citation reading, in part: '… however, the research work carried out by Black, Elion and Hitchings has had a more fundamental significance. While drug development had earlier mainly been built on chemical modification of natural products they introduced a more rational approach based on the understanding of basic biochemical and physiological processes.'

Black's work opened up the field of receptor pharmacology as an approach to drug discovery, and the pharmaceutical industry quickly followed his lead. Lookalike

---

[7]He was misled by the structural diversity of amines (including aliphatic as well as aromatic compounds) that provoke responses pharmacologically similar to those of adrenaline and noradrenaline, not having appreciated their capacity to act indirectly by releasing endogenous catecholamines.

[8]Ironically, propranolol had been made in 1959 in the laboratories of Boehringer Ingelheim, as part of a different, chemistry-led project. Only when linked to its target was its clinical potential appreciated—chemistry alone was not enough!

β-adrenoceptor antagonists and H_2-receptor antagonists followed rapidly during the 1970s and 1980s, and many other receptors were set up as targets for potential therapeutic agents, based on essentially the same approach—though with updated technology (Page et al., 2011; Walker, 2011).

Many other successful drugs have resulted from target-directed projects along the lines pioneered by Black and his colleagues. In recent years, of course, receptors have changed from being essentially figments in an operational scheme devised by pharmacologists to explain their findings to being concrete molecular entities that can be labelled, isolated, cloned and expressed just like many other proteins. As we shall see in later chapters, these advances have completely transformed the techniques employed in drug discovery research.

Accidental clinical discoveries

Another successful route to the discovery of new drugs has been through observations made in the clinic. Until drug discovery became an intentional activity, such serendipitous observations were the only source of knowledge. Withering's discovery in 1785 of the efficacy of digitalis in treating 'dropsy' (oedema, presumably caused by chronic cardiac failure) and Wenkebach's discovery in 1914 of the antidysrhythmic effect of quinine, when he treated a patient with malaria who also happened to suffer from atrial tachycardia are two of the many examples where a clinical effect of plant-derived agents has been discovered by highly observant clinicians. More recently, clinical benefit of unexpected kinds has been discovered with synthetic compounds developed for other purposes. In 1937, for example, Bradley tried *amphetamine* as a means of alleviating the severe headache suffered by children after lumbar puncture (spinal tap) on the grounds that the drug's cardiovascular effects might prove beneficial. The headache was not alleviated, but Bradley noticed that the children became much less agitated. From this chance observation, he went on to set up an observational clinical trial in children with behavioural disorders, which demonstrated that amphetamine had a calming effect—quite unexpected for a drug known to have stimulant effects in adults. From this developed the widespread use, validated by controlled clinical trials, of amphetamine-like drugs, particularly *methylphenidate* (Ritalin) to treat attention deficit hyperactivity disorder (ADHD) in children.

Other well-known examples include the discovery of the antipsychotic effects of phenothiazines by Laborit in 1949. Laborit was a naval surgeon, concerned that patients were dying from 'surgical shock'—circulatory collapse resulting in irreversible organ failure—after major operations. Thinking that histamine might be involved, he tested the antihistamine *promethazine* combined with autonomic blocking drugs to prevent this cardiovascular reaction. Although it was ineffective in treating shock, promethazine caused some sedation, and Laborit tried some chemically related sedatives, notably *promazine*, which had little antihistamine activity. Patients treated with it fared better during surgery, but Laborit particularly noticed that they appeared much calmer postoperatively. He therefore persuaded his psychiatrist colleagues to test the drug on psychotic patients, tests that quickly revealed the drug's antipsychotic effects and led to the development of the antipsychotic *chlorpromazine*. In a sequel, other phenothiazine-like tricyclic compounds were tested for antipsychotic activity but were found accidentally to relieve the symptoms of depression. After Bradley and Laborit, psychiatrists had become alert to looking for the unexpected, and further uses followed including the repurposing of certain anticonvulsant drugs as mood stabilizers (e.g., *carbamazepine*) or for neuropathic pain (e.g., *pregabalin*), as mentioned earlier. Such clinical insights remain valuable, despite their limitations (see the later section on clinical trials). A striking 21st century example is the observation that two severe cases of infantile haemangioma regressed strikingly during treatment with β-adrenoceptor antagonists prescribed because of coincidental cardiac disease, a therapeutic effect confirmed by a randomized controlled trial (Léauté-Labrèze et al., 2015).

The growth of biotechnology

In parallel with these developments in chemistry, pharmacology and medicine, fundamental advances in structural biology, microbiology and notably methods for the preparation of monoclonal antibodies (Galfré & Milstien, 1985) laid the scene for the arrival of molecular biology and its commercial wing, the biotechnology industry. This subsequently transformed the pharmaceutical industry, dramatically diversifying its products (see Chapters 8 and 9).

Biotechnology had its roots in brewing, baking and fermentation processes coupled with chemical engineering (see Bud, 1985). The first modern biotechnology companies (Cetus and Genentech) were founded in the United States in 1976; as of 2018, over 700 public companies and over 200,000 employees in the United States and Europe generate some $140 billion (US) of revenue annually. Biopharmaceutical products included the six top-costing medicines prescribed in the UK National Health Service (2015–16). Several of these (notably infliximab, the first anti-tumour necrosis factor (TNF) monoclonal and adalimumab, the first fully humanized monoclonal TNF antagonist) have held prominent positions for several years. Biopharmaceutical products have become commercially dominant—testament to their efficacy and safety and to the manufacturing and regulatory complexities of biopharmaceuticals in contrast to low-molecular-weight drugs.

The initial wave of biotech-derived products comprised therapeutic proteins, which now make up about 25% of newly registered medicines. Following on are the first wave of nucleic acid medicines, aimed at modifying the expression of specific genes, and of cell-based products, trends that are expected to take medicine (and the pharmaceutical industry) into a new era. As well as contributing directly in terms of products, biotechnology is transforming the ways in which conventional drugs are discovered, with rational design as opposed to trial-and-error empiricism now the norm.

Clinical trials

Despite the very real successes of clinical observation mentioned earlier, the unpredictable natural history of disease coupled with a limited understanding of pathophysiology makes the 'before-and-after' experience of the medical expert an uncertain guide to therapeutic efficacy. The idea that efficacy could best be tested scientifically dates to James Lind's experimental trial on the prevention of scurvy. Benjamin Franklin and other members of the Royal Commission into mesmerism discovered the powerful effects of suggestion on patient-reported outcome (what we would now refer to as 'placebo' effects), but it was not until the mid-20th century that formal scientifically based clinical trials came into their own. The Medical Research Council (MRC) trial of streptomycin (1948), enabled by post-war austerity, was a landmark: patients with tuberculosis were allocated via a randomization code prepared by the statistician Austin Bradford Hill to treatment with conventional care alone versus conventional care plus streptomycin. It confirmed efficacy but unexpectedly demonstrated a high rate of relapse with resistant organisms, underpinning the swift adoption of the highly effective strategy of triple therapy for tuberculosis. Subsequent trials of treatment of malignant and cardiovascular diseases focusing on clinical endpoints such as disease-free survival, stroke, death or myocardial infarction rapidly transformed clinical care.

While some intermediate endpoints such as blood pressure were shown to be reliable predictors of clinical outcome in hypertensive patients in terms of stroke prevention, others proved to be misleading. Such seemingly good candidates as drugs that inhibit cardiac dysrhythmias, or which increase cardiac contractile force (positive inotropes), not only failed to prolong the life of patients with, respectively, frequent ventricular ectopic beats or with low cardiac output heart failure, but actually shortened survival. Conversely, β-adrenoceptor antagonists used carefully have been repeatedly shown to improve survival in patients with chronic stable heart failure despite their negative inotropic effect. Such counterintuitive findings have had a salutary effect on physicians and regulators with stricter clinically relevant criteria now being required to support claims of efficacy. The impact on development time and cost has transformed drug development and the pharmaceutical industry, which is still adapting to the new landscape.

The regulatory process

In the mid-19th century, restrictions on the sale of poisonous substances were imposed in the United States and the UK, but it was not until the early 1900s that any system of 'prescription-only' medicines was introduced, requiring approval by a medical practitioner. Soon afterwards, restrictions began to be introduced on what 'cures' could be claimed in advertisements for pharmaceutical products and what information had to be given on the label, but legislation evolved at a leisurely pace. Most of the concern was with controlling frankly poisonous or addictive substances or contaminants, not with the efficacy and possible harmful effects of new drugs.

In 1937, the use of diethylene glycol as a solvent for a sulfonamide preparation caused 107 deaths in the United States, mainly in children, and a year later (1938), the 1906 Food and Drugs Act was revised, requiring safety to be demonstrated before new products could be marketed and allowing federal inspection of manufacturing facilities. The requirement for proven efficacy, as well as safety, was added in the Kefauver–Harris Amendment in 1962.

In Europe, it was not until the mid-1960s, in the wake of the thalidomide disaster that the UK began to follow the United States' lead in regulatory laws. The thalidomide disaster was averted in the United States by Frances Kelsey, then a junior officer at the FDA having worked previously on the mechanism of the toxicity of Elixir Sulfanilamide during her academic training and who used the provisions of the 1938 Food and Drugs Act to delay licensing approval. Until then, the ability of drugs to do harm—short of being frankly poisonous or addictive—was not really appreciated, most of the concern having been about contaminants. In 1959, when thalidomide was first put on the market by the German company Chemie Grünenthal, regulatory controls did not exist in Europe: it was up to the company to decide how much research was needed to satisfy itself that the drug was safe and effective. Grünenthal made a disastrously wrong judgement (see Sjöstrom & Nilsson, 1972, for a full account), which resulted in an estimated 10,000 cases of severe congenital malformation following the company's specific recommendation that the drug was suitable for use by pregnant women. This single event caused an urgent reappraisal, leading to the introduction of much tighter government

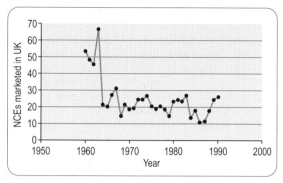

Fig. 1.3 Number of new chemical entities (NCEs) marketed in the UK 1960–90 showing the dramatic effect of the thalidomide crisis in 1961. (Data from Y Lis and S R Walker. [1989]. *Br J Clin Pharmacol*, 28[3]: 333–343.)

controls. The dramatic effect on the introduction of new drugs can be appreciated from Fig. 1.3, which shows new chemical entities marketed in the UK from 1960 to 1990. Thalidomide (or a derivative, lenalidomide) is now again used therapeutically but for the serious indication of multiple myeloma rather than as a hypnotic, and highly effective forms of contraception are co-prescribed where appropriate.

In the UK, the Committee on the Safety of Drugs was established in 1963 to be replaced, in turn, by the Committee on Safety of Medicines and the Medicines and Healthcare Products Regulatory Agency. For the first time, as in the United States, all new drugs (including new mixtures and formulations) had to be submitted for approval before clinical trials could begin, and before they could be marketed. Legally, companies could proceed even if the Committee did not approve, but very few chose to do so. This loophole was closed by the Medicines Act (1968), which made it illegal to proceed with trials to support a marketing application or the release of a drug without approval. Initially, safety alone was required, but in 1970, under the Medicines Act, evidence of efficacy was added to the criteria for approval. It was the realization that all drugs, not just poisons or contaminants, have the potential to cause harm that made it essential to seek proof of therapeutic efficacy to ensure that the net effect of a new drug, namely its balance of risk/benefit, was beneficial—official validation of the 16th century Swiss physician Paracelsus' dictum that 'only the dose makes the poison'.

In the decade leading up to 1970, the main planks in the regulatory platform—evidence of safety, efficacy and quality—were in place in most developed countries. Subsequently, the regulations have been adjusted in various minor ways and adopted with local variations in most countries.

A progressive tightening of the restrictions on the licensing of new drugs relating to the requirement for scientifically rigorous evidence of clinically relevant benefit has followed as public awareness of the harmful effects of drugs became heightened. Teratogenicity, albeit usually less predictable and dramatic than that caused by thalidomide, remains a major concern. Folate antagonists are teratogenic and anticonvulsant drugs, products of chemistry-led drug discovery as mentioned earlier, are a common cause of fetal abnormality. Neural tube defects in infants of mothers treated during pregnancy with valproate are particularly well documented. Newer agents, for example, *levetiracetam*, have been used less often so their risk is less well established than that of older agents. It is unclear if teratogenicity is an outcome of a shared drug discovery strategy leading to shared off-target effects versus possible downstream consequences of any effective anticonvulsant on neural development in the fetus. In practice, it appears that anticonvulsant drug use during pregnancy may cause less harm to the developing fetus than uncontrolled seizures, provided the number of drugs used is minimized and valproate avoided where possible.

The TeGenero disaster in 2006, when healthy volunteer subjects suffered from massive cytokine release in response to what in retrospect was recognized to have been a massive overdose of an antibody that activated an amplifying cascade (an effect not observed in animal tests), led to the introduction of tighter regulation of first-in-human and other phase I studies. The current state of licensing regulations is described in Chapter 20.

Concluding remarks

In this chapter, we have followed the evolution of ideas and technologies that have led to the present state of drug discovery research. The main threads, which came together, were:

- Clinical medicine, by far the oldest of the antecedents
- Pharmacy, which began with the apothecary trade in the 17th century, set up to serve the demand from clinical medicine for herbal preparations
- Organic chemistry, beginning in the mid-19th century and evolving into medicinal chemistry via dyestuffs
- Pharmacology, also beginning in the mid-19th century and setting out to explain the effects of pharmaceutical preparations in physiological and biochemical terms
- Bioengineering, accelerating from the latter half of the 20th century and leading to highly specific and efficacious biopharmaceutical products based on animal- rather than plant-derived molecules.

Some of the major milestones are summarized in Table 1.2.

Table 1.2 Milestones in the development of the pharmaceutical industry

Year	Event	Notes
c.1550 BCE	Ebers papyrus	The earliest known compendium of medical remedies
1540	Diethyl ether synthesized	'Sweet oil of vitriol', arguably the first synthetic drug
1668	Merck (Darmstadt) founded	The apothecary business, which later (1827) evolved into the first large-scale pharmaceutical company
1763	Lind shows that lack of fruit causes scurvy	
1775	Nitrous oxide synthesized	
1785	Withering describes use of digitalis extract to treat 'dropsy'	The first demonstration of therapeutic efficacy
1798	Jenner shows that vaccination prevents smallpox	
1799	Humphrey Davy demonstrates anaesthetic effect of nitrous oxide	
1803	Napoleon established examination and licensing scheme for doctors	
1806	Sertürner purifies morphine and shows it to be the active principle of opium	A seminal advance—the first evidence that herbal remedies contain active chemicals. Many other plant alkaloids isolated 1820–40
1846	Morton administers ether as anaesthetic at Massachusetts General Hospital	The first trial of surgical anaesthesia
1847	Chloroform administered to Queen Victoria to control labour pain	
1847	The first pharmacological institute set up by Buchheim	
mid-19th century	The first pharmaceutical companies formed: Merck (1827) Squibb (1858) Hoechst (1862) Parke-Davis (1866) Lilley (1876) Burroughs Wellcome (1880)	In many cases, pharmaceutical companies evolved from dyestuffs companies or apothecaries
1858	Virchow proposes cell theory	
1859	Amyl nitrite synthesized	
1865	Benzene structure elucidated (Von Kekulé), and first use of structural formulae to describe organic molecules	Essential foundations for the development of organic synthesis
1867	Brunton demonstrates use of amyl nitrite to relieve anginal pain	
1878	Pasteur proposes germ theory of disease	
1898	Heroin (diacetylmorphine) developed by Bayer	The first synthetic derivative of a natural product. Heroin was marketed as a safe and nonaddictive alternative to morphine
1899	Aspirin developed by Bayer	
1903	Barbital developed by Bayer	
1904	Elliott demonstrates biological activity of extracts of adrenal glands and proposes adrenaline release as a physiological mechanism	The first evidence for a chemical mediator—the basis of much modern pharmacology
1910	Ehrlich discovers Salvarsan	The first antimicrobial drug, which revolutionized the treatment of syphilis
1912	Starling coins the term 'hormone'	
1921	MacLeod, Banting and Best discover insulin	Produced commercially from animal pancreas by Lilly (1925)

Continued

Table 1.2 Milestones in the development of the pharmaceutical industry—cont'd

Year	Event	Notes
1926	Loewi demonstrates release of 'Vagusstoff' from heart	The first clear evidence for chemical neurotransmission
1929	Fleming discovers penicillin	Penicillin was not used clinically until Chain and Florey solved production problems in 1938
1935	Domagk discovers sulfonamides	The first effective antibacterial drugs, and harbingers of the antimetabolite era
1936	Steroid hormones isolated by Upjohn company	
1937	Bovet discovers antihistamines	Subsequently led to discovery of antipsychotic drugs
1946	Gilman and Philips demonstrate anticancer effect of nitrogen mustards	The first anticancer drug
1951	Hitchings and Elion discover mercaptopurine	The first anticancer drug from the antimetabolite approach
1961	Hitchings and Schwartz discover azathioprine	Also from the antimetabolite programme, immunosuppressant used to prevent transplant rejection
1962	Black and colleagues discover pronethalol	The first β-adrenoceptor antagonist to be used clinically
1972	Black and colleagues discover burimamide	The first selective H_2 antagonist
1975	Köhler and Milstein fused myeloma cells with B lymphocytes to create immortal hybridomas producing monoclonal antibodies specific to known antigens	
1976	Genentech founded	The first biotech company, based on recombinant DNA technology
1985	FDA approves OKT3 (muromonab-CD3)	The first monoclonal antibody to be approved anywhere as a drug for humans—for treatment of acute allogeneic transplant rejection
c.1990	Introduction of combinatorial chemistry	
2013	FDA approves mipomersen	The first antisense oligonucleotide to be approved. Used for homozygous familial hypercholesterolaemia. Possible forerunner of a family of anti-RNA drugs

FDA, US Food and Drug Administration.

The pharmaceutical industry as big business began around the beginning of the 20th century and for 60 or more years was dominated by chemistry. Gradually, from the middle of the century onwards, the balance shifted towards pharmacology until, by the mid-1970s, chemistry and pharmacology were evenly balanced. The maturation of the scientific and technological basis of the discovery process to its 1970s level coincided with the development of much more stringent regulatory controls, and an acceptable balance seemed to be struck between creativity and restraint.

Subsequently, there has been a trend away from me-too drugs with at best minor improvements from the patient perspective, towards fewer but more innovative products, a trend that has become more marked since the first edition of this book. The very substantial costs associated with meeting regulatory requirements, coupled with greater scientific agility in rational targeting of diseases for which there are major unmet clinical needs, have favoured a highly productive symbiotic relationship between pharmaceutical industry behemoths and smaller biotechnology companies.[9] Fig. 1.4 shows FDA approvals of new drugs (excluding vaccines and devices) from 2000–2018. There has been a trend of increasing numbers of approvals since a low in 2007. Fig. 1.4 also illustrates the increase in approvals of first-in-class drugs which account for approximately one-third of the total, reflecting innovation and of biopharmaceuticals, reflecting the growing impact of genomics on drug discovery.

[9]Less welcome has been extreme price and supply instability worldwide and over-pricing in the United States of old drugs with important niche uses (e.g., pyrimethamine for toxoplasmosis)—hopefully a trend that the industry will find a solution for that will not impede innovation.

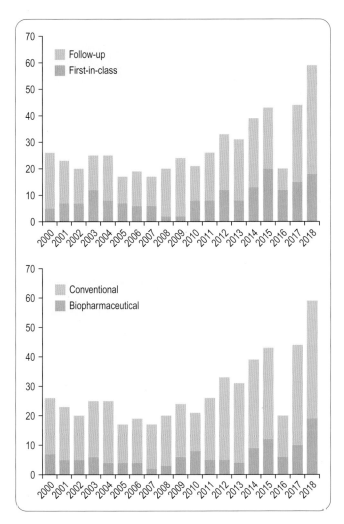

Fig. 1.4 Productivity and innovation. New registrations with the FDA since 2000, not including vaccines and diagnostic products. Upper panel separates first-in-class from follow-up products including 'first-in-class' drugs acting on a hitherto untargeted class of receptors or enzymes but excluding new agents with claimed selectivity for particular subtypes. Lower panel separates conventional from biopharmaceutical products.

Genomic approaches underpin two important trends, namely patient selection (personalized medicine) and target selection, both of which lead to fragmentation of what were hitherto seen as 'blockbuster' markets—in other words, more (but more expensive) drugs for smaller markets. The consequent major shift in drug discovery and development strategies is a theme that runs through much of this book.

The changes that are occurring in the first quarter of the 21st century show no sign of slowing down, and it is too soon to judge which developments will prove genuinely successful in terms of drug discovery and which will not. The present state of the art with respect to the science and technology of drug discovery is discussed in later chapters.

References

Bud, R. (1993). *The uses of life: A history of biotechnology*. United Kingdom: Cambridge University Press.

Caruthers, M. H. (1985). Gene synthesis machines: DNA chemistry and its uses. *Science, 230,* 281–285.

Drews, J. (2000). Drug discovery: A historical perspective. *Science, 287,* 1960–1964.

Drews, J. (2003). *In quest of tomorrow's medicines* (2nd ed.). New York: Springer.

Drews, J. (2004). Paul Ehrlich: Magister mundi. *Nature Reviews Drug Discovery, 3,* 797–801.

Galfré, G., & Milstein, C. (1981). Preparation of monoclonal antibodies: Strategies and procedures. *Methods in Enzymology, 73*(Part B), 3–46.

Griffin, J. P. (2004). Venetian treacle and the foundation of medicines regulation. *British Journal of Clinical Pharmacology, 58*, 317–325.

Hill, A. V. (1909). The mode of action of nicotine and curare determined by the form of the contraction curve and the method of temperature coefficients. *Journal of Physiology, 39*, 361–373.

Kassam, Z., Lee, C. H., Yuhong, Y., & Hunt, R. H. (2013). Fecal microbiota transplantation for Clostridium difficile infection: Systematic review and meta-analysis. *American Journal of Gastroenterology, 108*, 500–508.

Léauté-Labrèze, C., Hoeger, P., Mazereeuw-Hautier, J., Guibaud, L., Baselga, E., Posiunas, G., et al. (2015). A randomized, controlled trial of oral propranolol in infantile hemangioma. *New England Journal of Medicine, 372*, 735–746.

Lednicer, D. (Ed.). (1993). *Chronicles of drug discovery* (Vol. 3). Washington, DC: American Chemical Society.

Mann, R. D. (1984). *Modern drug use: An enquiry on historical principles.* Lancaster: MTP Press.

Maxwell, R. A., & Eckhardt, S. B. (1990). *Drug discovery: A casebook and analysis.* Clifton, NJ: Humana Press.

Oakley, H. (2015). *Pulmonaria officialis* and *Hepatica nobilis.* In H. Oakeley, J. Knowles, M. de Swiet, & A. Dayan (Eds.), *A garden of medicinal plants* (pp. 34–35, 33). Great Britain: Little Brown for the Royal College of Physicians.

Page, C., Schaffhausen, J., & Shankley, N. P. (2011). The scientific legacy of Sir James W Black. *Trends in Pharmacological Science, 32*, 181–182.

Porter, R. (1997). *The greatest benefit to mankind: A medical history of humanity from antiquity to the present.* London: Harper Collins.

Sjöstrom, H., & Nilsson, R. (1972). *Thalidomide and the power of the drug companies.* United Kingdom: Penguin, Harmondsworth.

Sneader, W. (1985). *Drug discovery: The evolution of modern medicines.* Chichester: John Wiley.

Walker, M. J. A. (2011). The major impacts of James Black's drug discoveries on medicine and pharmacology. *Trends in Pharmacological Science, 32*, 183–188.

Weatherall, M. (1990). *In search of a cure: A history of pharmaceutical discovery.* Oxford: Oxford University Press.

Yasiri, Z., & Shorvon, S. D. (2012). How phenobarbital revolutionized epilepsy therapy: The story of phenobarbital therapy in epilepsy in the last 100 years. *Epilepsia, 53*(Suppl. 8), 26–39.

Youyou, T. (December 7, 2015). *Artemisinin – A gift from traditional Chinese medicine to the world.* Nobel lecture. Retrieved from: http://www.nobelprize.org/uploads/2018/06/tu-lecture.pdf.

Chapter | 2 |

The nature of disease and the purpose of therapy

Duncan B Richards, Raymond G Hill

Introduction

In this book, we are concerned mainly with the drug discovery and development process, proudly regarded as the mainspring of the pharmaceutical industry. In this chapter, we consider the broader context of the human environment into which new drugs and medicinal products are launched, and where they must find their proper place. Most pharmaceutical companies place at the top of their basic mission statement a commitment to improve the public's health, to relieve the human burden of disease, and to improve the quality of life. Few would argue with the spirit of this commitment. Nevertheless, we need to look more closely at what it means, how disease is defined, what medical therapy aims to alter and how—and by whom—the effects of therapy are judged and evaluated. Here we outline some of the basic principles underlying these broader issues.

Concepts of disease

The practice of medicine predates by thousands of years the science of medicine, and the application of 'therapeutic' procedures by professionals similarly predates any scientific understanding of how the human body works, or what happens when it goes wrong. As discussed in Chapter 1, the ancients defined disease not only in very different terms but also on a quite different basis from what we would recognize today. The origin of disease and the measures needed to counter it were generally seen as manifestations of divine will and retribution, rather than of physical malfunction. The scientific revolution in medicine, which began in earnest during the 19th century and has been steadily accelerating since, has

changed our concept of disease quite drastically and continues to challenge it, raising new ethical problems and thorny discussions of principle. For the centuries of prescientific medicine, codes of practice based on honesty, integrity and professional relationships were quite sufficient: as therapeutic interventions were ineffective anyway, it mattered little to what situations they were applied. Now, quite suddenly, the language of disease has changed and interventions have become effective; not surprisingly, we have to revise our ideas about what constitutes disease, and how medical intervention should be used. In this chapter, we will try to define the scope and purpose of therapeutics in the context of modern biology. In reality, however, those in the science-based drug discovery business have to recognize the strong atavistic leanings of many healthcare professions,[1] whose roots go back much further than the age of science.

Therapeutic intervention, including the medical use of drugs, aims to prevent, cure or alleviate disease states. The question of exactly what we mean by disease, and how we distinguish disease from other kinds of human affliction and dysfunction, is of more than academic importance, because policy and practice with respect to healthcare provision depend on where we draw the line between what is an appropriate target for therapeutic intervention and what is not. The traditional systems have doctors at the centre of the decision-making process to define what is a disease; increasingly, however, patients and the public are demanding a greater say. Further complexity is added through the influence of political and commercial forces; the latter is not just the pharmaceutical industry but includes device manufacturers, insurance companies and

---

[1]The upsurge of 'alternative' therapies, many of which owe nothing to science—and, indeed, reject the relevance of science to what its practitioners do—perhaps reflects an urge to return to the prescientific era of medical history.

commercial healthcare providers. Much has been written on the difficult question of how to define health and disease, and what demarcates a proper target for therapeutic intervention (Caplan, 1993; Caplan et al., 2004; Reznek, 1987); nevertheless, the waters remain distinctly murky.

One approach is to define what we mean by health, and to declare the attainment of health as the goal of all healthcare measures, including therapeutics.

What is health?

In everyday parlance, we use the words 'health', 'fitness', 'wellbeing' on the one hand, and 'disease', 'illness', 'sickness', 'ill-health', etc., on the other, more or less interchangeably, but these words become slippery and evasive when we try to define them. The World Health Organization (WHO), for example, defines health as 'a state of complete physical, mental and social wellbeing and not merely the absence of sickness or infirmity'. On this basis, few humans could claim to possess health, although the majority may not be in the grip of obvious sickness or infirmity. Who is to say what constitutes 'complete physical, mental and social wellbeing' in a human being? Does physical wellbeing imply an ability to run a marathon? Does a shy and self-effacing person lack social wellbeing? Inhabitants of wealthy countries typically enjoy high levels of physical health but often high levels of stress and anxiety and substantial associated morbidity.

We also find health defined in functional terms, less idealistically than in the WHO's formulation: '. . . health consists in our functioning in conformity with our natural design with respect to survival and reproduction, as determined by natural selection . . .' (Caplan, 1993). Here the implication is that evolution has brought us to an optimal—or at least an acceptable—compromise with our environment, with the corollary that healthcare measures should properly be directed at restoring this level of functionality in individuals who have lost some important element of it. This has a fashionably 'greenish' tinge and seems more realistic than the WHO's chillingly utopian vision, but there are still difficulties in trying to use it as a guide to the proper application of therapeutics. The explosion in our understanding of genetics has highlighted how similar all humans are, but like all living creatures, we have evolved to our environment. A key feature of human history of the past couple of centuries has been migration (whether elective or enforced) of large numbers of people to environments very different from those their ancestors evolved to suit. The possession of a genetic abnormality of haemoglobin, known as sickle-cell trait, is advantageous in its heterozygous form in the tropics, as it confers resistance to malaria, whereas homozygous individuals suffer from a severe form of haemolytic anaemia (sickle-cell disease).

Health cannot, therefore, be regarded as a definable state—a fixed point on the map, representing a destination that all are seeking to reach. Rather, it seems to be a continuum, through which we can move in either direction, becoming more or less well adapted for survival in our particular environment. Perhaps the best current definition is that given by Bircher (2005) who states that 'health is a dynamic state of wellbeing characterized by physical, mental and social potential which satisfies the demands of life commensurate with age, culture and personal responsibility'. Although we could argue that the aim of healthcare measures is simply to improve our state of adaptation to our present environment, this is obviously too broad. Other factors than health—for example, wealth, education, peace and the avoidance of famine—are at least as important but lie outside the domain of medicine. What actually demarcates the work of doctors and healthcare workers from that of other caring professionals—all of whom may contribute to health in different ways—is that the former focus on *disease*.

What is disease?

Consider the following definitions of disease:
- A condition which alters or interferes with the normal state of an organism and is usually characterized by the abnormal functioning of one or more of the host's systems, parts or organs (*Churchill's Medical Dictionary*, 1989)
- A morbid entity characterized usually by at least two of these criteria: recognized aetiologic agents, identifiable groups of signs and symptoms or consistent anatomical alterations (elsewhere, 'morbid' is defined as diseased or pathologic) (*Stedman's Medical Dictionary*, 1990)
- 'Potential insufficient to satisfy the demands of life', as outlined by Bircher (2005) in his definition of health above.

We sense the difficulty that these thoughtful authorities found in pinning down the concept. The first definition emphasizes two aspects, namely *deviation from normality* and *dysfunction*; the second emphasizes *aetiology* (i.e., causative factors) and *phenomenology* (signs, symptoms, etc.), which is essentially the manifestation of dysfunction.

Deviation from normality does not define disease

The criterion of deviation from normality begs many questions. It implies that we know what the 'normal state' is and can define what constitutes an alteration of it. It suggests that if our observations were searching enough, we could unfailingly distinguish disease from normality. But we know, for example, that the majority of 50-year-olds will have atherosclerotic lesions in their arteries, or that some degree of osteoporosis is normal in postmenopausal women. These are not deviations from normality, nor do they in themselves cause dysfunction, and so they do not fall within these definitions of disease, yet both are seen as pathological and as legitimate—indeed important—targets for therapeutic intervention. Furthermore, as discussed later, deviations from normality are often beneficial and much prized.

Normal is also a concept that varies with time and age. Expectations of what those in their 60s would do 40 years ago are different from those today. It is also a feature of chronic illness that patients' expectations of what they can achieve narrow. The ability to undertake the routine activities of daily living is of course important, but we should not forget the important role that the ability to undertake social activities plays. Therapeutic targets fixed on the mechanics of life alone are incomplete but are often favoured by resource-limited healthcare systems.

Phenomenology and aetiology are important factors—the naturalistic view

Setting aside the normality criterion, the definitions quoted earlier are examples of the *naturalistic*, or observation-based, view of disease, defined by phenomenology and backed up in many cases by an understanding of aetiology. It is now generally agreed that this by itself is insufficient, for there is no *general* set of observable characteristics that distinguishes disease from health. Although individual diseases of course have their defining characteristics, which may be structural, biochemical or physiological, there is no common feature. Further, there are many conditions, particularly in psychiatry, but also in other branches of medicine, where such physical manifestations are absent, even though their existence as diseases is not questioned. Examples would include obsessive–compulsive disorder, schizophrenia, chronic fatigue syndrome and low back pain. In such cases, of which there are many examples, the disease is defined by symptoms of which only patients are aware, or altered behaviour of which they and those around them are aware: defining features at the physical, biochemical or physiological level are absent, or at least not yet recognized.

Harm and disvalue—the normative view

The shortcomings of the naturalistic view of disease, which is in principle value free, have led some authors to take the opposite view, to the extent of denying the relevance of any kind of objective criteria to the definition of disease. Crudely stated, this value-based (or *normative*) view holds that disease is simply any condition the individual or society finds disagreeable or harmful (i.e., *disvalues*). Taken to extremes by authors such as Szasz and Illich, this view denies the relevance of the physical manifestations of illness and focuses instead on illness only as a manifestation of *social* intolerance or malfunction. Although few would go this far—and certainly modern biologists would not be among them—it is clear that value-laden judgements play a significant role in determining what we choose to view as disease. 'Drapetomania', defined as a disease of American slaves, was characterized by an obsessional desire for freedom. This pseudoscientific medicalization of racism and other forms of prejudice have been common in the history of medicine and unfortunately remain common today. Homosexuality was seen as pathological, and determined attempts were made to treat it. An important feature of these issues is that the dependence on social attitudes means that circumstances vary across the world and can change, sometimes rapidly. While many countries have legislated to protect the rights of homosexuals, in others, legislative penalties have increased in recent years. There are many examples where healthcare professionals have used their knowledge to promote equality and understanding, but sadly there are also many examples where those skills have been used in quite the opposite way, often for personal advancement or financial gain.

A definition of disease which tries to combine the concepts of biological malfunction and harm (or disvalue) was proposed by Caplan et al. (1981):

> *States of affairs are called diseases when they are due to physiological or psychological processes that typically cause states of disability, pain or deformity, and are generally held to be below acceptable physiological or psychological norms.*

What is still lacking is any reference to aetiology, yet this can be important in recognizing disease, and, indeed, is increasingly so as we understand more about the underlying biological mechanisms. A patient who complains of feeling depressed may be reacting quite normally to a bereavement, or may come from a suicide-prone family, suggestive of an inherited tendency to depressive illness. The symptoms might be very similar, but the implications, based on aetiology, would be different.

In conclusion, disease proves extremely difficult to define (Scully, 2004). The closest we can get at present to an operational definition of disease rests on a combination of three factors: phenomenology, aetiology and disvalue, as summarized in Fig. 2.1.

Labelling human afflictions as diseases (i.e., 'medicalizing' them) has various beneficial and adverse

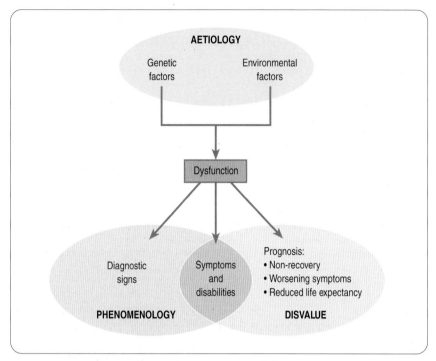

Fig. 2.1 Three components of disease.

consequences, both for the affected individuals and for healthcare providers. It is of particular relevance to the pharmaceutical industry, which stands to benefit from the labelling of borderline conditions as diseases meriting therapeutic intervention. Strong criticism has been levelled at the pharmaceutical industry for the way in which it uses its resources to promote the recognition of questionable disorders, such as female sexual dysfunction or social phobia, as diseases, and to elevate identified risk factors—asymptomatic in themselves but increasing the likelihood of disease occurring later—to the level of diseases in their own right. A pertinent polemic (Moynihan et al., 2004) starts with the sentence: 'there's a lot of money to be made from telling healthy people they're sick', and emphasizes the thin line that divides medical education from marketing (see Chapter 21). Current trends go beyond restoration to the 'norm'. The mean is often no longer the target; everyone wants to be above average. This is driving a medicalization of nutrition and endocrinology, with an explosion of isotonic drinks, protein shakes and testosterone 'boosters'. This is important because failure to achieve a supra normal result in one domain (e.g., muscle mass) may lead to very real morbidity in another domain, for example, in terms of mental health.

The aims of therapeutics

Components of disvalue

The discussion so far leads us to the proposition that the proper aim of therapeutic intervention is to minimize the disvalue associated with disease. The concept of disvalue is, therefore, central, and we need to consider what it comprises. The disvalue experienced by a sick individual has two distinct components[2] (Fig. 2.1), namely *present symp-*

---

[2]These concepts apply in a straightforward way to many real-life situations, but there are exceptions and difficulties. For example, in certain psychiatric disorders, the patient's judgement of his or her state of morbidity is itself affected by the disease. Patients suffering from mania, paranoid delusions or severe depression may pursue an extremely disordered and self-destructive lifestyle, while denying that they are ill and resisting any intervention. In such cases, society often imposes its own judgement of the individual's morbidity and may use legal instruments such as the Mental Health Act to apply therapeutic measures against the patient's will. Vaccination represents another special case. Here, the disvalue being addressed is the theoretical risk that a healthy individual will later contract an infectious disease such as diphtheria or measles. This risk can be regarded as an adverse factor in the prognosis of a perfectly normal individual. Similarly, a healthy person visiting the tropics will, if he is wise, take antimalarial drugs to avoid infection—in other words, to improve his prognosis.

toms and disabilities (collectively termed *morbidity*) and future *prognosis* (namely the likelihood of increasing morbidity or premature death). An individual who is suffering no abnormal symptoms or disabilities, and whose prognosis is that of an average individual of the same age, we call 'healthy'. An individual with a bad cold or a sprained ankle has symptoms and disabilities, but probably has a normal prognosis. An individual with asymptomatic lung cancer or hypertension has no symptoms but a poor prognosis. Either case constitutes disease and warrants therapeutic intervention. Very commonly, both components of disvalue are present, and both need to be addressed with therapeutic measures—different measures may be needed to alleviate morbidity and to improve prognosis. Of course, such measures need not be confined to physical and pharmacological approaches.

The proposition at the beginning of this section sets clear limits to the aims of therapeutic intervention, which encompass the great majority of noncontroversial applications. Real life is, of course, not so simple, and in the next section we consider some of the important exceptions and controversies that healthcare professionals and policymakers are increasingly having to confront.

Therapeutic intervention is not restricted to treatment or prevention of disease

The term 'lifestyle drugs' is a recent invention, but the concept of using drugs, and other types of interventions, in a medical setting for purposes unrelated to the treatment of disease is by no means new.

Pregnancy is not by any definition a disease, nor are skin wrinkles, yet contraception, abortion and plastic surgery are well established practices in the medical domain. Why are we prepared to use drugs as contraceptives or abortifacients but condemn using them to enhance sporting performance? The basic reason seems to be that we attach disvalue to unwanted pregnancy (i.e., we consider it harmful). We also attach disvalue to alternative means of avoiding unwanted pregnancy, such as sexual abstinence or using condoms. Other examples, however, such as cosmetic surgery to remove wrinkles or reshape breasts, seem to refute the disvalue principle: minor cosmetic imperfections are in no sense harmful, but society nonetheless concedes to the demand of individuals that medical technology should be deployed to enhance their beauty. In other cases, such as the use of sildenafil (Viagra)

to improve male sexual performance, there is ambivalence about whether its use should be confined to those with evidence for erectile dysfunction (i.e., in whom disvalue exists) or whether it should also be used to enhance sexual experience in men without erectile dysfunction.

It is obvious that departures from normality can bring benefit as well as disadvantage. Individuals with above-average IQs, physical fitness, ball-game skills, artistic talents, physical beauty or charming personalities have an advantage in life. Is it, then, a proper role of the healthcare system to try to enhance these qualities in the average person? Our instinct says not, because the average person cannot be said to be diseased or suffering. There may be value in being a talented footballer, but there is no harm in not being one. Indeed, the value of the special talent lies precisely in the fact that most of us do not possess it. Nevertheless, a magical drug that would turn anyone into a brilliant footballer would certainly sell extremely well; at least until footballing skills became so commonplace that they no longer had any value.[3]

Football skills may be a fanciful example; longevity is another matter. The 'normal' human lifespan varies enormously in different countries, and in the West, it has increased dramatically during our own lifetime (Fig. 2.2). Is lifespan prolongation a legitimate therapeutic aim? Our instinct—and certainly medical tradition—suggests that delaying premature death from disease is one of the most important functions of healthcare, but we are very ambivalent when it comes to prolonging life in the aged. Our ambivalence stems from the fact that the aged are often irremediably infirm, not merely chronologically old. In the future, we may understand better why humans become infirm, and hence more vulnerable to the environmental and genetic circumstances that cause them to become ill and die. And beyond that, we may discover how to retard or prevent aging, so that the 'normal' lifespan will be much

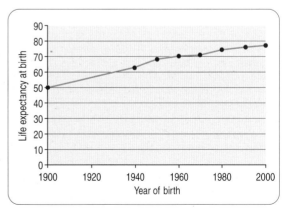

Fig. 2.2 Human lifespan in the United States. (Data from National Centre for Health Statistics, 1998.)

---

[3]The use of drugs to improve sporting performance is one of many examples of 'therapeutic' practices that find favour among individuals, yet are strongly condemned by society. We do not, as a society, attach disvalue to the possession of merely average sporting ability, even though the individual athlete may take a different view.

prolonged. Opinions will differ as to whether this will be the ultimate triumph of medical science or the ultimate social disaster.[4] A particular consequence of improved survival into old age is an increased incidence of dementia in the population. It is estimated that some 850,000 people in the UK have dementia and worldwide prevalence is thought to be over 24 million. The likelihood of developing dementia becomes greater with age, and 1.3% of people in the UK between 65 and 69 suffer from dementia, rising to 20% of those over 85. In the UK alone, it has been forecast that the number of individuals with dementia could reach 2 million by 2050 (Alzheimer's UK). The impact on healthcare systems is profound. Those with dementia will typically have 4–5 years of reduced quality of life (often substantially reduced) prior to death. The health and social costs during this time are huge and in a cost-constrained environment will inevitably divert resources from other areas of healthcare.

Conclusions

We have argued that disease can best be defined in terms of three components: aetiology, phenomenology and disvalue, and that the element of disvalue is the most important determinant of what is considered appropriate to treat. In the end, though, medical practice evolves in a more pragmatic fashion, and such arguments prove to be of limited relevance to the way in which medicine is actually practised, and hence to the therapeutic goals the drug industry sees as commercially attractive. Politics, economics and above all, social pressures are the determinants, and the limits are in practice set more by our technical capabilities than by issues of theoretical propriety.

Although the drug industry has so far been able to take a pragmatic view in selecting targets for therapeutic intervention, things are changing as technology advances. The increasing cost and sophistication of what therapeutics can offer mean that healthcare systems the world over are being forced to set limits, and have to go back to the issue of what constitutes disease. Furthermore, by invoking the concept of disease, governments control access to many other social resources (e.g., disability benefits, entry into the armed services, insurance pay-outs, access to life insurance, exemption from legal penalties, etc.).

So far, we have concentrated mainly on the impact of disease on individuals and societies. We now need to adopt a more biological perspective and attempt to put the concept of disease into the framework of contemporary ideas about how biological systems work.

Function and dysfunction: the biological perspective

The dramatic revelations of the last few decades about the molecular basis of living systems have provided a new way of looking at function and dysfunction, and the nature of disease. Needless to say, molecular biology could not have developed without the foundations of scientific biology that were built up in the 19th century. As we saw in Chapter 1, this was the period in which science came to be accepted as the basis on which medical practice had to be built. Particularly significant was cell theory, which established the cell as the basic building block of living organisms. In the words of the pioneering molecular biologist, François Jacob: 'With the cell, biology discovered its atom'. It is by focusing on the instruction sets that define the form and function of cells, and the ways in which these instructions are translated in the process of generating the structural and functional phenotypes of cells, that molecular biology has come to occupy centre stage in modern biology. Genes specify proteins, and the proteins a cell produces determine its structure and function. From a drug discovery perspective, genetic data provide a powerful indication that a target or system plays a part in the disease, but they do not tell us that the target is a key driver in our tissue of interest at the time we propose to intervene. The human cell atlas project (https://www.humancellatlas.org/) is providing vital insight into the precise cellular composition of tissues in health and disease.

From this perspective, deviations from the norm, in terms of structure and function at the cellular level, arise through deviations in the pattern of protein expression by individual cells, and they may arise either through faults in the instruction set itself (genetic mutations) or through environmental factors that alter the way in which the instruction set is translated (i.e., that affect gene expression). We come back to the age-old distinction between inherited and environmental factors (nature and nurture) in the causation of disease but with a sharper focus: altered gene expression, resulting in altered protein synthesis, is the mechanism through which all these factors operate. Conversely, it can be argued[5] that all therapeutic measures (other than physical procedures, such as surgery) also work at the cellular level, by influencing the same

---

[4]Jonathan Swift, in *Gulliver's Travels,* writes of the misery of the Struldbrugs, rare beings with a mark on their forehead who, as they grew older, lost their youth but never died, and who were declared 'dead in law' at the age of 80.

[5]This represents the ultimate reductionist view of how living organisms work, and how they respond to external influences. Many still hold out against it, believing that the 'humanity' of humans demands a less concrete explanation, and that 'alternative' systems of medicine, not based on our scientific understanding of biological function, have equal validity. Many doctors apparently feel most comfortable somewhere on the middle ground, and society at large tends to fall in behind doctors rather than scientists.

fundamental processes (gene expression and protein synthesis), although the link between a drug's primary target and the relevant effect(s) on gene expression that account for its therapeutic effect may be very indirect. We can see how it has come about that molecular biology and, in particular, genomics have come to figure so largely in the modern drug discovery environment. In the next phase, we anticipate that these will be mapped onto a more comprehensive understanding of cellular composition and architecture as a key step in target validation.

Levels of biological organization

Fig. 2.3 shows schematically the way in which the genetic constitution of a human being interacts with his or her environment to control function at many different levels, ranging from protein molecules, through single cells, tissues and integrated physiological systems, to the individual, the family and the population at large. For simplicity, we will call this the *bioaxis*. 'Disease', as we have discussed, consists of alterations of function sufficient to cause disability or impaired prognosis at the level of the individual. It should be noted that the arrows along the bioaxis in Fig. 2.3 are bidirectional—that is, disturbances at higher levels of organization will in general affect function at lower levels, and vice versa. Whereas it is obvious that genetic mutations can affect function further up the bioaxis (as in many inherited diseases, such as muscular dystrophy, cystic fibrosis or thalassaemia), we should not forget that environmental influences also affect gene function. Indeed, we can state that any long-term phenotypic change (such as weight gain, muscle weakness or depressed mood) *necessarily* involves alterations of gene expression. For example:

- Exposure to a stressful environment will activate the hypothalamopituitary system and thereby increase adrenal steroid secretion, which in turn affects gene transcription in many different cells and tissues, affecting salt metabolism, immune responses and many other functions
- Smoking, initiated as result of social factors such as peer pressure or advertising, becomes addictive as a result of changes in brain function, phenotypic changes which are in turn secondary to altered gene expression
- Exposure to smoke carcinogens then increases the probability of cancer-causing mutations in the DNA of the cells of the lung. The mutations, in turn, result in altered protein synthesis and malignant transformation, eventually producing a localized tumour and, later, disseminated cancer, with damage to the function of tissues and organs leading to symptoms and premature death.

The pathogenesis of any disease state reveals a similar level of complexity of such interactions between different levels of the bioaxis.

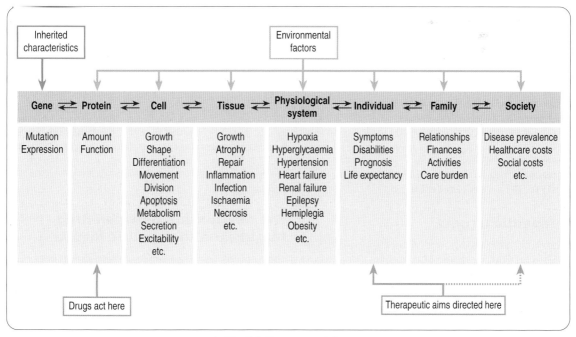

Fig. 2.3 The nature of disease.

There are two important conclusions to be drawn from the bidirectionality of influence between events at different levels of the bioaxis. One is that it is difficult to pinpoint the *cause* of a given disease. Do we regard the cause of lung cancer in an individual patient as the lack of control over tobacco advertising, the individual's susceptibility to advertising and peer pressure, the state of addiction to nicotine, the act of smoking, the mutational event in the lung epithelial cell or the individual's inherited tendency to lung cancer? There is no single answer, and the uncertainty should make us wary of the stated claim of many pharmaceutical companies that their aim is to correct the causes rather than the symptoms of disease. The truth, more often than not, is that we cannot distinguish them. Rather, the aim should be to intervene in the disease process in such a way as to minimize the disvalue (disability and impaired prognosis) experienced by the patient.

The second conclusion is that altered gene expression plays a crucial role in pathogenesis and the production of any long-term phenotypic change. If we are thinking of timescales beyond, at maximum, a few hours, any change in the structure and function of cells and tissues will be associated with changes in gene expression. These changes will include those responsible for the phenotypic change (e.g., upregulation of cytokine genes in inflammation, leading to leukocyte accumulation), and those that are consequences of it (e.g., loss of bone matrix following muscle paralysis); some of the latter will, in turn, lead to secondary phenotypic changes, and so on. The pattern of genes expressed in a cell or tissue (sometimes called the 'transcriptome', as distinct from the 'genome', which represents all of the genes present, whether expressed or not), together with the 'proteome' (which describes the array of proteins present in a cell or tissue), provides a uniquely detailed description of how the cell or tissue is behaving. Molecular biology is providing us with powerful methods for mapping the changes in gene and protein expression associated with different functional states—including disease states and therapeutic responses—and we discuss in more detail in Chapters 6 and 7 the way these new windows on function are influencing the drug discovery process (see Debouck & Goodfellow, 1999).

Therapeutic targets

Traditionally, medicine has regarded the interests of the individual patient as paramount, putting them clearly ahead of those of the community or general population. The primacy of the patient's interests remains the guiding principle for the healthcare professions; in other words, their aim is to address disvalue as experienced by the patient, not to correct biochemical abnormalities, nor to put right the wrongs of society. The principal aim of

therapeutic intervention, as shown in Fig. 2.3, is therefore to alleviate the condition of the individual patient. Genetic, biochemical or physiological deviations that are not associated with any disvalue for the patient (e.g., possession of a rare blood group, an unusually low heart rate or blood pressure or blood cholesterol concentration) are not treated as diseases because they neither cause symptoms nor carry an unfavourable prognosis. High blood pressure or high blood cholesterol, on the other hand, do confer disvalue because they carry a poor prognosis, and are targets for treatment—surrogate targets, in the sense that the actual aim is to remedy the unfavourable prognosis, rather than to correct the physiological abnormality per se.

Although the present and future wellbeing of the individual patient remains the overriding priority for medical care, the impact of disease is felt not only by individuals but also by society in general, partly for economic reasons but also for ideological reasons. Reducing the overall burden of disease, as measured by rates of infant mortality, heart disease or human immunodeficiency virus (HIV) infection, for example, is a goal for governments throughout the world, akin to the improvement of educational standards. The disease-related disvalue addressed in this case, as shown by the dotted arrow in Fig. 2.3, is experienced at the national, rather than the individual, level, for individuals will, in general, be unaware of whether or not they have benefited personally from disease prevention measures. As the therapeutic target has come to embrace the population as a whole, so the financial burden of healthcare has shifted increasingly from individuals to institutional providers of various kinds, mainly national agencies or large-scale commercial healthcare organizations. Associated with this change, there has been a much more systematic focus on assessment in economic terms of the burden of disease (disvalue, to return to our previous terminology) in the community and the economic cost of healthcare measures. The new and closely related disciplines of *pharmacoeconomics* and *pharmacoepidemiology*, discussed later, reflect the wish (1) to quantify disease-related disvalue and therapeutic benefit in economic terms and (2) to assess the impact of disease and therapy for the population as a whole, and not just for the individual patient.

The relationship between drug targets and therapeutic targets

There are very few exceptions to the rule, shown in Fig. 2.3, that protein molecules are the primary targets of drug molecules. We will come back to this theme repeatedly later, because of its prime importance for the drug discovery process. We should note here that many complex biological steps intervene between the primary drug target and the therapeutic target. Predicting, on the one hand, whether a drug that acts specifically on a particular protein will produce a worthwhile therapeutic effect, and in what disease state, or, on the other hand, what protein we should choose to target in order to elicit a therapeutic effect in a given disease state, are among the thorniest problems for drug discoverers. Molecular biology is providing new insights into the nature of genes and proteins and the relationship between them, whereas time-honoured biochemical and physiological approaches can show how disease affects function at the level of cells, tissues, organs and individuals. The links between the two nevertheless remain tenuous, a fact which greatly limits our ability to relate drug targets to therapeutic effects. Not surprisingly, attempts to bridge this Grand Canyon form a major part of the work of many pharmaceutical and biotechnology companies. Aficionados like to call themselves 'postgenomic' biologists; Luddites argue that they are merely coming down from a genomic 'high' to face once more the daunting complexities of living organisms. We patient realists recognize that a biological revolution has happened, but do not underestimate the time and money needed to bridge the canyon. More of this later.

Therapeutic interventions

Therapeutics in its broadest sense covers all types of intervention aimed at alleviating the effects of disease. The term 'therapeutics' generally relates to procedures based on accepted principles of medical science, that is, on 'conventional' rather than 'alternative' medical practice.[6] The account of drug discovery presented in this book relates exclusively to conventional medicine—and for this we make no apology—but it needs to be realized that the therapeutic landscape is actually much broader and includes many nonpharmacological procedures in the domain of conventional medicine, as well as quasipharmacological practices (e.g., homeopathy and herbalism) in the 'alternative' domain.

As discussed earlier, the desired effect of any therapeutic interventions is to improve *symptoms* or *prognosis* or both. From a pathological point of view, therapeutic interventions may be directed at *disease prevention, alleviation* of the effects of existing disease or permanent *cure* (i.e., restoration to a state of function and prognosis equivalent to those of a healthy individual of the same age, without the

need for continuing therapeutic intervention). In practice, there are relatively few truly curative interventions, and they are mainly confined to certain surgical procedures (e.g., removal of circumscribed tumours, fixing of broken bones) and chemotherapy of some infectious and malignant disorders. Most therapeutic interventions aim to alleviate symptoms and/or improve prognosis, and there is increasing emphasis on disease prevention as an objective.

It is important to realize that many types of interventions are carried out with therapeutic intent whose efficacy has not been rigorously tested. This includes not only the myriad alternative medical practices, but also many accepted conventional therapies for which a good scientific basis may exist but which have not been subjected to rigorous clinical trials. There have been a series of important surgical clinical trials recently showing that more 'modern' and complex techniques confer no meaningful benefit over simpler ones (Beard et al., 2018, 2019).

Measuring therapeutic outcome

Effect, efficacy, effectiveness and benefit

These terms have acquired particular meanings—more limited than their everyday meanings—in the context of therapeutic trials.

Pharmacological *effects* of drugs (i.e., their effects on cells, organs and systems) are, in principle, simple to measure in animals, and often also in humans. We can measure effects on blood pressure, plasma cholesterol concentration, cognitive function, etc., without difficulty. Such measures enable us to describe quantitatively the pharmacological properties of drugs but say nothing about their usefulness as therapeutic agents.

Efficacy describes the ability of a drug to produce a desired therapeutic effect in patients under carefully controlled conditions. The gold standard for measurements of efficacy is the randomized controlled clinical trial, described in more detail in Chapter 17. The aim is to discover whether, based on a strictly defined outcome measure, the drug is more or less beneficial than a standard treatment or placebo, in a selected group of patients, under conditions which ensure that the patients actually receive the drug in the specified dose. Proof of efficacy, as well as proof of safety, is required by regulatory authorities as a condition for a new drug to be licensed. Efficacy tests what the drug can do under optimal conditions, which is what the prescriber usually wants to know.

Effectiveness describes how well the drug works in real life, where the patients are heterogeneous, are not randomized, are aware of the treatment they are receiving and

---

[6]Scientific doctors rail against the term 'alternative', arguing that if a therapeutic practice can be shown to work by properly controlled trials, it belongs in mainstream medicine. If such trials fail to show efficacy, the practice should not be adopted. Paradoxically, whereas 'therapeutics' generally connotes conventional medicine, the term 'therapy' tends to be used most often in the 'alternative' field.

are prescribed different doses, which they may or may not take, often in combination with other drugs. The desired outcome is generally less well defined than in efficacy trials, related to general health and freedom from symptoms, rather than focusing on a specific measure. The focus is not on the response of individual patients under controlled conditions but on the overall usefulness of the drug in the population going about its normal business. Studies of effectiveness are of increasing interest to the pharmaceutical companies themselves, because effectiveness rather than efficacy alone ultimately determines how well the drug will sell, and because effectiveness may depend to some extent on the companies' marketing strategies (see Chapter 21). Effectiveness measures are also becoming increasingly important to the many agencies that now regulate the provision of healthcare, such as formulary committees, insurance companies, health management organizations and bodies such as the grandly titled National Institute for Health and Clinical Excellence (NICE), set up by the UK Government in 1999 to advise, on the basis of cost-effectiveness, which drugs and other therapeutic procedures should be paid for under the National Health Service.

Benefit comprises effectiveness expressed in monetary terms. It is popular with economists, as it allows cost and benefit to be compared directly, but treated with deep suspicion by many who find the idea of assigning monetary value to life and wellbeing fundamentally abhorrent.

Returning to the theme of Fig. 2.3, we can see that whereas *effect* and *efficacy* are generally measured at the level of cells, tissues, systems and individuals, *effectiveness* and *benefit* are measures of drug action as it affects populations and society at large. We next consider two growing disciplines that have evolved to meet the need for information at these levels, and some of the methodological problems that they face.

Pharmacoepidemiology and pharmacoeconomics

Pharmacoepidemiology (Strom, 2005) is the study of the use and effects of drugs in human populations, as distinct from individuals, the latter being the focus of clinical pharmacology. The subject was born in the early 1960s, when the problem of adverse drug reactions came into prominence, mainly as a result of the infamous thalidomide disaster. The existence of rare but serious adverse drug reactions, which can be detected only by the study of large numbers of subjects, was the initial stimulus for the development of pharmacoepidemiology, and the detection of adverse drug reactions remains an important concern. The identification of Reye's syndrome as a serious,

albeit rare, consequence of using aspirin in children is just one example of a successful pharmacoepidemiological study carried out under the auspices of the US Department of Health and published in 1987. The subject has gradually become broader, however, to cover aspects such as the variability of drug responses between individuals and population groups, the level of compliance of individual patients in taking drugs that are prescribed, and the overall impact of drug therapies on the population as a whole, taking all of these factors into account. The widely used antipsychotic drug *clozapine* provides an interesting example of the importance of pharmacoepidemiological issues in drug evaluation. Clozapine, first introduced in the 1970s, differed from its predecessors, such as haloperidol, in several ways, some good and some bad. On the good side, clozapine has a much lower tendency than haloperidol to cause extrapyramidal motor effects (a serious problem with many antipsychotic drugs), and it appeared to have the ability to improve not only the positive symptoms of schizophrenia (hallucinations, delusions, thought disorder, stereotyped behaviour) but also the negative symptoms (social withdrawal, apathy). Compliance is also better with clozapine, because the patient usually has fewer severe side effects. On the bad side, in about 1% of patients, clozapine causes a fall in the blood white cell count (leukopenia), which can progress to an irreversible state of agranulocytosis unless the drug is stopped in time. Furthermore, clozapine does not produce benefit in all schizophrenic patients—roughly one-third fail to show improvement, and there is currently no way of knowing in advance which patients will benefit. Clozapine is also more expensive than haloperidol. Considered from the perspective of an individual patient, and with hindsight, it is straightforward to balance the pros and cons of using clozapine rather than haloperidol, based on the severity of the extrapyramidal side effects, the balance of positive and negative symptoms that the patient has, whether clozapine is affecting the white cell count and whether the patient is a responder or a nonresponder. From the perspective of the overall population, evaluating the pros and cons of clozapine and haloperidol (or indeed of any two therapies) requires epidemiological data: how frequent are extrapyramidal side effects with haloperidol, what is the relative incidence of positive and negative symptoms, what is the incidence of agranulocytosis with clozapine, what proportion of patients are nonresponders and what is the level of patient compliance with haloperidol and clozapine?

It is a key feature of pharmacoepidemiological studies that they examine how a drug is actually used in practice. The populations in clinical trials and allowed co-medications are tightly controlled. Use in the 'real world' may be very different and lead to adverse effects that were not anticipated by the randomized controlled trial data.

Although pharmacoepidemiology has historically been primarily focused on drug safety, it may also be used to assess effectiveness, and this has been a focus of recent developments in the field.

The traditional toolkit of pharmacoepidemiology has included prospective and retrospective case–control and cohort studies. The utility and limitation of these methods are widely known. The rapid expansion in large healthcare databases (electronic health records, claims data, prescription data and patient registries) and the enormous costs of clinical trials have encouraged the increasing use of 'real world evidence' approaches. These types of data may be supplemented by data from wearables, m-health apps and environmental data, including data on social status, education and other lifestyle factors. These latter data offer much promise to deliver a holistic picture of an individual's health status. Advocates have suggested that these approaches may be able to replace the use of randomized controlled trials. The United States Twenty-First Century Cures Act mandated that the US Food and Drug Administration (FDA) should provide guidance about the circumstances under which manufacturers can use Real World Data (RWD) to support the approval of a medicine. More recently, investigators from the European Medicines Agency (EMA) detailed their views on this topic (Eichler et al., 2020). There are many complex methodological issues relating to real-world data, but the single most challenging is the lack of randomization. In the 'real world', both the severity of the disease being treated and the presence of other conditions may well affect the choice of treatment (often in ways that cannot be reliably quantified). Novel trial designs that involve randomization within a 'real-world' setting may go some way to addressing the issues.

In summary, pharmacoepidemiology is a special area of clinical pharmacology that deals with population, rather than individual, aspects of drug action and provides the means of quantifying *variability* in the response to drugs. Its importance for the drug discovery process is felt mainly at the level of clinical trials and regulatory affairs, for two reasons (Dieck et al., 1994). First, allowing for variability is essential in drawing correct inferences from clinical trials (see Chapter 17). Second, variability in response to a drug is per se disadvantageous, as drug A, whose effects are unpredictable, is less useful than drug B that acts consistently, even though the mean balance between beneficial and unwanted effects may be the same for both. From the population perspective, drug B looks better than drug A, even though for many individual patients the reverse may be true.

Pharmacoeconomics, a branch of health economics, is a subject that grew up around the need for healthcare providers to balance the ever-growing costs of healthcare against limited resources. The arrival of the welfare state, which took on healthcare provision as a national rather than an individual responsibility, was the signal for economists to move in. Good accounts of the basic principles and their application to pharmaceuticals are given by Gold et al. (1996), Johannesson (1996) and McCombs (1998). The aim of pharmacoeconomics is to measure the benefits and costs of drug treatments, and in the end, to provide a sound basis for comparing the value for money of different treatments. As might be expected, the subject arouses fierce controversy. Economics in general is often criticized for defining the price of everything but appreciating the value of nothing, and health economics particularly tends to evoke this reaction, as health and quality of life are such ill-defined and subjective, yet highly emotive, concepts. Nevertheless, pharmacoeconomics is a rapidly growing discipline and will undoubtedly have an increasing influence on healthcare provision.

Traditionally, there has been a distinction between the evidence required by regulatory authorities to license a drug which is focused on benefit/risk, and that required by payers to reimburse the cost of the drug within their system which is focused on pharmacoeconomics. There is increasing recognition that an absolute distinction between these types of information is unhelpful. Granting a license for a new drug will inevitably raise patients' expectations of receiving it. When that drug is then not made available in the health system because it is considered unaffordable or the data supporting its effectiveness are inadequate, these hopes may be dashed, and questions are asked about the regulatory process as a whole. Most of the major jurisdictions now offer processes by which scientific advice from regulatory agencies and feedback from payers can be obtained jointly. It would be wrong to assume, however, that seeking advice jointly will always mean that there is consensus between the parties as to what information is required.

Studies that generate data that can be used for pharmacoeconomic analysis are now a routine component of clinical trials programmes of new drugs. The trend can be seen as a gradual progression towards the right-hand end of the bioaxis in Fig. 2.3 in our frame of reference for assessing the usefulness of a new drug. Before 1950, new drugs were often introduced into clinical practice on the basis of studies in animals and a few human volunteers; later, formal randomized controlled clinical trials on carefully selected patient populations, with defined outcome measures, became the accepted standard, along with postmarketing pharmacoepidemiological studies to detect adverse reactions. Pharmacoeconomics represents the further shift of focus to include society in general and its provisions for healthcare. A brief outline of the main approaches used in pharmacoeconomic analysis follows. These analyses depend on the creation of a model through which to understand the data. At the simplest level, the model may describe how many people you need to treat, and the associated cost, in order to prevent one event. This may work well for an antibiotic for meningitis, but most modern treatments are more nuanced. A novel gene therapy may offer a young person many years of improved life, but early on in the treatment, it will not be known how many extra years will be added, and receiving the treatment involves 2 months of expensive inpatient hospital care. In addition, there is a long-term potential risk of malignancy that is not yet fully understood. Creating a pharmacoeconomic model for this setting is clearly much more complex, and there is ongoing debate as to how many aspects of the treatment and its implications need to be included in the model at the outset.

Pharmacoeconomics covers four levels of analysis:
- Cost identification
- Cost-effectiveness analysis
- Cost-utility analysis
- Cost–benefit analysis.

Cost identification consists of determining the full cost in monetary units of a particular therapeutic intervention, including hospitalization, working days lost, etc., as well as direct drug costs. It pays no attention to outcome, and its purpose is merely to allow the costs of different procedures to be compared. The calculation is straightforward, but deciding exactly where to draw the line (e.g., whether to include indirect costs, such as loss of income by patients and carers) is somewhat arbitrary. Nevertheless, cost identification is the least problematic part of pharmacoeconomics.

Cost-effectiveness analysis aims to quantify outcome as well as cost. This is where the real problems begin. The outcome measure most often used in cost-effectiveness analysis is based on prolongation of life, expressed as *life-years saved per patient treated*. Thus if treatment prolongs the life expectancy of patients, on average, from 3 years to 5 years, the number of life-years gained per patient is 2. Comparing cost and outcome for different treatments then allows the cost per life-year saved to be determined for each. For example, a study of various interventions in coronary heart disease, cited by McCombs (1998), showed that the cost per life-year saved was $5900 for use of a β-adrenoceptor blocker in patients who had suffered a heart attack, the corresponding figure for use of a cholesterol-lowering drug in patients with coronary heart disease was $7200, while coronary artery bypass surgery cost $34,000 per life-year saved. As these drugs have reached the end of their patent life and have become low-priced generic medicines, the cost difference changes in favour of their use. Any kind of all-or-nothing event, such as premature births prevented, hospital admissions avoided, etc., can be used for this kind of analysis. Its weakness is that it is a very crude measure, making no distinction between years of life spent in a healthy and productive mode and years of life spent in a state of chronic illness.

Cost-utility analysis is designed to include allowance for quality of life, as well as survival, in the calculation, and is yet more controversial, for it becomes necessary somehow to quantify quality—not an endeavour for the faint-hearted. What the analysis seeks to arrive at is an estimate known as *quality-adjusted life-years (QALYs)*. Thus if the quality of life for a given year, based on the results of the questionnaire, comes out at 70% of the value for an average healthy person of the same age, that year represents 0.7 QALYs, compared with 1 QALY for a year spent in perfect health, the assumption being that 1 year spent at this level of illness is 'worth' 0.7 years spent in perfect health.

Many different questionnaire-based rating scales have been devised to reflect different aspects of an individual's state of health or disability, such as ability to work, mobility, mental state, pain, etc. Some relate to specific disease conditions, whereas others aim to provide a general 'quality-of-life' estimate (Jaeschke & Guyatt, 1994), some of the best-known being the Sickness Impact Profile, the Nottingham Health Profile, the McMaster Health Index and a 36-item questionnaire known as SF-36. In addition to these general quality-of-life measures, a range of disease-specific questionnaires have been devised which give greater sensitivity in measuring the specific deficits associated with particular diseases. Standard instruments of this kind are now widely used in pharmacoeconomic studies.

To use such ratings in estimating QALYs, it is necessary to position particular levels of disability on a life/death scale, such that 1 represents alive and in perfect health and 0 represents dead. This is where the problems begin in earnest. How can we possibly say what degree of pain is equivalent to what degree of memory loss, for example, or how either compares with premature death? This problem has, of course, received a lot of expert attention (Drummond et al., 1997; Gold et al., 1996; Johannesson, 1996), and various solutions have been proposed, some of which, to the untrained observer, have a distinctly chilling and surreal quality. For example, the standard gamble approach, which is well grounded in the theory of welfare economics, involves asking the individual a question of the following kind:

> *Imagine you have the choice of remaining in your present state of health for 1 year or taking a gamble between dying now and living in perfect health for 1 year. What odds would you need to persuade you to take the gamble?*[7]

If the subject says 50:50, the implication is that he values a year of life in his present state of health at

---

[7]Imagine being asked this by your doctor! 'But I only wanted something for my sore throat', you protest weakly.

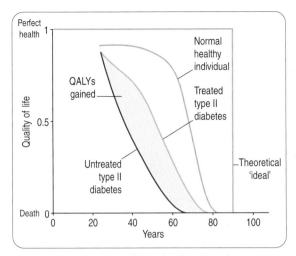

Fig. 2.4 Quality of life affected by disease and treatment.

0.5 QALYs. An alternative method involves asking the patient how many years of life in their present condition he or she would be prepared to forfeit in exchange for enjoying good health until they die. Although there are subtle ways of posing this sort of question, such an evaluation, which most ordinary people find unreal, is implicit in the QALY concept. Fig. 2.4 shows schematically the way in which quality of life, as a function of age, may be affected by disease and treatment, the area between the curves for untreated and treated patients representing the QALYs saved by the treatment. In reality, of course, continuous measurements spanning several decades are not possible, so the actual data on which QALY estimates are based in practice are much less than is implied by the idealized diagram in Fig. 2.4. Cost-utility analysis results in an estimate of monetary cost per QALY gained, and it is becoming widely accepted as a standard method for pharmacoeconomic analysis. Examples of cost per QALY gained range from £3700 for the use of sildenafil (Viagra) in treating erectile dysfunction (Stolk et al., 2000) to £328,000 for the treatment of multiple sclerosis with β-interferon (Parkin et al., 2000), this high value being accounted for by the high cost and limited therapeutic efficacy of the drug. 'Acceptable' thresholds for cost-effectiveness are suggested to be in the range of £8000–£30,000 per QALY gained (Hunter & Wilson, 2011). It is hard, if not impossible, to make sure that available funds are spent in the most appropriate way. Such has been the political pressure demanding access to novel therapies in cancer that the UK Government was moved to create a specific fund to support use of novel and expensive therapies, almost all of which did not meet the 'usual' or 'acceptable' limits per QALY. The debate still rages as to whether this is an important chance for UK patients to have access to novel therapies and so develop expertise to identify their optimal use or an abandonment of sound financial judgement, which will deny those with other conditions access to proven effective therapies.

In principle, cost-utility analysis allows comparison of one form of treatment against another, and this explains its appeal to those who must make decisions about the allocation of healthcare resources. It has been adopted as the method of choice for pharmacoeconomic analysis of new medicines by several agencies, such as the US Public Health Service and the Australian Pharmaceutical Benefits Advisory Committee.

Hard-line economists strive for an absolute scale by which to judge the value of healthcare measures compared with other resource-consuming initiatives that societies choose to support. *Cost–benefit* analysis fulfils this need in principle, by translating healthcare improvements into monetary units that can be directly balanced against costs, to assess whether any given procedure is, on balance, 'profitable'. The science of welfare economics has provided various tools for placing a monetary value on different experiences human beings find agreeable or disagreeable, based generally on the 'willingness-to-pay' principle. Not surprisingly, attempts to value human life and health in cash terms lead rapidly into an ethical and moral minefield, dangerous enough in the context of a single nation and its economy, but much more so in the global context. As a result, cost–benefit analysis has been largely shunned as a practical approach for evaluating medicines but may be unavoidable as more personalized and expensive medicines become available (Hunter & Wilson, 2011) (see Chapter 22).

Summary

In this chapter, we have discussed concepts of disease and the aims of therapeutics, the needs newly introduced drugs have to satisfy and the ways in which their ability to satisfy those needs are judged in practice. There are many uncertainties and ambiguities surrounding the definition of disease, and ideas are constantly shifting, but the two components that most satisfactorily define it are *dysfunction* and *disvalue*. Disvalue, which therapeutic interventions aim to mitigate, in turn has two main components, namely *morbidity* and *prognosis*.

We have described the bioaxis, which represents the various levels in the organizational hierarchy of living systems in general, and human beings in particular, and emphasized that disease inevitably affects all levels on the bioaxis. The drugs that we invent home in very specifically on one level, namely proteins, although the effects we want to produce are at another level, namely individuals.

31

Furthermore, we emphasize that healthcare issues are increasingly being viewed from the perspective of populations and societies, and so the impact of drugs at these levels—even further removed from their primary targets—has to be evaluated. With the exception of antimicrobial therapies, most drug treatment to date has not offered a definitive cure. Our tools and systems for the evaluation and assessment of new therapies are based on the premise that most drugs mitigate disease. New technologies and approaches offer the opportunity of cure from previously intractable conditions. Exciting though this prospect is, identifying a financially sustainable mechanism to fund these treatments will be a challenge.

In the next chapter, we will explore the range of therapeutic interventions available and how these are being employed to address human disease.

References

Alzheimer's UK. https://www.alzheimers.org.uk/about-us/policy-and-influencing/dementia-uk-report Accessed 08 Feb 2021

Beard, D. J., Davies, L. J., Cook, J. A., MacLennan, G., Price, A., Kent, S., et al.; TOPKAT Study Group. (2019). The clinical and cost-effectiveness of total versus partial knee replacement in patients with medial compartment osteoarthritis (TOPKAT): 5-year outcomes of a randomised controlled trial. *Lancet, 394*(10200), 746–756.

Beard, D. J., Rees, J. L., Cook, J. A., Rombach, I., Cooper, C., Merritt, N., et al.; CSAW Study Group. (2018). Arthroscopic subacromial decompression for subacromial shoulder pain (CSAW): A multicentre, pragmatic, parallel group, placebo-controlled, three-group, randomised surgical trial. *Lancet, 391*(10118), 329–338.

Bircher, J. (2005). Towards a dynamic definition of health and disease. *Medicine Health Care and Philosophy, 8,* 335–341.

Caplan, A. L. (1993). The concepts of health, illness, and disease. In W. F. Bynum & R. Porter (Eds.), *Companion encyclopedia of the history of medicine* (Vol. 1). London: Routledge.

Caplan, A. L., Engelhardt H. T., Jr., & McCartney, J. J. (Eds.). (1981). *Concepts of health and disease: Interdisciplinary perspectives.* London: Addison-Wesley.

Caplan, A. L., McCartney, J. J., & Sisti D. A. (Eds.). (2004). *Health, disease, and illness: Concepts in medicine.* Washington, DC: Georgetown University Press.

Debouck, C., & Goodfellow, P. N. (1999). DNA microarrays in drug discovery and development. *Nature Genetics, 21* (Suppl. 1), 48–50.

Dieck, G. S., Glasser, D. B., & Sachs, R. M. (1994). Pharmacoepidemiology: a view from industry. In B. L. Strom (Ed.), *Pharmacoepidemiology* (pp. 73–85). Chichester: John Wiley.

Drummond, M. F., O'Brien, B., Stoddart, G. I., Torrance, G. W., & Sculpher, M. J. (1997). *Methods for the economic evaluation of healthcare programmes.* Oxford: Oxford University Press.

Eichler, H. G., Koenig, F., Arlett, P., Enzmann, H., Humphreys, A., Pétavy, F., et al. (2020). Are novel, nonrandomised analytic methods fit for decision-making? The need for prospective, controlled, and transparent validation. *Clinical Pharmacology and Therapeutics, 107,* 773–779. doi:10.1002/cpt.1638.

Gold, M. R., Siegel, J. E., Russell, L. B., & Weinstein, M. C. (Eds.). (1996). *Cost-effectiveness in health and medicine.* New York: Oxford University Press.

Hunter, D., & Wilson, J. (2011). *Hyper-expensive treatments, background paper for forward look 2011* (p. 23). London: Nuffield Council on Bioethics.

Jaeschke, R., & Guyatt, G. H. (1994). Using quality-of-life measurements in pharmacoepidemiology research. In B. L. Strom (Ed.), *Pharmacoepidemiology* (pp. 495–505). Chichester: John Wiley.

Johannesson, M. (1996). *Theory and methods of economic evaluation of health care.* Dordrecht: Kluwer Academic.

McCombs, J. S. (1998). Pharmacoeconomics: What is it and where is it going? *American Journal of Hypertension, 11,* 112S–119S.

Moynihan, R., Heath, I., & Henry, D. (2004). Selling sickness: The pharmaceutical industry and disease mongering. *British Medical Journal, 324,* 886–891.

Parkin, D., Jacoby A., McNamee, P., Miller, P., Thomas, S., Bates, D. (2000). Treatment of multiple sclerosis with interferon beta: an appraisal of cost-effectiveness and quality of life. *Journal of Neurology, Neurosurgery and Psychiatry, 68,* 144–149.

Reznek, L. (1987). *The nature of disease.* New York: Routledge & Kegan Paul.

Scully, J. L. (2004). What is a disease? *EMBO Reports, 5,* 650–653.

Stolk, E. A., Busschbach, J. J., Caffa, M., Meuleman, E. J., & Rutten, F. F. (2000). Cost utility analysis of sildenafil compared with papaverine-phentolamine injections. *British Medical Journal, 320,* 1156–1157.

Strom, B. L. (Ed.). (2005). *Pharmacoepidemiology* (4th ed.). Chichester: John Wiley.

Chapter | 3 |

Therapeutic modalities

Duncan B Richards

Introduction

Therapeutics in its broadest sense covers all types of intervention aimed at alleviating the effects of disease. The term 'therapeutics' generally relates to procedures based on accepted principles of medical science, that is, on 'conventional' rather than 'alternative' medical practice.

The account of drug discovery presented in this book relates exclusively to conventional medicine—and for this we make no apology—but it needs to be realized that the therapeutic landscape is actually much broader and includes many nonpharmacological procedures in the domain of conventional medicine.

The evolution of therapeutic interventions

The earliest interventions were those aimed at alleviating the symptoms of a disease, for example, the use of opioids as analgesics. Relief of symptoms is an important therapeutic goal, and indeed the one the patient will thank the treating physician for most, but it does not address the underlying disease and so may be considered 'papering over the cracks'. In the worst cases, symptomatic treatment can mask or even accelerate disease progression. The pain associated with an arthritic joint in part protects against overuse; excessive analgesic use may hasten joint failure through overloading of the joint. As our understanding of pathophysiological processes has improved, interventions that modify disease processes have been developed. anti-inflammatory drugs address the inflammation that is at the centre of diseases such as rheumatoid arthritis. As inflammation resolves, the symptoms of fever, pain, redness and swelling also improve. In this case, the relief of symptoms is secondary to the modification of the disease process. Remember that relieving symptoms may not address the underlying disease, so addressing the underlying disease may not treat all the patient's symptoms. A substantial proportion of patients with rheumatoid arthritis have troubling ongoing pain despite achieving resolution of inflammation. When symptoms remain, always consider if they could be the result of another pathological process.

Some disease processes are asymptomatic, and therapy for these conditions is particularly challenging. Chronic hypertension markedly increases the risk of stroke, and lowering blood pressure reduces this risk. Other than in the most severe cases, however, hypertension is asymptomatic. The drugs used to treat hypertension are all associated with adverse effects. Cold extremities associated with use of β-blockers might be considered an acceptable inconvenience, but impotence would generally not be considered acceptable, even if the risk of stroke has been substantially reduced. It is therefore a key concept of therapeutics that the overall benefit risk be considered, and that the patient has the opportunity to have their views taken into account. 'Poor adherence' is often cited as a reason for therapeutic failure, but this terminology fails to take into account that if a patient is not aligned with the goals of a therapeutic intervention, they are unlikely to take it 'as directed'. For this reason, concordance is a better term to use, as it captures the concept that for a therapeutic intervention to be successful it should be based on a mutually agreed plan agreed between patient and treating clinician.

Although disease modification is the basis of most therapeutic interventions, and pharmaceutical interventions in particular, disease modification is not the same as cure. We are now entering an era when cure is becoming a realistic therapeutic target for many diseases. Our current standard of care is aimed at disease modification for those living with human immunodeficiency virus (HIV) infection. Combination triple and now dual antiviral therapy mean that those with access to standard of care can expect a normal life expectancy. Although the duration of life is now as long as the general population, it is important to remember that treatments still have adverse effects, so normal life-expectancy is not the same as a 'normal' life. The next generation of care is by contrast aimed at preexposure prophylaxis (PrEP) and might be considered a cure in that its intention is to avoid chronic HIV infection in the first place. Gene therapy for adenosine deaminase severe combined immunodeficiency (ADA–SCID) aims to correct the primary deficiency that causes this fatal condition. It is too early to say whether the currently available modalities offer a cure, that is, something that lasts a lifetime, but the principle of this type of therapy is an important one that we will likely see expand into other diseases over the coming years. The concept of risk–benefit assessment remains vital even when considering curative treatments. Childhood leukaemia may be cured by modern therapy, but the patient is left with an increased risk of other haematological malignancies in the long term. In this case, the benefit risk is generally considered acceptable given the likely fatal outcome of the initial disease, but it is important to consider whether a curative treatment for a mild condition could have serious sequelae later in life. Importantly, this information is very unlikely to be available for many years after the treatment is first marketed.

The range of therapeutic interventions

In the examples given so far, we have focused on pharmaceutical interventions, but other modalities, often used in combination with drug treatment, have a vital role to play in delivering an overall therapeutic intervention; examples include:

- Advice and counselling (e.g., genetic counselling)
- Psychological treatments (e.g., cognitive therapies for anxiety disorders, depression, etc.)
- Dietary and nutritional treatments (e.g., gluten-free diets for coeliac disease, diabetic diets, etc.)
- Physical treatments, including surgery and radiotherapy
- Pharmacological treatments—encompassing the whole of conventional drug therapy
- Biological and biopharmaceutical treatments, a broad category including vaccination, transplantation, blood transfusion, biopharmaceuticals (see Chapter 8), in vitro fertilization, etc.

The range of therapeutic interventions is expanding rapidly and includes many that look very different from conventional drugs (Fig. 3.1).

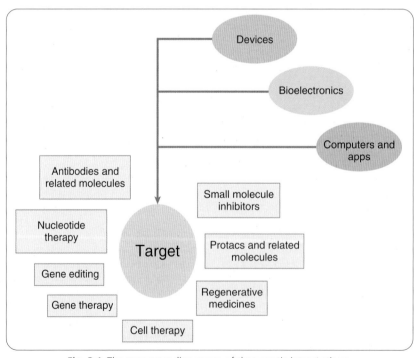

Fig. 3.1 The ever-expanding range of therapeutic interventions.

The fringes of conventional therapy are complex. Obesity is now a public health emergency and weight loss a valid therapeutic target. What is less clear is the contribution that the myriad of diets, dietary supplements and protein drinks make to this therapeutic target.

In this area, it is important to keep an open mind and to insist on evidence to support marketing claims. Some things that were once thought on the fringes are establishing a more sound scientific footing. For example, there is an increasing amount of evidence supporting an important role of the gut microbiome in inflammatory bowel disease—this could lead to important therapeutic advances in the future, but is not the same as saying that a yoghurt drink will cure Crohn's disease.

Adding more and more treatments is not always therapeutic, especially when the new treatments are aimed at addressing adverse effects of others. Sometimes the most therapeutic action can be to stop unnecessary and potentially interacting interventions.

This book is focused primarily on pharmaceutical interventions, that is, novel chemical or biological constructs with an intended therapeutic effect, but these should no longer be viewed in isolation; some of the most exciting advances are coming from the combination of drug and physical interventions in a single product. The most established of these are interventions such as the drug-eluting stent for coronary artery disease. In this case, the local delivery of an immunosuppressant reduces the risk of restenosis of the stented blood vessel. Like most physical interventions, its effectiveness remains dependent on the skill of the interventional cardiologist in placing the stent in the optimal position. Biomaterials may be conventional scaffolds, but some are in development that are designed to modify the body's response to their presence (e.g., induce fibrosis or prevent fibrosis). These types of properties are more drug-like and will require a different approach to development and evaluation from the traditional medical device approval process. The emerging field of bioelectronics seeks to modify organ responses through electrical stimulation—whether peripherally or centrally. Defining the appropriate body of evidence required to support commercial use of these kinds of intervention and the nature of the postmarketing follow-up present a considerable challenge to regulators. Disruptive innovations such as these require a novel and tailored approach—attempting to modify existing frameworks designed for pharmaceuticals or devices is unlikely to fulfil society's needs.

On the fringe of conventional medicine are preparations that fall into the category of 'nutriceuticals' or 'cosmeceuticals'. Nutriceuticals include a range of dietary preparations, such as slimming diets, and diets supplemented with vitamins, minerals, antioxidants, unsaturated fatty acids, fibre and so on. These preparations generally have some scientific rationale, although their efficacy has not, in most cases, been established by controlled trials. They are not subject to formal regulatory approval, so long as they do not contain artificial additives other than those that have been approved for use in foods. Cosmeceuticals is a fancy name for cosmetic products similarly supplemented with substances claimed to reduce skin wrinkles, promote hair growth and so on. These products achieve very large sales, and some pharmaceutical companies have expanded their business in this direction. We do not discuss these fringe 'ceuticals' in this book. Again, even in this area, we need not to be dismissive. If someone is frankly iron deficient, then treatment with iron would be considered therapeutic. Vitamins and minerals are widely administered in a therapeutic way, but most would not consider it necessary to routinely supplement a normal varied diet with a vitamin or mineral supplement.

Within each of the medical categories listed above lies a range of procedures: at one end of the spectrum are procedures that have been fully tried and tested and are recognized by medical authorities; at the other is outright quackery of all kinds. Somewhere between lie widely used 'complementary' procedures, practised in some cases under the auspices of officially recognized bodies, which have no firm scientific foundation. Here we find, among psychological treatments, hypnotherapy and analytical psychotherapy; among nutritional treatments, 'health foods', added vitamins and diets claimed to avoid ill-defined food allergies; among physical treatments, acupuncture and osteopathy; among chemical treatments, homeopathy, herbalism and aromatherapy. Biological procedures lying in this grey area between scientific medicine and quackery are uncommon (and we should probably be grateful for this)—unless one counts colonic irrigation and swimming with dolphins.

In this book, we are concerned with the last two treatment categories on the list, summarized in Table 3.1, and in this chapter, we consider the current status and future prospects of the three main fields; namely 'conventional' therapeutic drugs, biopharmaceuticals and various biological therapies.

Conventional therapeutic drugs

Small-molecule drugs, either synthetic compounds or natural products, have for a long time been the mainstay of therapeutics; however, biopharmaceuticals and related products have grown rapidly and represented nearly 40% of the US Food and Drug Administration (FDA) approvals in 2017. The daily 'white pill' has been a mainstay of therapeutics for most of the modern era, and it remains a straightforward and reliable way to deliver therapy,

Table 3.1 The main types of therapeutic intervention

Type	Source	Examples	Notes
Conventional small-molecule drugs	Synthetic organic compounds[a]	Most of the pharmacopoeia	The largest category of drugs in use, and of new registrations
	Natural products	Paclitaxel (Taxol), many antibiotics and anticancer drugs (e.g., penicillin, aminoglycosides, erythromycin), opiates (e.g., morphine), statins (e.g., lovastatin), ciclosporin, fujimycin	Continues to be an important source of new therapeutic drugs
	Semisynthetic compounds (i.e., compounds made by derivatizing natural products)	Penicillin derivatives (e.g., ampicillin), second-generation statins (e.g., simvastatin)	Strategy for generating improved 'second-generation' drugs from natural products
Protacs and related molecules	Heterobifunctional small molecule composed of two active domains and a linker capable of removing specific unwanted proteins	Several molecules in development	
Peptide and protein mediators	Synthetic	Somatostatin, calcitonin, vasopressin	Peptides up to approximately 20 residues can be reliably made by solid-phase synthesis
	Extracted from natural sources (human, animal, microbial)	Insulin, growth hormone, human γ-globulins, botulinum toxin	At one time, the only source of such hormones. Now largely replaced by recombinant biotechnology products. γ-Globulins still obtained from human blood
	Recombinant DNA technology	Human insulin, erythropoietin, human growth hormone, GM-CSF, TNF-α, hirudin	Many different expression systems in use and in development
Antibodies	Animal antisera, human immunoglobulins	Antisera used to treat infections such as hepatitis A and B, diphtheria, rabies, tetanus. Also poisoning by botulinum, snake and spider venoms, etc.	
	Monoclonal antibodies	Trastuzumab (directed against epidermal growth factor receptor), rituximab (directed against B-cell surface antigen)	A rapidly growing class of biopharmaceuticals, with many products in development
Enzymes	Recombinant DNA technology	Cerebrosidase, dornase, galactosidase	
Vaccines	Infecting organism (killed, attenuated or nonpathogenic strains)	Smallpox, diphtheria, measles, tuberculosis, tetanus, influenza and many others	The conventional approach, still widely used. Some risk of introducing viable pathogens
	Antigens produced by recombinant DNA technology	Many of the above vaccines now available as recombinant antigens	Advantages are greater consistency and elimination of risk of introducing pathogens
Nucleotide therapies	Recombinant DNA technology	Antisense and siRNA oligonucleotides (e.g., Vitravene; Inotersen (ASO); Patisiran (siRNA))	

Table 3.1 The main types of therapeutic intervention—cont'd

Type	Source	Examples	Notes
Gene therapy	Ex vivo and in vivo approaches, most with viral vectors, but nonviral approaches in development	Autologous CD34+ enriched cell fraction that contains CD34+ cells transduced with retroviral vector that encodes for the human ADA–cDNA sequence for severe combined immunodeficiency syndrome. Onasemnogene abeparvovec for spinal muscular atrophy	Gene editing therapies in development
Cells	Human donors	Blood and platelet transfusions	
	Engineered cell lines based on patient's own cells	Axicabtagene ciloleucel for large B-cell lymphoma. Tisagenlecleucel for acute lymphoblastic leukaemia	Intense research efforts to establish whether this therapy approach can be applied to solid tumours
Tissues	Human donors, animal tissues, engineered tissues	Apligraf	Bilayer of human skin cells
Organs	Human donors	Transplant surgery	

[a]Not considered here are many 'adjunct' therapies, such as oxygen, antiseptic agents, anaesthetic agents, intravenous salts, etc., which are outside the scope of this book.

ADA, Adenosine deaminase; *ASO*, antisense oligonucleotides; *GM-CSF*, Granulocyte macrophage colony-stimulating factor; *siRNA*, small interfering RNA; *TNF*, tumour necrosis factor.

especially for short periods. In an ageing population in which long-term polypharmacy is the norm, pill burden is, however, a genuine problem. New technologies offering long-term controlled release from a parenteral injection are increasingly employed to deliver long-term therapy without the need for daily injections or tablets.

There are important differences between small-molecule drugs and biopharmaceuticals, and these are summarized in Boxes 3.1 and 3.2.

In addition to the application of modified-release technology, the other key development in this field has been a substantial expansion in the range of targets and the chemical constructs employed. While G-protein coupled receptors remain a productive field of research, many small molecules are now directed against new types of target, such as proteins involved in the control of epigenetic coding.

New classes of drugs are emerging that make use of the cellular apparatus for degrading unwanted proteins. These molecules have one end that engages the E3 ubiquitin ligase complex, which then tags to the complex for intracellular proteolysis. The other end of the molecule can be designed to bind to the target protein of interest. This type of approach allows inhibition (functional knockdown) of proteins that are not amenable to conventional antagonist pharmacology; examples include CELMoD (Cereblon E3 Ligase Modulation Drugs) and PROTAC (proteolysis targeting chimera).

Therapies based on nucleotides are considered in the biological products section, see later, but in terms of their function, they have a lot in common with the protein-degrading technologies described immediately above.

Coupled with advances in technologies such as automated chemistry, high-throughput screening, the scope of small-molecule interventions continues to expand. While media focus has recently highlighted the potential of advanced therapies (see later), conventional therapy remains the mainstay of treatment for chronic conditions.

Biological products

Biological products, or biologics, encompass a very wide and expanding range of medicinal products. They may be made of sugars, proteins or nucleic acids or complex combinations of these substances, or may be living entities such as cells and tissues. The speed of technological advancement in this field is very rapid, and it is clear that there is substantial opportunity for breakthroughs in therapy. Remember, however, that some types of biological therapy are very new, and information on long-term safety is limited. It has been a feature of drug development over the past century that the therapeutic reach of novel modalities proves to be more restricted than originally envisaged, usually as a result of restricted

Box 3.1 **Advantages and disadvantages of small-molecule drugs**

Advantages

- 'Chemical space' is so vast that synthetic chemicals, according to many experts, have the potential to bind specifically to any chosen biological target: the right molecule exists; it is just a matter of finding it.
- Doctors and patients are thoroughly familiar with conventional drugs as medicines, and the many different routes of administration that are available. Clinical pharmacology in its broadest sense has become part of the knowledge base of every practising doctor, and indeed, part of everyday culture. Although sections of the public may remain suspicious of drugs, there are few who will refuse to use them when the need arises.
- Oral administration is often possible, as well as other routes where appropriate.
- Pharmaceutical companies have long experience in developing, registering, producing, packaging and marketing such products.

Disadvantages

- As emphasized elsewhere in this book, the flow of new small-molecule drugs seems to be diminishing, despite increasing R&D expenditure. There are many targets that are simply not tractable with a small molecule.
- Despite improved screening, toxicity remains a serious and unpredictable problem, causing failures in late development, or even after registration. Selectivity is always a relative term with drug molecules and is in general less good than with biopharmaceuticals.
- Humans and other animals have highly developed mechanisms for eliminating foreign molecules; achieving adequate exposure without toxicity is always a challenge.
- Oral absorption is poor for many compounds. Peptides cannot be given orally.

Box 3.2 **Advantages and disadvantages of biopharmaceuticals**

Advantages

- The main benefit offered by biopharmaceutical products is that they open up the scope of protein therapeutics, which was previously limited to proteins that could be extracted from animal or human sources.
- The discovery process for new biopharmaceuticals is often quicker and more straightforward than with synthetic compounds, as traditional screening and lead optimization approaches are not required.
- Unexpected toxicity is less common than with synthetic molecules.
- The risk of immune responses to nonhuman proteins—a problem with porcine or bovine insulins—may be mitigated by expressing the human sequence.
- The risk of transmitting virus or prion infections from extracts is avoided.

Disadvantages

- Producing biopharmaceuticals on a commercial scale has been expensive, requiring complex purification and quality control procedures.
- The products are not orally active. Achieving the desired exposure profile in a practical way can be complex. Like other proteins, biopharmaceutical products do not cross the blood–brain barrier.
- For the above reasons, development generally costs more and takes longer than it does for synthetic drugs.
- Many biopharmaceuticals are species specific in their effects, making tests of efficacy in animal models difficult or impossible.

therapeutic index. One of the key challenges for this field over the coming years will be to optimally align the various modalities with different types of disease. There will not be the resources to test each modality for every possible indication.

The earliest forms of biological drug were proteins and peptides that were extracted from animal or human sources in order to replace deficient production in humans. The principal examples of this were insulin and growth hormone. Extraction from another source will always carry a risk of transmission of infectious agents, and molecules derived from another species may induce immune responses that reduce the effectiveness of the agent. A breakthrough in this field happened in 1982 with

the development by Eli Lilly of recombinant human insulin (Humulin), made by genetically engineered *Escherichia coli*. Recombinant human growth hormone (also produced in *E. coli*), erythropoietin (Epogen) and tissue plasminogen activator (tPA) made by engineered mammalian cells followed during the 1980s. This was the birth of the biopharmaceutical industry, and since then, new bioengineered proteins have contributed an increasing proportion of new medicines to be registered (see Table 3.1 for some examples, and Chapters 8 and 9 for more details).

Monoclonal antibodies

Human immunoglobulin responses are polyclonal; this is associated with benefits in terms of efficacy and greater protection against mutation of the pathogen. Polyclonality is, however, a substantial challenge for a medicinal product because it has been a fundamental principle that the hallmarks of quality are definition and reproducibility.

The technological breakthroughs that led to our ability to produce monoclonal antibodies at scale have transformed modern therapeutics. The first monoclonal antibodies were produced by fusing an antibody-producing B cell with an immortal myeloma cell (Milstein and Köhler, 1975; awarded Nobel Prize in 1984). The first monoclonal antibody to be licensed was Orthoclone OKT3 (muromomab-CD3) in 1986 for use in prevention of kidney transplant rejection. This antibody is mouse IgG2a antibody whose cognate antigen is CD3 (murine antibodies include the stem 'mo'). The structure of mouse IgG is not the same as human, and this treatment is associated with a human anti-mouse antibody response, which can be treatment-limiting. The next generation of antibodies were chimeras in which the mouse variable region of the IgG was fused onto a human constant region, producing a more 'human' antibody. There are several examples of widely used antibodies in this category, including abciximab (ReoPro), basiliximab (Simulect), cetuximab (Erbitux), infliximab (Remicade) and rituximab (MabThera).

Several methods have been developed to produce fully human antibodies; of these, phage display is the best known (Smith and Winter, Nobel Prize 2018). Genetic information coding for the binding regions of antibodies is extracted from human B cells and inserted into bacteriophages. These then display the binding regions, and those that bind best to the target of choice can be selected. The selected binding regions are then inserted onto a human immunoglobulin scaffold.

The majority of therapeutic antibodies are used to bind to their target with the intention of blocking its action. A smaller proportion engage the immune system via their Fc region to induce antibody-dependent cellular cytotoxicity and/or complement-dependent cytotoxicity. These mechanisms are most commonly applied in cancer therapies, and examples of licensed drugs include trastuzumab and rituximab. The immunological response associated with these types of biopharmaceuticals is complex and may lead to treatment-limiting adverse effects such as cytokine release syndrome. In addition to engaging effector mechanisms, the Fc receptor is involved in recycling of antibodies, which may be an important determinant of their pharmacokinetic properties. Manipulation of the Fc region can lead to enhanced effector function or prolonged half-life.

Producing complex molecules such as monoclonal antibodies at scale and with the consistency and quality required of a medicinal product is highly complex and has been a rate-determining step for many biopharmaceutical development programmes. One of the most important advances of the last decade has been in manufacturing technology that allows molecules to be produced more quickly and cheaply than has been possible in the past.

The majority of current biopharmaceuticals are full-size monoclonal antibodies; advances in protein engineering allow the production of fragments, bi-specific molecules and other modified versions of monoclonal antibodies with the potential to confer novel pharmacological and pharmacokinetic properties.

While there is undoubtedly considerable scope for further enhancement of this modality, we now have a good general understanding of its strengths and weaknesses; we will now consider some of the emerging approaches about which much less is known.

Nucleotide-based therapies

The emergence of nucleotide therapies illustrates well the pattern for many new modalities. When the approach and the ability to silence specific gene products was first described, there was considerable hype, and it was hailed as the answer to a myriad of conditions. As development progressed, serious problems declared themselves: it proved very difficult to target these molecules to organs other than the liver, and some chemical constructs proved toxic. Development plans were reconsidered and focused on those areas most tractable, and we are now seeing the first wave of medicines for patients, most of which target the liver. The lessons learned from the first wave are informing the second wave as advances in our understanding of the science and improvements in technology allow the modality to be applied to a wider range of diseases.

Interfering with the process of translation of proteins is an attractive means to achieve a functional 'knockout' or downregulation of a pathological protein. There are two broad approaches: small interfering RNA (siRNA) and antisense oligonucleotides (ASO). ASO are single-stranded sections of RNA that bind to complementary messenger RNA and thus inhibit translation by steric hindrance, splicing alterations, initiation of target degradation or other mechanisms. Although ostensibly attractive, this approach has been challenging because the single strands can be very susceptible to nucleases and delivery of sufficient material to the target cells has proven difficult. siRNAs are double-stranded molecules of RNA, typically 20 to 25 nucleotides in length. Once in the cell, they are processed by Dicer proteins to single-stranded RNA molecules. These then become incorporated into the RNA-induced silencing complex (RISC), a multi-subunit protein that then also binds complementary messenger RNA and degrades it. The cellular machinery employed in this process is that by which naturally occurring micro-RNA molecules achieve gene silencing. This approach has faced two particular challenges in the development of effective therapeutics: achieving sufficient selectivity and the RNA protein complexes have proven to be immunogenic in some cases.

This is a field in which there has been intense activity to improve the chemical and pharmacokinetic characteristics of the molecules, and there are reasons to be optimistic that this will deliver substantial therapeutic advances in the coming years.

Cell-based therapies

Transplantation

Cell-based therapy has come to prominence recently, but it is important to remember that we have been using cells and indeed whole organs for some time in the field of organ transplantation. The principle of transplantation is to supplement or replace the function of a failing organ with a fully integrated alternative. The majority of human transplants are allografts, that is, from another human who is genetically distinct from the recipient. Despite advances in our understanding of the molecular mechanisms of rejection and improvements in drug treatment, rejection remains a major limitation to the widespread and long-term use of this technique. The treatment of haematological disorders and haematological malignancy in particular has been substantially altered by the regenerative properties of stem cells. The technique requires ablation of the existing bone marrow and replacement with stem cells derived from either a donor or the patient themselves (autograft). Bone marrow ablation carries substantial risks, and engraftment is not a certainty, both of which mean that despite substantial improvements, the technique continues to carry substantial risk and is not suitable for all patients. Harnessing the power of stem cells to regenerate other tissues remains an important therapeutic goal, and there are numerous development programmes seeking to derive a therapeutic effect in solid organs.

Whole organs and bone marrow are the most familiar transplants but groups of cells have also been tried. Islet cell transplantation for diabetes has been successful and is offered to small numbers of patients at specialist centres. Attempts to replace failing dopaminergic neurons in the substantia nigra of patients with Parkinson's disease have been made since the 1980s. Results have been very mixed, but there remains considerable interest in the approach. The most promising current one involves the use of embryonic neuronal cells that retain stem cell properties. The regenerative potential of stem cells is enormous, but achieving in situ differentiation and persistence has proven difficult to achieve. This is an area where there has been an explosion of activity in recent years as we better understand the basic mechanisms of cell control and differentiation. It is also unfortunately an area where the unscrupulous have taken advantage of patients claiming almost magical properties for cell preparations of dubious origin.

Modified T cells in cancer

The most important recent development in cell therapy has been the advent of modified T cells for the treatment of malignancy. The most advanced of these are the chimeric antigen receptor (CAR)-T cells; two examples have been licensed—axicabtagene ciloleucel for non-Hodgkin's lymphoma and tisagenlecleucel for acute lymphoblastic leukaemia and diffuse large B-cell lymphoma. In this intervention, T cells are harvested from the patient by apheresis. A CAR is then inserted (usually by lentivirus). The modified cells express this CAR on their surface. The cell pool proliferates and is then re-infused into the patient. The modified CAR-T cells recognize the cognate antigen (exclusive of major histocompatibility complex [MHC]) and engage the T-cell effector mechanisms. This approach has considerable potential, and in some cases, the effect has been dramatic, but adverse effects are common and can be severe (cytokine release syndrome). At present, we do not have a complete understanding of how to balance achieving a strong immunological response while avoiding potentially life-threatening adverse drug reactions. The second major approach is to introduce modified T-cell receptors that recognize antigen in the context of MHC—these have the potential to be able to target intracellular antigens and so treat a wider range of cancers.

The ability to modify the body's immune response to tumours shows considerable promise but at present is restricted to a small number of haematological malignancies and requires the infrastructure of highly specialized centres. The current approaches are in essence a form of gene therapy. In the next section, we will consider this approach more broadly.

Gene therapy

The contribution of our genes to the pathogenesis of disease is well recognized, so the concept of modifying our genes is an intrinsically attractive therapeutic approach.

There are three broad approaches:
- Replacing a mutated gene that causes disease with a healthy copy of the gene.
- Inactivating, or 'knocking out', a mutated gene that is functioning improperly.
- Introducing a new gene into the body to help fight a disease.

Although the concept of gene therapy has been around for some time, delivering it has proven difficult, and there remain few licensed treatments. Delivering sufficient gene product to the site of action and achieving a lasting effect have proven especially difficult problems to solve. Advances in vector technology, that is, the means by which the gene is delivered, are beginning to produce dividends, and it is likely we will see more licensed treatments in the near future.

The most widely investigated approach involves introducing new genes to replace missing or dysfunctional ones; this is most commonly done by engineering the new gene into a modified virus (the vector), which has the ability to enter the host cell, causing expression of the artificially introduced gene until the cell dies or expels the foreign DNA. Such nonintegrated DNA is usually eliminated quite quickly and is not passed on to the cell's progeny, and so this type of transfection is generally only appropriate in situations where transient expression is all that is required. Retroviral vectors are able to incorporate the new DNA into the host cell's chromosomes, where it will remain and be expressed during the lifetime of the cell and will be passed on to any progeny of that cell. More elaborate gene therapy protocols for treating single-gene disorders are designed actually to correct the disease-producing sequence mutation in the host genome, or to alter gene expression so as to silence dysfunctional genes.

At one time, gene therapy directed at germline cells was considered a possibility, the advantage being that an inherited gene defect could be prevented from affecting progeny, and effectively eliminated for good. The serious risks and ethical objections to such human genetic engineering, however, have led to a worldwide ban on germ-cell gene-therapy experiments, and efforts are restricted to somatic cell treatments.

Two approaches have emerged as offering real promise in the past few years. The first of these is to focus gene delivery by direct injection into the site of interest; this has proven most practical in the retina. The first disease to be treated in this way was choroideraemia, a rare X-linked recessive disorder caused by a loss-of-function mutation in the *CHM* gene. Preliminary results are encouraging and other retinal diseases are now being investigated in clinical trials. The ex vivo autologous approach has the following steps: cells are removed from the patient, modified ex vivo using a viral vector and then re-introduced to the patient. This approach lends itself most readily to haematological diseases and has resulted in licensing of Strimvelis (autologous CD34+ enriched cell fraction that contains CD34+ cells transduced with retroviral vector that encodes for the human ADA–cDNA sequence), a treatment for adenine deaminase deficiency that causes a severe combined immunodeficiency syndrome (ADA–SCID).

Gene editing

In many cases, the length of defective genetic code responsible for a disease is very short, and in some cases, it may only be one base pair. One could argue that replacing a whole chapter of a book when it only contains one typographical error is over complicating the situation. This has led to the development of gene editing as a therapeutic concept. The core technology here is clustered regularly interspaced short palindromic repeats, better known as CRISPR. In essence, these sequences are found in prokaryotes such as bacteria, and when coupled with the CAS9 enzyme, the complex recognizes and cleaves specific strands of DNA that are complementary to the CRISPR sequence. By creating artificial sequences, it is possible to induce highly specific editing of the genome. There is considerable excitement about this approach but it remains very early in development.

Other therapeutic approaches

Vaccines

Immunization against infectious diseases dates from 1796, when Jenner first immunized patients against smallpox by infecting them with the relatively harmless cowpox. Many other immunization procedures were developed in the 19th century, and from the 20th century onwards, pharmaceutical companies began producing standardized versions of the antigens, often the attenuated or modified organisms themselves, as well as antisera, which would give immediate passive protection against disease organisms. The core principle of vaccination for infectious disease has been to stimulate a cellular and/or humoral response by exposing an individual to the antigen such that if they subsequently encounter the infectious agent, it will be rapidly cleared. It is hard to overemphasize how important this approach has been to the mass control of infectious disease. It has delivered the eradication of small pox and the near eradication of tetanus and polio from large areas of the planet. The value has been highlighted recently by the reemergence of measles including fatal cases because of loss of herd immunity, as some parents withhold vaccination owing to concerns generated and promulgated by spurious claims of harm.

The concept of stimulating the human immune system to deliver a therapeutic effect has substantial parallels with the cellular therapies for cancer described earlier. Indeed, there are a number of efforts under way to use the principles of vaccination to stimulate immune responses in noninfectious disease, including cancer.

Biomaterials

Is a pig heart valve a transplant or a biomaterial? In broad terms, it is more of a material in that it is avascular and can be made acellular. The use of a full biological construct is, however, unusual; most work in the space involves the use of materials as scaffolds. The dangers of using synthetic durable materials in this were recently highlighted by polypropylene transvaginal mesh implants used for stress incontinence or vaginal prolapse. In some cases, these can erode tissue leading to scarring, fistula formation and pain. Efforts are underway to create biomaterials that form a temporary scaffold while tissues repair but are then absorbed so that no exogenous material remains long term.

Bioelectronics

Our bodies are a natural marvel of bioelectronics, and indeed, it is the electrical activity of our brains that makes us who we are. Our enhanced understanding of the nervous system now indicates that nerves have long-lasting effects on the tissues that go way beyond simple reflexes and include modification of immune responses. At the most extreme end, electroconvulsive therapy has been used to treat severe intractable depression, and deep brain stimulation has been used with some success for Parkinson's disease. The focus of current approaches is to use small implantable stimulators to stimulate nerves to induce a change in, for example, immune response or insulin secretion. This is an area of considerable promise, but the technical challenges are legion—achieving a good contact with the nerve, avoiding scarring, identifying an effective 'dose' and frequency of administration.

Summary

Our traditional view of therapeutics centres on the 'druggable target', typically an enzyme or transmembrane receptor that one tries to block, or less commonly simulate, with a chemical molecule. We have a robust understanding of physicochemical characteristics that confer a favourable developability profile, and we have established

methods to evaluate them preclinically. Familiar though this is, there are many therapeutic targets that cannot be addressed in this way, and identifying a synthetic chemical that has the required specificity and physicochemical properties without being highly toxic remains very challenging. Antibody therapy has made a huge contribution largely through its ability to bind to targets with very high specificity—off-target effects are rare. Immensely valuable though this approach has been, some targets are inaccessible, and antibodies still have to be given parenterally.

If the problem cannot be addressed by these approaches, the options have tended to be fairly drastic, with approaches such as organ and bone marrow transplantation and all their associated morbidities.

We now find ourselves in a very different environment. The explosion in biotechnology and molecular biology has delivered a huge range of new therapeutic approaches, including gene therapy, nucleotide drugs and cell therapies. For a long time, the key challenge in drug development was to be able to come up with something that adequately addressed a well-validated target. The range of modalities now available means that there are relatively few targets that cannot be addressed by one of them. The key challenge is to establish whether the target has the potential to be therapeutically useful. Competition between companies used to be within a drug class; success was based on the quality of the molecule and the ability to move quickly through development. Competition these days is often between modalities, for example, a nucleotide approach versus an antibody versus a gene therapy. Because many of these modalities are new, it can be challenging when a trial fails to establish whether it was the target or the technology. We have also seen that the costs of development have risen sharply, and it is unrealistic to expect that every modality will be tested in every possible disease. Identifying the best modality for a condition needs to be a critical objective for thoughtful drug research.

Further Reading

Classic papers on phage display

McCafferty, J., Griffiths, A. D, Winter, G., & Chiswell, D. J. (1990). Phage antibodies: filamentous phage displaying antibody variable domains. *Nature, 348*, 552–554.

Smith, G. P. (1985). Filamentous fusion phage: novel expression vectors that display cloned antigens on the virion surface. *Science, 228*, 1315–1317.

Nucleotide therapy for neurodegenerative disease

Wild, E. J., & Tabrizi, S. J. (2017). Therapies targeting DNA and RNA in Huntington's disease. *Lancet Neurology, 16*(10), 837–847.

A forward look for CAR-T therapy

Newick, K., O'Brien, S., Moon, E., & Albelda, S. M. (2017). CAR T cell therapy for solid tumors. *Annual Review of Medicine, 68*, 139–152.

Gene therapy overview

Gruntman, A. M., & Flotte, T. R. (2018). The rapidly evolving state of gene therapy. *FASEB Journal, 32*(4), 1733–1740.

CRISPR review

Fellmann, C., Gowen, B. G., Lin, P. C., Doudna, J. A., & Corn, J. E. (2017). Cornerstones of CRISPR-Cas in drug discovery and therapy. *Nature Reviews Drug Discovery, 16*(2), 89–100.

Chapter | **4** |

Target selection

Ricardo Macarrón, Duncan B Richards, Lea Sarov-Blat

Introduction

The landscape for drug discovery has altered substantially in the past 40 years. The 'golden' age of drug discovery in the 1980s was characterized by the identification of highly validated targets—often G-protein-coupled transmembrane receptors. For example, identification of the role of the histamine H_2 receptor in the control of stomach acid secretion led to development of highly successful drugs such as cimetidine and ranitidine. Acid secretion plays a key role in multiple clinical conditions:

- Dyspepsia
- Peptic ulcer disease
- As part of *Helicobacter pylori* eradication therapy
- Gastroesophageal reflux disease
- Barrett's oesophagus
- Eosinophilic oesophagitis
- Stress gastritis and ulcer prevention in critical care
- Gastrinomas and other conditions that cause hypersecretion of acid, including Zollinger–Ellison syndrome.

H_2 blockers (antagonists) are effective in all these conditions because of the fundamental link between the target, drug effect and pathophysiology. In this setting, drug development success is determined by the quality of the drug molecule and efficiency of the development process.

The situation today has altered substantially. The number of highly validated targets is relatively small and most have been exploited. Advances in genomics over the past decade have led to paradigm-shifting changes in the understanding of human diseases. The number of genes known to influence common diseases has exploded. Enabling technologies including DNA sequencing, genome editing, imaging and data analytics are revealing key insights into the processes by which genetic variation ultimately leads to human disease. Genomics has finally arrived at the point of translation, but not all genes are drug targets (and not all drug targets are genes). We now have a plethora of potential targets and modalities with which to prosecute them; the key challenge is to identify those targets that play a meaningful role in the disease process.

No matter how safe and innovative a newly developed drug might be, it will not be efficacious if the original pharmacological hypothesis was wrong and modulating the target protein has little or no effect on altering the course of disease. Unfortunately, this moment of truth comes often in late stages of clinical development after years of intense and expensive research. The most common reason for failure in phase II and phase III clinical trials is indeed lack of efficacy (Smietana et al., 2016). Targets must be selected with the best available information on their translational potential. Drug companies have often selected targets relying on publications connecting the targets to disease through preclinical models. This approach presents two fundamental challenges: the poor predictability of animal models of human disease (van der Worp et al., 2010) and the poor quality of published research (Hirsch & Schildknecht, 2019). In the last few years, a growing body of knowledge of the effect of coding and noncoding DNA variants in disease is providing new and nonbiased target connections to potential treatments (Plenge et al., 2013). This chapter describes current knowledge and methods for identification and early validation of new targets, with a focus on the use of human genetics for target selection.

General characteristics of drug targets

The term druggable genome was coined by Hopkins and Groom in 2002 (Hopkins & Groom, 2002) referring to *the* subset of the ~30,000 genes in the human genome that express proteins able to bind drug-like molecules. The current count of human genes that translate to proteins is closer to 20,000, although on top of these canonical genes, the genome encodes hundreds of small proteins and thousands of noncoding RNAs such as microRNAs and long noncoding RNAs with important functions that influence human health and disease in ways starting to be unveiled.

A recent analysis of drug targets points to 667 human proteins and 28 'other human biomolecules' (Santos et al., 2016). This latter category is growing with the advent of oligonucleotide-derived drugs (small interfering RNA [siRNA], antisense oligonucleotides [ASO]) that can modulate RNA (Crooke et al., 2018). Table 4.1 provides an overview of the modalities being pursued for phase II (typically clinical proof-of-concept) studies. This shows that while small molecules and biologics constitute the majority, novel modalities are an important minority. This chapter focuses on principles and methods for identifying human proteins that can be modulated with a biological or chemical ligand to treat disease.

With respect to the type of proteins associated with drug targets, traditional target classes include enzymes (with kinases as special case within this class), ion channels, G-protein-coupled receptors (GPCRs) and nuclear receptors. Table 4.2 contrasts the distribution of targets for all approved versus targets for novel experimental drugs in phase II. Traditional target classes are still being exploited, though new classes are taking off in part due to the shifts in therapeutic modalities (e.g., transcription factors that are not very tractable by small molecules can be targeted with nucleic acids such as ASO or emerging genome-editing therapies).

Table 4.1 Therapeutic modalities of unique agents in phase II clinical trials

	Number of drugs in phase II	
Biological (other)	106	5.4%
Biological (Ab)	304	15.4%
Biological (protein)	199	10.1%
Cell therapy	75	3.8%
Small molecule	1229	62.4%
Nucleic acid	57	2.9%
Total	1970	

Data from pharmaProjects database, https://pharmaintelligence. informa.com/ accessed on June 2019.

Target identification

There is a wide range of tools available to identify targets; each has its strengths and weaknesses. There is no recipe book for target identification, but a key concept is to put together an objective summary of data that represents a complete package of information.

There are essentially three mechanisms by which targets can be modulated: germline or somatic changes in the genome can increase or decrease the function of a protein through gain-of-function or loss-of-function mutations in the corresponding gene or its regulatory elements; drugs can pharmacologically increase or decrease target function and naturally occurring conditions may increase

Table 4.2 Target class distribution for drugs approved up to 2018

Target class	All	T_{clin}[a]	% of total drugs approved	Phase II targets	% of total drugs in phase II
Enzymes	4,146	186	31	129	20
Kinases	634	50	8	64	10
Ion channels	355	126	21	31	5
GPCRs (non-olfactory)	406	96	16	84	13
Nuclear receptors	48	18	3	15	2
Epigenetic proteins	280	12	2	24	4
Transporters	473	26	4	16	2
Others	11,957	87	14	283	44
Total	20,120	601		646	

[a]T_{clin} (clinic) proteins are drug targets linked to at least one approved drug (i.e., an active pharmaceutical ingredient) by mechanism of action. GPCRs, G-protein-coupled receptors.

T_{clin} (from Oprea, T. I., Bologa, C. G., Brunak, S., Campbell, A., Gan, G. N., Gaulton, A., et al. [2018]. Unexplored therapeutic opportunities in the human genome, Nature Reviews Drug Discovery, 17[5], 317–332.) and drugs in active clinical development as of June 2019 (from Informa Pharmaprojects https://pharmaintelligence.informa.com/).

or decrease the amount of a target, thereby increasing or decreasing its function.

Animal models have been called into question in the recent past, but the reason that they continue to be used is that they represent a tractable means to investigate a target. It is straightforward to design controlled experiments to establish a dose–response relationship between function and phenotype. This may involve pharmacological interventions or genetic ones (e.g., knockout models) to investigate how the biological process is altered. The key problem is that the results really apply to the animal species studies; they may have little relevance to human disease. By contrast, human genetics coupled with epidemiology is highly relevant to human disease, but on its own, it cannot prove causality.

We now discuss the main approaches to target identification.

Use of genetics for target identification

Technological and analytical advances in genomics and availability of large datasets have now made it possible to rapidly identify and interpret the genetic variation underlying individual predisposition or protection to many diseases, thereby providing a window into understanding biological mechanisms that cause or contribute to disease. Retrospective analysis of the progression of drugs in clinical development demonstrated that there is approximately a twofold increase in the success rate for targets with genetic evidence connecting to the disease intended to treat (Nelson et al., 2015). Encouraging though this is, it should be noted that the overall probability of success remains low.

The simplest and most direct association between genetics and disease is when the genetic difference has a direct effect in the coding region of the gene. This may alter the protein sequence, resulting in truncation or complete deletion of the protein. Changes in protein sequence may result in either a gain or loss of function. In many cases, the genetic variant is not in a coding region. In some cases, it is a region with a direct regulatory function, but in many cases, the functional consequence is not apparent. In other cases, mutations can alter splicing patterns, resulting in expression of unusual isoforms with subsequent gain or loss of function. Identifying the genetic association is only the start of the target validation process, as in most cases, the functional consequence of the genetic change is not readily apparent. Extensive in vitro work to establish both statistical associations and directions of effect is often required.

The simplest genetic association is one that is controlled by a single locus in an inheritance pattern. In such cases, a mutation in a single gene can cause a disease that is inherited according to Mendel's principles. Dominant diseases manifest in heterozygous individuals. Recessive ones are sometimes inherited unnoticeably by genetic carriers. The most dramatic genetic changes are observed in rare diseases. There are ∼7000 rare human diseases where the majority are characterized by Mendelian inheritance (Tambuyzer et al., 2020). This represents a robust target validation and a logical starting point to tackle these rare diseases.

For common diseases monogenic inheritance is very rare. Mutations in multiple genes (multifactorial inheritance disorder), a combination of gene mutations and environmental factors, or, in cancer, by damage to chromosomes are the norms. This complexity makes robust target validation more complex.

Genome-wide association studies (GWASs) and phenome-wide association studies (PheWASs) are currently the essential tools to explore new targets, particularly outside of oncology. GWAS is in essence a hypothesis-generating approach, while PheWAS provides a systematic approach to analyse the many phenotypes potentially associated with a specific genotype. The two approaches are complementary, providing a means to cross-validate findings.

A GWAS analysis incorporates all the genetic results of a phenotype of interest and systematically analyses variants across the entire genome (i.e., 'genome-wide') for association to the phenotype. As a result, GWAS identifies multiple genetic associations to a phenotype in complex or polygenic traits. The strength of the findings depends on the definition of the phenotype and the number of cases and controls. This method searches the genome for small variations, called single nucleotide polymorphisms or SNPs that occur more frequently in people with a particular disease than in people without the disease (Fig. 4.1). Each study can look at hundreds or thousands of SNPs at the same time. GWAS identifies common variants that tag a region of linkage disequilibrium (LD) containing causal variant(s). A P-value indicates the significance of the difference in frequency of the allele tested between cases and controls, that is, the probability that the allele is likely to be associated with the trait. GWAS results are often displayed in a Manhattan plot with $-\log_{10}$ (P-value) plotted against the position in the genome. Although stringent levels of statistical significance are used as the size of databases increases, the number of associations reaching this level also increases. A statistically significant result is not in itself clinically actionable. It should also be noted that most large databases are dominated by subjects of European descent and thus not all findings apply to the general human population. Additional or follow-on studies are usually required to narrow the region of association and identify the causal variant (commonly called quantitative

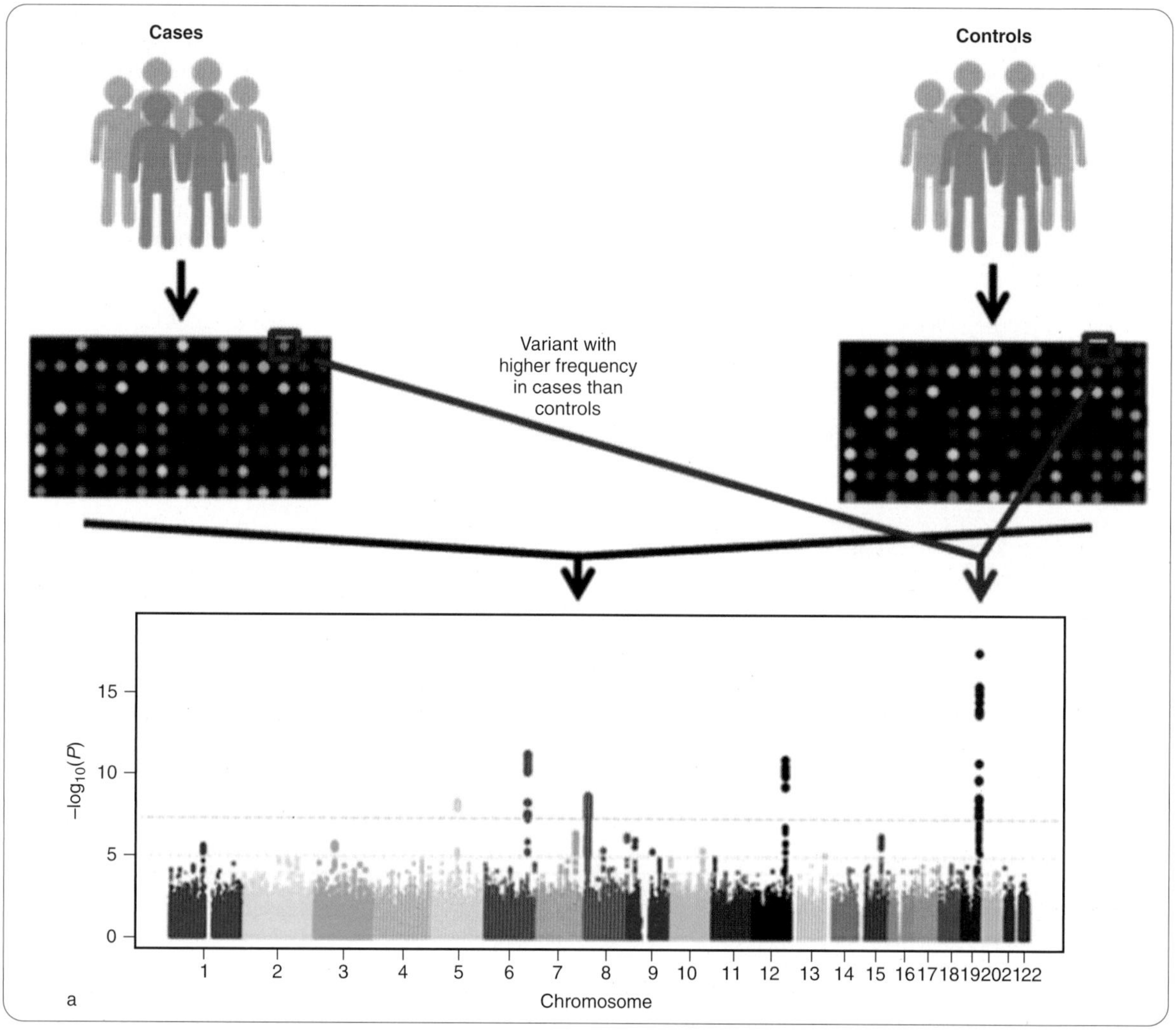

Fig. 4.1 The principles of a genome-wide association study (GWAS). The genome is searched for single nucleotide polymorphisms (SNPs) that occur more frequently in people with a particular disease than in people without the disease. A *P*-value indicates the significance of the difference in frequency of the allele tested between cases and controls, that is, the probability that the allele is likely to be associated with the trait. GWAS results are often displayed in a Manhattan plot with $-\log_{10}$ (*P*-value) plotted against the position in the genome. (Modified from Ikram, M. K., Xueling, S., Jensen, R. A., Cotch, M. F., Hewitt, A. W., Ikram, M. A., et al. [2010]. Four novel loci (19q13, 6q24, 12q24, and 5q14) influence the microcirculation in vivo. *PLoS Genetics, 6*[10], e1001184.)

trait locus or QTL). The complex architecture of complex diseases means that in most cases, the contribution of an individual variant to the risk of disease is small.

A PheWAS analysis starts with a genetic variant of interest and systematically analyses many phenotypes (i.e., 'phenome-wide') for association to the genotype. PheWAS has the ability to identify pleiotropy, or the finding of multiple independent phenotypes associated with a single genetic variant. PheWAS takes advantage of the large volume of clinical and epidemiological data with linked genotype data. Computational approaches allow identification of associations between a particular genetic variant(s) and a wide range of phenotypes (or traits) (Fig. 4.2).

The databases for GWAS and PheWAS analysis are developing rapidly; these include multiple international consortiums such as CKDGen for kidney disease (Köttgen & Pattaro, 2020), and country-wide initiatives such as UK Biobank (UKBB), which has collected patient information for 500,000 people and performed DNA analysis to connect disease and genetic data (Table 4.3).

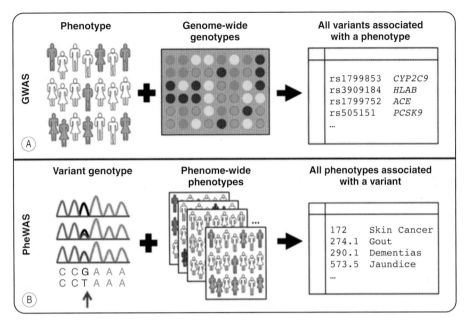

Fig. 4.2 Genome-wide association studies (GWASs) and phenome-wide association studies (PheWASs). (A) A GWAS begins with a phenotype of interest and systematically analyses variants across the entire genome (i.e., 'genome-wide') for association with the phenotype. GWAS can identify multiple genetic associations to a phenotype in complex or polygenic traits. (B) A PheWAS begins with a genetic variant of interest and systematically analyses many phenotypes (i.e., 'phenome-wide') for association to the genotype. PheWAS has the ability to identify pleiotropy, or the finding of multiple independent phenotypes associated with a single genetic variant. (From Robinson, J. R., Denny, J. C., Roden, D. M., & Van Driest, S. L. [2018]. Genome-wide and phenome-wide approaches to understand variable drug actions in electronic health records. *Clinical and Translational Science, 11*[2], 112–122.)

Table 4.3 Public databases to assist in target identification

Data type	Name of database	Information	Link
Target dossiers	Open targets	Target disease associations including genetics and mouse KO data	https://www.targetvalidation.org
	Pharos	Target, disease and ligand information	https://pharos.nih.gov
Genetic associations	UK Biobank	Genetic and phenotypic data for 500,000 subjects	https://www.ukbiobank.ac.uk
Rare disease	Orphanet	Rare/orphan disease-gene	http://www.orpha.net
	OMIM	Mendelian disease-gene associations	http://www.omim.org/
	GWAS catalog		https://www.ebi.ac.uk/gwas
Oncology	cBioPortal	Genetic alterations in cancer	https://www.cbioportal.org/
	DepMap	Susceptibility to gene KO of hundreds of cancer cell lines	https://depmap.org/portal/
Pathways	Reactome		https://reactome.org/
Gene ontology	UNIProt ID	Protein identifier from UniProt	https://www.uniprot.org
	ENSEMBL gene ID	Gene identifier from ENSEMBL	https://www.ensembl.org
	Entrez Gene ID	Gene identifier from NCBI	https://www.ncbi.nlm.nih.gov/gene
	HUGO symbol	Human gene nomenclature committee	https://www.genenames.org
Expression data	GTEx	Gene expression in human tissues	https://www.gtexportal.org
	Human Protein Atlas	Protein and RNA expression data	https://www.proteinatlas.org

GWAS, Genome-wide association study; *KO*, knock-out.

Illustrative examples

Genes involved in hearing loss

Loss of hearing is a complex but common phenomenon, and at present, we have no effective therapies. Wells et al. (2019) performed GWASs for two self-reported hearing phenotypes (hearing loss and use of a hearing aid) using more than 250,000 UKBB volunteers aged between 40 and 69 years. They identified 34 loci that are novel associations with hearing loss of any form. Gene sets from these loci are enriched in auditory processes such as synaptic activities, nervous system processes, inner ear morphology and cognition. These results provide insight into the genetic landscape underlying age-related hearing loss, opening up novel therapeutic targets for further investigation (Wells et al., 2019).

Mendelian randomization, PCSK9

Mendelian randomization is a rapidly emerging technique that uses genetic variation as a natural experiment to investigate the causal relations between potentially modifiable risk factors and health outcomes from observational data. It has advantages over purely observational approaches because it can address unmeasured confounding. For example, alcohol intake and blood pressure may be associated, but an unmeasured confounder such as smoking may limit the interpretation of the results.

The best known example of Mendelian randomization is PCSK9 (proprotein convertase subtilisin–kexin type 9). Variants of PCSK9 are associated with altered blood concentrations of low-density lipoprotein (LDL) cholesterol. A Mendelian randomization study showed that *PCSK9* and *HMGCR* (3-hydroxy-3-methylglutaryl–coenzyme A reductase—the target for statin drugs) variants were associated with approximately the same effect on the risk of cardiovascular disease per unit decrease in the LDL cholesterol level and suggests that treatment with a PCSK9 inhibitor should reduce the risk of cardiovascular events by approximately the same amount as treatment with a statin. Treatment with a PCSK9 inhibitor, used either alone or in combination with a statin, should reduce the risk of cardiovascular events by approximately 20% per decrease of 1.0 mmol/L (39 mg/dL) in the LDL cholesterol level (Ference et al., 2016). This effect was subsequently validated in large-scale clinical trials.

Genes associated with obesity

Obesity is considered a major contributor to morbidity and mortality, especially in Western societies; however, the data linking to specific conditions is weak. To understand the underlying genetic association with body mass index (BMI), Hyppönen et al. (2019) used PheWAS analysis from the UKBB to construct a genetic risk score of 76 variants related to BMI. Eligible UKBB participants were aged 37 to 73 years during recruitment, were White British, unrelated to each other and had available genetic information. After defining cases and controls, it was determined that the same variants of BMI were associated with endocrine disorders type 2 diabetes, circulatory diseases, congestive heart failure, hypertension and many other phenotypes as shown in Fig. 4.3 (Hyppönen et al., 2019).

Expression data of the target in tissues

A critical part of determining if a target is relevant to a disease is understanding the expression pattern of the target specifically in the relevant tissue in healthy and disease states. A systematic analysis to assess gene and protein expression for all targets of marketed and phase III drugs across a diverse collection of normal human tissues showed that for 87% of gene–disease pairs, the target is expressed in a disease-affected tissue under healthy conditions (Kumar et al., 2016). This observation links directly to the 'three pillars' of early clinical drug development. Candidates that demonstrate engagement of the target, drug at the site of action and evidence of pharmacology in the tissue of interest are much more likely to become medicines for patients (Morgan et al., 2012). Examples of public databases providing useful information continuously growing on expression of genes of interest include GTEx and The Human Protein Atlas (Table 4.3).

The advent of single-cell technology has opened up a powerful new approach to target validation. Oncostatin M (OSM) is a typical example of a contemporary drug target. OSM is a member of the interleukin (IL)-6 cytokine family and can signal through JAK-STAT, PI3K and MAPK. SNP analysis associates it with an increased risk of inflammatory bowel disease. There are multiple therapies for inflammatory bowel disease, but single-cell analysis provides powerful insight. This shows that OSM is upregulated in accordance with the severity of the disease in ulcerative colitis; it is upregulated in inflamed tissue but not uninflamed tissues in ulcerative colitis. In addition, it is upregulated in those who have not responded to first line anti–tumour necrosis factor (TNF) therapy. This type of insight is unique in that it defines the design of a proof-of-concept study: in this setting, the approach for an anti-OSM therapy would be aimed at those with active ulcerative colitis who are unresponsive to anti-TNF (West et al., 2017).

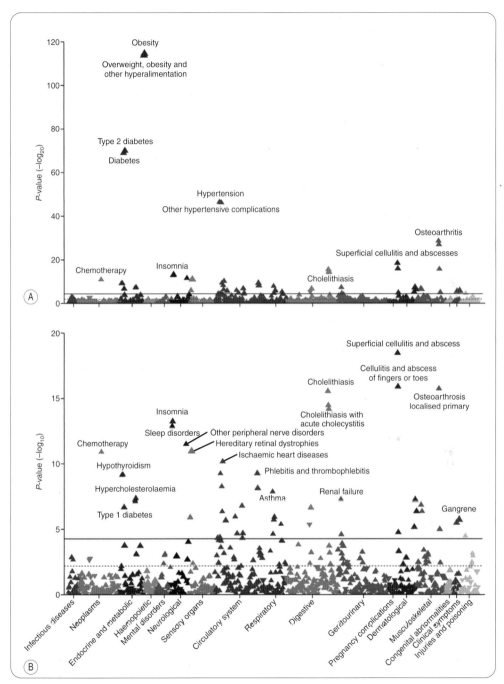

Fig. 4.3 Manhattan plot showing the phenome-wide association between body mass index (BMI) genetic risk score and disease outcomes. Bonferroni corrected threshold ($P < 0.0001$) is represented by the *red line* and false discovery rate-corrected threshold ($P < 0.0074$) by the *dashed line*. The direction of the arrow reflects whether variants increasing BMI were associated with increased (*up arrow*) or decreased (*down arrow*) odds of disease. (A) Global view with all disease outcomes. (B) Zoomed view, showing signals within the range of $P > 1 \times 10^{-20}$ to $P < 5.4 \times 10^{-5}$. (From Hyppönen, E., Mulugeta, A., Zhou, A., & Santhanakrishnan, V. K. [2019]. A data-driven approach for studying the role of body mass in multiple diseases: A phenome-wide registry-based case-control study in the UK Biobank. *Lancet Digital Health, 1*[3], e116–e126.)

Utilizing systematic literature searches to identify new targets

Our knowledge of human biology is constantly expanding and at an increasing rate. A thorough knowledge of the relevant literature has always been an important element of drug discovery. The sheer volume of material makes maintaining current knowledge more difficult. Additionally, the reproducibility of published results is particularly poor in the area of target selection. At the simplest level, emerging literature alerts can help researchers focus their reading time on the most relevant emergent information. Using the literature for drug discovery requires a more sophisticated and systematic approach.

It is perhaps inevitable that given the volume and complexity of the data, there has been an explosion of companies employing artificial intelligence (AI) techniques. It is too early to say whether these will deliver high-quality targets that will reach patients, but the concept is appealing. Any AI approach is only as good as the data it has available. While there is an enormous amount of literature data, their quality is highly variable. Curation of data is time-consuming and complex, as it requires a deep dive to understand the quality and reliability of the data before they are included in a database from which you will make decisions. A number of publically available databases have been harnessed for this purpose (Table 4.3). Many of these approaches have open access areas available to all but also the functionality to provide private areas to commercial clients where commercially sensitive data can be stored and analysed. Although much of the value of this approach is derived from the ability to examine very large amounts of data, size alone is a not a determinant of success. There is an important role for smaller databases, often focused on disease clusters with highly curated high-dimensional data to answer specific questions raised by initial screens conducted on a large dataset.

In addition to the genetic approaches outlined above, there are some specific approaches used on these platforms:

Pathway analysis

It is very important to understand a putative target in the context of the biological systems of which it forms a part. In many instances, a target that is highly expressed or has a genetic link is not the most tractable component of the pathway. Careful delineation of all of the components of a pathway may allow one to identify the optimal place to intervene. Targets that sit high up in the pathway may be ostensibly attractive as 'master controllers', but blocking them may have wide-raging effects, and toxicity is common. Intervening lower down the pathway may allow a more focused intervention with a better therapeutic index.

Several tools are available to map and visualize biological pathways. One such tool is Reactome (Table 4.3); this open access platform provides a set of online resources that use features of the electronic media to organize biological pathway information in ways that provide for more efficient access, and that allow new forms of analysis that were not possible with information stored in the traditional printed literature. As an example, pathway analysis has been applied to identify a novel target for liver fibrosis. GWASs have indicated that MerTK is a risk factor for liver fibrosis in nonalcoholic steatohepatitis (NASH), but it has an unknown mechanism. MerTK signalling in liver macrophages, which is enhanced in NASH owing to suppression of its cleavage by ADAM17, promotes transforming growth factor (TGF)-β1 production, hepatic stellate cells (HSC) activation and liver fibrosis in NASH. In this case, careful characterization of the pathway identified from a genetic screen has provided a mechanistic explanation that might form the basis for drug discovery.

Knockout databases

The ability to knock out the function of a specific gene has been an important tool in target identification and validation. The original technology introduces the knockout at the very earliest stages of embryonic development—the blastocyst. Approximately 15% of these knockouts are developmentally lethal, limiting their utility. Conditional knockouts allow control over when the knockout is activated or in which tissues. These are powerful tools but is time consuming and labour intensive; they involve making a large gene-targeting construct, transfecting and screening many embryonic stem (ES) cell clones, injecting positive ES clones into blastocysts to produce chimeric mice and breeding the chimeras to transmit the targeted gene through the germline. One of the most common approaches relies on the DNA recombinase Cre and its recognition (loxP) sites. For conditional mutagenesis, a target gene is modified by the insertion of two loxP sites that enable one to excise the flanked (floxed) gene segment through Cre-mediated recombination. Conditional mutant mice are obtained by crossing the floxed strain with a Cre transgenic line such that the target gene becomes inactivated in vivo within the expression domain of Cre. Most knockouts are in mouse strains and therefore caution must be exercised about the relevance of the observations to humans, especially when the target is a component of the immune system.

The field is being transformed by CRISPR–Cas9 (clustered regularly interspaced short palindromic repeats [CRISPR]–CRISPR-associated protein [Cas]) gene editing technology. This is a genetic manipulation tool derived from the defence system of certain types of bacteria against

Table 4.4 Examples of target selection projects using CRISPR KO on human cells

Disease area	Cellular system	Assay (technique)	References
Synthetic lethals for cancer	Cancer cell lines	Cell viability (RNAseq)	(Behan et al. (2019), Chan et al. (2019), Wang et al. (2015))
Lung fibrosis	Primary fibroblasts	Deposition of collagen (imaging)	Martufi et al. (2019)
Epithelial barrier for COPD	Primary lung epithelial cells	Cell differentiation (FACS)	Rapiteanu et al. (2019)
Regulators of immune function	Primary CD8+ T cells	Cell viability (RNAseq)	Shifrut et al. (2018)
HIV host dependency factors	CCRF–CEM & primary CD4+ T cells	HIV virus entry (FACS)	Park et al. (2017)

COPD, Chronic obstructive pulmonary disease; *CRISPR*, clustered regularly interspaced short palindromic repeats; FACS fluores; FACS fluorescence-activated cell sorting; CCRF-CEM T lymphoblastoid cell line

viruses and plasmids. The CRISPR–Cas9 system consists of directing the Cas9 nuclease to create a site-directed double-strand DNA break. The break activates repair through error-prone nonhomologous end joining (NHEJ) or homology-directed repair (HDR). In the absence of a template, NHEJ is activated, resulting in insertions and/or deletions (indels) that disrupt the target loci. In the presence of a donor template with homology to the targeted locus, the HDR pathway operates, allowing for precise mutations to be made. A recent example shows how this can be applied to target identification (Behan et al., 2019). In this case, genome-scale CRISPR–Cas9 screening was conducted in 324 human cancer cell lines from 30 cancer types. The focus was on genes associated with cell fitness. Genes required for cell fitness in specific molecular or histological contexts are likely to encode favourable drug targets, because of a reduced likelihood of inducing toxic effects in healthy tissues. Conversely, fitness genes that are common to the majority of tested cell lines or common within a cancer type (referred to as pan-cancer or cancer-type-specific core fitness genes, respectively) may be involved in essential processes in cells and have greater toxicity. Integration of cell fitness effects with genomic biomarkers and target tractability for drug development to systematically prioritize new targets in defined tissues and genotypes is being used. Some further examples of the use of this technology are provided in Table 4.4.

Tractability assessment

A highly validated target is not necessarily a highly tractable target. A key early step is to establish whether the protein target has, for example, a binding site that can be exploited for small-molecule binding or, alternatively, an accessible epitope for antibody-based therapy. Every target can be assessed for its tractability, that is, the probability of finding therapeutic modulators using a certain modality (Brown et al., 2018). This probability is not deterministic; however, it helps productivity of drug discovery efforts by favouring projects with higher probability of success.

The range of therapeutic modalities is now very wide, but companies and research institutes will have expertise in only a subset of these. It is important to establish early that your proposed target is tractable with a technology in which you have expertise. Public portals such as Open Targets (Koscielny et al., 2017) and Pharos (Nguyen et al., 2017) (links provided in Table 4.3) give access to up-to-date information of available tool molecules or drugs for any target of interest. Confidence in the initial tractability assessment will depend on the quality of data available. For example, a target that has been co-crystallized with a small molecule is clearly more tractable than one for which there is only a binding prediction. The availability of co-crystal data does, however, suggest that others are also evaluating the target, and so competition may be more intense than for a novel target that is less well characterized. Selection will always rely on a degree of judgement and an assessment of the acceptable level of risk.

Experimental validation of potential new targets

As we have described earlier, target identification often starts with analysis of genomic and genetic data from which susceptibility loci and lists of targets are identified with variable degree of confidence. Occasionally, a target rises clearly to the top and deserves immediate attention; a good example is PCSK9 for cardiovascular disease (Plenge et al., 2013). More often, there is a need to conduct an initial screening to understand the best potential targets/pathways for a disease indication or mechanism of action out of hundreds of potential genes.

There is a critical early step to translate genetic signals into drug targets. Most disease-associated SNPs cannot be associated with a single gene with high confidence. For example, SNPs located in an fat mass and obesity (FTO) gene intron that are strongly associated with obesity affect adipocyte differentiation not by changes in expression or splicing of FTO protein, but instead by altering distally the expression of transcription factors IRX3 and IRX5 (Clauss-nitzer et al., 2015). Therefore despite advances in statistical genetics and a growing body of expression data in human tissues and cells, the selection of target genes from genetic analysis might require experimental validation by functional genomics of the relationship between SNPs and putative genes derived by computational methods.

The development of genetic screens for experimental target selection starts by understanding molecular fingerprints of disease in relevant tissues. Additionally, any potential target is expected to be expressed in relevant tissues from patients (Kumar et al., 2016). Transcriptomics and single-cell technologies offer an early source of critical information about the molecular fingerprints of disease and will also provide data to help validate experimental models of disease. Proteomics and metabolomics technologies provide deeper insights and should be used whenever possible.

Ideally, all target selection and validation would take place in model systems fully predictive of human physiology. Traditionally, animal models have been used as the closer in vivo alternative. Scientific and ethical reasons have led to a conscious investment in human in vitro models to mimic human biology at this early stage whenever possible. Recent advances in cell engineering and material sciences are starting to deliver very promising in vitro human models (Ahadian et al., 2018; Ooft et al., 2019).

For any given disease of interest, there are typically several potential models in the following categories (in order of generic relevance): (1) ex vivo models (tissue slice), (2) complex in vitro models (e.g., organoids), (3) primary cells, (4) induced pluripotent stem cells (iPS)-derived cells and (5) cell lines. Cost, throughput and resource requirements decrease roughly in that same order. Pragmatic choices need to be made in the interest of speed. Typically, simple cellular models will be a first step. If primary cells from healthy and diseased donors can be used, that is the preferred choice. iPS-derived cell models are fast becoming the second alternative, with use of cell lines declining where possible.

Model validation, or in other words, definition of the predictive power of a model is an important step to understand the expected quality from the output of any experiment using it. Understanding of human physiology and pathobiology is a prerequisite to delineate the key biological elements needed such as biomarkers of disease and allow a determination of the domain of validity

(DoV), that is, what biological questions can and which ones cannot be explored with the model. If DoV for existing models is not appropriate, there is a need to develop new models until this minimal threshold is achieved. DoV always needs to be aligned with specific question and purpose—for target selection with hundreds of targets, simpler more limited models are appropriate, while for final stages of individual target validation, more complex models that mimic more aspects of pathobiology are sought.

Cellular models leverage our knowledge of key disease pathways/mechanisms and are employed to test the effect of target perturbation (e.g., siRNA, overexpression, knock-out (KO) and knock-in (KI) tool molecule) under different treatments (e.g., hormone exposure) for a disease-relevant phenotype (e.g., cytokine release) (Moffat et al., 2017). Examples of cellular models designed at GlaxoSmithKline to mimic specific mechanisms associated with chronic obstructive pulmonary disease (COPD) are depicted in Fig. 4.4.

Genome editing has become an excellent tool for genetic screens (Doench, 2018; Lu et al., 2017), overcoming the issues of off-target effects observed with siRNA screens (Housden & Perrimon, 2016; Kimberland et al., 2018). The applications of CRISPR have expanded rapidly beyond simple KO (Pickar-Oliver & Gersbach, 2019). Multiple genetic screens using a variety of cell models and assays have been published in recent years (Oughtred et al., 2019). A few illustrative examples of KO screens are shown in Table 4.4.

Understanding target mechanism of action

Genetic screens reveal the most promising targets for drug discovery with the limitations imposed by the model and assay employed. Additional target validation involves (1) early estimation of therapeutic window, that is, investigation of expected on-target toxicity (Nguyen et al., 2019), (2) understanding of specific target function that needs to be modulated to exert a therapeutic effect (e.g., what domain of the protein needs to be inhibited or activated) (Behan et al., 2019), (3) detailed expression analysis at the protein level (including isoforms, subcellular localization and histological variability across samples) and (4) understanding of target redundancy, that is, compensation mechanisms or feedback loops that will render target modulation less effective than observed in the genetic screen.

Some of these steps are often conducted in parallel with a commit-to-target decision, when a drug discovery organization agrees to pursue lead discovery activities for a specific mechanism of action (combination of biological target + biological action) with the intention to discover lead molecules (chemical or biological) for further optimization.

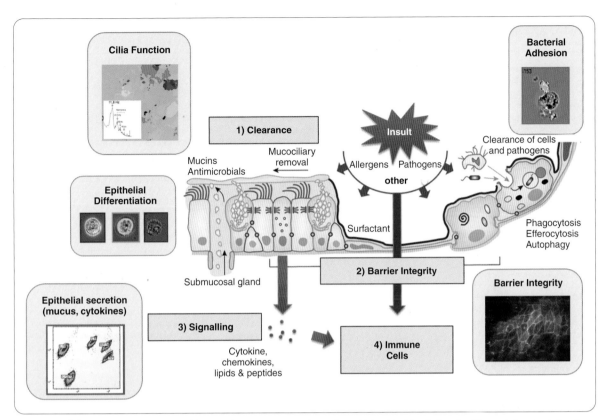

Fig. 4.4 Cellular models of lung epithelial barrier. These assays use primary bronchial epithelial cells from healthy and chronic obstructive pulmonary disease (COPD) patients to test relevant mechanisms of disease. (Courtesy Gareth Wayne, adapted from Whitsett, J. A., & Alenghat, T. [2015]. Respiratory epithelial cells orchestrate pulmonary innate immunity. *Nature Immunology, 16*[1], 27–35.)

Clinical context

The focus of this chapter has been on the scientific basis of target selection in order to have confidence in its validity and tractability. Critical though this first decision is, drug development is commonly a 10- to 20-year journey, and a clear vision for the potential medicine is vital.

The skillsets required to define a medicine vision include epidemiology, clinical medicine and commercial analysis. Large companies with an end-to-end portfolio can draw on this expertise from their late-stage divisions, but there is a very real challenge for small and emerging companies who may only have a handful of employees. Conducting this assessment early is, however, vital, as it will shape the pre-clinical package required to support clinical development. Examples of the types of question that should be considered at this early stage are outlined in Table 4.5.

Table 4.5 Clinical questions to ask early in target selection

What is the target patient population and how big is it (epidemiology)?

Is there an established diagnostic pathway?

What is the current standard of care?

Is this available to most patients?

What are the unmet needs in this patient population?

Based on the mechanism of action, what sort of clinical benefit is achievable? (e.g., symptomatic relief, preventative, curative, stop progression)

What is the competitive landscape?

Are there any specific development considerations? (e.g., need for a companion diagnostic, combination therapy)

What are the requirements for a medicine to be reimbursed/funded in this population?

References

Ahadian, S., Civitarese, R., Bannerman, D., Mohammadi, M. H., Lu, R. Wang, E., et al. (2018). Organ-on-a-chip platforms: A convergence of advanced materials, cells, and microscale technologies. *Advanced Healthcare Materials, 7*(2). doi:10.1002/adhm.201700506.

Behan, F. M., Iorio, F., Picco, G., Gonçalves, E., Beaver, C. M., Migliardi, G., et al. (2019). Prioritization of cancer therapeutic targets using CRISPR–Cas9 screens. *Nature, 568*(7753), 511–516. doi:10.1038/s41586-019-1103-9.

Brown, K. K., Hann, M. M., Lakdawala, A. S., Santos, R., Thomas, P. J., & Todd, K. (2018). Approaches to target tractability assessment-a practical perspective. *MedChemComm, 9*(4), 606–613. doi:10.1039/c7md00633k.

Chan, E. M., Shibue, T., McFarland, J. M., Gaeta, B., Ghandi, M., Dumont, N., et al. (2019). WRN helicase is a synthetic lethal target in microsatellite unstable cancers. *Nature, 568*(7753), 551–556. doi:10.1038/s41586-019-1102-x.

Claussnitzer, M., Dankel, S. N., Kim, K. H., Quon, G., Meuleman, W., Haugen, C., et al. (2015). FTO obesity variant circuitry and adipocyte browning in humans. *New England Journal of Medicine, 373*(10), 895–907. doi:10.1056/NEJMoa1502214.

Crooke, S. T., Witztum, J. L., Bennett, C. F., & Baker, B. F. (2018). RNA-targeted therapeutics. *Cell Metabolism, 27*(4), 714–739. doi:10.1016/j.cmet.2018.03.004.

Doench, J. G. (2018). Am I ready for CRISPR? A user's guide to genetic screens. *Nature Reviews Genetics, 19*(2), 67–80. doi:10.1038/nrg.2017.97.

Ference, B. A., Robinson, J. G., Brook, R. D., Catapano, A. L., Chapman, M. J., Neff, D. R. et al. (2016). Variation in PCSK9 and HMGCR and risk of cardiovascular disease and diabetes. *New England Journal of Medicine, 375*(22), 2144–2153. doi:10.1056/NEJMoa1604304.

Hirsch, C., & Schildknecht, S. (2019). In vitro research reproducibility: Keeping up high standards. *Frontiers in Pharmacology, 10*, 1484. doi:10.3389/fphar.2019.01484.

Hopkins, A. L., Groom, C. R. (2002). The druggable genome. *Nature Reviews. Drug Discovery, 1*(9), 727–730. doi:10.1038/nrd892.

Housden, B. E., & Perrimon, N. (2016). Comparing CRISPR and RNAi-based screening technologies. *Nature Biotechnology, 34*(6), 621–623. doi:10.1038/nbt.3599.

Hyppönen, E., Mulugeta, A., Zhou, A., & Santhanakrishnan, V. K. (2019). A data-driven approach for studying the role of body mass in multiple diseases: A phenome-wide registry-based case-control study in the UK Biobank. *Lancet Digital Health, 1*(3), e116–e126. doi:10.1016/S2589-7500(19)30028-7.

Ikram, M. K., Xueling, S., Jensen, R. A., Cotch, M. F., Hewitt, A. W., Ikram, M. A., et al. (2010). Four novel loci (19q13, 6q24, 12q24, and 5q14) influence the microcirculation in vivo. *PLoS Genetics, 6*(10), e1001184. doi:10.1371/journal.pgen.1001184.

Kimberland, M. L., Hou, W., Alfonso-Pecchio, A., Wilson, S., Rao, Y., Zhang, S., et al. (2018). Strategies for controlling CRISPR/Cas9 off-target effects and biological variations in mammalian genome editing experiments. *Journal of Biotechnology, 284*, 91–101. doi:10.1016/j.jbiotec.2018.08.007.

Koscielny, G., An, P., Carvalho-Silva, D., Cham, J. A., Fumis, L., Gasparyan, R., et al. (2017). Open targets: A platform for therapeutic target identification and validation. *Nucleic Acids Research, 45*(D1), D985–D994. doi:10.1093/nar/gkw1055.

Köttgen, A., & Pattaro, C. (2020). The CKDGen Consortium: Ten years of insights into the genetic basis of kidney function. *Kidney International, 97*(2), 236–242. doi:10.1016/j.kint.2019.10.027.

Kumar, V., Sanseau, P., Simola, D. F., Hurle, M. R., & Agarwal, P. (2016). Systematic analysis of drug targets confirms expression in disease-relevant tissues. *Scientific Reports, 6*. doi:10.1038/srep36205.

Lu, Q., Livi, G. P., Modha, S., Yusa, K., Macarrón, R., & Dow, D. J. (2017). Applications of CRISPR genome editing technology in drug target identification and validation. *Expert Opinion on Drug Discovery, 12*(6), 541–552. doi:10.1080/17460441.2017.1317244.

Martufi, M., Good, R. B., Rapiteanu, R., Schmidt, T., Patili, E., Tvermosegaard, K., et al. (2019). Single-step, high-efficiency CRISPR-Cas9 genome editing in primary human disease-derived fibroblasts. *CRISPR Journal, 2*, 31–40. doi:10.1089/crispr.2018.0047.

Moffat, J. G., Vincent, F., Lee, J. A., Eder, J., & Prunotto, M. (2017). Opportunities and challenges in phenotypic drug discovery: An industry perspective. *Nature Reviews. Drug Discovery, 16*(8), 531–543. doi:10.1038/nrd.2017.111.

Morgan, P., Van Der Graaf, P. H., Arrowsmith, J., Feltner, D. E., Drummond, K. S., Wegner, C. D., et al. (2012). Can the flow of medicines be improved? Fundamental pharmacokinetic and pharmacological principles toward improving phase II survival. *Drug Discovery Today, 17*(9-10), 419–424. doi:10.1016/j.drudis.2011.12.020.

Nelson, M. R., Tipney, H., Painter, J. L., Shen, J., Nicoletti, P., Shen, Y., et al. (2015). The support of human genetic evidence for approved drug indications. *Nature Genetics, 47*(8), 856–860. doi:10.1038/ng.3314.

Nguyen, D. T., Mathias, S., Bologa, C., Brunak, S., Fernandez, N., Gaulton, A., et al. (2017). Pharos: Collating protein information to shed light on the druggable genome. *Nucleic Acids Research, 45*(D1), D995–D1002. doi:10.1093/nar/gkw1072.

Nguyen, P. A., Born, D. A., Deaton, A. M., Nioi, P., & Ward, L. D. (2019). Phenotypes associated with genes encoding drug targets are predictive of clinical trial side effects. *Nature Communications, 10*(1), 1579. doi:10.1038/s41467-019-09407-3.

Ooft, S. N., Weeber, F., Dijkstra, K. K., McLean, C. M., Kaing, S., van Werkhoven, E., et al. (2019). Patient-derived organoids can predict response to chemotherapy in metastatic colorectal cancer patients. *Science Translational Medicine, 11*(513), eaay2574. doi:10.1126/scitranslmed.aay2574.

Oprea, T. I., Bologa, C. G., Brunak, S., Campbell, A., Gan, G. N., Gaulton, A., et al. (2018). Unexplored therapeutic opportunities in the human genome. *Nature Reviews. Drug Discovery, 17*(5), 317–332. doi:10.1038/nrd.2018.14.

Oughtred, R., Stark, C., Breitkreutz, B. J., Rust, J., Boucher, L., Chang, C., et al. (2019). The BioGRID Interaction Database: 2019 update. *Nucleic*

Acids Research, 47(D1), D529–D541. doi:10.1093/nar/gky1079.

Park, R. J., Wang, T., Koundakjian, D., Hultquist, J. F., Lamothe-Molina, P., Monel, B., et al. (2017). A genome-wide CRISPR screen identifies a restricted set of HIV host dependency factors. *Nature Genetics, 49*(2), 193–203. doi:10.1038/ng.3741.

Pickar-Oliver, A., & Gersbach, C. A. (2019). The next generation of CRISPR–Cas technologies and applications. *Nature Reviews. Molecular Cell Biology, 20*(8), 490–507. doi:10.1038/s41580-019-0131-5.

Plenge, R. M., Scolnick, M., & Altshuler, D. (2013). Validating therapeutic targets through human genetics. *Nature Reviews Drug Discovery, 12*(8), 581–594. doi:10.1038/nrd4051.

Rapiteanu, R., Karagyozova, T., Zimmermann, N., Singh, K., Wayne, G., Martufi, M., et al. (2020) Highly efficient genome editing in primary human bronchial epithelial cells differentiated at air-liquid interface. Eur Respir J. 2020 May 21;55(5):1900950. doi: 10.1183/13993003.00950-2019. Print 2020 May.

Robinson, J. R., Denny, J. C., Roden, D. M., & Van Driest, S. L. (2018). Genome-wide and phenome-wide approaches to understand variable drug actions in electronic health records. *Clinical and Translational Science, 11*(2), 112–122. doi:10.1111/cts.12522.

Santos, R., Ursu, O., Gaulton, A., Bento, A. P., Donadi, R. S., Bologa, C. G., et al. (2016). A comprehensive map of molecular drug targets. *Nature Reviews. Drug Discovery, 16*(1), 19–34. doi:10.1038/nrd.2016.230.

Shifrut, E., Carnevale, J., Tobin, V., Roth, T. L., Woo, J. M., Bui, C. T., et al. (2018). Genome-wide CRISPR screens in primary human T cells reveal key regulators of immune function. *Cell, 175*(7), 1958–1971.e15. doi:10.1016/j.cell.2018.10.024.

Smietana, K., Siatkowski, M., & Møller, M. (2016). Trends in clinical success rates. *Nature Reviews Drug Discovery, 15*(6), 379–380. doi:10.1038/nrd.2016.85.

Tambuyzer, E., Vandendriessche, B., Austin, C. P., Brooks, P. J., Larsson, K., Miller Needleman, K. I., et al. (2020). Therapies for rare diseases: Therapeutic modalities, progress and challenges ahead. *Nature Reviews Drug Discovery, 19*(2), 93–111. doi:10.1038/s41573-019-0049-9.

van der Worp, H. B., Howells, D. W., Sena, E. S., Porritt, M. J., Rewell, S., O'Collins, V., et al. (2010). Can animal models of disease reliably inform human studies? *PLoS Medicine, 7*(3), 1–8. doi:10.1371/journal.pmed.1000245.

Wang, T., Birsoy, K., Hughes, N. W., Krupczak, K. M., Post, Y., Wei, J. J. et al. (2015). Identification and characterization of essential genes in the human genome. *Science, 350*(6264), 1096–1101. doi:10.1126/science.aac7041.

Wells, H. R. R., Freidin, M. B., Zainul Abidin, F. N., Payton, A., Dawes, P., Munro, K. J., et al. (2019). GWAS identifies 44 independent associated genomic loci for self-reported adult hearing difficulty in UK Biobank. *American Journal of Human Genetics, 105*(4), 788–802. doi:10.1016/j.ajhg.2019.09.008.

West, N. R., Hegazy, A. N., Owens, B. M. J., Bullers, S. J., Linggi, B., Buonocore, S., et al. (2017). Oncostatin M drives intestinal inflammation and predicts response to tumor necrosis factor–neutralizing therapy in patients with inflammatory bowel disease. *Nature Medicine, 23*, 579–589. doi:10.1038/nm.4307.

Whitsett, J. A., & Alenghat, T. (2015). Respiratory epithelial cells orchestrate pulmonary innate immunity. *Nature Immunology, 16*(1), 27–35. doi:10.1038/ni.3045.

Chapter | 5 |

From drug target to drug discovery

Jeremy Griggs

Introduction

In this chapter, we assume that a molecular target has been identified against which a de novo drug discovery effort is proposed. To have arrived at this point, there must have been compelling evidence—perhaps drawn from in vitro, in vivo, genetic and clinical sources—that pharmacological modulation of the target would be beneficial in human disease (see Chapter 4). There must also have been a favourable assessment of the risks associated with modulating the target's normal physiological role, that is, the potential for 'on-target' toxicity.

However, these considerations alone are not sufficient to justify the substantial investment of resources and time required for successful drug discovery. As we will discuss in this chapter, a variety of other key project selection criteria should be satisfied in advance of starting the project, including favourable assessments of the unmet medical need, the predicted tractability of modulating the target with an available modality and the feasibility ultimately of evaluating the proposed new medicine efficiently in patients. Once these criteria have been satisfactorily met, attention can turn to planning the project. Although beyond the scope of this discussion, much attention will also be given to the strength of the commercial proposition of the new medicine and the extent to which the project is a good strategic fit to the company (e.g., in terms of therapeutic area focus and the relative probability of success compared with other projects in the portfolio).

Key project selection criteria

Companies may have a plethora of potential targets to choose from, all of which will have relative strengths and weaknesses. These must be weighed against each other to assess the relative probability of success of each potential project ultimately reaching a medicine. Given the extraordinarily high cost of drug discovery and the reality that pharmaceutical and biotechnology companies increasingly operate within stringently constrained R&D budgets, not all attractive projects can be pursued. Rather, opportunities must be rigorously assessed such that, overall, a strong drug discovery portfolio, balanced with respect to risk and potential reward, can be built.

When making these choices, a useful approach is to start with the vision of the medicine to which the new target ultimately relates—this enables the clear articulation of the proposed patient population and the definition of their unmet medical need. From there, one can essentially work backwards—assessing how such a potential medicine might be tested in the clinic, what its mechanism of action will be, the most appropriate modality to effect this mechanism and the likelihood of discovering a molecule suitable for clinical progression—thereby arriving at the starting point of how the project should be planned and operationalized.

Unmet medical need

A compelling case must be presented that an unmet need exists for the target patient population. Importantly, it is not sufficient merely that the current standard of care is inadequate, but also that the current unmet need will remain by the time a new drug is launched (which is likely to be more than a decade following the start of drug discovery). This requires an awareness of the preclinical and clinical development activities happening elsewhere and a judgement of how likely they are to be successful (and if they are, the extent to which the need for a further medicine will still exist).

The unmet need for a given disease may be readily apparent and easily quantifiable (e.g., diseases for

All contributions to this chapter were undertaken in a personal capacity, and do not reflect GSK in any way.

which there are currently no effective treatments and where an easily identifiable patient population exists). However, perhaps more frequently, there may be some benefit offered by the current standard of care, but this is inadequate for some or all patients, and there is reason to believe that it could be improved upon. This may be because the degree of response is inadequate, responsive patients become refractory to treatment over time or a subpopulation of patients fail to respond to the current standard of care. It is increasingly recognized that patients themselves have a key role in helping to identify and define the unmet need, as evidenced by the increased impact achieved by charities and patient advocacy groups on drug discovery efforts for both common and rare diseases. Occasionally, a highly effective standard of care may exist, but there may be the potential to improve upon it further, even by modulating the same molecular target (e.g., replacing an intravenously administered medicine with an orally available equivalent, or improving the pharmacokinetics of a monoclonal antibody such that its dosing interval is significantly extended.

Importantly, assessing the unmet need is not simply a commercial exercise through which a likely return on investment can be calculated. Rather, building a strong understanding of the target patient population as early as possible in the project can also play a critical role in defining the project plan, and identifying the biological studies that should progress in parallel with drug discovery to further strengthen both the therapeutic hypothesis and the commercial proposition.

Clinical tractability

It may seem premature at the beginning of drug discovery to focus on how clinical development will be performed, but in fact, this is a key criterion. An early assessment of clinical tractability does not require a detailed plan of each phase of clinical development, but it is important to understand that, in principle at least, clinical development is feasible. Furthermore, this analysis can serve to identify key capability and knowledge gaps (e.g., diagnostic methods, biomarker discovery) that may be remedied in parallel with drug discovery efforts, hence enabling a seamless transfer from drug discovery to clinical development later in the project.

A key starting point for assessing clinical tractability is understanding how the patient population will be identified. This is particularly relevant in the era of target-based therapies, since—unless the molecular basis of the disease in question is identical in all patients—it will be necessary to identify the subpopulation of patients for whom the new medicine is most relevant.

For example, only 15–30% of patients with metastatic breast cancer express Her2, the molecular target of

trastuzumab and the related antibody–drug conjugate trastuzumab-emtansine, among others. In this case, the subpopulation of breast cancer patients for whom trastuzumab may be appropriate can readily be identified using a companion diagnostic, typically, either an immunohistochemical or fluorescent in situ hybridisation assay to detect Her2 amplification. In the absence of such a companion diagnostic (i.e., if the diagnosis of metastatic breast cancer was the sole criterion for patient selection), it follows that up to 70% of clinical trial subjects might receive a drug for which there was no biological rationale for achieving clinical benefit. Such an approach would not only severely jeopardize the likelihood of successful clinical development (since the apparent efficacy rate would likely be very low) but would also unnecessarily expose some patients to an experimental medicine and possibly deprive them of alternative treatment options that might be more successful.

Such relatively straightforward means of patient selection tend to predominate in therapeutic areas such as oncology and genetically defined diseases, since the target's overexpression, mutational status or other aberrant activity can often be readily detected. Conversely, in diseases where this target profile does not apply, successful identification of patient (sub-)populations may rely more heavily on clinical presentation (and careful differential diagnosis), disease biomarkers distinct from the therapeutic target or even selection based on nonresponsiveness to existing therapies. In these cases, informed clinician input early in the project can be particularly useful in building confidence that the optimal patient population will be identifiable.

Once it is clear that the patient population can be identified, it is important to build confidence that efficient routes will exist to establish whether the new medicine engages with and modulates its molecular target in humans and, ultimately, achieves efficacy against the disease. The risk associated with relying solely on efficacy as a clinical endpoint varies significantly depending on the disease setting. In acute diseases, where the proposed intervention is expected rapidly to have a measurable benefit, proving target engagement and resulting pharmacodynamic effects in patients may be important but not critical, since one can rely on efficacy as a primary measure of success. Conversely, in chronic conditions, where disease modification may only be apparent over a protracted time course, or where disease *prevention* is the aim, it is necessary to confirm successful engagement and modulation of the target as early as possible, to give confidence that pursuing further and prolonged late-stage development may be worthwhile.

While the feasibility of determining the pharmacokinetics of an investigational drug is rarely a major risk when considering clinical tractability (it is typically investigated as part of early [Phase I] clinical trials, which assess safety and tolerability), the feasibility of confirming target engagement can vary substantially depending on the disease setting and the therapeutic target. It may involve direct detection of the drug engaging with its target or may rely on detecting the biological consequence of this engagement (i.e., a pharmacodyamic effect). To illustrate this, consider a hypothetical example where, within a clearly defined patient population, the therapeutic target is a cytokine which acts on B cells. The therapeutic approach is to neutralise it with a monoclonal antibody. Confirming *target engagement* may be readily achieved by detecting decreased levels of free cytokine in the circulation (assuming there is no added complexity, for example, upregulation of cytokine expression in response to neutralisation). Importantly, this does not speak to whether a *pharmacodynamic* effect is being achieved but this could be assessed assessing the activation status of the cytokine's cognate receptor on B cells, for example, by measuring the activity of downstream signalling mediators, expression of genes responsive to the pathway being modulated or other phenotypic readouts.

Conversely, greater challenges and risks around clinical tractability would be apparent in an example where the therapeutic target is at a poorly accessible site (e.g., in the CNS), and there are no known biomarkers in the peripheral circulation that would inform on target engagement or pharmacodynamic effect. This may place a heavy reliance on noninvasive means of detecting target engagement (e.g., by using a radiolabelled drug) or interim readouts of disease modulation (e.g., by using diagnostic imaging techniques, if available), or may mandate a clinical development pathway that contains few, if any, opportunities for interim evaluation of success until the clinical efficacy endpoint is reached. The latter scenario is clearly undesirable, particularly in diseases that follow a very protracted clinical course, since substantial time and resource will be invested without any accompanying change to the overall level of risk of failure. If drug discovery did proceed against such a backdrop, there would doubtless be strong motivation aggressively to pursue biomarker discovery early in the project.

As with the assessment of unmet need, early investment in understanding clinical tractability can inform the design of the overall drug discovery path such that the therapeutic hypothesis is continually strengthened and key risks discharged as effectively as possible as the project progresses. Not only will an early assessment of clinical tractability identify the need (or otherwise) to invest effort in biomarker discovery and companion diagnostic development in advance of clinical studies, it should also help to define the goal preclinical data package that offers the best prospects for translation into humans, particularly with respect to pharmacodynamic markers and interim and endpoint efficacy measures. As clinical development progresses, convincing evidence of a pharmacokinetic–pharmacodynamic relationship (i.e., drug exposure correlating with target engagement and a detectable pharmacodynamic effect) that is consistent with preclinical data and the therapeutic hypothesis will help to provide support to proceed with further clinical development and give confidence in the overall approach.

A further consideration relevant to clinical tractability is selection of the preferred lead indication (i.e., the first/principal disease in which the medicine will be evaluated clinically). Because it is common for a given therapeutic target to play a role in the pathogenesis of more than one disease, there may be several potential diseases from which to select a lead indication. Although they may share a common therapeutic target, they may differ significantly in their clinical tractability profiles. Hence, the optimal lead indication may not necessarily be that which has the greatest commercial potential. Rather, it may be more appropriate to select an alternative—if smaller—indication with a superior clinical tractability profile and potentially, therefore, a greater probability of success. The development of the medicine for the larger indication may then follow in due course and can leverage much of the pharmacokinetic, pharmacodynamic, safety and tolerability data obtained through the initial clinical development activities. However, this approach is not without its hazards and, if pursued, it is important that the selected lead indication for clinical development is *bona fide* with respect to the therapeutic hypothesis, since failure here will jeopardize the prospects for progressing to the indication of greatest interest. As with all assessments of clinical tractability, there must be confidence that the relevant 'gateway indication' patient population will be available for recruitment into clinical trials—some diseases are commonly selected as gateway indications (e.g., Sjogren's syndrome as a 'prototypical' immuno-inflammatory disease), and hence there may be 'competition' for available patients.

The potential for 'on-target' toxicity (i.e., that arising specifically from affecting the target's normal physiological role) folds into the assessment of unmet need, clinical tractability and potential lead indications. It is the clinical context of a medicine's use that determines the risk/benefit posed by modulating the target's pathogenic activity versus interfering with its normal physiological function. A critical analysis of the degree to which on-target hazards are offset by potential therapeutic benefits should have been completed during target identification and validation efforts. It is relevant not only to the intended patient population, but also to how clinical development should be pursued (for example whether it is appropriate to expose healthy volunteers to the candidate in Phase I clinical trials. From both a drug discovery and development perspective, the focus should therefore be on assessing how and when these risks will be mitigated or discharged as the project progresses.

Modality selection

Assuming that the tests of unmet need and clinical tractability have been met, we now turn our attention to selecting the most appropriate pharmacological modality. For the purposes of this chapter, we will focus only on conventional small-molecule and biopharmaceutical modalities, since these are by far the most prevalent among marketed drugs. However, this is not to undermine the (growing) importance of alternative modalities, including cell and gene therapies, which are described in Chapter 9. Notwithstanding the restricted focus of this chapter, it is important to note that as a guiding principle, drug discovery should be 'modality agnostic', that is, the target has primacy, and modality selection should be based on which approach will most effectively achieve its modulation in patients. In practice, adherence to this principle is variable—for example, the optimal modality may be outside of the core expertise of the company or may be commercially nonviable (e.g., due to a prohibitively high cost-of-goods).

For some therapeutic targets, the specific cellular or tissue location of the target mandates which modality should be selected. In general terms, intracellular targets are considered inaccessible to biopharmaceuticals, and hence this modality is typically only appropriate for cell surface and circulating therapeutic targets. Moreover, some compartments are considered inaccessible to biopharmaceuticals—for example, the blood-brain barrier (BBB) is poorly permeable to monoclonal antibodies, and successful targeting of the CNS is more likely to be achieved by small molecules, except in diseases where the BBB is compromised.

Therefore for intracellular targets or for those located at sites inaccessible to antibodies, the decision to pursue a small-molecule modality is relatively straightforward, and attention can turn to the target's chemical tractability. Conversely, for target classes known to have poor chemical tractability with small-molecule intervention (e.g., neutralizing circulating growth factors, cytokines and chemokines), a biopharmaceutical approach may be the default choice, with little consideration given to small-molecule approaches.

For targets that could (in principle, at least) be modulated by either a small molecule or a biopharmaceutical, selecting the most appropriate modality depends on a wide variety of factors, both scientific and commercial, which are often inter-linked. Scientific considerations will include the target's pharmacological tractability, the proposed medicine's intended mechanism of action, the normal physiological role of the target, the proposed route of administration and the clinical setting. These will overlay considerations of pharmacoeconomics and the available technical expertise, capabilities and strategy of the company.

The potential for on-target toxicity is also a relevant consideration when assessing modality choices, since pharmacokinetic and other features of particular modalities may have an important impact on the therapeutic window of a medicine. For example, effects on normal physiology resulting from a short-lived exposure to a small-molecule drug may be tolerable, whereas sustained exposure to a biopharmaceutical (which typically has a half-life of approximately 3 weeks) may not. Conversely, features specific to particular modalities may be exploited to reduce the on-target toxicity risk. For example, in a scenario where a therapeutic target's activity in the periphery is pathogenic but it fulfils an important normal function in the brain, a biopharmaceutical modality may be selected on the basis that CNS penetrance will be low, or a small-molecule approach may be pursued but with a specific medicinal chemistry approach to minimize BBB penetrance.

Mechanism of action

An integral element of both modality selection and assessing pharmacological tractability of the target (see later) is an understanding of the desired mechanism(s) of action of the proposed medicine based on knowledge of the target's biological role in disease. The starting point for this analysis is commonly straightforward, that is, whether the aim is to agonize or antagonize the biological function of the target. Indeed, there are scenarios where this simplistic approach may be sufficient. For example, if the target is an oncogenic kinase overexpressed in a particular cancer type, it is credible to assume that the mechanism of action may be the adenosine triphosphate (ATP)-competitive inhibition of the kinase domain, and attention can turn to assessing the chemical tractability of the target (including, for example, the potency that would be required of an inhibitor to successfully compete intracellular ATP and the likelihood of achieving the required degree of selectivity over other kinases). Similarly, if the target is a circulating proinflammatory cytokine involved in autoimmune pathogenesis, it may be credible to assume that the mechanism of action will be the inhibition of the target's binding to its cognate receptor(s). However, more complex scenarios are commonplace. For example, the therapeutic hypothesis may be based on achieving more complex modulation of the target's activity (e.g., functional selectivity/biased agonism) or the target's biology may mandate indirect targeting of the active site (e.g., by allosteric modulation). Of course, many targets are biologically multifunctional, and it is important carefully to define which biological activity of the target is intended for modulation (e.g., whether it is the catalytic activity of an enzyme, or a protein–protein interaction interface of a nonenzymatic domain of the same target). Alternatively, the target may have no known catalytic or otherwise 'target-able' activity, and hence there may be very little granularity to the initial description of the proposed mechanism of action, other than that project seeks to modulate the target's overall contribution to a pathogenic effect.

Ultimately, consideration of the proposed mechanism of action should drive two key areas of analysis: (1) Are the available target validation data sufficiently robust to help define the most appropriate mechanism of action? (2) What impact does the proposed mechanism of action have on the design of the drug discovery process?

When considering the former, a critical analysis of the target validation data must be undertaken to give confidence that they are being correctly interpreted and therefore that the correct mechanistic approach is being pursued. To take a simplistic example, where human expression data implicated an enzymatic target in disease, the therapeutic hypothesis to inhibit the enzyme's catalytic activity may be predicated on beneficial phenotypic effects observed both in vitro and in vivo following genetic knockdown of the target. In fact, such data would be insufficient for defining whether the mechanism of action of the proposed drug should be the inhibition of the target's catalytic activity or the modulation of some other biological function of the target, since genetic knockdown will have abolished both. As such, further target validation work (e.g., interrogating the effect of specifically inactivating the active site) may be required.

The proposed mechanism of action will impact many aspects of the drug discovery process, but most importantly, it will dictate the screening approach required in the early stages of the project and will influence the probability of success. For example, screening for an enzymatic inhibitor may require a relatively straightforward biochemical screen, readily miniaturized for high-throughput screening. Conversely, screening for a protein–protein interaction inhibitor may be possible only with a complex cell-based screen requiring sophisticated downstream assays to deconvolute the targets of initial hits.

Individual medicines can achieve their effects through multiple mechanisms of action, and the choice of modality is relevant to whether this potential is exploited. For example, in a hypothetical case where the proposed therapeutic target in oncology is a cell surface receptor tyrosine kinase implicated in mitogenic signalling, the therapeutic hypothesis proposes that inhibiting this signalling pathway will decrease tumour cell proliferation. A priori, a small-molecule inhibitor of the receptor's kinase domain or a monoclonal antibody that blocks the binding of the receptor's cognate ligand might be predicted to be equally valid approaches. However, selecting a biopharmaceutical modality would afford the opportunity additionally to incorporate additional mechanisms of action to effect cell death, including antibody-directed cell cytotoxicity (ADCC), complement-directed cytotoxicity (CDC) and/or the delivery of a cytotoxic payload following internalization (antibody–drug conjugates) and indeed, Fc-mediated mechanisms contribute to the efficacy of some approved drugs. Conversely, Fc functionality can be disabled if such mechanisms of action are not desirable (e.g., if killing the target-expressing cell is not the goal).

Pharmacological tractability

Intertwined with considerations of mechanism of action and modality selection is the formal assessment of the pharmacological tractability of the target, that is, the probability of successfully identifying a small molecule or biopharmaceutical that will bind to the target and modulate it in the desired way. Importantly, a distinction may be drawn between tractability and druggability—the latter describing the likelihood of such a small molecule or biopharmaceutical being a precursor to a therapeutically useful drug. This is important because it encompasses not only the binding and modulation of the target but also the ability to achieve this safely, with adequate potency, selectivity and efficacy.

An initial assessment of target tractability may be somewhat generic and based on the target's particular class and whether historically such target classes (or homologues of specific targets) have been proven to be amenable to targeting. This can at least help to begin to assign the level of risk associated with this selection criterion. For example, there are multiple small-molecule inhibitors of kinases and G-protein-coupled receptors (GPCRs) and, similarly, numerous monoclonal antibody inhibitors of circulating cytokines, growth factors and cell-surface proteins, and these classes are hence generally considered highly tractable. Conversely, phosphatases and transcription factors are among target classes that have historically been associated with poor chemical tractability.

Following such a superficial triage, a more detailed and bespoke analysis of the target should be undertaken, even when it falls into what is ostensibly a 'low-risk' target class. Typically, chemical tractability assessments for small-molecule approaches are based around the integrated in silico assessment of a variety of data sources, particularly structural information, and many of these are in the public domain. Where structural information is available (or can credibly be modelled), tractability analysis typically focuses on identifying potential *accessible* binding pockets for drug-like molecules (and where appropriate, assessing how different they are from closely related protein domains, and hence the likelihood of achieving selectivity). As described earlier, the relevance of potential binding sites to the proposed mechanism of action of the medicine is paramount, that is, it is clearly not sufficient merely to achieve binding of a small molecule to satisfy the test of pharmacological tractability.

Although it is important to maintain a strong focus on data-led objectivity when assessing tractability, there will frequently be an element of subjectivity—for better or worse, since tractability prediction remains an inexact science and ultimately usually requires a judgement call. This subjectivity can be born of past experience of screening the same or similar targets, or may derive from institutional bias or unreasonable aversion to risk. The former can be useful insofar as it helps to avoid fruitless endeavours but should be tempered by knowing that past failures do not always predict future outcomes. Well-managed screening collections (typically at the scale of 1–2 million compounds in large pharmaceutical companies) continually evolve and should improve in quality—hence, a contemporary screening effort may yield a better outcome than a screen a decade or more ago. Similarly, better success against previously intractable targets of classes may be achieved based on new data (e.g., structural insights) and/or approaches other than high-throughput screening (e.g., fragment-based methods). With regard to risk aversion, in the 'omics' era, with an ever-increasing number of potential novel targets emerging, it must be accepted that with novelty comes risk, and that there will be occasions when the only way to determine pharmacological tractability is to move forwards and invest fully in a comprehensive drug discovery programme.

In practice, for all but the most precedented target classes, it is important to remember that tractability assessments provide neither certainty nor guarantees, and that their outcomes should be integrated with the analysis of other project selection criteria. For example, in scenarios where all other target selection criteria (e.g., unmet need, clinical tractability, etc.) are compellingly met but the predicted tractability is poor, the decision may nonetheless be made to progress the project 'at risk', on the grounds that chemical tractability is a risk that can be assessed, and potentially discharged, relatively early in the project. Of course, the same cannot be said for the reverse scenario, where predicted tractability is very high, but the clinical case is weak—in which case the project should not proceed.

Route of administration and clinical setting

To illustrate why criteria such as unmet need, clinical and chemical tractability, modality selection and mechanism of action should be assessed in an integrated way, it is useful to consider a scenario where a target pathway is known to be highly tractable to both small-molecule and biopharmaceutical modalities, but where only one modality has thus far proven successful in the clinic.

Wet age-related macular degeneration (AMD) is an ocular disease affecting around 2% of the population over 50 and 12% of those over 80 (https://www.nice.org.uk/guidance/ng82/chapter/Context). It is most prevalent in the elderly and is an important cause of central vision loss. The disease is characterized by pathogenic neovascularization driven principally by vascular endothelial growth factor (VEGF), a potent proangiogenic factor, acting primarily through the activation of one of its cognate receptors VEGFR2, a receptor tyrosine kinase. From a biological perspective, a credible hypothesis might be that neutralizing VEGF with a biopharmaceutical and inhibiting VEGFR2's kinase activity with a small molecule would be equivalent in preventing further neovascularization. Both approaches are known to be tractable (bevacizumab is an anti-VEGF monoclonal antibody approved for use in a variety of cancers and a variety of small-molecule VEGFR2 inhibitors exist (e.g., pazopanib and sunitinib—albeit with varying degrees of promiscuity for other kinases). At the time of writing, all approved therapies for wet AMD in Europe and the United States are VEGF-targeting biopharmaceuticals, administered by intravitreal injection.

Given the known chemical tractability for targeting VEGFR2, a credible 'medicine vision' in this setting might have originally described a small-molecule kinase inhibitor, administered topically (eye drops). In principle, there should be several benefits to this approach: eye drops can conveniently be self-administered by the patient, the small-molecule inhibitor should have a relatively low cost-of-goods, exposure to other sites in the body (with attendant on- and off-target liabilities) should be minimal, and there is no biological basis for concern that this modality would be inferior to a biopharmaceutical. These advantages could reasonably be expected to offset the likely requirement for frequent dosing given the expected pharmacokinetic and pharmacodynamic profile of the small molecule. Yet, in practice, this pathway is targeted using a biopharmaceutical with a high cost-of-goods (and therefore a high drug cost) that must be administered by a clinician through a relatively invasive route. These disadvantages are offset—at least in part—by the relatively infrequent dosing, enabled by the extended pharmacokinetics of the biopharmaceutical.

The principal driver for the development of a biopharmaceutical over a kinase inhibitor in this setting is in fact the difficulty in achieving sufficient bioavailability of small molecules at the required ocular site of action following topical administration (and the unacceptably high systemic exposure that would likely be required to achieve sufficient ocular bioavailability from oral or parenteral dosing).

Hence, this example illustrates the benefits of a 'modality agnostic' approach when considering targets that could ostensibly be modulated by either a small-molecule or biopharmaceutical approach. Here, clinical and commercial success was realized by an integrated analysis of unmet need, tractability and so on, all within the context of the clinical setting. It is an obvious point that this now presents the potential opportunity for the eventual development of medicines differentiated from those currently approved (whether they are topically administered small-molecule inhibitors overcoming current shortfalls in bioavailability, or biopharmaceutical formulations with a further extended half-life and hence requiring less frequent dosing), and this is currently an area of active interest.

Target product profile

As part of forming the "medicine vision", a target product profile (TPP) is typically generated. The TPP will highlight the most key features of the medicine, inter alia the patient population(s) who will benefit, its mechanism of action, the route and frequency of administration and its expected tolerability and safety profile. In addition to being a useful means of articulating the need for and vision of the proposed medicine, the TPP can be an invaluable tool for helping to plan and manage the project, since it essentially forms a list of specifications required of the new medicine. Understanding the relative importance of each of these specifications (and the flexibility around them) is crucial, which helps to define key go/no-go criteria for various stages of the project. Critically, although beyond the scope of this discussion, the TPP will reference the current (or potentially emerging) standard of care for the disease of interest, will define the features of the new medicine that are required for successful differentiation (its key value drivers) and will describe the thresholds that have been set for the medicine being considered commercially viable. incorporate aspects of the commercial proposition.

Planning the project

It is important to appreciate that all drug discovery projects start with a variety of risks that combine to give a low overall probability of successfully discovering and developing a new medicine. At a scientific level, the most important risks in the early stages of drug discovery are those associated with the target's biology, its pharmacological tractability and the overarching therapeutic hypothesis. As the project progresses to clinical development, usually several years later, risks involving changes in the clinical landscape (e.g., a reduced unmet medical need due to successful competitor activity) and payer behaviours (affecting the commercial viability of the proposed medicine) may, in addition, be realized. In other words, almost every aspect of a drug discovery project has attendant risks. A well-designed drug discovery project seeks to identify these risks at the outset and discharge or mitigate as many of them as possible, as early as possible. Some of these challenges may prove to be insurmountable, but if failure is inevitable, it is always better to fail early and avoid the intense financial and opportunity costs of late-stage attrition.

Careful planning of drug discovery projects is required to ensure the optimal use of finite resources, achieve the aim of discharging risks and define staged success criteria to prevent the continued pursuit of projects that are destined to fail. Because all potential targets (and therapeutic hypotheses) are unproven until they are successful in the clinic, ongoing target validation and biological studies should continue in parallel with drug discovery activities.

Project phases

Early-stage drug discovery projects (defined here as activities leading to the generation of a molecule that is ready for clinical development) can usefully be divided into several generic stages: assay development, hit identification and lead optimization. Although drug discovery and development overall should be viewed as a continuum, dividing the early stages of drug discovery projects into specific phases is a useful means of defining key success criteria that should be met to progress to the next project phases and helps to articulate how and whether key risks to the project will be mitigated or discharged over time. This approach should also ensure that assays, models and other analytical tools are in place when they are required, such that the drug discovery process can progress relatively seamlessly. Phasing the project in this way and setting clear go/no-go criteria for project progression should not be intended to impose unreasonable rigidity on the process, since science is unpredictable and new data relating to the target's biology or the therapeutic hypothesis may come to light that require the project plan to be modified or the approach to be changed. Discipline is needed to ensure that drug discovery projects do not persist beyond the point at which they should be terminated. Otherwise, they may continue perhaps due to a loss of objectivity in recognizing 'no-go' decision points, a failure to acknowledge that the case for pursuing the project has diminished since its initiation or an unrealistic expectation that issues encountered may be overcome by further investment of time and resources. Within and beyond the pharmaceutical industry, some of these challenges are as much cultural as they are scientific, and it should be acknowledged that rigorous, timely and data-driven decisions to terminate projects (and hence liberate resources for other efforts) can be as legitimate a measure of success for project teams as progressing an asset to the clinic.

Assay development

The primary purpose of the assay development phase is to establish the screening assays that will support the hit generation (screening) phase. This will likely include both the primary screen and any secondary or counter screens required for hit validation efforts, and hence its design requires a clearly defined screening cascade. For projects following a high-throughput approach, the general features of such screening cascades are common for small-molecule and biopharmaceutical projects—both aim to triage a large library of molecules as efficiently as possible, to derive a smaller number of 'hits' and for further evaluation and possible progression as leads. Cascades will typically comprise the primary screen against the target itself, followed by secondary or counter-screens that aim to exclude hits based on specific criteria (e.g., undesirable activity against closely related targets, lack of binding to target orthologues from critical species intended for use in toxicology and efficacy testing, etc.).

The format of the screens will be influenced by inter alia the target, the modality, the mechanism of action and the screening platforms/technologies being employed. Screens vary widely in complexity and the degree of effort required to develop them to a point of being fit-for-purpose. A relatively simple example may be a scenario where the target is a cytosolic enzyme that can readily be purified as an active recombinant protein, the proposed modality is a small molecule and the intended mechanism of action is inhibition of the enzyme's ATPase activity. Here, the development of a high-throughput (e.g., 1536-well scale) primary biochemical assay of ATP turnover by the recombinant enzyme is likely to be relatively straightforward, and the focus of secondary screens in this case may be limited in the first instance to counter-screens against closely related ATPases. Conversely, a more complex example would be a scenario where the target is a nuclear protein, the proposed modality is a small molecule and the intended mechanism of action is the inhibition of a protein–protein interaction between the target and a binding partner. Here, a more complex cell-based primary screen may need to be constructed (e.g., a proximity ligation assay), and the focus of secondary screens may be to build confidence in the validity of emerging hits.

An important alternative to screening directly against a target is to undertake a phenotypic screen, in which a cell-based assay is developed that reports on changes in a phenotype considered to be relevant to the target, pathway or—even more broadly—the disease process of interest. Where the desired target is known, the assay should ideally be formatted such that it is biased as much as possible in favour of identifying only those hits that are relevant to the target of interest (as opposed to those that may effect the same phenotypic change but through an alternative, irrelevant mechanism). The phenotypic screening approach may also be an advantage where a novel pathway has been identified, but it is unclear which specific node on the pathway is most appropriate for targeting. In both cases, the assay development phase should include

constructing assays aimed at deconvoluting the target(s) of emerging hits, to enable later lead optimization efforts to proceed efficiently.

Key success criteria for the assay development phase will likely include provision for assays being sufficiently robust and reproducible for use in screening, having an acceptable assay window (signal/noise) and being miniaturized sufficiently to be compatible with the scale of the intended screening library. These criteria may differ between the primary screen (against which millions of compounds may be screened) and secondary counter screens, which may be employed in the analysis of far fewer molecules emerging from the primary screen. Importantly, successful conclusion of this phase should not be taken to imply that no further assays will be needed during the lifetime of the project. On the contrary, it is likely that further assay development may be required to support later-stage lead optimization (e.g., in vitro biological assays using primary human samples, analytical techniques to support pharmacodynamic and efficacy studies, etc.), but it may be prudent to withhold investment in developing these assays until hit discovery efforts have been successful, and it is therefore clear that they will be needed.

Hit/lead identification

This phase of the project employs the assays developed in the preceding stage to identify initial hits, that is, the earliest precursors to the eventual medicine, identified based on their activity in the primary screening assay. During this phase, hits are typically triaged through secondary screening assays with a view to their validation and to enable the selection of preferred leads for further progression. For both small-molecule and biopharmaceutical projects, it is important to highlight that hits and leads emerging at this stage of the project are—at best—early precursors to the eventual medicine and are far from being suitable for clinical development. It is typical for several years of optimization to be required before a clinical candidate can formally be designated (as described later). Because sources of attrition during the lead optimization phases of the project cannot necessarily be predicted, it is useful if some diversity of hits can be maintained at this early stage of the project (e.g., several diverse molecular series for small-molecule projects and multiple complementarity-determining region (CDR) sequence families/epitope bins for biopharmaceuticals). Importantly, the successful identification of hits during this phase of the project constitutes an important *first stage* in discharging risks related to chemical tractability of the target. Whether this risk proves to be fully discharged will be determined in the subsequent phases of the project since, for example, it may not prove possible to improve upon the (invariably inadequate) potency or other properties of the initial hit.

Lead optimization

Assuming that there is sufficient confidence that leads have been identified that are worthy of progression, the lead optimization phase(s) of the project seek to optimize the molecules to arrive at a candidate molecule for clinical progression. It should do so with reference to the TPP, giving due attention to identifying an optimal molecule that complies as closely as possible to the desired 'specifications' of the molecule, whether in relation to potency, pharmacokinetic profile, efficacy in preclinical models of disease and so on. In the case of small-molecule projects, this will likely require very extensive medicinal chemistry effort, as structure–activity relationships (SARs) are defined, and lead series are iteratively improved upon with respect to the plethora of properties required of a clinical candidate. For biopharmaceutical molecules, the scope for iteratively improving individual lead molecules will be dictated by the technical platform being employed (e.g., conventional hybridoma methods, humanized in vivo platforms or in vitro libraries). In all cases, triaging molecules based on their suitability for large-scale manufacture is a critical stage, and the development of a manufacturing cell line is commonly a prerequisite for candidate selection (see Chapter 8).

It is important to appreciate that a proposed clinical candidate will rarely fully satisfy all the goal criteria defined at the outset of the project. Rather, it is likely that there would have been a trade-off between those properties for which there proved to be some degree of mutual exclusivity. For example, achieving optimal potency of a small molecule may come at the expense of, say, cell permeability or homologue selectivity. Conversely, the highest affinity antibody identified may not bind at the most appropriate epitope for catalysing complement-dependent cytotoxicity or may have an inferior immunogenicity prediction. It is important, therefore, to view the properties of the clinical candidate collectively, when objectively assessing whether the project should proceed to clinical development. This principle is as important for the molecular features of the potential candidate as it is for the overarching vision of the medicine. This underscores the utility of defining the TPP in advance, understanding the key drivers for pursuing the project and hence the degree of tolerance for noncompliance for particular aspects of the intended medicine. For example, if the TPP described a medicine suitable for both intravenous and oral administration, the impact of arriving at a molecule that shows exquisite efficacy in preclinical models following intravenous administration but has poor oral availability should be understood. Similarly, the effect on the commercial proposition for a proposed broad-spectrum novel antibiotic that achieves efficacy against only a subset of target bacterial species should have been evaluated, as such data emerged during drug discovery.

Target validation and biological studies

As discussed previously, it is rare to embark on a drug discovery project with full confidence in the validity of the target and the strength of the therapeutic hypothesis, particularly as it relates to clinical translation and tractability. Typically, there is a balance between taking the time to amass sufficient evidence to justify embarking on the project versus delaying drug discovery (and possibly losing competitive advantage) until a more definitive dataset can be built. It is important, therefore, to recognize that studies supporting target validation and clinical translation should proceed in parallel with formal drug discovery activities. For example, it may be appropriate to strengthen the therapeutic hypothesis (and better define the patient population) by evaluating greater numbers of patient-derived samples (potentially from a range of possible disease indications) to interrogate target overexpression and relevance. Alternatively, the (time-consuming) generation of transgenic models to evaluate the safety implications of modulating the target or to undertake more detailed mechanistic studies may be appropriate. Importantly, such studies should not be viewed as mere corollaries to the drug discovery effort, but central to it, inasmuch as data emerging from them, whether serving to strengthen or undermine the project, should carry as much weight as those emerging from drug discovery activities.

Chapter | 6 |

High-throughput screening

David Cronk, Joanne Shearer

Introduction: a historical and future perspective

Systematic drug research began about 100 years ago, when chemistry had reached a degree of maturity that allowed its principles and methods to be applied to problems outside the field, and when pharmacology had in turn become a well-defined scientific discipline. A key step was the introduction of the concept of selective affinity through the postulation of 'chemoreceptors' by Paul Ehrlich. He was the first to argue that differences in chemoreceptors between species may be exploited therapeutically. This was also the birth of chemotherapy. In 1907, Ehrlich identified compound number 606, Salvarsan (diaminodioxy-arsenobenzene) (Ehrlich & Bertheim, 1912), which was brought to the market in 1910 by Hoechst for the treatment of syphilis, and hailed as a miracle drug (Fig. 6.1).

This was the first time extensive pharmaceutical screening had been used to find drugs. At that time, screening was based on phenotypic readouts (antimicrobial effect), a concept that has since led to unprecedented therapeutic triumphs in antiinfective and anticancer therapies, based particularly on natural products. In contrast, today's screening is largely driven by distinct molecular targets and modulation of specific biochemical reactions, cellular effects attributed to modulation of specific pathways or phenotypic readouts, although the latter most commonly use high-resolution imaging platforms now rather than the cell death readouts applied by Ehrlich.

In the further course of the 20th century, drug research became influenced primarily by biochemistry. The dominant concepts introduced by biochemistry were those of enzymes and receptors, which were empirically found to be drug targets. In 1948, Ahlquist made a crucial, further step by proposing the existence of two types of adrenoceptor (α and β) in most organs. The principle of receptor classification has been the basis for a large number of diverse drugs, including β-adrenoceptor agonists and antagonists, benzodiazepines, angiotensin antagonists and ultimately monoclonal antibodies.

Today's marketed drugs target a range of human biomolecules, ranging from various enzymes and transporters to G-protein-coupled receptors (GPCRs) and ion channels (Santos et al., 2017). At present, the GPCRs are the predominant target family, with around 700 approved drugs targeting 134 receptors out of a total of approximately 360 druggable GPCRs (Sriram & Insel, 2018). It should be recognized that there are approximately 800 GPCRs identified in the human genome; however, it is predicted that less than half are druggable, as they are implicated in sensory signal transduction (taste, olfaction and vision), and in reality, enzymes, transporters and modulation of protein interactions may represent the more potential as targets for pharmaceutical products (Santos et al., 2017). Although the target portfolio of a pharmaceutical company can change from time to time, the newly chosen targets are still likely to belong to one of the main therapeutic target classes. The selection of targets and target families (see Chapter 4) plays a pivotal role in determining the success of today's lead molecule discovery.

Over the last 20 years, significant technological progress has been achieved in genomic sciences (Chapter 4), high-throughput medicinal chemistry (Chapter 7), cell-based assays and high-throughput screening (HTS). These have led to a 'new' concept in drug discovery, whereby targets with therapeutic potential are incorporated into biochemical or cell-based assays that are exposed to large numbers of compounds, each representing a given chemical structure space. Massively parallel screening, called HTS, was first introduced by pharmaceutical companies in the early 1990s and is now employed routinely as the most widely applicable technology for identifying chemistry starting

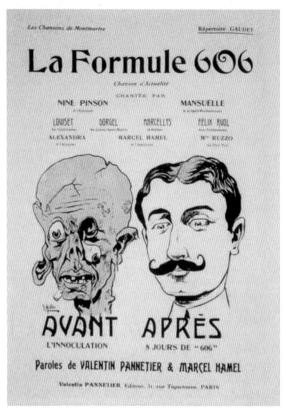

Fig. 6.1 In France, where Salvarsan was called 'Formule 606', true miracles were expected from the new therapy.

points for drug discovery programmes, and it is regarded that many of the clinical development candidates in pharmaceutical companies have their origins in HTS (Macarron et al., 2011).

Nevertheless, HTS remains just one of a number of possible lead discovery strategies (see Chapter 4). In the best case, it can provide an efficient way to obtain useful data on the biological activity of large numbers of test samples by using high-quality assays and high-quality chemical compounds. Today's lead discovery departments are typically composed of the following units: (1) compound logistics; (2) assay development and screening (which may utilize automation); (3) tool (reagent) production; and (4) profiling. While most HTS projects focus on the use of synthetic molecules typically within a molecular weight range of 250–600 Da based on the properties of marketed drugs as defined by Lipinski et al. (1997), natural products are still regarded as being a valuable source for identification of therapeutics agents (Coma et al., 2014). To support this, some companies, for example, Venomtech and Analyticon, specialize in the use of

naturally occurring material such as venoms, plant extracts or molecules based on natural product structures and have dedicated research departments for this purpose. These groups work closely with the HTS groups to curate the natural products, which are typically stored as complex mixtures, and provide the necessary analytical skills to isolate the single active molecule.

Compared with HTS in the 1990s, there is now much more focus on quality-oriented output. At first, screening throughput was the main emphasis, but it is now only one of many performance indicators. In the 1990s, the primary concern of a company's compound logistics group was to collect all its historical compound collections in sufficient quantities and of sufficient quality to file them by electronic systems, and store them in the most appropriate way in compound archives. This resulted in huge collections that range from several hundred thousand to a few million compounds (Macarron et al., 2011). Due to the different historical disease interest between most pharmaceutical companies, there was surprisingly little overlap in compounds between collections. In order to limit the time and expense of building collections to introduce different compounds in screening libraries, some pharmaceutical companies are working collaboratively to allow reciprocal screening of their collections against a target of interest to another company (Kogej et al., 2013). Overall, the drive for increasing numbers of compounds in a screening library has waned, and today's focus has shifted to the application of defined electronic or physical filters, computational chemistry and artificial intelligence for compound selection before they are assembled into a library for testing. The result is a customized ensemble of either newly designed or historic compounds for use in screening, otherwise known as 'cherry picking', or in silico screening prior to conducting focused 'wet laboratory' screens. However, it is often the case that the HTS departments have sufficient infrastructure to enable routine screening of the entire compound collection, and it is only where the assay is complex or relatively expensive that the time to create 'cherry picked', focused compound sets is invested (Valler & Green, 2000). That said, as the targets entering into HTS diversify, there is renewed drive for the ability to generate and screen larger compound numbers with less effort. This has led to the evolution of technologies to allow multiple compounds to be screened in the same well and the target/compound association to be effectively decoded. Examples of this approach included DNA-encoded libraries (DEL) (Kunig et al., 2018) and affinity selection mass spectrometry (Thomas et al., 2014).

In assay development, there is a clear trend towards mechanistically driven high-quality assays that capture the relevant biochemistry (e.g., stoichiometry, kinetics) or cell biology. Homogeneous assay principles, along with sensitive detection technologies, have enabled the miniaturization of assay formats producing a concomitant reduction of reagent usage and cost per data point. With this evolution of HTS formats, it is becoming increasingly common to gain more than one set of information from the same assay well either through multiparametric analysis or multiplexing, for example, cellular function response and toxicity (Beske & Goldbard, 2002; Hallis et al., 2007; Hanson, 2006). The drive for information-rich data from HTS campaigns is no more evident than through the use of imaging technology to enable subcellular resolution, a methodology broadly termed high content screening (HCS), or the use of flow cytometry. Both HCS and flow cytometry platforms facilitate the study of intracellular pharmacology through spatiotemporal resolution, and/or the quantification of cell surface markers, signalling and regulatory pathways. Both techniques increasingly use cells that are more phenotypically representative of disease states and may include patient-derived primary cells or stem cells with an appropriate genotype (Clemons, 2004; Eglen, 2009), in an effort to add further value to the information provided. The drawback of using primary cells or stem cells is that they tend to be more difficult to produce in larger numbers than immortalized cell lines, which may result in either screening fewer compounds or extended screening timelines.

Screening departments in large pharmaceutical companies utilize automated screening platforms, which in the early days of HTS were large linear track systems, typically 5 m or more in length. The more recent trends have been towards integrated networks of workstation-based instrumentation which may be placed on removable docking stations, which themselves may form small automated workstations, typically arranged around the circumference of a static, rotating robotic arm which offers greater flexibility and increased efficiency in throughput due to reduced plate transit times within the automated workcell. Typically, the screening unit of a large pharmaceutical company will generate tens of millions of single point determinations per year, with fully automated data acquisition and processing. Following primary screening, there has been an increased need for secondary/complementary screening to confirm the primary results, provide information on test compound specificity and selectivity and to refine these compounds further. Typical data formats include half-maximal concentrations at which a compound causes a defined modulatory effect in functional assays, or binding/inhibitory constants. Post-HTS, broader selectivity profiling may be required, for active compounds against panels of related target families. As HTS technologies continue to be adopted into other related disciplines, compound potency and selectivity are no longer the only parameters to be optimized during hit-finding. With this broader acceptance of key technologies, harmonization and standardization of data across disciplines are crucial to facilitate analysis and mining of the data. Important information such as compound purity and its associated physicochemical properties such as solubility can be derived very quickly on relatively large numbers of compounds and thus help prioritize compounds for progression based on overall suitability, not just potency (Fligge & Schuler, 2006). These quality criteria, and quality assessment at all key points in the discovery process, are crucial. Late-stage attrition of drug candidates, particularly in development and beyond, is extremely expensive, and such failures must be kept to a minimum. This is typically done by an extensive assessment of chemical integrity, synthetic accessibility, functional properties, structure–activity relationship (SAR) and biophysicochemical properties, and related absorption, distribution, metabolism and excretion (ADME) characteristics, as discussed further in Chapter 10.

In summary, significant technological progress has been made over the last 20 years in HTS. Major concepts such as miniaturization and parallelization have been introduced in almost all areas and steps of the lead discovery process. This, in turn, has led to a great increase in screening capacity, significant savings in compound or reagent consumption and ultimately to improved cost-effectiveness. More recently, stringent quality assessment in library management and assay development, along with consistent data formats in automated screening, has led to much higher-quality screening outcomes. The perception of HTS has also changed significantly in the past decade and is now recognized as a multidisciplinary science, encompassing biological sciences, engineering and information technology. HTS departments generate huge amounts of data that can be used in computational chemistry tools to drive compound SARs and aid selection of focused compound sets for further testing from larger compound libraries. Where information-rich assays are used, complex analysis algorithms may be required to ensure the relevant data are extracted. Various statistical, informatics and filtering methods have recently been introduced to foster the integration of experimental and in silico screening, and so maximize the output in lead discovery. As a result, lead-finding activities continue to benefit greatly from a more unified and knowledge-based approach to biological screening, in addition to the many technical advances towards even higher-throughput screening.

Lead discovery and high-throughput screening

A lead compound is generally defined as a new chemical entity that could potentially be developed into a new drug by optimizing its beneficial effects and minimizing its side effects (see Chapters 4 and 5 for a more detailed discussion of the criteria). HTS is currently the main approach for the identification of lead compounds, that is, large numbers of compounds (the 'compound library') are assembled to give a broad coverage of available molecular scaffolds, so-called chemical diversity, and tested for their biological activity against a disease-relevant target without making any assumption as to which scaffold will demonstrate biological activity. However, there are other techniques in place for lead discovery that are complementary to HTS.

Besides the conventional literature search (identification of compounds already described for the desired activity), structure-based virtual screening is a frequently applied technique (Ghosh et al., 2006; Waszkowycz, 2008). Molecular recognition events are simulated by computational techniques based on knowledge of the molecular target, thereby allowing very large 'virtual' compound libraries (> 4 million compounds) to be screened in silico and, by applying this information, pharmacophore models can be developed. These allow the identification of potential leads in silico, without experimental screening and the subsequent construction of smaller sets of compounds ('focussed libraries') for testing against a specific target or family of targets (Muegge & Oloff, 2006; Stahura et al., 2002). Similarly, X-ray analysis of the target can be applied to guide the de novo synthesis and design of bioactive molecules. In the absence of computational models, very-low-molecular-weight compounds (typically 150–300 Da), so-called fragments, may be screened using biophysical methods to detect low affinity interactions. The use of protein crystallography and X-ray diffraction techniques allows elucidation of the binding mode of these fragments, and these can be used as a starting point for developing higher affinity leads (Congreve et al., 2008; Hartshorn et al., 2005; Rees et al., 2004). Alongside these established methods, there is a growing application of artificial intelligence in the field of hit finding and drug discovery (Fleming, 2018). This topic is too broad to cover within this chapter other than to make the reader aware that its application reaches into the identification of new targets, design of new molecules, selection of molecules to be screened and interpretation of screening data.

Typically, in HTS, large compound libraries are screened ('primary' screen), and numerous bioactive compounds ('primary hits' or 'positives') are identified. These compounds are taken through successive rounds of further screening ('secondary' screens) to confirm their activity, potency and, where possible, gain an early measure of specificity for the target of interest. A typical HTS activity cascade is shown in Fig. 6.2, resulting in the identification of hits, usually with multiple members of a similar chemical core or chemical series. These hits then enter into the 'hit-to-lead' process, during which medicinal chemistry teams synthesize specific compounds or small arrays of compounds for testing to develop an understanding of the SAR of the underlying chemical series. The result of the hit-to-lead phase is a group of compounds (the lead series) which has appropriate drug-like properties such as specificity, pharmacokinetics or bioavailability. These properties can then be further improved by medicinal chemistry in a 'lead optimization' process (Fig. 6.3). Often the HTS group will provide support for these hit-to-lead and lead optimization stages through ongoing provision of reagents, provision of assay expertise or execution of the assays themselves.

Assay development and validation

The target validation process (see Chapter 5) establishes the relevance of a target in a certain disease pathway. In the next step, an assay has to be developed, allowing the quantification of the interaction of molecules with the chosen target. This interaction can be inhibition, stimulation or simply binding. There are numerous different assay technologies available, and the choice for a specific assay type will always be determined by factors such as type of target, the required sensitivity, robustness, ease of automation and cost. Assays can be carried out in different formats based on 96-, 384-, 1536- or 3456-well microtitre plates. The format to be applied depends on various parameters, for example, readout, desired throughput or existing hardware in liquid handling and signal detection with 384- (either standard volume or low volume) and 1536-well formats being the most commonly applied. In all cases, the homogeneous type of assay is preferred, as it is quicker, easier to handle and cost-effective, allowing 'mix and measure' operation without any need for further separation steps.

Next to scientific criteria, cost is a key factor in assay development. The choice of format has a significant effect on the total cost per data point: the use of 384-well low-volume microtitre plates instead of a 96-well plate format results in a significant reduction of the reaction volume (see Table 6.1). This reduction correlates directly with reagent costs per well. The size of a typical screening library is between 500,000 and 1 million compounds. Detection reagent costs per well can easily vary between US$0.05 and more than US$0.5 per data point, depending on the type and format of the assay. Therefore screening an assay with a 500,000 compound library may cost either US$25,000 or US$250,000, depending on the selected assay design—a significant difference! It should also be borne in mind that these costs are representative for reagents only, and the cost of consumables (assay plates and disposable liquid handling tips) and carbon footprint (amount of single use plastic per assay plate)

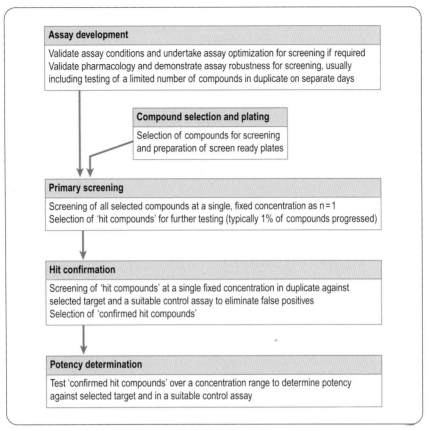

Assay development

Validate assay conditions and undertake assay optimization for screening if required
Validate pharmacology and demonstrate assay robustness for screening, usually including testing of a limited number of compounds in duplicate on separate days

Compound selection and plating

Selection of compounds for screening and preparation of screen ready plates

Primary screening

Screening of all selected compounds at a single, fixed concentration as n = 1
Selection of 'hit compounds' for further testing (typically 1% of compounds progressed)

Hit confirmation

Screening of 'hit compounds' at a single fixed concentration in duplicate against selected target and a suitable control assay to eliminate false positives
Selection of 'confirmed hit compounds'

Potency determination

Test 'confirmed hit compounds' over a concentration range to determine potency against selected target and in a suitable control assay

Fig. 6.2 The typical high-throughput screening process.

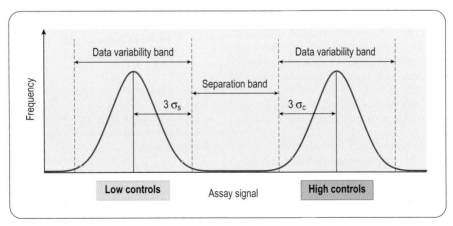

Fig. 6.3 Illustration of data variability and the signal window, given by the separation band between high and low controls.

Table 6.1 Impact of miniaturization, based on screening of 150,000 compounds

Plate format	Number of plates	Assay volume (μL)	Reagent volume (L)	Compound required (μL)	Time to screen (50 plates/day) (days)	Compounds per day
96-well	1875	10–200	18	1	38	4,000
384-well	427	25–50	8.2	0.5	9	17,600
Low volume 384-well	427	5–20	2.6	0.15	9	17,600
1536-well	107	2–10	1.3	0.08	2	70,400

may be additional considerations. While the consumables costs are higher for the higher density formats, the saving in reagent costs and increased throughput associated with miniaturization usually result in assays being run in the highest density format the HTS department has available.

Once a decision on the principal format and readout technology is taken, the assay has to be validated for its sensitivity and robustness. Biochemical parameters, reagents and screening hardware (e.g., detectors, microtitre plates) must be optimized. To give a practical example, in a typical screen designed for inhibitors of protease activity, test compounds are mixed together with the enzyme and finally substrate is added. The substrate consists of a cleavable peptide linked to a fluorescent label, and the reaction is quantified by measuring the change in fluorescence intensity that accompanies the enzymic cleavage. In the process of validation, the best available labelled substrate (natural or synthetic) must be selected, the reaction conditions optimized (e.g., reaction time, buffers and temperature), enzyme kinetic measurements performed to identify the linear range and the response of the assay to known inhibitors (if available) tested. Certain types of compound or solvent (which in most cases will be dimethylsulfoxide [DMSO]) may interfere with the assay readout, and this has to be checked. The stability of assay reagents is a further important parameter to be determined during assay validation, as some assay formats require a long incubation time.

At this point, other aspects of screening logistics have to be considered. If the enzyme is not available commercially, it has to be produced in-house by process development, and batch-to-batch reproducibility and timely delivery have to be ensured. With cell-based screens, it must be guaranteed that the cell production facility is able to deliver sufficient quantities of consistently functioning, physiologically intact cells during the whole screening campaign, and that there is no degradation of signal or loss of protein expression from the cells with extended periods of subculture.

The principal goal of developing HTS assays is the fast and reliable identification of active compounds ('positives' or 'hits') from chemical libraries. Most HTS programmes test compounds at only one concentration. In most instances, this approximates to a final test concentration in the assay of 10 μM. This may be adjusted depending on the nature of the target but in all cases must be within the bound of the solvent tolerance of the assay determined earlier in the development process. In order to identify hits with confidence, only small variations in signal measurements can be tolerated. The statistical parameters used to determine the suitability of assays for HTS are the calculation of standard deviations, the coefficient of variation (CV), signal-to-noise (S/N) ratio or signal-to-background (S/B) ratio. The inherent problem with using these last two is that neither takes into account the dynamic range of the signal (i.e. the difference between the background [low control] and the maximum [high control] signal), or the variability in the sample and reference control measurements. A more reliable assessment of assay quality is achieved by the Z'-factor equation (Zhang et al., 1999):

$$Z' = 1 - \frac{[3(\text{SD of high control}) + 3(\text{SD of low control})]}{(\text{Mean of high control} - \text{Mean of low control})}$$

where SD is the standard deviation and the maximum possible value of Z is 1. For biochemical assays, a value greater than 0.5 represents a good assay, whereas a value less than 0.5 is generally unsatisfactory for HTS. A lower Z' threshold of 0.4 is usually considered acceptable for cell-based assays.

This equation takes into account that the quality of an assay is reflected in the variability of the high and low controls, and the separation band between them (Fig. 6.3). Z'-factors are obtained by measuring plates containing 50% low controls (in the protease example: assay plus reference inhibitor, minimum signal to be measured) and 50% high controls (assay without inhibitor; maximum signal to be measured). In addition, inter- and intra-plate CVs are determined to check for systematic sources of variation. All measurements are normally made in triplicate.

Once an assay has passed these quality criteria, it can be transferred to the robotic screening laboratory. A reduced number of control wells can be employed to monitor Z'-values when the assay is progressed to HTS mode, usually 16 high- and 16 low-controls on a 384-well plate, with the removal of no more than two outlying controls to achieve an acceptable Z'-value. The parameter can be further modified to calculate the Z-value, whereby the average signal and standard deviation of test compound wells are compared to the high-control wells (Zhang et al., 1999). Due to the variability that will be present in the compound wells, and assuming a low number of active compounds, the Z-value is usually lower than the Z'-value.

While there are several alternatives to Zhang's proposal for assessing assay robustness, such as power analysis (Sui & Wu, 2007), the simplicity of the equation still makes the Z'-value the primary assessment of assay suitability for HTS.

The Assay Guidance Website hosted by the NIH Chemical Genomics Center (https://ncats.nih.gov/expertise/preclinical/agm) provides comprehensive guidance of factors to consider for a wide range of assay formats.

Biochemical and cell-based assays

There is a wide range of assay formats that can be deployed in the drug discovery arena (Hemmilä & Hurskainen, 2002), although they broadly fall into two categories, *biochemical* and *cell-based*. The reader should be aware, however, that there are some technologies such as high-throughput mass spectrometry (discussed later in the chapter) that can be deployed in either the biochemical or cellular scenario to detect a specific reaction product.

Biochemical assays (Fig. 6.4) involve the use of cell-free in vitro systems to model the biochemistry of a subset of cellular processes. The assay systems vary from simple interactions, such as enzyme/substrate reactions, receptor binding or protein–protein interactions, to more complex models such as in vitro transcription systems. In contrast to cell-based assays, biochemical assays give direct information regarding the nature of the molecular interaction (e.g., kinetic data) and tend to have increased solvent tolerance compared to cellular assays, thereby permitting the use of higher compound screening concentration if required. However, biochemical assays lack the cellular context, and are insensitive to properties such as membrane permeability, which determine the effects of compounds on intact cells.

Unlike biochemical assays, cell-based assays (Fig. 6.5) mimic more closely the in vivo situation, particularly where disease-relevant primary cells or stem cells (which may themselves be patient derived) are used and can be adapted for targets that are unsuitable for screening in

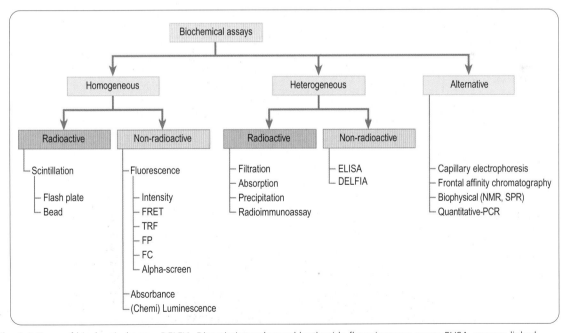

Fig. 6.4 Types of biochemical assay. *DELFIA*, Dissociation-enhanced lanthanide fluoroimmuno assay; *ELISA*, enzyme-linked immunosorbent assays; *FC*, fluorescence correlation; *FP*, fluorescence polarization; *FRET*, fluorescence resonance energy transfer; *NMR*, nuclear magnetic resonance; *PCR*, polymerase chain reaction; *SPR*, surface plasmon resonance; *TRF*, time-resolved fluorescence.

biochemical assays, such as those involving signal transduction pathways, membrane transport, cell division cytotoxicity or antibacterial actions. Parameters measured in cell-based assays range from growth, transcriptional activity, changes in cell metabolism or morphology to changes in the level of intracellular messengers such as cAMP, intracellular calcium concentration and changes in membrane potential for ion channels (Moore & Rees, 2001). Importantly, cell-based assays are able to distinguish between receptor antagonists, agonists, inverse agonists and allosteric modulators, which cannot be done by measuring binding affinity in a biochemical assay.

Many cell-based assays have quite complex protocols, for example, removing cell culture media, washing cells, adding compounds to be tested, prolonged incubation at 37°C and finally reading the cellular response. Therefore screening with cell-based assays requires a sophisticated infrastructure in the screening laboratory (including cell cultivation facilities and robotic systems equipped to maintain physiological conditions during the assay procedure) and the throughput is generally lower.

Cell-based assays frequently lead to higher hit rates, because of non-specific and 'off-target' effects of test compounds that affect the readout. Primary hits therefore need to be assessed by means of secondary assays such as non- or control-transfected cells to determine the mechanism of the effect (Moore & Rees, 2001).

Although cell-based assays are generally more time-consuming than cell-free assays to set up and run in high-throughput mode, there are many situations in which they are needed. For example, assays involving GPCRs, membrane transporters and ion channels generally require intact cells if the functionality of the test compound is to be understood, or at least membranes prepared from intact cells for determining compound binding. In other cases, the production of biochemical targets such as enzymes in sufficient quantities for screening may be difficult or costly compared to cell-based assays directed at the same targets. The main pros and cons of cell-based assays are summarized in Table 6.2.

Assay readout and detection

Ligand binding assays

Assays to determine direct interaction of the test compound with the target of interest through the use of

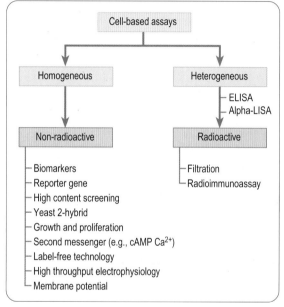

Fig. 6.5 Types of cell-based assay. *cAMP*, cyclic adenosine monophosphate; *ELISA*, Enzyme-linked immunosorbent assay.

Table 6.2 Advantages and disadvantages of cell-based assays	
Advantages	**Disadvantages**
Cytotoxic compounds can be detected and eliminated at the outset	Require high-capacity cell culture facilities and more challenging to fully automate
In receptor studies, agonists can be distinguished from antagonists	Often require specially engineered cell lines and/or careful selection of control cells
Detection of allosteric modulators	Reagent provision and control of variability of reagent batches
Binding and different functional readouts can be used in parallel—high information content	Cells liable to become detached from support
Phenotypic readouts are enabling when the molecular target is unknown (e.g., to detect compounds that affect cell division, growth, differentiation or metabolism)	High rate of false positives due to non-specific effects of test compounds on cell function
More disease relevant than biochemical assays	Assay variability can make assays more difficult to miniaturize
No requirement for protein production/scale up	Assay conditions (e.g., use of solvents, pH) limited by cell viability

radiolabelled compounds are sensitive and robust and are widely used for ligand-binding assays. The assay is based on measuring the ability of the test compound to inhibit the binding of a radiolabelled ligand to the target and requires that the assay can distinguish between bound and free forms of the radioligand. This can be done by physical separation of bound from unbound ligand (*heterogeneous* format) by filtration, adsorption or centrifugation. The need for several washing steps makes it unsuitable for fully automated HTS and generates large volumes of radioactive waste, raising safety and cost concerns over storage and disposal. Such assays are mainly restricted to 96-well format due to limitations of available multiwell filter plates and achieving consistent filtration when using higher density formats. Filtration systems do provide the advantage that they allow accurate determination of maximal binding levels and ligand affinities at sufficient throughput for support of hit-to-lead and lead optimization activities.

In the HTS arena, filtration assays have been superseded by *homogeneous* formats for radioactive assays. These have reduced overall reaction volume and eliminate the need for separation steps, largely eliminating the problem of waste disposal and provide increased throughput.

The majority of homogeneous radioactive assay types are based on the scintillation proximity principle. This relies on the excitation of a scintillant incorporated in a matrix, in the form of either *microbeads* ('SPA') or *microplates* (FlashPlates, PerkinElmer) (Sittampalam et al., 1997), to the surface of which the target molecule is also attached (Fig. 6.6). Binding of the radioligand to the target brings it into close proximity to the scintillant, resulting in light emission, which can be quantified. Free radioactive ligand is too distant from the scintillant and no excitation

takes place. Isotopes such as ^{3}H or ^{125}I are typically used, as they produce low-energy particles that are absorbed over short distances (Cook, 1996). Test compounds that bind to the target compete with the radioligand and thus reduce the signal.

With bead technology (Fig. 6.6), polymer beads of ~5 μm diameter are coated with antibodies, streptavidin, receptors or enzymes to which the radioligand can bind (Beveridge et al., 2000; Bosworth & Towers, 1989). Ninety-six- or 384-well plates can be used. The emission wavelength of the scintillant is in the range of 420 nm and is subject to limitations in the sensitivity due to both colour quench by yellow test compounds and the variable efficiency of scintillation counting, due to sedimentation of the beads. The homogeneous platforms are also still subject to limitations in throughput associated with the detection technology via multiple photomultiplier tube-based detection instruments, with a 384-well plate taking in the order of 15 minutes to read.

The drive for increased throughput for radioactive assays led to the development of scintillants, containing europium yttrium oxide or europium polystyrene, contained in beads or multiwell plates with an emission wavelength shifted towards the red-end of the visible light spectrum (~560 nm) and suited to detection on charge-coupled device (CCD) cameras (Ramm, 1999) to allow quantitative imaging to scan the whole plate, resulting in a higher throughput and increased sensitivity. Imaging instruments provide a read time typically in the order of a few minutes or less for the whole plate irrespective of density, representing a significant improvement in throughput, along with increased sensitivity. The problem of compound colour quench effect remains, although blue compounds now provide false hits rather than yellow. As CCD detection is independent of plate density, the use of imaging-based radioactive assays has been adopted widely in HTS and adapted to a 1536-well format and higher (see Bays et al., 2009, for example), but the availability of imaging instruments has become increasingly limited due to environmental regulation of refrigerant gases and components of the instrument. As a result, the ability to execute radiometric screening is arguably the only area of screening where we are becoming less able to reduce volumes and increase throughput.

In the microplate form of scintillation proximity assays, the target protein (e.g., an antibody or receptor) is coated onto the floor of a plate well to which the radioligand and test compounds are added. The bound radioligand causes a microplate surface scintillation effect (Brown et al., 1997). FlashPlate has been used in the investigation of protein–protein (e.g., radioimmunoassay) and receptor–ligand (i.e., radioreceptor assay) interactions (Birzin & Rohrer, 2002), and in enzymatic (e.g., kinase) assays (Braunwaler et al., 1996).

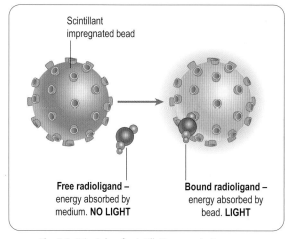

Scintillant impregnated bead

Free radioligand – energy absorbed by medium. **NO LIGHT**

Bound radioligand – energy absorbed by bead. **LIGHT**

Fig 6.6 Principle of scintillation proximity assays.

Due to the level of sensitivity provided by radioactive assays, they are still widely adopted within the HTS setting. However, environmental safety and local legislative considerations have led to the necessary development of alternative formats, in particular those utilizing fluorescent-ligands (Lee et al., 2008; Leopoldo et al., 2009). Through careful placement of a suitable fluorophore in the ligand via a suitable linker, the advantages of radioligand-binding assays in terms of sensitivity can be realized without the obvious drawbacks associated with the use of radioisotopes. The use of fluorescence-based technologies is discussed in more detail in the following section.

Fluorescence technologies

The application of fluorescence technologies is widespread, covering multiple formats (Gribbon & Sewing, 2003), and yet in the simplest form involves excitation of a sample with light at one wavelength and measurement of the emission at a different wavelength. The difference between the absorbed wavelength and the emitted wavelength is called the *Stokes shift*, the magnitude of which depends on how much energy is lost in the fluorescence process (Lakowicz, 1999). A large Stokes shift is advantageous, as it reduces optical crosstalk between photons from the excitation light and emitted photons.

Fluorescence techniques currently applied for HTS can be grouped into six major categories:

- Fluorescence intensity
- Fluorescence resonance energy transfer (FRET)
- Time-resolved fluorescence (TRF)
- Fluorescence polarization (FP)
- Fluorescence correlation
- AlphaScreen (amplified luminescence proximity homogeneous assay)

Fluorescence intensity. In fluorescence intensity assays, the change of total light output is monitored and used to quantify a biochemical reaction or binding event. This type of readout is frequently used in enzymatic assays (e.g., proteases, lipases). There are two variants: *fluorogenic assays* and *fluorescence quench assays*. In the former type, the reactants are not fluorescent, but the reaction products are, and their formation can be monitored by an increase in fluorescence intensity.

In fluorescence quench assays, a fluorescent group is covalently linked to a substrate. In this state, its fluorescence is quenched. Upon cleavage, the fluorescent group is released, producing an increase in fluorescence intensity (Haugland, 2002).

Fluorescence intensity measurements are easy to run and cheap. However, they are sensitive to fluorescent interference resulting from the colour of test compounds,

organic fluorophores in assay buffers and even fluorescence of the microplate itself (Comley, 2003).

Fluorescence resonance energy transfer. In this type of assay, a *donor* fluorophore is excited, and most of the energy is transferred to an *acceptor* fluorophore or a quenching group; this results in measurable photon emission by the acceptor. In simple terms, the amount of energy transfer from donor to acceptor depends on the fluorescent lifetime of the donor, the spatial distance between donor and acceptor (10–100 Å) and the dipole orientation between donor and acceptor. The transfer efficiency for a given pair of fluorophores can be calculated using the equation of Förster (Clegg, 1995).

Usually the emission wavelengths of donor and acceptor are different, and FRET can be determined either by the quenching of the donor fluorescence by the acceptor (as shown in Fig. 6.7) or by the fluorescence of the acceptor itself. Typical applications are for protease assays based on quenching of the uncleaved substrate, although FRET has also been applied for detecting changes in membrane potential in cell-based assays for ion channels (Gonzalez & Maher, 2002). With simple FRET techniques, interference from background fluorescence is often a problem, which is largely overcome by the use of TRF techniques, described below.

Time resolved fluorescence. TRF techniques (Comley, 2006) use lanthanide chelates (samarium, europium, terbium and dysprosium) that give an intense and long-lived

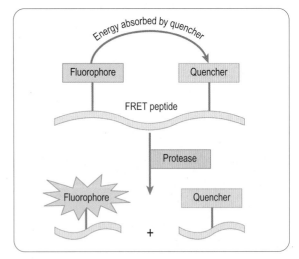

Fig. 6.7 Protease assay based on fluorescence resonance energy transfer (FRET). The donor fluorescence is quenched by the neighbouring acceptor molecule. Cleavage of the substrate separates them, allowing fluorescent emission by the donor molecule.

fluorescence emission (>1000 μs). Fluorescence emission is elicited by a pulse of excitation and measured after the end of the pulse, by which time short-lived fluorescence has subsided. This makes it possible to eliminate the short-lived autofluorescence and reagent background, and thereby enhance the S/N ratio. Lanthanides emit fluorescence with a large Stokes shift when they coordinate to specific ligands. Typically, the complexes are excited by ultraviolet (UV) light and emit light of a wavelength longer than 500 nm.

Europium (Eu^{3+}) chelates have been used in immunoassays by means of a technology called DELFIA (dissociation-enhanced lanthanide fluoroimmuno assay). DELFIA is a heterogeneous time-resolved fluorometric assay based on *dissociative fluorescence enhancement*. Cell- and membrane-based assays are particularly well suited to the DELFIA system because of its broad detection range and extremely high sensitivity (Valenzano et al., 2000).

High sensitivity—to a limit of about 10^{-17} moles/well—is achieved by applying the dissociative enhancement principle. After separation of the bound from the free label, a reagent is added to the bound label which causes the weakly fluorescent lanthanide chelate to dissociate and form a new highly fluorescent chelate inside a protective micelle. Though robust and very sensitive, DELFIA assays are not ideal for HTS, as the process involves several binding, incubation and washing steps.

The need for homogeneous ('mix and measure') assays led to the development of homogeneous time-resolved Förster resonance energy transfer fluorescence (TR-FRET) methods such as LANCE (PerkinElmer Life Sciences) and HTRF (homogeneous time-resolved fluorescence; cisbio). LANCE, like DELFIA, is based on chelates of lanthanide ions but in a homogeneous format. The chelates used in LANCE can be measured directly without the need for a dissociation step; however, in an aqueous environment, the complexed ion can spontaneously dissociate and increase background fluorescence (Alpha et al., 1987).

In HTRF (Fig. 6.8), these limitations are overcome by the use of a *cryptate* molecule, which has a cage-like structure, to protect the central ion (e.g., Eu^+) from dissociation. HTRF uses two separate labels, the donor (Eu)K and the acceptor APC/XL665 (a modified allophycocyanine from red algae), and such assays can be adapted for use in plates up to a 1536-well format.

In both LANCE and HTRF, measurement of the ratio of donor and acceptor fluorophore emission can be applied to compensate for non-specific quenching of assay reagents. As a result, the applications of both technologies are widespread, covering detection of kinase enzyme activity (Jia et al., 2006), protease activity (Karvinen et al., 2002), second messengers such as cAMP and inositol tri-phosphate ($InsP_3$) (Titus et al., 2008; Trinquet et al., 2006), epigenetic modifications of proteins such as methylation of histone proteins and numerous biomarkers such as

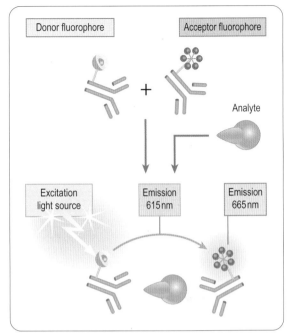

Fig. 6.8 Homogeneous time-resolved fluorescence (HTRF) assay type: the binding of a europium-labelled ligand (= donor) to the allophycocyanine (APC = acceptor)-labelled receptor brings the donor–acceptor pair into close proximity and energy transfer takes place, resulting in fluorescence emission at 665 nm.

interleukin 1β (IL-1β) and tumour necrosis factor alpha (TNF-α) (Achard et al., 2003).

Fluorescence polarization. When a stationary molecule is excited with plane-polarized light, it will fluoresce in the same plane. If it is tumbling rapidly, in free solution, so that it changes its orientation between excitation and emission, the emission signal will be depolarized. Binding to a larger molecule reduces the mobility of the fluorophore so that the emission signal remains polarized, and so the ratio of polarized to depolarized emission can be used to determine the extent of binding of a labelled ligand (Nasir & Jolley, 1999). The rotational relaxation speed depends on the size of the molecule, the ambient temperature and the viscosity of the solvent, which usually remain constant during an assay.

The method requires a significant difference in size between labelled ligand and target, which is a major restriction to its application (Nosjean et al., 2006), and the reliance on a single, non-TRF output makes the choice of fluorophore important to minimize compound interference effects (Turek-Etienne et al., 2003). FP-based assays can be used in 96-well up to 1536-well formats.

Other fluorescence methods. Although an uncommon technique in most HTS departments, due to the requirement for specific and dedicated instrumentation, there are several fluorescence technologies that provide highly sensitive metrics using very low levels of detection reagents and are very amendable to ultra-high-throughput screening (uHTS) (Eggeling et al., 2003). These include *fluorescence correlation spectroscopy*, allowing molecular interactions to be studied at the single-molecule level in real time, and *fluorescence intensity distribution analysis* (FIDA and 2-dimensional FIDA [Kask et al., 2000] also fall into this grouping, sharing the common theme of the analysis of biomolecules at extremely low concentrations). In contrast to other fluorescence techniques, the parameter of interest is not the emission intensity itself but rather intensity fluctuations. By confining measurements to a very small detection volume, achieved by the use of confocal optics, and low reagent concentrations, the number of molecules monitored is kept small, and the statistical fluctuations of the number contributing to the fluorescence signal at any instant become measurable.

Fluorescence lifetime analysis (Moger et al., 2006) is a relatively straightforward assay methodology that overcomes many of the potential compound interference effects achieved through the use of TRF but without the requirement for expensive fluorophores. The technique utilizes the intrinsic lifetime of a fluorophore, corresponding to the time the molecule spends in the excited state. This time is altered upon binding of the fluorophore to a compound or protein and can be measured to develop robust assays that are liable to minimum compound interference using appropriate detection instrumentation.

AlphaScreen technology. The proprietary bead-based technology from PerkinElmer is a proximity-based format utilizing a donor bead which, when excited by light at a wavelength of 680 nm, releases singlet oxygen that is absorbed by an acceptor bead, assuming it is in sufficiently close proximity (<200 nm), resulting in the emission of light between 520 and 620 nm (Fig. 6.9). This phenomenon is unusual in that the wavelength of the emitted light is shorter and therefore has higher energy than the excitation wavelength. This is of significance since it reduces the potential for compound inner filter effects; however, reactive functionality may still inhibit the energy transfer.

As with other bead-based technologies, the donor and acceptor beads are available with a range of surface treatments to enable the immobilization or capture of a range of analytes. The range of immobilization formats and the distance over which the singlet oxygen can pass to excite the donor bead provide a suitable format for developing homogeneous antibody-based assays similar to enzyme-linked immunosorbent assays (ELISA), which are generally

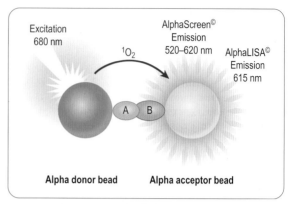

Fig. 6.9 Principle of AlphaScreen assays.

avoided in the HTS setting due to multiple wash, addition and incubation steps. These bead-based ELISA assays such as AlphaLISA (PerkinElmer) provide the required sensitivity for detection of biomarkers in low concentration and can be configured to a 1536-well format without loss of signal window.

Cell-based assays

Readouts for cell-based assays

Readouts that can be used for cell-based assays are many and varied. In some cases, such as radioligand binding or enzyme activity, the readouts are essentially the same as those described above. Here, we describe five cell-based readout technologies that have found general application in many types of assays, namely *fluorometric methods, reporter gene assays, yeast complementation assays, high-throughput electrophysiology assays, bioluminescence resonance energy transfer (BRET) and label-free detection platforms.* Some informative case histories of cell-based assays based on different readout principles have been presented by Johnston and Johnston (2002).

Fluorometric assays are widely used to monitor changes in the intracellular concentration of ions or other constituents such as cAMP. A range of fluorescent dyes has been developed which have the property of forming reversible complexes with ions such as Ca^{2+}, Na^+ or Tl^+ (as a surrogate for K^+). Their fluorescent emission intensity changes when the complex is formed, thereby allowing changes in the free intracellular ion concentration to be monitored, for example, in response to activation or block of membrane receptors or ion channels, other membrane-bound dyes are available whose fluorescence signal varies according to the cytoplasmic or mitochondrial membrane potential. Membrane-impermeable dyes which bind to intracellular structures can be used to monitor cell death, as only dying cells with leaky membranes are stained. In addition to dyes, ion-sensitive proteins such as the jellyfish photoprotein *aequorin* (see below), which emits a strong fluorescent signal when complexed with Ca^{2+}, can also be used to monitor changes in $[Ca^{2+}]_i$. Cell lines can be engineered to express this protein, or it can be introduced by electroporation. Such methods find many applications in cell biology, particularly when coupled with confocal microscopy to achieve a high level of spatial resolution. For HTS applications, the development of the fluorescence imaging plate reader (FLIPR, Molecular Devices Inc., described by Schroeder & Negate, 1996), allowing the simultaneous application of reagents and test compounds to multiwell plates and the capture of the fluorescence signal from each well was a key advance in allowing cellular assays to be utilized in the HTS arena. Early instruments employed an argon laser to deliver the excitation light source, with the emission measured using a CCD imaging device. In more recent models, the laser has been replaced with light emitting diode (LED) light source (https://www.moleculardevices.com) and overcomes some of the logistical considerations for deploying these instruments in some laboratories. Repeated measurements can be made at intervals of less than 1 second to determine the kinetics of the cellular response, such as changes in $[Ca^{2+}]_i$ or membrane potential, which are often short-lasting, so that monitoring the time profile rather than taking a single snapshot measurement is essential.

Reporter gene assays

Gene expression in transfected eukaryotic cells can be quantified by linking a promoter sequence to a reporter gene, whose level of expression is readily monitored, and reflects the degree of activation or inhibition of the promoter (Naylor, 1999). Compounds activating or inhibiting the promoter itself, or interfering with a signal pathway connected to that promoter, can thus be detected. By using two different reporter constructs, for example, firefly and *Renilla* luciferase, different targets can be screened simultaneously (Kent et al., 2005) or used to normalize for transfection efficiency. The principle of a reporter gene assay for GPCR activity, based on luciferase, is shown in Fig. 6.10. Reporter readouts can also be duplexed with more immediate readouts of cell signalling, such as calcium sensitive dyes, to reduce the false-positive liability associated with using a single assay readout (Hanson, 2006).

Commonly used reporter genes are CAT (chloramphenicol acetyltransferase), GAL (β-galactosidase), LAC (β-lactamase) (Zlokarnik et al., 1998), LUC (luciferase; Kolb & Neumann, 1996) and GFP (green fluorescence protein; Kain, 1999), usually employing a colorimetric or fluorescent readout and each having relative merits (Suto & Ignar, 1997). The number of reporter genes is dwarfed compared to the range of promoters that can be employed in this format, covering a diversity of signalling events.

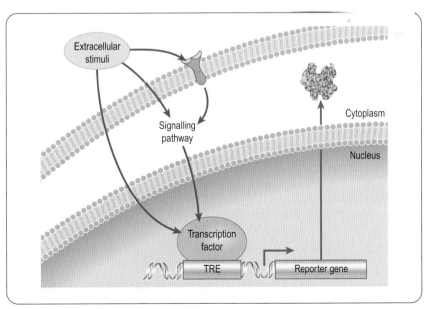

Fig. 6.10 Reporter gene assay principle for the detection of a ligand-mediated signalling event in a cell-based assay. Upon binding of a small molecule to the receptor, the signalling cascade is initiated, resulting in the binding of a signalling mediator to a specific transcription factor response element, controlling the expression of the reporter protein.

While having been widely deployed in the drug discovery process, there are several limitations of reporter gene technology, not least because of the measurement of a response distal to the ligand interaction and the longer compound incubation times required, increasing the potential for cytotoxic events (Hill et al., 2001).

Yeast complementation assay

Yeast is a well-characterized organism for investigating mammalian systems, and particularly convenient for genetic engineering (Tucker, 2002). The yeast two-hybrid assay is a powerful genetic screening technique for measuring the protein–protein and protein–DNA interactions that underlie many cellular control mechanisms (reviewed in Brückner et al., 2009). Widely used in cell and systems biology to study the binding of transcription factors at the sequence level, the yeast two-hybrid system can also be used to screen small molecules for their interference with protein–protein and protein–DNA interactions and has recently been adapted for other types of drug–target interactions (Fields & Song, 1989; Serebriiskii et al., 2001; Young et al., 1998). Conventional in vitro measurements, such as immunoprecipitation or chromatographic co-precipitation (Phizicky & Fields, 1995), require the interacting proteins in pure form and at high concentrations, and therefore are often of limited use.

The yeast two-hybrid system uses two separated peptide domains of transcription factors: a DNA-specific binding part (DNB) and a transcription activation domain (AD). The DNB moiety is coupled to one protein (the 'bait'), and the AD moiety to another (the 'prey'). If the prey protein binds to the bait protein, the AD moiety is brought into close association with the reporter gene, which is thereby activated, producing a product (e.g., GAL or LAC, as described above, or an enzyme which allows the yeast to grow in the presence of cycloheximide). The addition of a test compound that blocks the specific protein–protein interaction prevents activation of the reporter gene. Serbriiskii and colleagues (2001) describe a project in which lead compounds able to block the activation of a specific N-type voltage-gated Ca^{2+} channel have been identified with a yeast two-hybrid assay. The bait and prey proteins contained domains of two different channel subunits which need to associate to form a functional channel.

High-throughput electrophysiology assays

The progression of ion channels, and in particular voltage-gated ion channels, as druggable targets using screening approaches was severely limited by the throughput of conventional electrophysiology techniques and lack of suitable higher throughput assay platforms. Although

fluorescence methods using membrane potential sensitive dyes such as $DiBAC_4(3)$ and the FLIPR variants of this and the FRET-based voltage sensor probes (Gonzalez & Maher, 2002) were widely used, the methodology could not provide accurate voltage control and the temporal resolution of the evoked responses was poor. The introduction of planar patch-clamp instruments, particularly systems such as IonWorks Quattro, which record using multihole planar substrate consumables (Finkel et al., 2006; Southan & Clark, 2009) (see Fig. 6.11 for the operating principle), initially overcame the throughput hurdle, yet fell short of non-electrophysiology methods in terms of throughput (a maximum of approximately 3000 data points per day per instrument compared with $> 20,000$ per day for a FLIPR) and also higher cost per data point due to highly engineering consumables. These platforms offered were highly suited to screening of targeted libraries, diverse compound decks up to around 100,000 compounds and the confirmation of a large number of hits identified in less physiologically relevant platforms. Technological advances have led to the development of truly high-throughput electrophysiology platforms to allow screening in a 384-well format, thus enabling primary screening of ion channels under physiologically relevant conditions (Bell & Dallas, 2018).

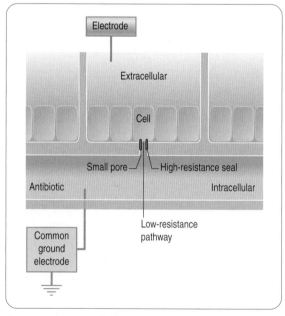

Fig. 6.11 Planar patch clamp, the underlying principle of high-throughput electrophysiology.

Bioluminescence resonance energy transfer

The challenge with many FRET-based systems that rely on the use of excitation light is that they can be cytotoxic and have limited applicability in cell-based assay systems. While BRET-based systems utilize the energy transfer between two proteins in proximity to each other, typically < 10 nm to allow energy transfer, the key difference is the donor is luminescent and does not require an excitatory light source, thereby circumventing phototoxicity. The principle is that a bioluminescent protein, the donor, is tagged to one binding partner of the assay and a fluorescent protein, the acceptor, is associated with the other binding partner. For example, the donor photoprotein may be aequorin with GFP as the acceptor. During the assay, provision of coelenterazine and calcium will allow emission of light from aequorin, which in turn excites GFP, and the resultant emitted light can be measured without the need for a potentially cytotoxic light source (Shen, 2018). As the methodology has become more established, there has been a drive to establish smaller, brighter proteins for use with BRET assays and expand the applicability of the technique further for utility in cell-based protein–protein interactions (Dale et al., 2019).

Label-free detection platforms

Many of the assay systems described above rely on knowledge of the cellular response or signalling pathway modulation the target will elicit. The drawback in the study of targets is where the signalling mechanism is unknown, for example, orphan GPCRs, multiple assay systems would need to be developed which would be time-consuming and costly or highly engineered cells would be required, moving away from physiological relevance. Consequently, the application of assay platforms which detect gross cellular responses, usually cell morphology due to actin cytoskeleton remodelling, to physiological stimuli have been developed. These fall into two broad categories, those that detect changes in impedance through cellular dielectric spectroscopy (Ciambrone et al., 2004), for example, xCelligence (Roche Diagnostics), or the use of optical biosensors (Fang, 2006), for example, Epic (Corning Inc.), Octet (ForteBio), or Bind (SRU Biosystems). The application of these platforms in the HTS arena had limited update due to lower throughput, relatively high cost per data point and complexity of data interpretation compared to established methods. However, the assay development time is quite short, a single assay may cover a broad spectrum of cell signalling events, and these methods are considered to be more sensitive than many existing methods enabling the use of endogenous receptor expression and even the use of primary cells in many instances (Fang et al., 2007; Minor, 2008).

High-content screening and flow cytometry

HCS is a further development of cell-based screening in which multiple fluorescence readouts are measured simultaneously in intact cells by means of imaging techniques. Repetitive scanning provides temporally and spatially resolved visualization of cellular events. HCS is suitable for monitoring such events as changes in cell morphology, neurite outgrowth, nuclear translocation, apoptosis, GPCR activation, receptor internalization, changes in $[Ca^{2+}]_i$, nitric oxide production, apoptosis, gene expression, neurite outgrowth and cell viability in immortalized primary and stem cells (Zock, 2009). Whereas HCS detects changes in cell morphology or proteins in cells immobilized onto the surface of a microtitre plate, flow cytometry allows the researcher to analyse heterogeneous populations of cells in suspension. For flow cytometry, cells are treated in wells with test compound and stained for the required cell markers. The wells are then processed via an autosampler through the flow cytometer to assess the cell population (Buckman, 2010; Ding et al., 2017)

Although flow cytometry may have lagged behind HCS in drug discovery terms, the underlying principle remains the same, namely to quantify and correlate drug effects on cellular events or targets by simultaneously measuring multiple signals from the same cell population, yielding data with a higher content of biological information than is provided by single-target screens (Liptrot, 2001).

Current instrumentation is based on automated digital microscopy and flow cytometry in combination with hard and software systems for the analysis of data. Within the configuration, a fluorescence-based laser scanning plate reader (96- to 1536-well format), able to detect fluorescent structures against a less fluorescent background, acquires multicolour fluorescence image datasets of cells at a preselected spatial resolution. The spatial resolution is largely defined by the instrument specification and whether it is optical confocal or widefield. Confocal imaging enables the generation of high-resolution images by sampling from a thin cellular section and rejection of out of focus light, thus giving rise to improved signal:noise than the more commonly applied epi-fluorescence microscopy. There is a powerful advantage in confocal imaging for applications, such as subcellular localization and membrane translocation; however, for many biological assays, confocal imaging is not ideal (e.g., phototoxicity issues or applications that have a need for a larger focal depth).

HCS relies heavily on powerful image pattern recognition software in order to provide rapid, automated and unbiased assessment of experiments.

The concept of gathering all the necessary information about a compound at one go has obvious attractions, but the very sophisticated instrumentation and software produce problems of reliability. Furthermore, the principle of 'measure everything and sort it out afterwards' has its drawbacks: interpretation of such complex datasets often requires complex algorithms and significant data storage capacity. While the complexity of the analysis may seem daunting, HCS allows the study of complex signalling events and the use of phenotypic readouts in highly disease relevant systems. Inevitably, the application of machine learning or artificial intelligence is likely to impact how the industry approaches HCS data, and rather than measuring patterns observable to the human eye, computing power will be exploited to solve complex problems and improve accuracy with which decisions are made from information-rich assays platforms (Kusumoto et al., 2018).

Biophysical methods in high-throughput screening

Conventional bioassay-based screening remains a mainstream approach for lead discovery. However, during recent years, alternative biophysical methods such as nuclear magnetic resonance (NMR) (Hajduk & Burns, 2002), surface plasmon resonance (SPR) (Gopinath, 2010) and X-ray crystallography (Carr & Jhoti, 2002) have been developed and/or adapted for drug discovery whose main purpose is the detection of low-affinity low-molecular-weight compounds in a different approach to HTS, namely *fragment-based screening*. Hits from HTS usually already have drug-like properties, for example, a molecular weight of ~400 to 500 Da. During the following lead optimization synthesis programme, an increase in molecular weight is very likely, leading to poorer drug-like properties with respect to solubility, absorption or clearance. Therefore it may be more effective to screen small sets of molecular fragments (<10,000) of lower molecular weight (100–250 Da), which can then be chemically linked to generate high-affinity drug-like compounds. Typically, such fragments have much weaker binding affinities than drug-like compounds and are outside the sensitivity range of a conventional HTS assay. NMR-, SPR- or X-ray crystallography-based assays are better suited for the identification of weak binders, as these methodologies lend themselves well to the area of fragment-based screening. As the compound libraries screened are generally of limited size, throughput is less important than sensitive detection of low-affinity interactions. Once the biophysical interactions are determined, further X-ray protein crystallographic studies can be undertaken to understand the binding mode of the fragments, and this information can then be used to rapidly drive the fragment-to-hit or fragment-to-lead chemistry programme (Carr et al., 2005).

As discussed in Chapter 7, the chemical linkage of weak binding fragments can generate a high-affinity lead without violating the restrictions in molecular weight. The efficiency of this strategy has been demonstrated by several groups (Lesuisse et al., 2002; Nienaber et al., 2000).

Mass spectrometry–based screening methods

The reader will have realized that many of the techniques utilized in HTS rely on the use of a surrogate marker of enzyme activation or cellular activation. The key differentiator for mass spectrometry–based methods is detection of the precise mass of the product of the reaction product or depletion of a substrate, be that through modification of a protein, lipid or a cellular metabolite. As such, provided appropriate assay conditions and, in the case of cellular assays, suitable extraction methods determined analyte detection using mass spectrometry is applicable to both biochemical and cellular assays. Mass spectrometry is traditionally associated with requiring higher sample volume and being a low-throughput detection system, by separation of reactants using liquid chromatography, followed by injection into the mass spectrometer. The key advance for the adaption of this technique was the development of high-throughput autosamplers and associated chromatography columns to allow processing of samples in a relatively high-throughput manner (<15 seconds per injection) and in low volume (~20 μL per injection) (Ozbal et al., 2004). This is achieved through the use of very small solid phase extraction cartridges to 'trap' the analyte of interest with buffer salts and other reagent components passing through to waste. Rapid buffer or solvent switching results in step-wise elution of the analyte for injection of the sample into the mass spectrometer for detection of the appropriate mass of interest. Development of the RapidFire instrument by Agilent Technologies, and then the ADDA platform by Apricot Designs enabled the introduction of high-throughput mass spectrometry into the HTS arena. Even though at throughputs typically of less than 20 384-well plates per day undertaking very large screens is challenging, the techniques can be enabling where direct detection of the analyte is the only option or where more traditional label-based methods have failed to provide confirmed hits through interference with the detection system (Adam et al., 2015).

The challenge for the 'trap and elute' systems remains the limitation to a 384-well format and associated sample processing time. This can be overcome using Matrix-assisted laser desorption/ionization time-of-flight mass spectrometry (MALDI-TOF), where the samples for analysis are prepared onto a target, and through a series of drying and washing steps, the sample is ready for analysis. The use of a 1536-well format sample preparation and analysis is routine, and potentially higher densities up to 6144 samples per target are reported with a sample time of 1.2 samples per second (Haslam et al., 2016). As one would expect to prepare the targets and analyse the samples at such a rate, dedicated instrumentation has been developed including the rapifleX platform from Bruker. While MALDI-TOF offers truly impressive throughput very much aligned with uHTS, one should remember that 1.2 seconds per sample is only for the analysis time, and preparation of the MALDI target also needs to be factored in.

The most recent development in this field, acoustic mist injection mass spectrometry (AMI-MS) (Sinclair et al., 2016, 2019), utilizes acoustic droplet dispensing technology to directly inject low-volume assay samples directly into the mass spectrometer (Fig. 6.12). In so doing, this approach overcomes the sampling processing and injection volumes associated with the 'trap and elute' platforms and the sample preparation requirements of the MALDI-TOF systems. These systems are still in their infancy and not fully commercialized at the time of this manuscript, and although limited to a 384-well plate format, initial data suggest samples' throughput times of less than 1 sample per second without the need for extensive sample processing, which would clearly meet the requirements for placing mass spectrometry–based screening methods in HTS.

Perhaps the most interesting part of all these mass spectrometry–based approaches is that they demonstrate the collaboration in advancing HTS techniques through

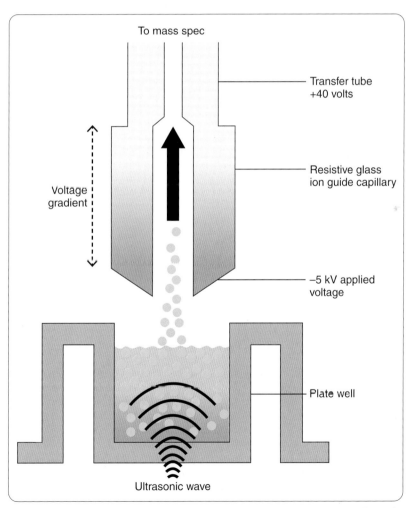

Fig. 6.12 Schematic of acoustic mist injection mass spectrometry demonstrating direct injection of sample into the mass spectrometer.

the application of established screening technology (liquid handling), biological assay knowledge and analytical chemistry to facilitate drug discovery.

Assay formats—miniaturization

Multiwell plates began to be used for screening in the early 1980s, before which time tube-based assays were routinely used in a low-throughput mode. The introduction of 96-well plates allowed the automation and miniaturization of biochemical experiments and was rapidly followed by the transition of many cell-based assays into the same density formats. The drive to increase throughput and reduce associated reagent costs has seen great advances in liquid handling and detection technologies since the 1990s, with most vendors basing their approach on adaptation of the 96-well format to reduce the space between wells (the pitch), while maintaining an overall standard footprint and depth for the plate for the ease and constancy of instrument design (see Society for Laboratory Automation and Screening, www.slas.org/education/microplate.cfm). Reducing the pitch by one-half yields a fourfold increase in density to 384 wells per plate and a further twofold reduction gives rise to 1536-well format plates. In both cases, the wells of these increased density plates can still be addressed using standard 96-well technology, although for liquid handling, the reduced volumes and well area associated with the 1536-well formats present challenges for tip-based, displacement dispensing. To overcome this, the low-volume 384-well plate (Garyantes, 2002) has emerged as an important format, offering lower reagent usage per well, while overcoming the issues of well access. In turn, the liquid handling technologies to support 1536-well plates has developed significantly through the use of fixed tips or non-contact dispensing using piezo-electric dispensers or acoustic dispensing. These latter formats do not rely on tip-based technology and can dispense volumes as low as 2.5 nL (Dunn & Feygin, 2000; Ellson et al., 2003).

Outside of the 96-, 384- and 1536-well arena, there remains a drive for further increased density to a 3456-well format (Kornienko et al., 2004) and micro-fluidics/lab-on-a-chip (Pihl et al., 2005) approaches to further reduce reagent usage.

Regardless of the microplate format adopted by a screening laboratory, the advances in microplates, liquid handling, plate stacking and handling devices, and sensitive reagents and detection instrumentation (such as CCD imagers) have advanced to the point where execution of a high-throughput screen is rarely the bottleneck in drug discovery. Although as the density increases, the time to develop a robust assay with low variability can also increase as the challenges of reagent evaporation and mixing are overcome.

Robotics in high-throughput screening

In many dedicated HTS facilities, automation is employed to varying degrees to facilitate execution of the screen. This varies from the use of automated workstations with some manual intervention to the use of fully automated robotic platforms. During the assay development phases, the key pieces of automation present in the automated platform will be used to ensure the assay is optimized correctly, followed by transfer of the assay to a robotic workstation that can operate in high-throughput mode (typically up to 100,000 compounds per day at a single concentration). The robotic system consists of devices for storage, incubation and transportation of plates in different formats; instruments for liquid transfer and a series of plate readers for the various detection technologies. In many instances, these devices will be replicated on the same system to allow the screen to continue, albeit at lower throughput, should one device fail mid-run. The key for automation in most HTS laboratories is to be highly versatile, with as small a footprint as possible. To this end, the trend is for a centralized robotic arm to transfer plates between different stations to carry out specific tasks.

A typical robotic system is illustrated in Fig. 6.13. Robotic arms and/or automated transport systems move plates to the various stations around the platform. Importantly, the stations, or carts, around the robotic arm can be undocked from the central platform and either replaced with carts containing different functionality and/or used as automated workstations in isolation. The stations themselves contain plate storage devices ('hotels'), and incubators are used for storage and incubation of microplates. Incubators can be cooled or heated; for mammalian cell cultivation, they can also be supplied with CO_2 and are designed to facilitate automatic transfer of plates in and out. Compound plates are typically supplied with seals that can be perforated by the liquid handling devices to allow easy dilution and compound transfer to the assay plates. The assay plates themselves may either have removable lids or be sealed automatically once all reagents have been added. Stackers are sequential storage units for microtitre plates, connected to automated pipetting instruments and are equally common in laboratories where HTS is conducted without the large-scale application of automation, as they allow the scientists to walk away and return when the pipetting steps are complete. Various detection devices (enabling different modes of detection) are located at the output of the system before the assay plate, and usually the compound plate as well, and are automatically discarded to waste. Central to the platform is the control (scheduling) software, which controls the overall process including correct timing of different steps during the assay. This is critical and co-ordination of the use of the different

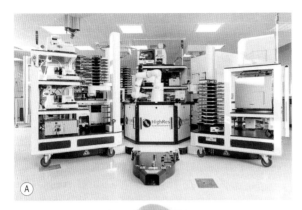

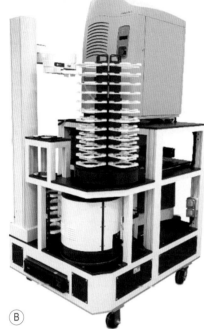

(A)

(B)

Fig. 6.13 Typical layout of fully automated high-throughput screening platform. (A) High-throughput screening platform showing central robotic arm with associated stations arranged in circumference and (B) individual station or cart undocked from the automation system showing integrated arm to the left of the image allowing the cart to be used as a standalone automated workstation. (Courtesy HighRes BioSolutions.)

devices (pipetters, incubators, readers, etc.) ensures maximum efficiency. This software will also control recovery and/or continued operation of the platform in the event of an error without manual intervention. As one can imagine, programming and testing of the different process steps for individual screens can be a time-consuming part of the operation, and frequently, dedicated automation teams exist in large HTS departments to expedite this.

Before primary screening can start, sample plates have to be prepared, which is usually done offline by separate automated liquid transfer systems (384-tip pipettors or acoustic dispensing devices). Compound storage plates, containing the library to be screened prepared as DMSO solutions, are delivered from the compound library warehouse, and samples are further diluted with aqueous buffer to reach the desired compound and DMSO concentration for the assay. Samples are usually transferred to the assay plates by the robot during the assay run.

During the screening itself, all processes have to be monitored online to ensure the quality of the data obtained. The performance of the assay is continuously measured by calculating Z' values for each plate (see earlier section). For this purpose, each screening plate includes high and low controls for quality analysis, in addition to the compounds for screening.

For the selection of positives, a variety of methods may be applied based upon the control wells present on the assay plate. This hit threshold may be an arbitrary activity cut-off set across the screen or statistically based on a plate-by-plate or screen-wide basis and is then usually set at least three standard deviations away from the mean of the library signal (Brideau et al., 2003).

Data analysis and management

Owing to the large volume of data generated in HTS, efficient data management is essential. Software packages for HTS (e.g., ActivityBase, Spotfire, Genedata) are available to carry out the principal tasks:

- Storage of raw data
- Association of raw data with compound information
- Quality control
- Transformation of data into information
- Visualization
- Documentation
- Reporting.

In HTS, each biochemical experiment in a single well is analysed by an automated device, typically a plate reader or other kind of detector. The output of these instruments comes in different formats depending on the type of reader. Where possible, the HTS favours the use of a single 'end point' read rather than more time-consuming multiple or kinetic readings. However, the instrument itself may perform some initial calculations, and these heterogeneous types of raw data are automatically transferred into the data management software. Assay plates are typically identified by a unique barcode to relate the data to the compound plate layout. Ideally, the plate reader will have an integral barcode reader, and the data file will be automatically named with the barcode to provide an error-free association of the correct data file with the compounds tested.

In a next step, raw data are translated into contextual information by calculating results. Data on percentage inhibition or percentage of control are normalized with values obtained from the high and low controls present in each plate. In secondary screening, IC_{50}/EC_{50} and K_i values are also calculated. The values obtained depend on the method used (e.g., the fitting algorithm used for concentration–response curves) and have to be standardized for all screens within a company. Once the system captures the data, it is then necessary to apply validation rules and techniques, such as trimmed means, to eliminate outliers (ideally using automated an algorithm) and to apply predetermined acceptance criteria to the data, for example, the S/N ratio, the Z'-value or a test for Gaussian distribution of the data. All plates that fail against one or more quality criteria are flagged and discarded.

The process may also involve a step to monitor visually the data that have been flagged, as a final check on quality. This is to ensure the system has performed correctly, that is, no missed reagent dispense or patterns indicative of blocked dispenser tips or edge effects which may lead to false positives or negatives (Gunter et al., 2003). While this inspection may be performed manually, there are a number of software packages available, for example, the GeneData Assay Analyzer (www.genedata.com), which flag such errors and, in the case of edge effects, apply mathematical corrections to overcome them. Examples of validation data obtained in a typical screening of 100,000 compounds and some common data patterns revealed by tracking such parameters are shown Fig. 6.14. In addition to tracking high and low control values, most HTS departments also include

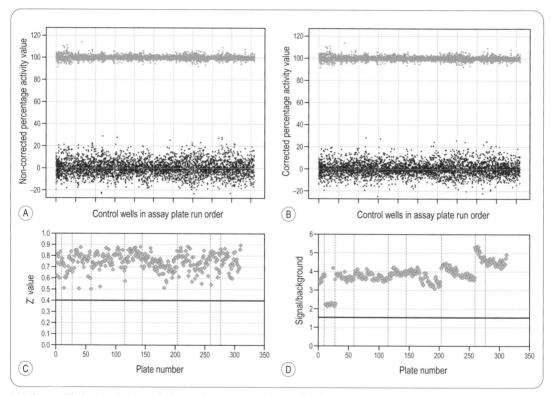

Fig. 6.14 Data validation checks in a typical screening assay. Distribution of high (*green symbols*) and low controls (*red symbols*) (% inhibition) in a set of screening plates. Each marker represents one well. Panel (A) shows the original data and (B) shows the same data following treatment with a GeneData Assay Analyzer to take account of spatially induced effects. Note the reduction in variability of the low-control well data. (C) Z' values and (D) signal-to-background ratios from a high-throughput screening campaign. The plate run order is shown on the *x*-axis, and vertical *dashed lines* divide each screening run, the horizontal lines at $Z' = 0.5$ and $S/B = 1.5$ represent the quality control pass levels, and each data point represents an assay plate. The data demonstrate a decline in assay performance during each screening day. The marked change in rate of assay performance deterioration after plate 150 correlates with a change in the batch of a key assay component. (C) Well-based pipetting artefacts. The *y*-axis shows the number of 'positive' compounds as a function of the well position, in an assay involving many plates. With randomly distributed compounds, there should be an equal chance of finding positives at each well address. The high values in wells A3, B3 and F3 therefore represent artefacts due to mechanical failure. "Data kindly supplied by Charles River Laboratories, with permission"

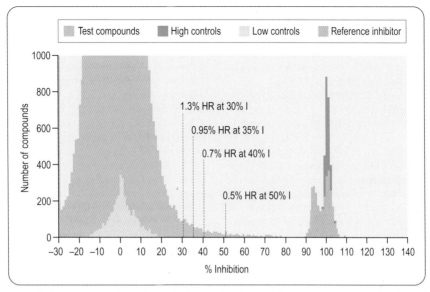

Fig. 6.15 Histogram analysis of compound activity against control well populations from a screen to identify antagonists of a G-protein-coupled receptor. The median of the compound wells is in line with the null control population. The hit rate (% HR) associated with selecting each of the percentage inhibition value (% I) is as indicated. As the percentage inhibition is lowered, the confidence in the reality of the hit is reduced; however, these compounds can provide useful information on the hit series being identified. Note the reference compound controls appear to fall into two populations. This is associated with the change in reagent batch as described in Fig. 6.13. "Data kindly supplied by Charles River Laboratories, with permission"

quality control plates at regular intervals throughout an assay run which contain standard compounds to allow target pharmacology to be monitored.

On completion of the screen, it is advisable to plot a distribution histogram of the compound data against the control well populations and any other quality-control wells that have been included (Fig. 6.15). The median of the test wells should be the same as the null control population and, if the assay is robust as demonstrated by the Z' value, there will be good separation between the two control well populations. The variability of the null control population can be used to determine an acceptable cut-off level for selecting the hit compounds for further progression.

In addition to registering the test data, all relevant information about the assay has to be logged, for example, the supplier and batch of reagents, storage conditions, a detailed assay protocol, plate layout and algorithms for the calculation of results. Each assay run is registered, and its performance documented. If assay performance is charted, any significant change in assay quality can be reviewed and, if caused by reagent change, readily identified.

HTS will initially deliver hits in targeted assays. Retrieval of these data has to be simple, and the data must be exchangeable between different project teams to generate knowledge from the mass of data.

Screening libraries and compound logistics

Compound logistics

In the drug discovery value chain, the effective management of compound libraries is a key element and is usually handled by a dedicated compound logistics group, either within the screening organization or at a specialist outsourcing provider, and exchanged widely with other parts of the drug discovery organization. The compound management facility is the central port for transshipment of compounds in lead discovery, not only for primary screening, but also during the hit-to-lead phase. It is the unit responsible for registration of samples, their preparation, storage and retrieval. This facility has to ensure global compound accessibility, both individually and in different formats; maintain compound integrity (quality control and proper storage); guarantee error-free compound handling; guarantee efficient compound use and guarantee a rapid response to compound requests.

Many pharmaceutical companies have greatly increased both the size and quality of their compound collection. Screening libraries frequently exceed 1,000,000 compounds and originate from many different sources with variable quality, although there has been great attention to how the assays themselves are impacted by poor compound quality, particularly solubility (Di & Kerns, 2006). This has necessitated both hardware and software automation of compound management to cope with the increasing demands of HTS and lead discovery.

Most advanced systems use fully automated robotics for handling compounds (Fig. 6.16). Compounds used for screening are stored as liquids in microtitre plates in a controlled environment (temperature −4 °C to −20 °C; low humidity or storage under an inert atmosphere and control of freeze–thaw cycles), and numerous studies have been undertaken to identify the most appropriate conditions to maintain compound stability (e.g., Blaxill et al., 2009). The most appropriate conditions for compound storage is a subject of much debate, and one in which it is difficult to reach consensus other than the two key contributory factors are the humidity and the nature of the compounds themselves. With regard to the latter, most companies undertake regular reviews of their libraries and exclude chemical structures identified as being unstable for prolonged storage in DMSO or frequently being active in specific assay formats (e.g., Pan-Assay Interference Compounds (PAINS) filters; Baell & Nissink, 2018).

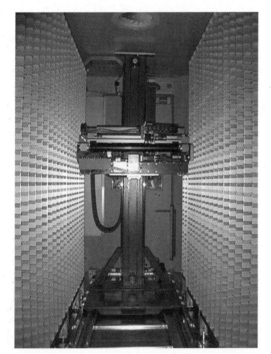

Fig. 6.16 Storage of a compound screening collection in 384-well plates at −4°C. A robot is able to move around and collect the plates or individual samples specified in the compound management software.

Splitting the collection into a number of copies in different formats secures a balance between fast response times to the various compound requests and optimal storage conditions. Different sets of compound libraries are needed, depending on the target and project specifications, with the preferred storage format of the compound collection being dictated by the chosen screening plate density, that is, a 384- or 1536-well.

Because library sets are not static, as new compounds are continuously being added, samples in the repository need to be individually addressable to allow a flexible and quick rearrangement of existing libraries to more specific, focused collections. Advanced compound logistic systems store compound libraries in a single tube system so that individual tubes can be accessed without the need to take out a whole plate from the storage facility.

This functionality is a prerequisite for efficient 'cherry picking'. After primary screening, positive compounds have to be confirmed in secondary assays and concentration–response curves determined. The individual active compounds have to be located and reformatted in microtitre plates. With a large number of targets and projects running at any one time, a highly automated compound handling systems is needed to do this efficiently.

Profiling

HTS, the subject of this chapter, has as its first objective the identification of a few 'validated hits' (defined in Chapters 5 and 7) within large compound libraries. The decision as to whether a particular hit is worth pursuing as a chemical lead in a drug discovery project depends on several factors, important ones being its chemical characteristics and its pharmacodynamic and pharmacokinetic properties. These aspects, broadly covered by the term 'compound profiling', are discussed in detail in the next three chapters.

The technology involved in miniaturization, automation and assay readouts required for HTS has developed rapidly and continues to do so. As this technology evolves, the laboratory set-ups installed in HTS facilities are steadily broadening their capabilities beyond their primary function of identifying hits to apply HTS techniques to more diverse compound profiling assays relating not only to the target selectivity of compound libraries, but also to their pharmacokinetic characteristics. Increasingly, therefore, early compound profiling tasks on 'hit' compounds are being carried out in HTS laboratories where the necessary technological expertise is concentrated. Such assays are also very helpful in the 'lead identification' stage of a project, where focused synthetic compound libraries based on the initial hits need to be assessed. As this work generally involves testing small compound libraries, usually fewer than 1000 compounds at a time, in several different assays, small dedicated robotic workstations are needed, rather than the fast but inflexible factory-style robotic assemblies used for large-scale HTS.

In vitro pharmacokinetic assays (see Chapter 10), which are not generally project specific and can be automated to run in medium-throughput fashion, are very suitable for running in this environment. This extension of the work of HTS laboratories beyond the primary task of finding hits is a clear and continuing trend, for which the term 'high-throughput profiling' (HTP) has been coined. It brings the work of HTS laboratories into a close

and healthy relationship with drug discovery teams. The highly disciplined approach to assay formats and data logging that is essential for HTS, but not second nature to many laboratory scientists, brings the advantage that profiling data collected over a wide range of projects and drug targets is logged in standard database formats, and is therefore a valuable company-wide tool for analysing SARs. This necessity to handle and visualize such data has driven the development software packages such as Spotfire (https://www.spotfire.tibco.com).

In summary, it is clear that pharmacological profiling will be an increasing activity of HTS units in the future and will help to add further value in the drug discovery chain.

References

Achard, S., Jean, A., Lorphelin, D., Amoravain, M., & Claret, E. (2003). Homogeneous assays allow direct "in well" cytokine level quantification. *Assay and Drug Development Technologies, 1*(Suppl. 2), 181–185.

Adam, G. C., Meng, J., Joseph, M., Rizzo, J. M., Amoss, A., Lusen, J. W., et al. (2015). Use of high-throughput mass spectrometry to reduce false positives in protease uHTS screens. *Journal of Biomolecular Screening, 20*(2), 212–222.

Alpha, B., Lehn, J. M., & Mathis, G. (1987). Energy-transfer luminescence of europium(III) and terbium(III) with macrobicyclic polypyridine ligands. *Angewandte Chemie. 99*, 259–261.

Baell, J. B., & Nissink, J. W. M. (2018). Seven year itch: Pan-assay interference compounds (PAINS) in 2017—utility and limitations. *ACS Chemical Biology, 13*(1), 36–44.

Bays, N., Hill, A., & Kariv, I. (2009). A simplified scintillation proximity assay for fatty acid synthase activity: Development and comparison with other FAS activity assays. *Journal of Biomolecular Screening, 14*, 636–642.

Bell, D. C., & Dallas, M. L. (2018). Using automated patch clamp electrophysiology platforms in pain-related ion channel research: Insights from industry and academia. *British Journal of Pharmacology, 175*, 2312–2321.

Beske, O., & Goldbard, S. (2002). High-throughout cell analysis using multiplexed array technologies. *Drug Discovery Today, 7*, S131–S135.

Beveridge, M., Park, Y. E., Hermes, J., Marenghi, A., Brophy, G., & Santos, A. (2000). Detection of p56(lck) kinase activity using scintillation proximity

assay in 384-well format and imaging proximity assay in 384- and 1536-well format. *Journal of Biomolecular Screening, 5*, 205–212.

Birzin, E. T., & Rohrer, S. P. (2002). High-throughput receptor-binding methods for somatostatin receptor 2. *Analytical Biochemistry, 307*, 159–166.

Blaxill, Z., Holland-Crimmen, S., & Lifely, R. (2009). Stability through the ages: The GSK experience. *Journal of Biomolecular Screening, 14*, 547–556.

Bosworth, N., & Towers, P. (1989). Scintillation proximity assay. *Nature, 341*, 167–168.

Braunwaler, A. F., Yarwood, D. R., Hall, T., Missbach, M., Lipson, K. E., & Sills, M. A. (1996). A solid-phase assay for the determination of protein tyrosine kinase activity of c src using scintillating microtitration plates. *Analytical Biochemistry, 234*, 23–26.

Brideau, C., Gunter, B., Pikounis, B., & Liaw, A. (2003). Improved statistical methods for hit selection in high-throughput screening. *Journal of Biomolecular Screening, 8*, 634–647.

Brown, B. A., Cain, M., Broadbent, J., Tompkins, S., Henrich, G., Joseph, R. S., et al. (1997). FlashPlate technology. In P. J. Devlin (Ed.), *High-throughput screening: The discovery of bioactive substances* (pp. 317–328). New York: Marcel Dekker.

Brückner, A., & Polge, C., Lentze, N., Auerbach, D., & Schlattner, U. (2009). Yeast two-hybrid, a powerful tool for systems biology. *International Journal of Molecular Sciences, 10*, 2763–2788.

Buckman, D. (2010). Application of flow cytometry in drug discovery. *European Pharmaceutical*

Review, (6). https://www.europeanpharmaceuticalreview.com/article/4818/application-of-flow-cytometry-in-drug-discovery/

Carr, R., Congreve, M., Murray, C., & Rees, D. (2005). Fragment-based lead discovery: Leads by design. *Drug Discovery Today, 10*, 987–992.

Carr, R., & Jhoti, H. (2002). Structure-based screening of low-affinity compounds. *Drug Discovery Today, 7*, 522–527.

Ciambrone, G., Liu, V., Lin, D., McGuiness, R., Keung, G., & Pitchford, S. (2004). Cellular dielectric spectroscopy: A powerful new approach to label-free cellular analysis. *Journal of Biomolecular Screening, 9*, 467–480.

Clegg, R. M. (1995). Fluorescence resonance energy transfer. *Current Opinion in Biotechnology, 6*, 103–110.

Clemons, P. (2004). Complex phenotypic assays in high-throughput screening. *Current Opinion in Chemical Biology, 8*, 334–338.

Coma, I., Bandyopadhyay, D., Diez, E., Ruiz, E. A., de los Frailes, M. T., & Colmenarejo, G. (2014). Mining natural-products screening data for target-class chemical motifs. *Journal of Biomolecular Screening, 19*(5), 749–757.

Comley, J. (2003). Assay interference a limiting factor in HTS? *Drug Discovery World Summer*, 91–98.

Comley, J. (2006). TR-FRET based assays—getting better with age. *Drug Discovery World Spring*, 22–37.

Congreve, M., Chessari, G., Tisi, D., & Woodhead, A. (2008). Recent developments in fragment-based drug discovery. *Journal of Medicinal Chemistry, 51*, 3661–3680.

Cook, N. D. (1996). Scintillation proximity assay: A versatile high-throughput screening technology. *Drug Discovery Today*, 1, 287–294.

Dale, N. C., Johnstone, E. K. M., White, C. W., & Pfleger, K. D. G. (2019). NanoBRET: The bright future of proximity-based assays. *Frontiers in Bioengineering and Biotechnology*, 7, 56.

Di, L., & Kerns, E. (2006). Biological assay challenges from compound solubility: Strategies for bioassay optimization. *Drug Discovery Today*, 11, 446–451.

Ding, M., Kaspersson, K., Murray, D., Bardelle, C. (2017) High-throughput flow cytometry for drug discovery: principles, applications, and case studies. *Drug Discovery Today*, 22, 1844–1850.

Dunn, DA & Feygin, I (2000). Challenges and solutions to ultra-high-throughput screening assay miniaturization: submicroliter fluid handling. *Drug Discovery Today*, Vol. 5(12): pp. S84–S91.

Eggeling, C., Brand, L., Ullmann, D., & Jäger, S. (2003). Highly sensitive fluorescence detection technology currently available for HTS. *Drug Discovery Today*, 8, 632–641.

Eglen, R. (2009). High throughput screening, high content screening, primary and stem cells new techniques now converging. *Drug Discovery World Online*, 25–31.

Ehrlich, P. and Bertheim, A., (1912) Über das salzsaure 3.3´-Diamino-4.4´-dioxy-arsenobenzol und seine nächsten Verwandten. *Berichte*, 45, 756–766.

Ellson R, Mutz M, Browning B, Lee L, Miller MF, Papen R. (2003) Transfer of Low Nanoliter Volumes between Microplates Using Focused Acoustics—Automation Considerations. *Journal of the Association for Laboratory Automation*, 8(5), 29–34.

Fang, Y. (2006). Label-free cell-based assays with optical biosensors in drug discovery. *Assay and Drug Development Technologies*, 4, 583–595.

Fang, Y., Guangshan, L., & Ferrie, A. (2007). Non-invasive optical biosensor for assaying endogenous G protein-coupled receptors in adherent cells. *Journal of Pharmacological and Toxicological Methods*, 55, 314–322.

Fields, S. and Song, O. 1989. A novel genetic system to detect protein-protein interactions. *Nature* 340 (245–246).

Finkel, A., Wittel, A., Yang, N., Handran, S., Hughes, J., & Costantin, J. (2006). Population patch clamp improves data consistency and success rates in the measurement of ionic currents. *Journal of Biomolecular Screening*, 11, 488–496.

Fleming, N. (2018). How artificial intelligence is changing drug discovery. *Nature*, 557, S57.

Fligge, T., & Schuler, A. (2006). Integration of a rapid automated solubility classification into early validation of hits obtained by high throughput screening. *Journal of Pharmaceutical and Biomedical Analysis*, 42, 449–454.

Garyantes, T. K. (2002). 1536-well assay plates: When do they make sense? *Drug Discovery Today*, 7, 489–490.

Ghosh, S., Nie, A., An, J., & Huang, Z. (2006). Structure-based virtual screening of chemical libraries for drug discovery. *Current Opinion in Chemical Biology*, 10, 194–202.

Gonzalez, J., & Maher, M. (2002). Cellular fluorescent indicators and voltage/ion probe reader (VIPR): Tools for ion channel and receptor drug discovery. *Receptors Channels*, 8, 283–295.

Gopinath, S. (2010). Biosensing applications of surface plasmon resonance-based Biacore technology. *Sensors and Actuators B*, 150, 722–733.

Gribbon, P., & Sewing, A. (2003). Fluorescence readouts in HTS: No gain without pain? *Drug Discovery Today*, 8, 1035–1043.

Gunter, B., Brideau, C., Pikounis, B., & Liaw, A. (2003). Statistical and graphical methods for quality control determination of high-throughput screening data. *Journal of Biomolecular Screening*, 8, 624–633.

Hallis, T., Kopp, A., Gibson, J., Lebakken, C., Hancock, M., & Van Den Heuvel-Kramer, K., et al. (2007). An improved beta-lactamase reporter assay: Multiplexing with a cytotoxicity readout for enhanced accuracy of hit identification. *Journal of Biomolecular Screening*, 12, 635–644.

Hajduk, P. J., & Burns, D. J. (2002). Integration of NMR and high-throughput screening. *Combinatorial Chemistry & High Throughput Screening*, 5, 613–621.

Hanson, B. (2006). Multiplexing Fluo-4 NW and GeneBLAzer® transcriptional assay for high-throughput screening of G-protein-coupled receptors. *Journal of Biomolecular Screening*, 11, 644–651.

Hartshorn, M., Murray, C., Cleasby, A., Frederickson, M., Tickle, I., & Jhoti, H. (2005). Fragment-based lead discovery using X-ray crystallography. *Journal of Medicinal Chemistry*, 48, 403–413.

Haslam, C., Hellicar, J., Dunn, A., Fuetterer, A., Hardy, N., Marshall, P., et al. (2016). The evolution of MALDI-TOF mass spectrometry toward ultra-high-throughput screening: 1536-well format and beyond. *Journal of Biomolecular Screening*, 21(2), 176–186.

Haugland, R. P. (2002). *Handbook of fluorescent probes and chemical research* (9th ed.). Molecular Probes. Retrieved from www.probes.com/handbook.

Hemmilä, I. A., & Hurskainen, P. (2002). Novel detection strategies for drug discovery. *Drug Discovery Today*, 7, S150–S156.

Hill, S., Baker, G., & Rees, S. (2001). Reporter-gene systems for the study of G-protein-coupled receptors. *Current Opinion in Pharmacology*, 1, 526–532.

Jia, Y., Quinn, C., Gagnon, A., & Talanian, R. (2006). Homogeneous time-resolved fluorescence and its applications for kinase assays in drug discovery. *Analytical Biochemistry*, 356, 273–281.

Johnston, P. A., & Johnston, P. A. (2002). Cellular platforms for HTS: Three case studies. *Drug Discovery Today*, 7, 353–363.

Kain, R. K. (1999). Green fluorescent protein (GFP): Applications in cell-based assays for drug discovery. *Drug Discovery Today*, 4, 304–312.

Karvinen, J., Hurskainen, P., Gopalakrishnan, S., Burns, D., Warrior, U., & Hemmilä, I. (2002). Homogeneous time-resolved fluorescence quenching assay (LANCE) for Caspase-3. *Journal of Biomolecular Screening*, 7, 223–231.

Kask, P., Palo, K., Fay, N., Brand, L., Mets, U., Ullmann, D., et al. (2000). Two-dimensional fluorescence intensity distribution analysis: Theory and applications. *Biophysical Journal*, 78, 1703–1713.

Kunig, V., Potowski, M., Gohla, A., Brunsschweiger, A. (2018). DNA-encoded libraries—an efficient small molecule discovery technology for the biomedical sciences. *Biological Chemistry*, 399, 691–710.

Kusumoto, S., Lachmann, M., Kunihiro, T., Yuasa, S., Kishino, Y., Kimura, M., et al. (2018). Automated deep learning-based system to identify endothelial cells derived from induced pluripotent stem cells. *Stem Cell Reports*, 10, 1687–1695.

Kent, T., Thompson, K., & Naylor, L. (2005). Development of a generic dual-reporter gene assay for screening G-protein-coupled receptors. *Journal of Biomolecular Screening*, 10, 437–446.

Kogej, T., Blomberg, N., Greasley, P. J., Mundt, S., Vainio, M. J., Schamberger, J., et al. (2013). Big pharma screening collections: More of the same or unique libraries? The AstraZeneca-Bayer Pharma AG case. *Drug Discovery Today, 18* (19–20), 1014–1024.

Kolb, A. J., & Neumann, K. (1996). Luciferase measurements in high throughput screening. *Journal of Biomolecular Screening, 1*, 85–88.

Kornienko, O., Lacson, R., Kunapuli, P., Schneeweis, J., Hoffman, I., Smith, T., et al. (2004). Miniaturization of whole live cell-based GPCR assays using microdispensing and detection systems. *Journal of Biomolecular Screening, 9*, 186–195.

Lakowicz, J. R. (1999). *Principles of fluorescence spectroscopy.* New York: Plenum Press.

Lee, P., Miller, S., Van Staden, C., & Cromwell, E. (2008). Development of a homogeneous high-throughput live-cell G-protein-coupled receptor binding assay. *Journal of Biomolecular Screening, 13*, 748–754.

Leopoldo, M., Lacivita, E., Berardi, F., & Perrone, R. (2009). Developments in fluorescent probes for receptor research. *Drug Discovery Today, 14*, 706–712.

Lesuisse, D., Lange, G., Deprez, P., Bénard, D., Schoot, B., Delettre, G., et al. (2002). SAR and X-ray. A new approach combining fragment-based screening and rational drug design: Application to the discovery of nanomolar inhibitors of Src SH2. *Journal of Medicinal Chemistry, 45*, 2379–2387.

Lipinski, C. A., Lombardo, F., Dominy, B. W., & Feeney, P. J. (1997). Experimental and computational approaches to estimate solubility and permeability in drug discovery and development settings. *Advanced Drug Delivery Reviews, 23*(1–3), 3–25.

Liptrot, C. (2001). High content screening— from cells to data to knowledge. *Drug Discovery Today, 6*, 832–834.

Macarron, R., Banks, M. N., Bojanic, D., Burns, D. J., Cirovic, D. A., Garyantes, T., et al. (2011). Impact of high-throughput screening in biomedical research. *Nature Reviews. Drug Discovery, 10*, 188–195.

Minor, L. (2008). Label-free cell-based functional assays. *Combinatorial Chemistry & High Throughput Screening, 11*, 573–580.

Moger, J., Gribon, O., Sewing, A., & Winlover, C. (2006). The application of fluorescence lifetime readouts in high-throughput screening. *Journal of Biomolecular Screening, 11*, 765–772.

Moore, K., & Rees, S. (2001). Cell-based versus isolated target screening: How lucky do you feel? *Journal of Biomolecular Screening, 6*, 69–74.

Muegge, I., & Oloff, S. (2006). Advances in virtual screening. *Drug Discovery Today. Technologies, 3*, 405–411.

Nasir, M. S., & Jolley, M. E. (1999). Fluorescence polarization: An analytical tool for immunoassay and drug discovery. *Combinatorial Chemistry & High Throughput Screening, 2*, 177–190.

Naylor, L. (1999). Reporter gene technology: The future looks bright. *Biochemical Pharmacology, 58*, 749–757.

Nienaber, V. L., Richardson, P. L., Klighofer, V., Bouska, J. J., Giranda, V. L., & Greer, J. (2000). Discovering novel ligands for macromolecules using X-ray crystallographic screening. *Nature Biotechnology, 18*, 1105–1108.

Nosjean, O., Souchaud, S., Deniau, C., Geneste, O., Cauquil, N., & Boutin, J. (2006). A simple theoretical model for fluorescence polarization binding assay development. *Journal of Biomolecular Screening, 11*, 949–958.

Thomas, N., O'Connell, T. N., Ramsay, J., Rieth, S. F., Shapiro, M. J., & Stroh, J. G. (2014). Solution-based indirect affinity selection mass spectrometry—a general tool for high-throughput screening of pharmaceutical compound libraries. *Analytical Chemistry, 86*(15), 7413–7420.

Ozbal, C. C., LaMarr, W. A., Linton, J. R., Green, D. F., Katz, A., Morrison, T. B., et al. (2004). High throughput screening via mass spectrometry: A case study using acetylcholinesterase. *Assay and Drug Development Technologies, 2*(4), 373–381.

Phizicky, E.M., and Fields, S. (1995). Protein-protein interactions: methods for detection and analysis. *Microbiological Reviews, 59* (1), 94–123.

Pihl, J., Karlsson, M., & Chiu, D. (2005). Microfluidics technologies in drug discovery. *Drug Discovery Today, 10*, 1377–1383.

Ramm, P. (1999). Imaging systems in assay screening. *Drug Discovery Today, 4*, 401–410.

Rees, D., Congreve, M., Murray, C., & Carr, R. (2004). Fragment-based lead discovery. *Nature Reviews. Drug Discovery, 3*, 660–672.

Santos, R., Ursu, O., Anna Gaulton, A., Bento, P., Donadi, R. S., Bologa, C. G., et al. (2017). A comprehensive map of molecular drug targets. *Nature Reviews. Drug Discovery, 16*(1), 19–34.

Schroeder, K. S., & Negate, B. D. (1996). FLIPR, a new instrument for accurate high-throughput optical screening. *Journal of Biomolecular Screening, 1*, 75–80.

Serebriiskii, Ilya & Mitina, Olga & Chernoff, Jonathan & Golemis, Erica. (2001). Two-hybrid dual bait system to discriminate specificity of protein interactions in small GTPases. *Methods in enzymology, 332*, 277–300.

Shen, M. (2018). Principles of bioluminescence resonance energy transfer (BRET). Retrieved from https://blog.benchsci.com/principles-of-bioluminescence-resonance-energy-transfer-bret.

Sinclair, I., Stearns, R., Pringle, S., Wingfield, J., Datwani, S., Hall, E., et al. (2016). Novel acoustic loading of a mass spectrometer: Toward next-generation high-throughput MS screening. *Journal of Laboratory Automation, 21*(1), 19–26.

Sinclair, I., Bachman, M., Addison, D., Rohman, M., Murray, D. C., Davies, G., et al. (2019). Acoustic mist ionization platform for direct and contactless ultrahigh-throughput mass spectrometry analysis of liquid samples. *Analytical Chemistry, 91*, 3790–3794.

Sittampalam, G. S., Kahl, S. D., & Janzen, W. P. (1997). High-throughput screening: Advances in assay technologies. *Current Opinion in Chemical Biology, 1*, 384–391.

Southan, A., & Clark, G. (2009). Recent technological advances in electrophysiology based screening technology and the impact upon ion channel discovery research. *Methods in Molecular Biology, 565*, 187–208.

Sriram, K., Insel, P. A. (2018). GPCRs as targets for approved drugs: How many targets and how many drugs? *Molecular Pharmacology, 93*(4), 251–258.

Stahura, F., Xue, L., Godden, J., & Bajorath, J. (2002). Methods for compound selection focused on hits and application in drug discovery. *Journal of Molecular Graphics & Modelling, 20*, 439–446.

Sui, Y., & Wu, Z. (2007). Alternative statistical parameter for high-throughput screening assay quality assessment. *Journal of Biomolecular Screening, 12*, 229–234.

Suto, C., & Ignar, D. (1997). Selection of an optimal reporter gene for cell-based high throughput screening assays. *Journal of Biomolecular Screening, 2*, 7–9.

Titus, S., Neumann, S., Zheng, W., Southall, N., Michael, S., Klumpp, C., et al. (2008). Quantitative high-throughput screening using a live-cell cAMP assay identifies small-molecule agonists of the TSH receptor. *Journal of Biomolecular Screening, 13*, 120–127.

Trinquet, E., Fink, M., Bazin, H., Grillet, F., Maurin, F., Bourrier, E., et al. (2006). D-*myo*-Inositol 1-phosphate as a surrogate of D-*myo*-inositol 1,4,5-tris phosphate to monitor G protein-coupled receptor activation. *Analytical Biochemistry, 358*, 126–135.

Tucker, C. (2002). High-throughput cell-based assays in yeast. *Drug Discovery Today, 7*, S125–S130.

Turek-Etienne, T., Small, E., Soh, S., Xin, T., Gaitonde, P., Barrabee, E., et al. (2003). Evaluation of fluorescent compound interference in 4 fluorescence polarization assays: 2 kinases, 1 protease and 1 phosphatase. *Journal of Biomolecular Screening, 8*, 176–184.

Valenzano, K. J., Miller, W., Kravitz, J. N., Samama, P., Fitzpatrick, D., Seeley, K. (2000). Development of a fluorescent ligand-binding assay using the AcroWell filter plate. *Journal of Biomolecular Screening, 5*, 455–461.

Valler, M. J., & Green, D. (2000). Diversity screening versus focussed screening in drug discovery. *Drug Discovery Today, 5*, 286–293.

Waszkowycz, B. (2008). Towards improving compound selection in structure-based virtual screening. *Drug Discovery Today, 13*, 219–226.

Young, K., Lin, S., Sun, L., Lee, E., Modi, M., Hellings, S., Ozenberger, B., Franco, R. (1998) Identification of a calcium channel modulator using a high throughput yeast two-hybrid screen. *Nature Biotechnology, 16*(10):946–950.

Zhang, J. H., Chung, T. D., & Oldenburg, K. R. (1999). A simple statistical parameter for use in evaluation and validation of high-throughput screening assays. *Journal of Biomolecular Screening, 4*, 67–73.

Zlokarnik, G., Negulescu, P. A., Knapp, T. E., Mere, L., Burres, N., Feng, L., et al. (1998). Quantitation of transcription and clonal selection of single living cells with beta-lactamase as reporter. *Science, 279*, 84–88.

Zock, J. M. (2009). Applications of high content screening in life science research. *Combinatorial Chemistry & High Throughput Screening, 12*(9), 870–876.

Chapter | 7 |

The role of medicinal chemistry in the drug discovery process

Paul Beswick

Introduction

The level of clinical unmet need has never been higher, and continues to rise due to increasing longevity in the developed world and the consequential increased prevalence of age-related diseases such as cancer and dementia. While few would dispute that the role of the medicinal chemist is pivotal to the discovery of new medicines to address this growing need, and will continue so for the foreseeable future, the environment in which the medicinal chemist operates has continued to change over the last decade. Following several decades of decreasing productivity within the pharmaceutical industry, the period between 2015 and 2018 saw a much awaited increase in new drug approvals, with 59 in 2018 and 46 in 2017 (Jarvis, 2019). This compares favourably with the situation 10 years earlier. In 2009, only 19 new chemical entities (NCEs) were approved by the US Food & Drug Administration (FDA), two less than in 2008 (Hughes, 2010). The approval of six biological licence applications in 2009, compared with three in 2008, was perhaps the first indication of the greater emphasis that Pharma was placing on the discovery of biological therapeutic agents, a trend that has continued, and now biological agents are an important part of the therapeutic armoury available to clinicians. Small-molecule discovery is likely to remain the mainstay of therapeutic innovation for at least the next 20 years.

The reason for the recent improvement in clinical success is attributed to the increased importance that biomarkers play in drug discovery projects, allowing the generation of informed translational science packages that provide additional confidence of success at the preclinical stage and allow early determination of target engagement in the clinic. Additionally, the increase in availability of genetic data has been highlighted as a second key contributor to the recent success. However, despite the recent encouraging trends, it is important that drug discovery scientists do not become complacent, and there remain a number of key challenges to be overcome that can potentially further increase the success level. The medicinal chemist might play a role in addressing these challenges in the future. There remains a level of attrition in the clinic due to lack of sufficient efficacy, despite the increased use of biomarkers, and it reflects an inadequate understanding of disease pathophysiology in humans and the poor predictability of many of the preclinical animal models of human disease. Thus there is a pressing need to improve the quality of validation of novel targets, placing less emphasis on preclinical in vivo models and single gene 'knock-outs', and a greater emphasis on cellular pathways, genetically associated targets and innovative clinical trial design. This approach will require the availability of selective chemical tools with which to validate targets in human tissue, and thus the role of the medicinal chemist in the future may incorporate a greater component of chemical biology. The increasing trend towards academic target and drug discovery is also likely to place greater emphasis on chemical biology skills.

Despite stringent toxicity evaluation during the discovery phase, an unacceptable level of failure due to safety issues remains. The present situation is arguably worse than 30 years ago, as there has been a trend towards molecules failing later in the safety evaluation process, incurring greater cost and time. If significant impact is to be made on this source of attrition, it will be important for the medicinal chemist to develop a rational understanding of possible structural and physicochemical determinants of toxicity in much the same way as the determinants of oral bioavailability have been recognized. However, this objective is likely to be much more challenging due to the diverse and complex nature of the multiple pathologies. Preliminary studies to evaluate this approach have been recently reported and will be discussed later in the chapter.

It is clear that addressing the challenges described earlier and raising productivity will require long-term investment and persistence. However, due to the immediate financial pressures, the industry has responded to the productivity challenge by minimizing costs, shifting focus to cheaper sources of chemistry, predominantly in the Far East, and in-licensing assets. Thus today's medicinal chemist is required to optimally integrate a network of both internal and external resources to prosecute the identification of development candidates.

While medicinal chemistry is facing unprecedented pressures due to the volatility of the sector, it is clear that small-molecule therapeutics will be required for the foreseeable future, and that, whatever infrastructure evolves within the industry, the medicinal chemist will have a key role to play. This chapter will discuss some of the recent scientific advances in the field which will enable the medicinal chemist to rise to the challenges ahead.

Target selection and validation

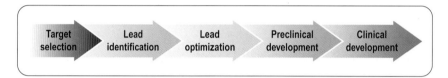

A key challenge in increasing the industry's productivity will be the selection of targets that have compelling validation in terms of both efficacy and safety in the human context, and that consequently have a greater probability of achieving a successful clinical proof of concept (Gashaw et al., 2012). The role of the medicinal chemist has previously focused primarily on ensuring the quality of preclinical candidate molecules in terms of potency, selectivity and physicochemical properties such as those highlighted initially by Lipinski et al. (1997) and, more recently, by Leeson and Springthorpe (2007). As a result, the level of attrition due to poor absorption, distribution, metabolism and excretion (ADME) properties fell dramatically between 1991 and 2000 (Kola & Landis, 2004), but the level of clinical success with new mechanisms remains poor. However, chemists are now increasingly becoming engaged, along with their biology and clinical counterparts, in the process of selecting and prioritizing future protein targets. In particular, the development of an in-depth understanding of the structural biology of the target and the biophysics of its interaction with low-molecular-weight ligands is a critical component at the outset of a project and very much in the chemist's domain. The necessity for a rigorous analysis of potential targets cannot be overemphasized since this occurs at the start of the 12- to 15-year period of intensive effort and investment required to achieve the launch of a new medicine into large-scale clinical usage. The postgenomic era has provided the industry with a plethora of potential drug targets; however, the selection of tractable targets with a high probability of delivering safe and effective treatments represents a huge challenge requiring a multidisciplinary approach.

While a detailed discussion of the complex facets of target validation is beyond the scope of this chapter, it is clear that targets with strong genetic associations such as the chemokine CCR_5 receptor (Westby & van der Ryst, 2005), which has led to the discovery of treatments for HIV infection, and the Kv7.2 (Corbin-Leftwich et al., 2016) voltage-gated ion channel, which has led to a treatment for benign familial neonatal convulsions type 1 (BFNC1) and the cystic fibrosis transmembrane conductance regulator (Dechecchi, 2018), exemplify an aspirational level of target validation. It is, however, important to exercise caution when considering genetic target validation as not all data have led to successful outcomes, a good example being the voltage-gated sodium channel $NaV_{1.7}$ (Waxman et al., 2007), identified to have potential utility in the treatment of pain, and was the subject of intense interest for many years; however, to date, no selective agent acting via this mechanism has produced positive effects in the clinic. An elegant study from Pfizer suggested that mutations of this channel that produce a similar disease phenotype cause a diverse range of effects on channel function, hence thus explain the lack of efficacy seen in their clinical studies (Cao et al., 2016). The perils of taking genetic target validation evidence in isolation were highlighted recently by an Australian neuroscientists who proposed a robust strategy for full validation targets highlighted by genetic studies (Oyrer et. al., 2018). While genetic disease-association data can provide strong evidence of target involvement, target modulation, ideally within a human cellular pathway, provides compelling validation, and the identification of early chemical probes in addition to subsequent lead molecules will be an important challenge for the medicinal chemist in the future. It is important to stress that many chemical probes are not suitable for target validation studies due to poorly understood pharmacology and inadequate physical properties, and there still remains a need for major improvements in this area.

Frye (2010) has described essential features of a quality chemical probe, which are summarized below.

Molecular profiling. Sufficient in vitro potency and selectivity data to confidently associate its in vitro profile to its cellular or in vivo profile.

Mechanism of action. Activity in a cell-based or cell-free assay influences a physiologic function of the target in a dose-dependent manner.

Identity of the active species. Has sufficient chemical and physical property data to interpret results as due to its intact structure or a well-characterized derivative.

Proven utility as a probe. Cellular activity data available to confidently address at least one hypothesis about the role of the molecular target in a cell's response to its environment.

Availability. Is readily available to the academic community with no restrictions on use.

The first four criteria attempt to describe ideal properties of a probe, while the latter point addresses a more philosophical viewpoint on the sharing of precompetitive information. Unfortunately, workers failed to take notice of these guidelines, and despite global initiative (Arrowsmith et al., 2015), the quality of currently available chemical probes remains at best unreliable (Antolin et al., 2018), and great caution should be exercised when considering the use of these agents.

It is well known that target classes are associated with different levels of tractability with respect to the probability of being able to identify quality lead molecules. For example, the G-protein-coupled receptor (GPCR) superfamily is generally considered to be one of the most tractable target classes, with approximately 40% of prescription drugs in current practice producing efficacy via modulation of a GPCR (Santos, 2017). In contrast, voltage-gated ion channels are generally regarded as one of the more challenging variety of protein targets to modulate, particularly with respect to subunit specificity. Progress in this area was for many years limited by lack of suitable screening platforms to facilitate drug discovery. In the period 2000–2010, technological developments offered the potential to more fully explore this target class (Kaczorowski et al., 2008); however, despite promising preclinical data, a large number of candidates have progressed to the clinic and failed to demonstrate adequate efficacy, possibly highlighting the need for a better understanding of disease biology.

Various criteria for the selection and prioritization of targets are utilized within major Pharma in the process of building sustainable portfolios of viable potential targets

for the discovery scientists to address. An illustration published by the University Medicine Mannheim (Wehling, 2009) highlighted one such approach that objectively applies weighted scores to available target information.

With the emergence of exciting new insights into disease pathologies, the importance of rigorous target selection will become even more important in the future. The availability of the human genome sequence coupled with impressive advances in biology is uncovering challenging targets for the medicinal chemist to address. As an example, epigenetic phenomena became increasingly recognized as a potentially important area in the development of chronic diseases (Gluckman & Heindel, 2008), and the discovery and characterization of specific histone-modifying enzyme subfamilies (Cole, 2008) offered the medicinal chemist the opportunity to design specific enzyme modulators with which to regulate gene expression. The promise of this area was illustrated by the successful discovery of the histone deacetylase (HDAC) inhibitor vorinostat (McGuire & Lee, 2010; Fig. 7.1).

Historically, natural products have been considered as a source of both new drugs and potential targets. More recently, this approach has suffered demise due to its disappointing productivity. However, there have been a number of recent success stories, which are illustrated by the following examples. Ziconotide (Prialt; Schmidtko et al., 2010) is a potent and selective N-type calcium channel blocker approved by the FDA in December 2004 for the treatment of severe chronic pain. Ziconotide has subsequently demonstrated efficacy in patients with refractory pain, that is, pain that has proven difficult to control using conventional analgesics. Ziconotide is a synthetic peptide derived from a toxin extracted from the marine snail *Conus magus*. The success of ziconotide has highlighted the potential of natural toxins in drug discovery and has stimulated renewed interest from a number of groups in the area (Halai & Craik, 2009). Peptides offer high levels of both potency and selectivity that make them valuable tools for target validation, and the toxins of a number of venomous species have proved to be a rich source of such molecules. The identification of the endogenous

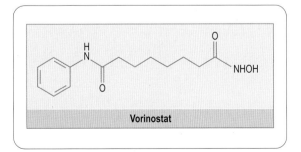

Fig. 7.1 The histone deacetylase (HDAC) inhibitor vorinostat.

peptide hormone ghrelin (Hellström, 2009), and subsequent understanding of its function, has highlighted the potential clinical value of ghrelin receptor agonists in a number of conditions such as gastroparesis (Ejskjaer et al., 2009) and postoperative ileus (Popescu et al., 2010) in which the ghrelin receptor agonist TZP-101 (Fig. 7.2) has recently demonstrated clinical efficacy. These are just two examples of the resurgence of interest in peptides as therapeutics that has occurred during recent years such that there is now a rich pipeline of peptide-based drugs in development to support those that have already made it to market (Henniot et al., 2018). Several of the major disease challenges facing society, such as Alzheimer's disease, cancer and heart disease and so on, have been shown to be associated, at least in part, with aberrant protein folding and/or protein–protein interactions, and the identification of both small-molecule and peptidic therapeutics to address these pathologies will require significant innovation.

Encouragingly, great strides have recently been made in our understanding of the factors that cause proteins to misfold, primarily through the use of biophysical and computational techniques that enable systematic and quantitative analysis of the effects of a range of different perturbations in proteins (Fry, 2015; Luheshi et al., 2008). Notable advances in the design of small-molecule inhibitors that inhibit protein–protein interactions have been amply demonstrated by the discovery of the serum amyloid P cross-linking agent CPHPC (Pepys et al., 2002; Fig. 7.3A) and the C-reactive protein inhibitor 1,6-bis(phosphocholine)-hexane (Pepys et al., 2006; Fig. 7.3B).

It is clear from the above selected examples that there is likely to be a plethora of novel biological targets to challenge the innovation of medicinal chemists for the foreseeable future.

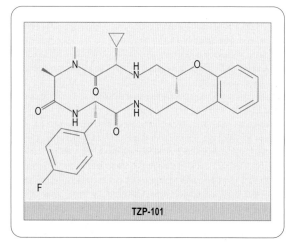

Fig. 7.2 The ghrelin receptor agonist TZP-101.

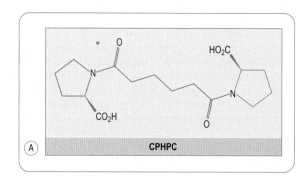

Fig. 7.3. The serum amyloid P cross-linking agent CPHPC (A) and the C-reactive protein inhibitor 1,6-bis(phosphocholine)-hexane (B).

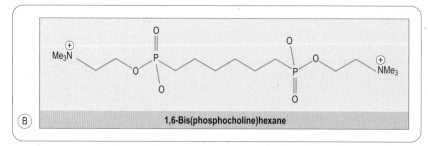

Lead identification/generation

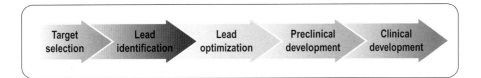

The identification of high-quality lead molecules is a critical phase in the discovery of drug candidates since decisions made at this point in the process are likely to have a significant impact on the outcome of the project, as it sets the framework for future lead optimization and development (Bleicher et al., 2003; Hughes et al., 2011).

Reducing attrition has already been alluded to as a major challenge in the discovery of new therapeutic agents, and the lead generation phase is the earliest point in the drug discovery process where the incorporation of appropriate physicochemical properties can be addressed. It is important to establish a clear target lead profile at this early stage of the process that takes into account the critical properties required of the ultimate preclinical candidate and extrapolates back into an appropriate minimum acceptable profile for a lead series. Such a profile should not simply take into account target potency and selectivity but should also include consideration of a wide range of physicochemical characteristics that would facilitate favourable ADMET properties later in the process.

The initial aim at the lead identification/generation stage is to identify 'hits' that are molecules that interact with the chosen biological target in an initial screen, often carried out at a high concentration, to elicit a measurable response in a reproducible assay. Once validated by establishing the molecular integrity of the hit molecule(s), and confirming the robustness of the biological response, a 'validated hit' may be further investigated to establish whether it possesses the potential to be regarded as a lead series.

Several strategies have been adopted to identify these early hits as listed below:

- Existing drugs
- Natural ligands
- Natural products
- Focused screens
- Rational structure-based design
- Knowledge-based design
- Fragment screening
- Virtual screening
- High-throughput screening (including phenotypic screens).

The widespread use of high-throughput screening has generally been reported to have enabled the identification of leads for approximately 50% of the projects addressed by this approach (Fox et al., 2006), although a 2011 review suggests that the success rate had increased to approximately 60% (Macarron et al., 2011). However, it was noteworthy that, despite the massive growth in the numbers of compounds screened over the 20 years leading to 2011, no corresponding increase in the number of successful NCEs had resulted. It has been argued that, in view of increasing development times, it is still too early to evaluate the true success of high-throughput screening (Macarron et al., 2011). More recent studies have suggested that it is the quality and diversity of a screening collection that are the key drivers for success, as opposed to large numbers of compounds, and that the optimal number of diverse molecules is approximately 300,000 (Boss et al., 2017). Nevertheless, there has been continued focus on improving the 'drug and lead-like' properties and the structure/property diversity of screening collections. 'Drug-likeness' can be broadly defined as the overall profile of biophysicochemical properties of a molecule that facilitate its access to and effective mode of interaction at the site of action at a biologically relevant and safe concentration for sufficient duration to elicit the desired therapeutic effect. Leeson discusses the importance of considering the properties conferring 'drug-likeness', particularly lipophilicity, in a survey of selected development candidates in leading drug companies (Leeson & Springthorpe, 2007). An analysis of the structural relationship of launched drugs to their corresponding lead molecules revealed that, in general, the structure of the marketed molecule was very closely related to the lead series (Proudfoot, 2002). Thus one could infer that the apparent disappointing success rate of high-throughput screening has been related to the lack of 'drug-likeness' in the compound collections, and significant effort is now being devoted to address this. Another development in recent years is in the diverse nature of organizations offering screening services, including contract research organizations (CROs) and groups such as the European Lead Factory (Karawajczyk et al., 2016).

Screening providers have therefore filtered their screening collections to exclude constituents that do not possess physicochemical properties that are generally accepted to confer 'drug-like' attributes (Bleicher et al., 2003; Boss et al., 2017). However, it should be noted that, although the discovery of drug-like preclinical development candidates requires the initial identification of quality leads, the properties that confer 'drug-likeness' and those associated with 'lead-likeness' are not the same (Rishton, 2003). It is therefore important to understand the components conferring 'lead-likeness' when assessing screening collections. A publication from the AstraZeneca group addressed the design of lead-like combinatorial libraries and suggested that leads suitable for further optimization are most likely to be relatively polar, low molecular weight (MW = 200–350) and of relatively low lipophilicity (clogP approx. 1.0–3.0) (Teague et al., 2001). The authors point out that when beginning from such a tractable low-molecular-weight lead molecule, subsequent optimization to increase potency and selectivity is likely to increase molecular weight and lipophilicity to values in the order of the accepted 'drug-likeness' parameters.

While significant progress is being made in improving the quality of compound collections with respect to the enrichment of 'lead-like' components and the elimination of potentially toxic or undesirable functionality, improving chemical diversity is an ongoing preoccupation since the concept of diversity is open to a variety of interpretations. While in its original conception, combinatorial chemistry aimed to generate large numbers of molecules providing a high level of diversity, the early libraries tended to be bolstered with molecules having significant molecular complexity and only modest diversity due to the limitations of the synthetic methodologies that could be utilized in a high-throughput mode. Furthermore, compound collections with less than optimal physicochemical properties were previously employed in high-throughput screening campaigns. Thus more attention is now being paid to the generation of focused libraries containing subsets of compounds having so-called 'privileged scaffolds' for specific target classes.

High-throughput screening continues to be a valuable strategy where there is little information around the structure of the biological target or ligands; however, where such knowledge exists, it has generally been more successful to utilize this information to identify potential molecular starting points. For example, structural information on ligands that are known to interact with a target can be used to construct a pharmacophore that may be used in an initial virtual screening programme of proprietary or commercial compound collections to enrich the sample ultimately selected for actual screening. A critical review assessing the past effectiveness of virtual screening and proposing considerations for future improvements has been published (Schneider, 2010). Computational tools are widely used to generate in silico pharmacophores, using either molecular or electronic overlays. The introduction of electronic field overlay technology has allowed chemists to interrogate electronic properties in a relatively accessible manner. Similarly, the latter technology may be usefully applied to 'scaffold hopping', where a structurally distinct compound class has been derived from an active series via application of a field pharmacophore (Cheeseright et al., 2008). An extreme example of utilizing structural information is where an existing known drug molecule is used as the starting point to discover an improved agent (Naik et al., 2010).

Although the majority of high-throughput screens are aimed at known biological targets with supporting target validation in the disease of interest, there has been significant activity in establishing screens based on the cell phenotype, that is, where biochemical pathways are targeted as opposed to specific proteins within the pathway. The major challenge associated with this approach is the subsequent identification of the specific molecular target or targets with which the agents interact to produce the desired cellular response (Hart, 2005). While in some cases further optimization of leads has been carried using the phenotypic assay itself, because of the numerous variables involved, for example, multiple targets and cellular distribution and so on, precise structure–activity relationships (SARs) can be difficult to obtain from the phenotypic assay. Thus a detailed analysis and elucidation of the mechanism of action is often required to enable rapid progress to be achieved using a protein-specific assay.

Established a decade ago, fragment-based drug discovery has become an established technique for lead generation, often in conjunction with other strategic approaches (Whittaker et al., 2010) and is now a mainstay in lead generation practices (Jacquemard, 2019), having produced two drugs currently on the market. Fragment-based screening consists of screening a chemical library of low-molecular-weight compounds, usually at high concentration, using sensitive assay methods. In addition to biochemical assays, such campaigns often incorporate biophysical methodology such as nuclear magnetic resonance (NMR), surface plasmon resonance (SPR), isothermal titration calorimetry (ITC) and X-ray crystallography (Carr & Jhoti, 2002; Orita et al., 2009; Rees et al., 2004). The considerable progress achieved with in silico design of fragment libraries using a variety of techniques has been reviewed (Konteatis, 2010). Essentially the fragment-based approach aims to identify ligands for the target protein that have relatively low affinity but high ligand/ligand-lipophilicity efficiency (LLE). Ligand efficiency (LE) is a measure of the binding energy of a molecule normalized by its size. This is often calculated by dividing the pK_i or IC$_{50}$ by the molecular weight or number of heavy atoms. Similarly, LLE can be calculated by determining the difference between the pK_i or pIC$_{50}$ value and the clogP, which provides a measure of the binding energy of a molecule normalized by its lipophilicity (Smith, 2009). Thus compounds with high LE and LLE interact highly efficiently with the biological target. Subsequent optimization is then focused on increasing potency while maintaining high LE/LLE, thus avoiding the pitfall of increasing potency by increasing size and lipophilicity, which often leads to promiscuous 'off-target' interactions and subsequent toxicity. Although the concepts of LE and LLE have been particularly applied in fragment-based design, they are now widely applied across all lead generation strategies. There are now numerous examples of a fragment-based approach being employed in drug discovery projects and several have been reviewed (Congreve et al., 2008).

In stark contrast to the fragment-based approach to lead generation, natural products have been, and arguably continue to be, a fruitful source of lead molecules and drugs over the past 25−30 years (Cragg & Newman, 2013; Newman & Cragg, 2007). However, despite the demonstrable historical successes of natural product research, major Pharma largely ceased its investment in natural product screening in favour of the small-molecule library approaches described earlier, during the early part of this century. The anticipation that combinatorial chemistry would provide an excess of small-molecule leads for most biological targets was partly responsible for the demise of this strategy. Furthermore, the technical challenges associated with the deconvolution of multicomponent natural product mixtures and subsequent chemical simplification of large and complex structures have also deterred continued investment in this field. There has seen a resurgence in the use of natural products in early stage drug discovery (Harvey, 2008; Harvey et al., 2010). This change in strategy is starting to demonstrate success, with a number of success stories starting to emerge. An excellent example is the identification of a new antibiotic less likely to generate resistance than existing agents (Ling et al., 2015).

Despite the relative demise and subsequent reemergence of natural product screening over the past few years, natural products have inspired the development of new strategies in the identification of privileged structures from which small-molecule libraries have

been constructed. Herbert Waldman has received notable acclaim for his biology-oriented synthesis (BIOS) strategy, which encompasses the development of small molecular entities derived from natural product and drug families, the so-called 'structural classification of natural products' (SCONP) (Waldmann et al., 2008) and an associated 'scaffold hunter' approach (Waldmann et al., 2009).

X-ray crystallography has been effectively applied over many years to optimize small-molecule ligands primarily for soluble enzyme targets. With the introduction of fragment-based screening, high-throughput X-ray crystallography has over the past decade also assumed an important role in the identification of lead molecules (Carr & Jhoti, 2002). Similarly, NMR is proving to be an effective, accessible, complementary technique in identifying ligand–protein interactions, particularly for membrane-bound proteins such as GPCRs for which detailed X-ray structures are relatively rare (Bartoschek et al., 2010).

Developments in the acquisition of bioengineered protein and subsequent X-ray crystal structures of stabilized GPCRs (Tate & Schertler, 2009) may provide exciting future opportunities for medicinal chemists to actively use ligand-bound co-crystal structures of GPCRs in an analogous fashion to the enzyme co-crystallization structures that have greatly facilitated the discovery of selective enzyme inhibitors.

Transmission electron cryomicroscopy (CryoTEM), a technique that allows the structural determination of large membrane proteins such as GPCRs and ion channels in their natural state, has recently been developed such that it is starting to be used as a tool in lead generation (Quentin & Raunser, 2018).

Industry pressure to improve productivity and efficiency in the identification of NCEs has added stimulus to the exploration of new technologies in the identification of lead molecules. In particular, miniaturization and automation of chemical synthesis and biological screening assays are currently under intense focus (Lombardi & Dittrich, 2010).

The identification of screening platforms which obviate the requirement for artificial labels or reporter systems is also receiving considerable attention (Shiau et al., 2008). Biophysical methods such as SPR and impedance-based technologies are developing rapidly and will become more widely used, particularly since these approaches are less likely to identify false positives that result from labelling artefacts and aggregation phenomena (Giannetti et al., 2008). The successful development of these new technologies has the potential to transform the lead identification process and address in part the challenge of improving productivity (see Chapter 6).

Lead optimization

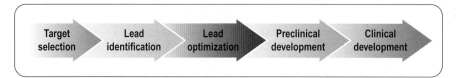

The lead optimization stage of drug discovery is at the pivotal interface between lead identification and the early development phase of a molecule. The ultimate aim of the lead optimization phase is the identification of a compound that possesses the required properties of the targeted preclinical development candidate. Thus the medicinal chemist must be cognizant of the wide range of parameters that will need to be optimized in the lead, thus ensuring a high probability of success during subsequent development. It is important that the desired candidate profile is clearly defined as early as possible, ideally before the initiation of a programme, thus giving the medicinal chemist and the programme team a clear focus. From the candidate profile a focused screening strategy can be developed and should only contain screens that are decision-making. Careful consideration should be given to the components and order of assays within the screening cascade that should include higher throughput assays, for which high attrition can be expected, early in the triage, and lower throughput and more discerning assays, including those involving animals, later in the cascade. A major consideration in constructing an effective screening cascade is the choice of selectivity assays that need to be included. The selectivity panel normally consists of proteins both within the target family and selected 'off-target' proteins that, if modulated, would result in undesirable toxicity or side-effects, discussed later in more detail.

In addition to fulfilling potency and selectivity criteria, a potential development candidate should possess appropriate ADME properties to deliver acceptable exposure of the compound at the target site by the preferred route of administration, allowing data obtained from subsequent in vivo profiling in preclinical disease models to be interpreted with confidence and facilitate predictions for future clinical efficacy. Much of this section will focus on molecules intended for oral administration, but a brief discussion on the different requirements for drugs intended for administration via other routes will also be included.

A number of excellent reviews have appeared that describe the lead optimization process in detail (Baringhaus & Matter, 2005; Lindsley et al., 2009). This section will focus on recent discoveries and developments that have enhanced or have the potential to further improve the traditional process.

The process commences with the careful selection of lead series which, as previously stated, is of great importance since this selection has consequences for the future lengthy and expensive discovery and development programme. It is essential that great attention is paid to selecting robust leads with the appropriate physicochemical properties. Analyses (Keserü & Makara, 2009; Kola & Landis, 2004; Leeson, 2016) have clearly shown that leads chosen from the 'wrong' area of chemical space have a much higher probability of failure than those from the 'correct' area. Often failure occurs late in development and can be extremely costly. Far too often, medicinal chemists have been seduced by high levels of potency in 'non-drug-like' lead molecules only to find that the physical properties of the molecule are incompatible with the desired candidate profile.

Lipinski has highlighted (Lipinski et al., 1997) the importance of the physical properties of a molecule and, while this paper is often quoted, the guidelines contained within are too often disregarded.

It is important to measure key physical properties such as $\log D$, solubility and pK_a (where appropriate), and so on of novel compounds throughout the drug discovery process to ensure that molecules continue to reside within 'drug-like' chemical space and to regularly analyse data to investigate potential correlations between physicochemical properties, ADME parameters and biological activities.

In addition to having the desired physicochemical properties, a lead molecule should also have the following characteristics: (1) be a member of a distinct structural series with confirmed SARs, (2) show evidence of the desired selectivity profile, (3) have activity in cellular systems if necessary, (4) have acceptable metabolic stability in vitro, (5) be free of any structural toxicity alerts and (6) not have any major cytotoxicity issues. It is highly advantageous for a lead to demonstrate some evidence of activity after oral administration even at this early stage.

It is important also to consider how many lead series should be investigated in the early stages of the optimization process and the requisite level of structural diversity in order to mitigate against failure of a particular series. Ideally, three structurally distinct lead series would be selected for lead optimization at the commencement of the process.

A lead molecule will have a predefined level of potency at the chosen target, together with the initial target selectivity for both related targets and common 'off-target' liabilities that are considered important to avoid. The primary assays in most screening cascades focus on activity at the target protein and selectivity to allow the medicinal chemist to quickly optimize these important parameters early in the process. At this stage, rudimentary SARs will have already been established during the lead identification phase, providing an insight as to which moieties of the lead compound may be modified to achieve the desired result. Furthermore, the availability of other information, such as protein X-ray crystal structures or docking predictions from target protein homology models, can provide strategic guidance for the optimization process. In addition to considering selectivity within the target protein family, it is important to consider selectivity more broadly (Bass et al., 2009) since a growing number of 'liability targets' are being identified as being potentially responsible for safety issues that are often only detected later in the development process.

Screening compounds against recombinant proteins has become widely accepted since this allows the configuration of robust high-throughput assays that perform consistently over time. However, caution should be exercised when interpreting data generated from such assays since the biological activity data from these assays does not necessarily correlate well with activity from native tissue systems (Eglen et al., 2008). It is therefore important, where feasible, to periodically interrogate the relationship between activities derived from each assay system. Ideally, the native tissue used should be closely related to the target tissue and from the relevant disease situation wherever possible.

A further consideration when designing a screening cascade is the potential for species differences to exist in which the biological activity at the target protein varies between different species. Species differences can lead to problems in the extrapolation of in vitro to in vivo data and the interpretation of data from in vivo efficacy and safety studies (Swanson & Beasley, 2010). While an indication of potential species differences can be obtained by performing a bioinformatics analysis early in the project, differences in activity can occur even when there is a high degree of homology between proteins. It is therefore important to consider the incorporation of animal orthologue assays in the screening cascade that would typically be the species of choice for the primary animal model.

Much of the focus in lead optimization is on optimization of ADME parameters that are clearly important to (1) select the most appropriate compounds for evaluation in in vivo disease models, (2) ensure that the drug is optimally delivered to its intended site of action, (3) allow a prediction of the human pharmacokinetics and estimation of clinical dose, (4) minimize the potential for drug–drug interaction, (5) avoid selecting compounds with the potential to form reactive metabolites and thus reduce the potential for idiosyncratic toxicity and (6) provide confidence that safety studies can be performed in several species (see Chapter 10).

Several in vitro ADME screens feature early in virtually all screening strategies employed by major Pharma. The introduction of cytochrome P450 (CYP450) inhibition assays has allowed potent inhibitors of these key metabolizing enzymes to be identified early in the optimization process. The elucidation of crystal structures of a number of CYP450 enzymes has alerted medicinal chemists to specific chemical modifications with which to mitigate such liabilities from candidate molecules, thus reducing the risk of drug–drug interactions in the clinic (Ekroos & Sjögren, 2006; Foti et al., 2010). For most CYP450 isoforms, a strong correlation exists between the lipophilicity of a compound and its CYP450 inhibitory potential (Lewis et al., 2007).

In addition to determining the potential of a molecule to inhibit CYP450 enzymes, it is also important to assess the potential of a compound to induce CYP450 expression. CYP450 induction can potentially lead to increased clearance of the compound on chronic dosing and toxicity due to the possible formation of reactive oxygen species. For some years, the pregnane X receptor (PXR), a nuclear hormone receptor assay, has been used to determine the potential of a compound to induce CYP3A4. More recently, additional assays have become available for mechanisms by which other CYP isoforms are induced (Chu et al., 2009) and could enter more routine use in the future. Currently, such CYP450 induction assays are not commonly included early in the screening cascade unless the particular liability has been identified, but are employed in the later stages of lead optimization, particularly if the level of systemic exposure falls following chronic dosing.

Much attention is currently being given to the role of transporter proteins (Chu et al., 2009) that have been implicated in the unfavourable disposition of drugs, either by active efflux from target tissue, potentially limiting efficacy, or through accumulation leading to toxicity and potential drug–drug interactions (Lai et al., 2010). For many years only P-glycoprotein (Pgp) assays were used in routine screening; however, studies have identified and demonstrated many other transporters potentially implicated in drug disposition and drug–drug interactions, and scientists often incorporate these in routines screening (Colas et al., 2016). Examples include organic anion transporters, organic cation transporters and amino acid transporters. The assessment of potential metabolic instability is also an important early evaluation in a screening cascade. Thus typically compounds are incubated with human and/or rodent liver microsomes, and their metabolic stability is expressed as the percentage of compound remaining after a given time or, more commonly, as an intrinsic clearance parameter (Nagai, 2010). For a more thorough evaluation of in vitro metabolic turnover, human and rodent hepatocytes may be used that possess the capacity to carry out both phase 1 and 2 metabolic processing. In addition, an assessment of plasma protein binding is often included since the degree to which a molecule binds to plasma proteins can influence both the efficacy and the tissue distribution of the compound (Chang et al., 2010).

As molecules progress to the later stages of lead optimization, an understanding of the route and specific sites of metabolism of the compounds can be important information to assist the medicinal chemist to further improve the metabolic stability of the compound. For example, the introduction of blocking groups at sites of metabolism or electron withdrawing substituents at appropriate sites on the molecule which will reduce electrophilicity can significantly reduce the rate of metabolic turnover. An early assessment of the potential of a compound to form reactive, and therefore potentially toxic, metabolites is also valuable and can be achieved by using a combination of time-dependent CYP450 inhibition (Howard et al., 2010) and trapping experiments, typically with either glutathione or cyanide (Riley et al., 2007). For molecules with the potential for reactive metabolite formation, additional in vitro and in vivo studies to detect covalent binding to tissue protein, using radiolabelled compound, may be required (Evans et al., 2004).

A preclinical pharmacokinetic (PK) study (see Chapter 10) is often the first occasion at which a compound is tested in an in vivo experiment. These studies are normally performed in rats since this is the species of choice for the majority of disease models and for rodent safety assessment studies. Compounds targeted as oral therapies are administered by both intravenous (i.v.) and oral (p.o.) routes, each experiment providing valuable information for the medicinal chemist. An i.v. PK study allows the clearance (the rate by which the drug is eliminated from the system) of the drug to be measured together with the volume of distribution (a measure of how well the drug distributes into tissue). Both the clearance and the volume of distribution determine the half-life of the drug (Doss & Baillie, 2006). A p.o. study is used to determine the circulating levels that can be achieved after a given p.o. dose. Studies frequently use both i.v. and p.o. routes of administration to gain a full profile of a compound and allow the absolute bioavailability to be determined (White, 2009).

The volume of distribution is a parameter that quantifies the distribution of the drug between the plasma and body tissue, and ideal molecules should have low clearance from the blood and a volume of distribution indicative of distribution into total body water (i.e. >1). It is thus important to understand the properties that affect the volume of distribution of a compound. Common factors that can affect this parameter are plasma protein binding, the physical properties (particularly the presence or absence of either an acidic or basic centre) and the involvement of transporters (Grover & Benet, 2009). Common strategies to increase the volume of distribution include the introduction of a basic centre to increase the pK_a, if appropriate, and to increase the logD. However, unless the lead molecule is hydrophilic in nature, increasing lipophilicity can result in increased metabolism and CYP450 inhibition as discussed earlier, and thus the identification of the optimal properties is often a tradeoff of physicochemical properties. In addition to blocking sites of metabolism to reduce clearance, reducing the lipophilicity of a molecule is often effective at reducing the rate of metabolism. Drugs that are specifically aimed at targets within the central nervous system (CNS) require more stringent control of their physicochemical properties to facilitate passive permeation of the blood–brain barrier, which comprises endothelial tight junctions. In comparison with Lipinski guidelines, molecules designed to cross the blood–brain barrier would typically have a lower molecular weight (<450), lower clogP (1–3), reduced hydrogen bond acceptors (<6) and donors (<2) and lower total polar surface area (TPSA) (<60 Å^2). The blood–brain barrier also contains efflux transporters, such as Pgp that serve to prevent access of substrates into the CNS. The free fraction of the compound, that is, that proportion that is not bound to plasma protein, has also been reported to have a profound effect on both access to the CNS and subsequent distribution to the site of action (Jeffrey & Summerfield, 2010). The recent introduction of multiparameter optimization approaches has streamlined and enhanced the use of calculated physical properties in this area (Wager et al., 2016).

The desired PK profile of a drug will depend on the site of action and the nature of the target. Most commonly, drugs are required to penetrate tissue to reach their target protein and to be present at therapeutically efficacious concentrations for long enough to support once, or at most twice, daily dosing.

The majority of discovery programmes have targeted orally well-absorbed molecules with high metabolic stability to maintain high circulating blood levels for sufficient time to deliver the required duration of action. Thus the duration of action for these agents is related to their PK properties, particularly the rate of clearance from the plasma. An alternative approach has been to identify molecules that have an extended residence time, due to a slow 'off rate', at the target protein that is significantly longer than the time over which an efficacious plasma concentration of the compound is maintained. In such cases, there is a clear mismatch between the PK and pharmacodynamic (PD) half-lives for the compounds, thus obviating the need to maintain high drug levels in the plasma over an extended time period to produce an efficacious response. A potential key advantage of these so-called 'tight binders' is that they may possess an improved safety profile (Vauquelin et al., 2010).

Molecules that fulfil the targeted potency, selectivity and ADME properties will usually progress to in vivo studies in animal models to assess their potential for in vivo efficacy. The relevance of animal models for both efficacy and, in some cases, safety is a matter of much debate within the drug discovery community. With an increasing number of compounds failing to demonstrate clinical efficacy, despite having shown excellent results in preclinical models of disease, it is clear that the animal models are not totally predictive, and a better understanding of the translation of data from animal model to human disease for a particular mechanism is required. Within areas where validated predictive models exist for specific mechanisms, in vivo data can be very powerful both in aiding the selection of advanced molecules as potential development candidates and in predicting the efficacious clinical dose through the use of PK/PD studies that correlate the systemic exposure of the compound with the degree of efficacy.

In addition to the optimization of ADME properties during the lead optimization phase, compounds are also evaluated for potential toxicity, with subsequent chemical modification being applied to mitigate potential risks. A detailed discussion of toxicological evaluation in drug discovery is beyond the scope of this section; however, it is pertinent to mention the function of such assays in the process. Cytotoxicity assays are commonly used alongside cellular functional screens to identify molecules that produce biological activity by virtue of cellular toxicity. An area of intense current interest is that of the potential for compounds to produce adverse cardiovascular effects in the clinic, since cardiovascular toxicity is responsible for a significant number of drug withdrawals. An increasing number of targets, currently confined to ion channels, have been identified and are now commonly included in 'off-target' selectivity panels during lead optimization, the most well characterized of these being the hERG channel (Hancox et al., 2008). The panel of cardiac liability channels being incorporated into screening cascades is increasing, with many groups routinely including other channels, such as Nav1.5, Kv1.5, Cav1.2, KCNQ1 (hmink) among others (Cao et al., 2010). Later in the optimization phase, when potential candidates have been identified, assays to detect genotoxicity are routinely employed. Typically, compounds are tested in both a bacterial mutagenicity assay, such as the Ames test initially, and also in a mammalian screen such as the mouse micronucleus assay (Imbrici

et al., 2018; Reifferscheid & Buchinger, 2010). Prior to being accepted into preclinical development, it is usual to conduct a preliminary in vivo safety study, typically dosing for 7 or 14 days, to provide an initial assessment of the maximum tolerated dose in preparation for subsequent more precise regulatory safety studies (see Chapter 12).

Much of this section has focused on the lead optimization process for oral drugs, and it is important to recognize other routes of administration where the molecule profiles will be significantly different, particularly with respect to ADME and physical properties. Other common routes of administration are inhaled or intranasal, intravenous and topical.

For inhaled drugs, whose site of action is in the lung, a poorly soluble molecule that is highly metabolized in the circulation and of low membrane permeability is often the preferred profile. This profile is aimed at ensuring maximum residence time in the lung for optimal efficacy and minimal systemic exposure, thus reducing the potential for any systemic side-effects (Ritchie et al., 2009; Strong et al., 2018). A similar profile is desirable for topical drugs for application to the skin (Sloan et al., 2006).

For intravenously administered drugs, a very different profile is required, where a highly soluble molecule is preferred (Shi et al., 2009) to allow a low dose volume to be employed. In the latter case, the focus of optimization is generally on the identification of highly potent agents (to facilitate low dose), with high metabolic stability and an acceptable duration of action. For drugs projected to be administered via routes other than the oral route, considerations such as Lipinski guidelines, which address oral bioavailability, are inappropriate.

Addressing attrition

Attrition is currently the major issue facing scientists engaged in the drug discovery process. During the 1990s, the pharmaceutical industry took great steps to identify the reasons responsible for the high attrition rate in development and introduced measures to overcome the issues (Kola & Landis, 2004). The incorporation of both in vitro and in vivo ADME assays in discovery screening cascades significantly reduced the subsequent level of attrition due to poor PK properties during clinical evaluation between 1990 and 2000. However, in 2000, an increased number of molecules were failing due to toxicity (Kola & Landis, 2004). Ten years later, the level of attrition due to toxicity is still high in the discovery phase and much effort is currently being devoted to identifying the key reasons responsible for this.

Of more concern is the level of late-stage attrition, that is, that occurring subsequent to the discovery and development phase, and a worrying number of registered drugs continue to be withdrawn from the market at an unacceptable level. In the last 10 years 17, drugs have been withdrawn (http://en.wikipedia.org/wiki/List_of_withdrawn_drugs) due to adverse drug reactions. Furthermore, adverse drug reactions have been estimated to account for approximately 5% of deaths among hospital patients and 3% of the general population (Wester et al., 2008). The most common toxicities are associated with the liver, the cardiovascular system, skin and blood. Significant efforts are being made to understand the reasons responsible for these toxicities and thus to develop assays capable of identifying molecules possessing the potential to cause these adverse events.

There are four main factors that can give rise to organ toxicities: the overall physical properties of a drug molecule, the primary pharmacology, the secondary or 'off-target' pharmacology and the presence of structural elements known to cause toxicity. The medicinal chemist needs to consider all of these factors when designing potential drug molecules.

Medicinal chemists have long been aware of the relationship between physical properties and 'drug-likeness' (Lipinski et al., 1997); however, reviews (Leeson & Springthorpe, 2007) suggest that a significant percentage of compounds being prepared by major pharmaceutical companies are too highly lipophilic, and it has been proposed that high lipophilicity is likely to be a major cause of toxicity. A study by Pfizer (Price et al., 2009) that investigated potential correlations between physical properties and observed in vivo toxicity for 245 of their preclinical development compounds showed a marked correlation between clogP and toxicity and an inverse correlation between TPSA and toxicity. They concluded that, ideally, a molecule should have a clogP < 3 and TPSA > 75 to reduce the probability of producing toxicity. The importance of reducing lipophilicity cannot be overemphasized, as it has been shown to influence all parameters that the medicinal chemist needs to control in discovering an orally bioavailable drug, including solubility, membrane permeability, plasma protein binding, metabolism (Waring, 2010) and the potential to cause drug–drug interactions (Lewis & Ito, 2010). High lipophilicity has been postulated to increase the probability for promiscuous binding of the compound to 'off-target' proteins thus increasing the likelihood of toxicity (Leeson & Springthorpe, 2007). Despite these analyses performed during the first decade of the century, it appears that chemists have largely ignored them (Leeson, 2016; Leeson & Young, 2015) based on the analysis of recent patents. The reasons are not clear, and it may be that chemists are working more in areas where attrition is less of an issue, for example, oncology or more on indications that require non-oral administration.

Adverse drug reactions have been characterized into three groups (Park et al., 1998). Type A (augmented) adverse reactions are the so-called target-mediated toxicities and are related to the pharmacological effect of the drug, and such adverse events are predictable and dose-related. Type B (idiosyncratic) adverse reactions are unpredictable, often non-dose related, less common but frequently more severe than Type A. Type C (chemical) adverse reactions are related to structural elements in the drug molecule and may be predictable from the molecular structure. This classification is still used today (Kaufmann, 2016).

Type A, augmented or target-mediated, toxicity is an important factor to take into account, particularly when choosing a target or during a target validation exercise. If interacting with the target is likely to cause an adverse event, then the implications of the adverse event in the context of the disease require careful consideration based on the potential benefit of the entity versus its risk. For example, many anticancer agents are cytotoxic and would not be considered suitable treatments for less serious conditions.

Type B, idiosyncratic, toxicity is a growing area of considerable interest (Ulrich, 2007) and the major cause of drug withdrawals. This type of toxicity is often severe and can result in hospitalization and, in extreme cases, death. Data suggest that some of the mechanisms responsible are becoming better understood, but there is still a need for much further work. In particular, the formation of reactive metabolites that may bind covalently to cellular protein and precipitate an immunological response is currently a leading hypothesis to explain at least some of the idiosyncratic toxicity (Kaplowitz, 2005). The potential for a compound to form reactive metabolites can be assessed by a combination of time-dependent CYP450 inhibition studies and electrophile trapping experiments with an agent such as glutathione (Kalgutkar and Didiuk, 2009), followed, if necessary, by detailed covalent protein binding studies (Evans et al., 2004). The major organs affected by idiosyncratic toxicity are the heart, liver, kidneys and skin (Caldwell et al., 2006). It is important that any potential for idiosyncratic toxicity should be considered in the context of the predicted efficacious plasma concentration of the drug and the targeted indication. Empirically, it is assumed that if the dose is 10 mg or less, then the probability of idiosyncratic toxicity is reduced significantly (Uetrecht, 2001).

Cardiovascular toxicity still remains one of the major causes of drug withdrawal, and the removal of clobutinol from clinical usage as a result of cardiac QT interval prolongation (Takahara et al., 2009) highlights the need to study potential drug molecules carefully to assess the risk of this phenomenon. The hERG channel, a potassium channel involved in the repolarization phase of the heart, has been known for some time to be associated with cardiac QT interval prolongation, and there is a good correlation between compounds that have high hERG binding activity and clinical arrhythmogenic activity, particularly the torsade des pointes syndrome (Polak et al., 2009). A variety of assays are available to assess the potential of compounds to inhibit the hERG channel, but it is important to choose the most appropriate in vitro assay and not to rely on data from one assay in isolation (Pollard et al., 2010). It is advisable, for advanced compounds, to obtain data in both in vitro and in vivo assays to allow an informed decision on the potential progression of the molecule. The hERG channel is one of several ion channels (Witchel, 2010) involved in the repolarization phase of the heart, interference with any of which could lead to an adverse cardiovascular effect. Many groups are now screening compounds against a panel of cardiac ion channels throughout the discovery process (see the 'Lead optimization' section).

A number of medicinal chemistry strategies have been adopted to reduce the potential for hERG inhibition that include reducing lipophilicity, modulating the pK_a to reduce π–cationic interactions and reducing the potential for $\pi-\pi$ interactions. The relative success of these strategies has been reviewed (Jamieson et al., 2006). There is currently no available X-ray crystal structure of the hERG channel; however, the value of homology models using known potassium channel structures to guide structural modifications has been effectively demonstrated in the discovery of the CCR5 receptor antagonist, maraviroc (Price et al., 2006).

Drug-induced liver injury is also a major cause of compound attrition, often through the formation of reactive metabolites, and this will be discussed later in this section. A greater understanding is emerging of the possible role of drug–transporter interactions in the development of hepatotoxicity (Lai et al., 2010) that may result in cellular accumulation, impaired efflux, alteration of nutrient transport and altered drug disposition leading to drug–drug interactions. For example, the toxicity of troglitazone has been partially attributed to its interaction with the bile salt export pump (BSEP) (Funk et al., 2001). The number of known transporters is currently growing, and assays are being developed to assess the potential of drugs to cause toxicity through interaction with these proteins (Greer et al., 2010).

Another area of current growing interest, which has been implicated in liver toxicity, and indeed other organs, is the potential of a drug to impair mitochondrial function (Dykens & Will, 2010). This is a complex and developing area that is beyond the scope of this chapter; however, 80% of drugs that have received FDA 'Black Box Warnings' for hepatotoxicity and cardiovascular toxicity have been shown to inhibit mitochondrial function (Dykens & Will, 2007). Assay systems are currently available and a suggested protocol for their use in drug discovery has been published (Dykens & Will, 2010).

Studies have suggested biomarkers that are potentially predictive of liver injury that could be used both preclinically and clinically. Two such biomarkers are the High Mobility Group Box 1 and Keratin 18 proteins (Antoine et al., 2009).

While renal toxicity has not been responsible for a large number of drug withdrawals, it is still a major cause for concern. Interaction with transporter proteins has been implicated in the renal toxicity of a number of substances. Rosuvastatin (Crestor) was shown to cause proteinuria at a dose of dose related proteinuria in phase 3 etc clinical trials. This phenomenon has subsequently been shown to be due to a combination of the target pharmacology of the drug (inhibition of protein endocytosis) and the fact that it is a substrate for the organic anion transporter 3 (OAT3) that causes it to accumulate in the kidney (Windass et al., 2007). Until recently, there has been a lack of predictive biomarkers for renal toxicity; however, a study by an international consortium has identified seven biomarkers that can be used both preclinically and in human studies (Hewitt & Herget, 2009).

Type C or structural-based toxicity is clearly an area that the medicinal chemist should particularly consider before embarking on a chemical modification. Structural alerts, of which the chemist should be aware, can be divided into four groups: chemically reactive functionality, structural elements that present a risk following metabolic activation, DNA binders and CYP450 inhibitors. There are several excellent reviews in the literature covering this area (Blagg, 2006; Kalgutkar & Didiuk, 2009) in detail and describe many structural features that should be given careful consideration before incorporation within a drug molecule. The medicinal chemist is advised to read these carefully and to be aware of new toxicophores as they appear in the literature.

Despite the increasing volume of information, the theoretical prediction of toxicity is still imprecise. It is therefore important to incorporate 'predictive' assays early in screening strategies. Despite recent progress, current in vitro safety testing is conducted in animal cells or, at best, in recombinant human cell lines. It would be preferable to conduct these studies in native human cells, and advances in stem cell research facilitate this opportunity in the future (Balls, 2010). While toxicity is a major cause of compound failure, the failure of potential drug molecules to demonstrate efficacy upon clinical evaluation is a more difficult issue to address since the factors that contribute to these failures are complex. Inadequate target validation, poor predictability of animal models, poor clinical trial design and patient selection are potential causes. While the medicinal chemist cannot address all of these issues, it is important that potent, selective and safe molecules with appropriate physical properties are identified for such studies to ensure that it is the mechanism of action of the drug that is being tested and not the quality of the molecule. Greater involvement of the medicinal chemist at the initial target identification and validation stage may provide better tool or probe compounds (see the 'Target selection and validation' section) with which to validate novel targets.

Summary

The environment in which drug discovery is taking place is currently undergoing considerable change and will continue to do so for some time to come. The downsizing of major Pharma and the increased focus on academic drug discovery are attempts to deal with the escalating costs, high attrition rate and patent expiries that are threatening the viability of the current discovery model.

This chapter is intended to convey the message that the medicinal chemist has an extremely important role to play in all aspects of the discovery process to address the challenges of increasing efficiency and productivity and reducing attrition. While traditionally the medicinal chemist has not become engaged with the drug discovery process until the lead identification phase, there is a compelling argument for their involvement at the target selection and validation stage. The identification of high-quality chemical probes as early as possible will enable robust target validation and the selection of those biological targets that are more likely to succeed.

Furthermore, an increasing array of technological advances are becoming available that will enable the chemist to develop a detailed understanding of the biophysics associated with compound-target engagement that can be effectively incorporated into the design of suitable preclinical candidates.

While significant progress has been made over the past 10 to 15 years in reducing attrition due to poor ADME properties, toxicity remains a major source of attrition and the chemist has an important role to play in reducing the late-stage attrition due to compound-related toxicity. While the current predictive packages are imperfect, there is a developing understanding of the impact of chemical structure and physicochemical properties on toxicity. It is anticipated that an increasing number of screening assays will become available for incorporation into project screening cascades that will help to identify potential risks as early as possible in the discovery process.

Thus while the industry is entering uncharted territory, there is an unprecedented opportunity for the medicinal chemist to make a major contribution to the future success of the discovery of new and important medicines to meet the growing level of unmet clinical need.

References

Antoine, D. J., Williams, D. P., Kipar, A., Jenkins, R. E., Regan, S. L., Sathish, J. G., et al. (2009). High-Mobility Group Box-1 Protein and Keratin-18, circulating serum proteins informative of acetaminophen-induced necrosis and apoptosis in vivo. *Toxicological Sciences, 112*(2), 521–531.

Antolin, A. A., Tym, J. E., Komianou, A., Collins, I., Workman, P., Al-Lazikani, B. (2018). Objective, quantitative, data-driven assessment of chemical probes. *Cell Chemical Biology, 25*(2), 194–205.

Arrowsmith, C. H., Audia, J. E., Austin, C., Baell, J., Bennett, J., Blagg, J., et al. (2015). The promise and peril of chemical probes. *Nature Chemical Biology, 11*(8), 536–541.

Balls, M. (2010). Adult human stem cells and toxicity—realising the potential. *Alternatives to Laboratory Animals, 38*(2), 91–92.

Baringhaus, K. H., & Matter, H. (2005). Efficient strategies for lead optimization by simultaneously addressing affinity, selectivity and pharmacokinetic parameters. In R. Mannhold, H. Kubinyi, G. Folkers, & T. I. Oprea (Eds.), *Chemoinformatics in drug discovery*, 333–79.

Bartoschek, S., Klabunde, T., Defossa, E., Dietrich, V., Stengelin, S., Griesinger, C., et al. (2010). Drug design for G-protein-coupled receptors by a ligand-based NMR method. *Angewandte Chemie (International Ed. in English), 49*(8) 1426–1429.

Blagg, J. (2006). Structure-activity relationships for in vitro and in vivo toxicity. *Annual Reports in Medicinal Chemistry, 41*, 358.

Bleicher, K. H., Boehm, H. J., Mueller, K., & Alanine, A. I. (2003). A guide to drug discovery: Hit and lead generation: Beyond high-throughput screening. *Nature Reviews. Drug Discovery, 2*(5), 369–378.

Boss, C., Hazemann, J., Kimmerlin, T., von Korff, M., Lüthi, U., Peter, O., et al. (2017). The screening compound collection: A key asset for drug discovery. *Chimia (Aarau), 71*(10), 667–677.

Caldwell, G. W., & Yan, Z. (2006). Screening for reactive intermediates and toxicity assessment in drug discovery. *Current Opinion in Drug Discovery & Development, 9*(1), 47–60.

Cao, X., Lee, Y. T., Holmqvist, M., Lin, Y., Ni, Y., Mikhailov, D., et al. (2010). Cardiac ion channel safety profiling on the IonWorks Quattro automated patch clamp system. *Assay and Drug Development Technologies, 8*(6), 766–780.

Cao, L., McDonnell, A., Nitzsche, A., Alexandrou, A., Saintot, P. P.,

Loucif, A. J., et al. (2016). Pharmacological reversal of a pain phenotype in iPSC-derived sensory neurons and patients with inherited erythromelalgia. *Science Translational Medicine*, 8(335), 335ra56.

Carr, R., & Jhoti, H. (2002). Structure-based screening of low-affinity compounds. *Drug Discovery Today*, 7(9), 522–527.

Bass, A. S., Cartwright, M. E., Mahon, C., Morrison, R., Snyder, R., McNamara, P., et al. (2009). Exploratory drug safety— a drug discovery strategy to reduce attrition in development. *Journal of Pharmacological and Toxicological Methods*, 60(1), 69–78.

Chang, G., Steyn, S. J., Umland, J. P., & Scott, D. O. (2010). Strategic use of plasma and microsome binding to exploit in vitro clearance in early drug discovery. *ACS Medicinal Chemistry Letters*, 1(2), 50–53.

Cheeseright, T. J., Mackey, M. D., Melville, J. L., & Vinter, J. G. (2008). FieldScreen: Virtual screening using molecular fields. Application to the DUD data set. *Journal of Chemical Information and Modeling*, 48(11), 2108–2117.

Colas, C., Ung, P. M., & Schlessinger, A. (2016). SLC transporters: Structure, function, and drug discovery. *Medchemcomm*, 7, 1069–1081.

Chu, V., Einolf, H. J., Evers, R., Kumar, G., Moore, D., Ripp, S., et al. (2009). In vitro and in vivo induction of cytochrome P450: A survey of the current practices and recommendations: A pharmaceutical research and manufacturers of America perspective. *Drug Metabolism and Disposition*, 37(7), 1339.

Cole, P. A. (2008). Chemical probes for histone-modifying enzymes. *Nature Chemical Biology*, 4(10), 590–597.

Congreve, M., Chessari, G., Tisi, D., & Woodhead, A. J. (2008). Recent developments in fragment-based drug discovery. *Journal of Medicinal Chemistry*, 51(13), 3661–3680.

Corbin-Leftwich, A., Mossadeq, S. M., Ha, J., Ruchala, I., Le, A. H., Villalba-Galea, C. A. (2016). Retigabine holds KV7 channels open and stabilizes the resting. *Journal of General Physiology*, 147(3), 229–241.

Cragg, G. M., & Newman, D. J. (2013). Natural products: A continuing source of novel drug leads. *Biochimica et Biophysica Acta*, 1830(6), 3670–3695.

Dechecchi, M. C. (2018). Molecular basis of cystic fibrosis: From bench to bedside. *Annals of Translational Medicine*, 6(17), 334.

Luheshi, L. M., Crowther, D. C., & Dobson, C. M. (2008). Protein misfolding and disease: From the test tube to the organism. *Current Opinion in Chemical Biology*, 12(1), 25–31.

Doss, G. A., & Baillie, T. A. (2006). Addressing metabolic activation as an integral component of drug design. *Drug Metabolism Reviews*, 38(4), 641–649.

Dykens, J. A., & Will, Y. (2007). The significance of mitochondrial toxicity testing in drug development. *Drug Discovery Today*, 12(17-18), 777–785.

Dykens, J. A., & Will, Y. (2010). Drug-induced mitochondrial dysfunction: An emerging model of idiosyncratic drug toxicity. *International Drug Discovery*, 5(3), 32–36.

Eglen, R. M., Gilchrist, A., & Reisine, T. (2008). The use of immortalized cell lines in GPCR screening: The good, bad and ugly. *Combinatorial Chemistry & High Throughput Screening*, 11(7), 560–565.

Ekroos, M., & Sjögren, T. (2006). Structural basis for ligand promiscuity in cytochrome P 450 3A4. *Proceedings of the National Academy of Sciences of the United States of America*, 103(37), 13682–13687.

Ejskjaer, N., Vestergaard, E. T., Hellström, P. M., Gormsen, L. C., Madsbad, S., Madsen, J. L., et al. (2009). Ghrelin receptor agonist (TZP-101) accelerates gastric emptying in adults with diabetes and symptomatic gastroparesis. *Alimentary Pharmacology & Therapeutics*, 29(11), 1179–1187.

Evans, D. C., Watt, A. P., Nicoll-Griffith, D. A., & Baillie, T. A. (2004). Drug-protein adducts: An industry perspective on minimizing the potential for drug bioactivation in drug discovery and development. *Chemical Research in Toxicology*, 17(1), 3–16.

Foti, R. S., Wienkers, L. C., & Wahlstrom, J. L. (2010). Application of cytochrome P450 drug interaction screening in drug discovery. *Combinatorial Chemistry & High Throughput Screen*, 13(2), 145–158.

Fox, S., Farr-Jones, S., Sopchak, L., Boggs, A., Nicely, H. W., Khoury, R., et al. (2006). High-throughput screening: Update on practices and success. *Journal of Biomolecular Screening*, 11(7), 864–869.

Fry, D. C. (2015). Targeting protein-protein interactions for drug discovery. *Methods in Molecular Biology*, 1278, 93–106.

Frye, S. V. (2010). The art of the chemical probe. *Nature Chemical Biology*, 6(3), 159–161.

Funk, C., Ponelle, C., Scheuermann, G., & Pantze, M. (2001). Cholestatic potential of troglitazone as a possible factor contributing to troglitazone-induced hepatotoxicity: In vivo and in vitro interaction at the canalicular bile salt export pump (BSEP) in the rat. *Molecular Pharmacology*, 59(3), 627–635.

Gashaw, I., Ellinghaus, P., Sommer, A., & Asadullah, K. (2012). What makes a good drug target? *Drug Discovery Today*, 17, S24–S30.

Giannetti, A. M., Koch, B. D., & Browner, M. F. (2008). Surface plasmon resonance based assay for the detection and characterization of promiscuous inhibitors. *Journal of Medicinal Chemistry*, 51(3), 574–580.

Gluckman, P. D., & Heindel, J. J. (2008). In utero and early-life conditions and adult health and disease—in reply. *New England Journal of Medicine*, 359(14), 1524.

Greer, M. L., Barber, J., Eakins, J., & Kenna, J. G. (2010). Cell based approaches for evaluation of drug induced liver injury. *Toxicology*, 268(3), 125.

Grover, A., & Benet, L. Z. (2009). Effects of drug transporters on volume of distribution. *AAPS Journal*, 11(2), 250–261.

Halai, R., & Craik, D. J. (2009). Conotoxins: Natural product drug leads. *Natural Product Reports*, 26(4), 526–536.

Hancox, J. C., McPate, M. J., El Harchi, A., & Zhang, Y. H. (2008). The hERG potassium channel and hERG screening for drug-induced torsades de pointes. *Pharmacology & Therapeutics*, 119(2), 118–132.

Hart, C. P. (2005). Finding the target after screening the phenotype. *Drug Discovery Today*, 10(7), 513–519.

Harvey, A. L. (2008). Natural products in drug discovery. *Drug Discovery Today*, 13(19/20), 894–901.

Harvey, A. L., Clark, R. L., Mackay, S. P., & Johnston, B. F. (2010). Current strategies for drug discovery through natural products. *Expert Opinion on Drug Discovery*, 5(6), 559–568.

Hellström, P. M. (2009). Faces of ghrelin— research for the 21st century. *Neurogastroenterology and Motility*, 21(1), 2.

Henniot, A., Collins, J. C., & Nuss, J. M. (2018). The current state of peptide drug discovery: Back to the future. *Journal of Medicinal Chemistry*, 61(4), 1382–1414.

Hewitt, P., & Herget, T. (2009). Value of new biomarkers for safety testing in drug development. *Expert Review of Molecular Diagnostics*, 9(6), 531–536.

Howard, M. J., Hill, J. J., Galluppi, G. R., & McLean, M. A. (2010). Plasma protein binding in drug discovery and development. *Combinatorial Chemistry & High Throughput Screening, 13*(2), 170–187.

Hughes, B. (2010). 2009 FDA drug approvals. *Nature Reviews. Drug discovery, 9*(2), 89–92.

Hughes, J. P., Rees, S., Kalindjian, S. B., & Philpott, K. L. (2011). Principles of early drug discovery. *British Journal of Pharmacology, 162*(6), 1239–1249.

Imbrici, P., Nicolotti, O., Leonetti, F., Conte, D., & Liantonio, A. (2018). Ion channels in drug discovery and safety pharmacology. *Methods in Molecular Biology, 1800*, 313–326.

Jacquemard, C. (2019). A bright future for fragment-based drug discovery: What does it hold? *Expert Opinion on Drug Discovery, 14*(5), 413–416.

Jamieson, C., Moir, E. M., Rankovic, Z., & Wishart, G. (2006). Medicinal chemistry of hERG optimizations: Highlights and hang-ups. *Journal of Medicinal Chemistry, 49*(17), 5029–5046.

Jarvis, L. M. (2019). The new drugs of 2018. *Chemical Engineering News, 9*(3), 33–37.

Jeffrey, P., & Summerfield, S. (2010). Assessment of the blood–brain barrier in CNS drug discovery. *Neurobiology of Disease, 37*(1), 33–37.

Kaczorowski, G. J., McManus, O. B., Priest, B. T., & Garcia, M. L. (2008). Ion channels as drug targets: The next GPCRs. *Journal of General Physiology, 131*(5), 399–405.

Kalgutkar, A. S., & Didiuk, M. T. (2009). Structural alerts, reactive metabolites, and protein covalent binding: How reliable are these attributes as predictors of drug toxicity? *Chemistry & Biodiversity, 6*(11), 2115–2137.

Kaplowitz, N. (2005). Idiosyncratic drug hepatotoxicity. *Nature Reviews. Drug Discovery, 4*(6), 489–499.

Karawajczyk, A., Orrling, K. M., de Vlieger, J. S., Rijnders, T., & Tzalis, D. (2016). The European Lead Factory: A blueprint for public–private partnerships in early drug discovery. *Frontiers in Medicine, 3*, 75.

Kaufmann, G. (2016). Adverse drug reactions: Classification, susceptibility and reporting. *Nursing Standard, 30*(50), 53–63.

Keserü, G. M., & Makara, G. M. (2009). The influence of lead discovery strategies on the properties of drug candidates. *Nature Reviews. Drug Discovery, 8*(3), 203–212.

Kola, I., & Landis, J. (2004). Opinion: Can the pharmaceutical industry reduce attrition rates? *Nature Reviews. Drug discovery, 3*(8), 711–716.

Konteatis, Z. D. (2010). In silico fragment-based drug design. *Expert Opinion on Drug Discovery, 5*(11), 1047–1065.

Lai, Y., Sampson, K. E., & Stevens, J. C. (2010). Evaluation of drug transporter interactions in drug discovery and development. *Combinatorial Chemistry & High Throughput Screening, 13*(2), 112–134.

Leeson, P. D., & Springthorpe, B. (2007). The influence of drug-like concepts on decision-making in medicinal chemistry. *Nature Reviews. Drug discovery, 6*(11), 881–890.

Leeson, P. D., & Young, R. J. (2015). Molecular property design: Does everyone get it? *ACS Medicinal Chemistry Letters, 6*(7), 722–725.

Leeson, P. D. (2016). Molecular inflation, attrition and the rule of five. *Advanced Drug Delivery Reviews, 101*, 22–33.

Lewis, D., & Ito, Y. (2010). Human CYPs involved in drug metabolism, structures, substrates and binding affinities. *Expert Opinion on Drug Metabolism & Toxicology, 6*(6), 661–674.

Lewis, D. F., Lake, B. G., & Dickins, M. (2007). Quantitative structure-activity relationships (QSARs) in inhibitors of various cytochromes P450: The importance of compound lipophilicity. *Journal of Enzyme Inhibition and Medicinal Chemistry, 22*(1), 1–6.

Lindsley, C. W., Weaver, D., Bridges, T. M., & Kennedy, J. P. (2009). Lead optimization in drug discovery. *Wiley Encyclopedia Chem Biol, 2*, 511–519.

Ling, L. L., Schneider, T., Peoples, A. J., Spoering, A. L., Engels, I., Conlon, B. P., et al. (2015). A new antibiotic kills pathogens without detectable resistance. *Nature, 517*, 455–459.

Lipinski, C. A., Lombardo, F., Dominy, B. W., & Feeney, P. J. (1997). Experimental and computational approaches to estimate solubility and permeability in drug discovery and development settings. *Advanced Drug Delivery Reviews, 23*(1–3), 3–25.

Lombardi, D., & Dittrich, P. S. (2010). Advances in microfluidics for drug discovery. *Expert Opinion on Drug Discovery, 5*(11), 1081–1094.

Macarron, R., Banks, M. N., Bojanic, D., Burns, D. J., Cirovic, D. A., Garyantes, T., et al. (2011). Impact of high-throughput screening in biomedical research. *Nature Reviews. Drug discovery, 10*(3), 188–195.

McGuire, C., & Lee, J. (2010). Brief review of vorinostat. *Clinical Medicine Insights Therapeutics, 2*, 83–88.

Nagai, N. (2010). Drug interaction studies on new drug applications—current situation and regulatory view in Japan. *Drug Metabolism and Pharmacokinetics, 25*(1), 3–15.

Naik, P., Murumkar, P., Giridhar, R., & Yadav, M. R. (2010). Angiotensin II receptor type 1 (AT1) selective nonpeptidic antagonists—A perspective. *Bioorganic & Medicinal Chemistry, 18*(24), 8418–8456.

Newman, D. J., & Cragg, G. M. (2007). Natural products as sources of new drugs over the last 25 years. *Journal of Natural Products, 70*(3), 461–477.

Orita, M., Warizaya, M., Amano, Y., Ohno, K., & Niimi, T. (2009). Advances in fragment-based drug discovery platforms. *Expert Opinion on Drug Discovery, 4*(11), 1125–1144.

Oyrer J, Maljevic S, Scheffer IE, Berkovic SF, Petrou S, Reid CA. Ion Channels in Genetic Epilepsy: From Genes and Mechanisms to Disease-Targeted Therapies. *Pharmacol Rev*, 2018 Jan; *70*(1), 142–173.

Park, K. B., Breckenridge, A. M., Kitteringham, N. R., & Park, B. K. (1998). Adverse drug reactions. *BMJ, 316*(7140), 1295–1298.

Pepys, M. B., Herbert, J., Hutchinson, W. L., Tennent, G. A., Lachmann, H. J., Gallimore, J. R., et al. (2002). Targeted pharmacological depletion of serum amyloid P component for treatment of human amyloidosis. *Nature, 417*(6886), 254–259.

Pepys, M. B., Hirschfield, G. M., Tennent, G. A., Gallimore, J. R., Kahan, M. C., Bellotti, V., et al. (2006). Targeting C-reactive protein for the treatment of cardiovascular disease. *Nature, 440*(7088), 1217–1221.

Polak, S., Wiśniowska, B., & Brandys, J. (2009). Collation, assessment and analysis of literature in vitro data on hERG receptor blocking potency for subsequent modeling of drugs' cardiotoxic properties. *Journal of Applied Toxicology, 29*(3), 183–206.

Pollard, C. E., Abi Gerges, N., Bridgland-Taylor, M. H., Easter, A., Hammond, T. G., & Valentin, J. P. (2010). An introduction to QT interval prolongation and non-clinical approaches to assessing and reducing risk. *British Journal of Pharmacology, 159*(1), 12–21.

Popescu, I., Fleshner, P. R., Pezzullo, J. C., Charlton, P. A., Kosutic, G., & Senagore, A. J. (2010). The Ghrelin agonist TZP-101 for management of postoperative ileus after partial colectomy: A randomized, dose-ranging, placebo-controlled clinical trial. *Diseases of the Colon and Rectum*, 53(2), 126–134.

Price, D. A., Blagg, J., Jones, L., Greene, N., & Wager, T. (2009). Physicochemical drug properties associated with toxicological outcomes—a review. *Expert Opinion on Drug Metabolism & Toxicology*, 5(8), 921–931.

Price, D. A., Armour, D., de Groot, M., Leishman, D., Napier, C., Perros, M., et al. (2006). Overcoming HERG affinity in the discovery of the CCR5 antagonist maraviroc. *Bioorganic & Medicinal Chemistry Letters*, 16(17), 4633–4637.

Proudfoot, J. R. (2002). Drugs, leads, and drug-likeness: An analysis of some recently launched drugs. *Bioorganic & Medicinal Chemistry Letters*, 12(12), 1647–1650.

Quentin, D., & Raunser, S. (2018). Electron cryomicroscopy as a powerful tool in biomedical research. *Journal of Molecular Medicine (Berlin, Germany)*, 96(6), 483–493.

Rees, D. C., Congreve, M., Murray, C. W., & Carr, R. (2004). Fragment-based lead discovery. *Nature Reviews. Drug discovery*, 3(8), 660–672.

Reifferscheid, G., & Buchinger, S. (2010). Cell-based genotoxicity testing. Genetically modified and genetically engineered bacteria in environmental genotoxicology. *Advances in Biochemical Engineering/Biotechnology*, 118, 85–112.

Riley, R. J., Grime, K., & Weaver, R. (2007). Time-dependent CYP inhibition. *Expert Opinion on Drug Metabolism & Toxicology*, 3(1), 51–66.

Rishton, G. M. (2003). Reactive compounds and in vitro false positives in HTS. *Drug Discovery Today*, 8(2), 86–96.

Ritchie, T. J., Luscombe, C. N., & Macdonald, S. J. (2009). Analysis of the calculated physicochemical properties of respiratory drugs: Can we design for inhaled drugs yet? *Journal of Chemical Information and Modeling*, 49(4), 1025–1032.

Santos, R. (2017). A comprehensive map of molecular drug targets. *Nature Reviews. Drug Discovery*, 16(1), 19–34.

Schmidtko, A., Lötsch, J., Freynhagen, R., & Geisslinger, G. (2010). Ziconotide for treatment of severe chronic pain. *Lancet*, 375(9725), 1569–1577.

Schneider, G. (2010). Virtual screening: An endless staircase? *Nature Reviews. Drug Discovery*, 9(4), 273–276.

Shi, Y., Porter, W., Merdan, T., & Li, L. C. (2009). Recent advances in intravenous delivery of poorly water-soluble compounds. *Expert Opinion on Drug Delivery*, 6(12), 1261–1282.

Shiau, A. K., Massari, M. E., & Ozbal, C. C. (2008). Back to basics: Label-free technologies for small molecule screening. *Combinatorial Chemistry & High Throughput Screening*, 11(3), 231–237.

Sloan, K. B., Wasdo, S. C., & Rautio, J. (2006). Design for optimized topical delivery: Prodrugs and a paradigm change. *Pharmaceutical Research*, 23(12), 2729–2747.

Smith, G. F. (2009). Medicinal chemistry by the numbers: The physicochemistry, thermodynamics and kinetics of modern drug design. *Progress in Medicinal Chemistry*, 48, 1–29.

Strong, P., Ito, K., Murray, J., & Rapeport, G. (2018). Current approaches to the discovery of novel inhaled medicines. *Drug Discovery Today*, 23(10), 1705–1717.

Swanson, R., & Beasley, J. R. (2010). Pathway-specific, species, and sub-type counterscreening for better GPCR hits in high throughput screening. *Current Pharmaceutical Biotechnology*, 11(7), 757–763.

Takahara, A., Sasaki, R., Nakamura, M., Sendo, A., Sakurai, Y., Namekata, I., et al. (2009). Clobutinol delays ventricular repolaraisation in the guinea pig heart—comparison UIT cardiac effects of hERG K+ channel inhibitor E-4031. *Journal of Cardiovascular Pharmacology*, 54(6), 552–559.

Tate, C. G., & Schertler, G. F. X. (2009). Engineering G protein-coupled receptors to facilitate their structure determination. *Current Opinion in Structural Biology*, 19(4), 386–395.

Teague, S. J., Davis, A. M., Teague, S. J., & Leeson, P. D. (2001). (2001). Is there a difference between leads and drugs? A historical perspective. *Journal of Chemical Information and Computer Sciences*, 41(5), 1308–1315.

Uetrecht, J. (2001). Prediction of a new drug's potential to cause idiosyncratic reactions. *Current Opinion in Drug Discovery & Development*, 4(1), 55–59.

Ulrich, R. G. (2007). Idiosyncratic toxicity: A convergence of risk factors. *Annual Review of Medicine*, 58, 17–34.

Vauquelin, G., Wennerberg, M., Balendran, A., Packeu, A. (2010). Estimation of the dissociation rate of unlabelled ligand-receptor complexes by a 'two-step' competition binding approach. *British Journal of Pharmacology*, 161(6), 1311–1328.

Wager, T. T., Hou, X., Verhoest, P. R., & Villalobos, A. (2016). Central nervous system multiparameter optimization desirability: Application in drug discovery. *ACS Chemical Neuroscience*, 7(6) 767–775.

Waldmann, H., Kaiser, M., Wetzel, S., & Kumar, K. (2008). Biology-inspired synthesis of compound libraries. *Cellular and Molecular Life Sciences*, 65(7–8), 1186–1201.

Waldmann, H., Wetzel, S., Klein, K., Renner, S., Rauh, D., Oprea, T. I., et al. (2009). Interactive exploration of chemical space with Scaffold Hunter. *Nature Chemical Biology*, 5(8), 581–583.

Waring, M. J. (2010). Lipophilicity in drug discovery. *Expert Opinion on Drug Discovery*, 5(3), 235–248.

Waxman, S. G., Dib-Hajj, S. D., Cummins, T. R., & Black, J. A. (2007). From genes to pain: Nav1.7 and human pain disorders. *Trends in Neurosciences*, 30(11), 555–563.

Wehling, M. (2009). Assessing the translatability of drug projects: What needs to be scored to predict success? *Nature Reviews. Drug Discovery*, 8(7), 541–546.

Westby, M., & van der Ryst, E. (2005). CCR5 antagonists: Host-targeted antivirals for the treatment of HIV infection. *Antiviral Chemistry & Chemotherapy*, 16(6), 339–354.

Wester, K., Jönsson, A. K., Spigset, O., Druid, H., & Hägg, S. (2008). Incidence of fatal adverse drug reactions: A population based study. *British Journal of Clinical Pharmacology*, 65(4), 573–579.

White, R. E. (2009). Pharmacokinetics of drug candidates. *Wiley Encyclopedia of Chemical Biology*, 3, 652–661.

Whittaker, M., Law, R. J., Ichihara, O., Hesterkamp, T., & Hallett, D. (2010). Fragments: Past, present and future. *Drug Discovery Today Technologies*, 7(3), E163–E171.

Windass, A. S., Lowes, S., Wang, Y., & Brown, C. D. (2007). The contribution of organic anion transporters OAT1 and OAT3 to the renal uptake of rosuvastatin. *Journal of Pharmacology and Experimental Therapeutics*, 322(3), 1221–1227.

Witchel, H. J. (2010). Emerging trends in ion channel-based assays for predicting the cardiac safety of drugs. *IDrugs*, 13(2), 90–96.

Chapter | 8 |

Therapeutic Antibodies

Steven D Grant

Introduction:

Monoclonal antibodies (mAbs) and biopharmaceuticals derived from antibody fragments are one of the largest and most rapidly growing classes of therapeutics. Since the first mAb muromonab-CD3 (trade name Orthoclone OKT3) was licensed for human use by the US Food and Drug Administration (FDA) in 1985 as an antirejection treatment for renal transplantation (Smith, 1996), the antibody therapeutic market has grown to at least US$95.1 billion in 2017 and is expected to reach a value of US$131.3 billion by 2023 (Global Monoclonal Antibodies Market, 2018). As of March 2021, there are 95 therapeutic antibody drugs approved in the European Union (EU) or the United States (Antibody Society; see https://www.antibodysociety.org) treating a diverse range of disease indications, including oncology, autoimmunity and inflammation, respiratory, vascular, infection, metabolic and neurological/migraine. Table 8.1 provides examples of marketed therapeutic antibodies and associated indications. Prior to the advent of mAb therapeutics, serotherapy (pioneered by Emil Behring in the 1890s [Simon, 2007], in which polyclonal antibodies from blood or, more recently, plasma from convalescent donors is administered to patients) has been used to treat a range of diseases including diphtheria, Spanish flu, tetanus, measles, poliovirus, severe acute respiratory syndrome (SARS), Ebola and a phase II clinical trial for severe influenza (Beigel et al., 2017).

Successfully launching a therapeutic antibody onto the clinical market is a hugely complex undertaking typically involving hundreds of individuals from multiple companies and government agencies. Developing an antibody therapy is at least as expensive ($1–$2.5 billion; DiMasi et al., 2016) and time-consuming (10–15 years) as developing other forms of treatment. Antibodies are highly selective binding agents; their effect may be to simply bind the target or to modulate ligand–receptor signalling through antagonizing or agonizing the target receptor. There are some key factors that should be taken into account when considering a therapeutic antibody discovery project:

- Can the antibody access the target to mediate a therapeutic effect? Antibody therapeutic targets are typically extracellular or cell surface–associated proteins (or carbohydrates). Not all therapeutic targets are easily addressed using antibodies. Full-length antibodies cannot traverse cell membranes of viable cells. If the therapeutic target is located in the cytosol, it is unlikely that an antibody will be successful in reaching the intended target (companies and researchers are working on technologies to enable intracellular antibody targeting; Choi et al., 2014).

- Antibodies are complex molecules, and the different regions of the molecule contribute different properties. A number of questions need to be considered at the design intent stage, all of which can influence the antibody selection criteria. These include: what is the anticipated dose and dosing frequency of the therapeutic antibody? Factors that influence this include the systemic molar concentration of the target, or the number of target molecules displayed on the surface of a given cell type, the location of the target in the body and whether the target is recycled back onto the cell surface/extracellular space or internalized into the cell. What is the biological mechanism the antibody is interfering with—is the antibody binding, antagonizing or agonizing the target? What antibody affinity is required for efficacy, for example, to inhibit a receptor–ligand interaction?

- Antibodies are unique molecules derived from specific cell lines. Any change to the sequence of the antibody will require an entirely new cell line and development programme. For this reason, it is especially important

Table 8.1 Therapeutic antibody examples

International non-proprietary name	Brand name	Target; antibody format	Indication first approved or reviewed	First EU/US approval year
Rituximab	MabThera, Rituxan	CD20; chimeric IgG1	Non-Hodgkin's lymphoma	1998/1997
Infliximab	Remicade	TNF; chimeric IgG1	Crohn's disease	1999/1998
Palivizumab	Synagis	RSV; humanized IgG1	Prevention of respiratory syncytial virus infection	1999/1998
Adalimumab	Humira	TNF; human IgG1	Rheumatoid arthritis	2003/2002
Omalizumab	Xolair	IgE; humanized IgG1	Asthma	2005/2003
Bevacizumab	Avastin	VEGF; humanized IgG1	Colorectal cancer	2005/2004
Ranibizumab	Lucentis	VEGF; humanized IgG1 Fab	Macular degeneration	2007/2006
Ofatumumab	Arzerra	CD20; human IgG1	Chronic lymphocytic leukaemia	2010/2009
Belimumab	Benlysta	BLyS; human IgG1	Systemic lupus erythematosus	2011/2011
Ipilimumab	Yervoy	CTLA-4; human IgG1	Metastatic melanoma	2011/2011
Pembrolizumab	Keytruda	PD1; humanized IgG4	Melanoma	2015/2014
Evolocumab	Repatha	PCSK9; human IgG2	High cholesterol	2015/2015
Mepolizumab	Nucala	IL-5; humanized IgG1	Severe eosinophilic asthma	2015/2015
Benralizumab	Fasenra	IL-5Rα; humanized IgG1	Asthma	2018/2017
Dupilumab	Dupixent	IL-4Rα; human IgG4	Atopic dermatitis	2017/2017
Ocrelizumab	OCREVUS	CD20; Humanized IgG1	Multiple sclerosis	2018/2017
Erenumab	Aimovig	CGRP receptor; human IgG2	Migraine prevention	2018/2018

BLyS, B Lymphocyte Stimulator; *CGRP*, Calcitonin gene-related peptide; *CTLA4*, cytotoxic T-lymphocyte-associated protein-4; *Fab*, antigen-binding fragment; *IgG*, immunoglobulin G; *IL*, interleukin; *PCSK9*, Proprotein convertase subtilisin/kexin type 9; *PD1*, Programmed cell death protein 1; *RSV*, respiratory syncytial virus; *TNF*, tumour necrosis factor; *VEGF*, vascular endothelial growth factor. Data from the Antibody Society (https://www.antibodysociety.org/news/approved-antibodies/).

to ensure that the selected molecule has all of the desired properties, as subsequent changes are very difficult to implement.

- Antibodies need to be given parenterally, in many cases intermittently, but, nonetheless, this may make this approach less suitable for the treatment of some conditions.
- Will the drug be first to market/launch? Development of biopharmaceuticals is especially complex. If not first to market, the new drug must have a clear differentiating advantage over competing drugs, such as improved safety, fewer or less severe side-effects, improved route of administration or significantly lower cost.

The focus of this chapter will primarily be on how the pharmaceutical industry discovers, optimizes and develops mAbs into therapeutics drugs.

Antibody structure and properties

Almost all therapeutic mAbs are based on the immunoglobulin G (IgG) isotype class of antibodies. Natural IgG is a complex bivalent Y-shaped glycoprotein, composed of four protein chains (two identical heavy chains

and two identical light chains) with N-linked carbohydrates attached to the heavy chain Fc region (Fig. 8.1). Each heavy and light chain is composed of variable and constant domains (the light chain possesses one variable domain and one constant domain; the heavy chain possesses one variable domain and three constant domains). The variable domains are at the top of the Y-shaped structure and bind the target antigen. The constant domains comprising the Fc region (base of the Y-shaped structure) of the antibody elicit effector functions through engagement of the Fc gamma receptors (FcγR), the neonatal Fc-receptor (FcRn) or complement. The heavy and light chains are linked together via disulfide bonds that help to stabilize the IgG. The biological mechanisms of how antibodies are created *in vivo* are not covered, as this is reviewed extensively elsewhere (Male et al., 2012).

Several properties of antibody molecules (particularly IgG) make them particularly useful as therapeutics. For example, they can be selected or engineered to bind with high affinity (nM to pM) to their target antigen; they typically have very low or no detectable off-target binding (nonspecific target binding); they can bind to the FcγR (CD16, CD32, CD64) (Takai, 2005) to activate and recruit

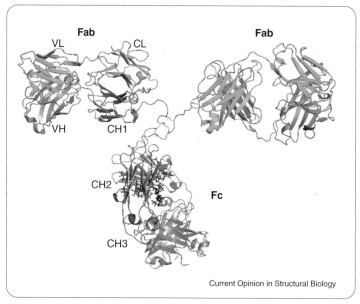

Fig. 8.1 Structural model of a human IgG$_1$. The Fab region is composed of the interaction between the variable heavy chain and CH1 domains with the variable light chain and constant light (CL) domains. The light chain is coloured in *green*, with the variable region coloured in *bright green*. The heavy chain is coloured *brown*, with the corresponding variable region coloured in *orange*. The CH2 domain contains N-linked glycosylation sites (carbohydrate residues depicted in *blue*) that orient between the two heavy chains in the Fc region. *VH*, Variable heavy chain; *VL*, variable light chain. (From Chiu, M. L., & Gilliland, G. L. [2016]. Engineering antibody therapeutics. *Current Opinion in Structural Biology, 38*, 163–173.)

immune cells and thereby bridge the adaptive and innate functions of the immune system; they can activate the complement cascade; their molecular mass (~150 kDa) is above the renal clearance cutoff, so they are not excreted and they bind to the neonatal receptor under acidic pH so are rescued from lysosomal proteolytic degradation, resulting in mAbs typically possessing a half-life ($T_{1/2}$) in human serum that is of sufficient duration to enable dosing once every 2 to 4 weeks (depending on the target class and the *in vivo* concentration of the target). Since mAbs are glycoproteins, composed of amino acids and carbohydrates, they are broken down and catabolized, and there are no synthetic byproducts to be eliminated from the body (unless conjugated to a synthetic immunotoxin, for example).

There are also disadvantages to using antibodies as therapeutics: mAbs are complex multichain proteins containing carbohydrate groups that are added post-translationally so require expensive eukaryotic manufacturing and extensive quality control. For some diseases, engaging with cells via the FcγR may be undesirable or detrimental (so non-binding Fc mutants or IgG4 isotype may be more desirable). mAbs are too large to pass efficiently across the blood–brain barrier (BBB) to enter the brain when injected systemically, only between 0.1% and 1% of systemically

injected mAbs pass into the cerebrospinal fluid (CNS is incorrect, should be (CSF)). (Boado et al., 2010).

Therapeutic antibody discovery

To initiate a therapeutic antibody campaign, a suitable therapeutic target needs to be identified that is implicated in the disease pathway and is accessible to antibody engagement. Typically, this restricts therapeutic targets to those that are cell surface expressed or released into the systemic circulation or interstitial space. To enable *in vivo* immunization or *in vitro* antibody selections, a supply of therapeutic target (ideally purified) is required against which to select antibodies. The therapeutic target can be purified from *in vivo* sources (i.e., soluble protein/carbohydrates, cell membrane preparations) or manufactured recombinantly (i.e., soluble proteins, truncated protein fragments, amino acid peptides, cell lines expressing recombinant cell surface proteins, virus-like particles displaying the protein of interest on their surface, DNA for *in vivo* immunization/transfection).

Once a supply of therapeutic target has been generated, researchers utilize their antibody discovery platform(s) to generate a panel of *in vivo*–derived mAbs or a panel of *in vitro* clones for subsequent screening to identify hit molecules possessing desirable biological and biophysical properties using a variety of assays. The ideal strategy would be to screen a panel of antibody clones (hundreds to several thousands) as early as possible in a suitable functional assay. However, in practice, this is difficult to implement, and so strategies are used to identify clones that bind the target by various techniques such as enzyme-linked immunosorbent assay (ELISA), kinetic off-rate ranking (which is concentration independent) and flow cytometry against a recombinant cell line expressing the target of interest or primary cells. Once a panel of binding clones has been identified, unique antibody clones based on their DNA sequence are expressed, purified and tested in various functional cell assays to determine their biological potency. Further triaging of the clones takes place, and ultimately, tens to hundreds of clones are tested in a primary cell assay using blood cells or tissue derived from healthy donors or patients. For *in vitro*–derived hit clones, a subsequent affinity maturation campaign may be required to increase the affinity of the lead clones to therapeutically relevant levels. Likewise, antibodies derived from wild-type mice (or other species) would need to undergo humanization to make the antibody amino acid sequence more human-like to reduce the chance of patient-derived antidrug antibodies being generated following repeated administration of the antibody drug. Following humanization or affinity maturation, kinetic and functional assays are repeated to identify improved variants or to demonstrate that the humanization procedure did not adversely impact the potency of the antibodies compared with the mouse parental clones (biophysical assessment is covered in more detail later in this chapter). From this panel of clones, a lead antibody sequence and potentially a backup molecule(s) would be advanced into cell line development.

The following paragraphs describe in more detail *in vivo* and *in vitro* platforms and technologies used to identify potential therapeutic lead antibody molecules.

Antibody discovery using *in vivo* technologies

For therapeutic use, researchers have developed multiple approaches to exploit the natural immune response of an animal (typically mice) through repeated injection with the desired antigen, followed by generating hybridomas and screening the resulting antibodies for the required activity. More recently, advances in technology have allowed direct screening of individual B cells or plasma cells from immunized animals to identify antibodies with the required activity and specificity. An advantage of these *in vivo* approaches is that the animal can generate high-affinity antibodies that typically do not require affinity

maturation, unlike *in vitro*–derived antibodies that generally need to have their binding affinities enhanced to be of therapeutic use. Additionally, *in vivo* antibodies are subjected to natural cellular selection processes in the host organism, therefore the resulting antibodies tend to have superior biophysical and drug development properties compared with *in vitro* derived antibodies (particularly earlier generations of *in vitro* libraries). There are also disadvantages to using animals for antibody discovery. One concern is the use of animals for this initial drug discovery approach. Second, *in vivo*–derived antibodies from nonhuman immune repertoires contain exogenous amino acid sequences and therefore will likely be recognized as xenogeneic proteins by patients when repeatedly injected, causing the patient to mount an immune response against the antibody drug. These antibodies can be neutralizing and can dramatically reduce the drug's efficacy. This problem can be addressed by humanizing the antibody (discussed later).

Hybridoma generation

When the immune system is exposed to a foreign antigen, naive B cells expressing a B-cell receptor that binds serendipitously to the foreign antigen are stimulated, divide and mature to generate populations of related B-cell-derived plasma cells producing secreted mAbs. Each plasma cell produces large amounts of secreted antibody with a unique amino acid composition and a defined target antigen specificity. In 1975, George Köhler and César Milstein published a revolutionary technique enabling the generation of mAbs ex vivo (Köhler & Milstein, 1975) through fusing the short-lived antibody-producing B cells with myeloma cells to generate stable immortalized antibody-producing hybrid cells called hybridomas. Hybridomas can be grown in cell culture to produce mAbs that can be purified in substantial amounts from the culture supernatant, paving the way for the exploitation of mAbs in basic research and medicine.

A well-established technique to generate mAbs for both laboratory and clinical (diagnostic and therapeutic) use is to immunize mice with the desired antigen repeatedly, in conjunction with an adjuvant, to stimulate the immune system to generate antibodies against the injected antigen. Following initial immunization, subsequent booster immunizations (typically 2–4) are administered at intervals of 14 to 28 days. The immune titre of the mice is assessed by ELISA through testing a small volume of blood serum (~20 μL) to determine the strength of the immune response. Typically, an increase compared to preimmunization serum samples of 100- to 1000-fold in the antibody titre is observed. Considerations for *in vivo* immunization conditions are reviewed by Leenaars and Hendriksen (2005). When a mouse with the desired immune response is identified, its B cells are recovered and fused with myeloma cells. The resulting hybridoma cells secreting the desired antibody specificity are cloned using limited dilution until a monoclonal hybridoma is identified. Limited dilution is one of several approaches used to identify hybridomas; see Hanack et al. (2016) for additional information.

Direct screening of B cells and plasma cells

mAb discovery using hybridoma fusion technology is a powerful technique that has enabled the identification of numerous antibodies that have been developed into therapeutics. However, hybridoma technology is inefficient, is both time and labour intensive and, in practice, only a few thousand clones can be physically screened. To address these limitations, researchers have over the past decade developed or adapted technologies to enable the high-throughput analysis of individual cells, for example, B cells recovered from the spleen of immunized mice or immunized rabbit peripheral blood mononuclear cells (PBMCs) using fluorescence activated cell sorting (FACS) (Carbonetti et al., 2017; Starkie et al., 2016) or microfluidic encapsulation technologies (Eyer et al., 2017; Köster et al., 2008) that enable the screening of proteins secreted from individual cells (i.e., antibodies secreted from plasma cells). Microfluidic encapsulation technologies involve the compartmentalization of individual cells in picolitre volume emulsion droplets that are assayed for antibody binding or activity at rates of hundreds of droplets per second (Mazutis et al., 2013). Microfluidic encapsulation is ideally suited to *in vivo* antibody discovery, enabling hundreds of thousands of individual B cells or plasma cells to be screened during a single experimental run. Combining binding or functional data with DNA sequencing of the antibody variable genes can enable the rapid identification of a diverse panel of lead antibody molecules, including rare antibodies with unique and desirable characteristics.

Antibody chimerization and humanization

The human immune system is highly tuned to identify and react to exogenous 'foreign' proteins and carbohydrate antigens. When mouse mAbs were initially administered to humans, their clinical efficacy was compromised by an antidrug antibody (ADA) reaction generated by the patients in response to the xenogeneic antibody. These human anti-mouse antibody (HAMA) immune reactions against the therapeutic molecule (Tjandra et al., 1990) reduce or inhibit the activity of the therapeutic antibody through preventing binding to its target or by increasing clearance of the therapeutic antibody from the circulation, thus rapidly decreasing the systemic concentration.

A further disadvantage of using mouse antibodies as human therapeutics is the lack of sufficient effector function *in vivo*. To address the immunogenicity of mouse antibodies and lack of or suboptimal effector function, scientists exploited molecular biology to initially substitute the constant regions of the mouse antibody with human constant regions to generate chimeric molecules (Morrison et al., 1984). A further refinement called 'CDR grafting' enabled the mouse complementarity-determining regions (CDRs) to be cloned onto a human antibody variable region, resulting in humanized antibodies (Jones et al., 1986) containing fewer non-human T-cell epitopes, thereby reducing the likelihood of an ADA reaction (Fig. 8.2). Approximately half of all mAbs marketed in the United States or EU are humanized, the remainder are either fully human or chimeric molecules.

Transgenic mice

With the increasing understanding of human and mouse humoral antibody immune responses, researchers in the 1990s were able to exploit advances in genetic engineering to create transgenic mice expressing human antibodies. The benefit of these mice is that the resulting hybridomas express fully human antibodies, eliminating the requirement to humanize the antibodies for therapeutic use. An additional potential advantage is that fully human antibodies can be expressed directly from the hybridoma cell line (Green, 2014), although most mAbs are currently expressed using Chinese hamster ovary (CHO) cell systems. The first generation of genetically engineered mice, including the XenoMouse (Gerpharm Inc./Medarex Inc./BMS) and HuMAb-Mouse (Cell Genesys Inc./Abgenix Inc./Medarex) (Green, 2014), expressed fully human antibodies *in vivo*, including a human Fc region that potentially results in suboptimal B-cell development due to the human Fc domains possessing xenogenic sequences and cytoplasmic domains when interacting with native mouse immune receptors and intracellular signalling components. Second generation transgenic mice, such as the VelocImmune mouse (Regeneron), expressed chimeric antibody molecules, with human variable regions fused to mouse constant regions, allowing for native immune signalling and immune cell development *in vivo*. Transgenic mice yield antibodies that have undergone natural affinity maturation and typically possess desirable biophysical characteristics, making them an excellent starting point for therapeutic antibody development. Transgenic mice have been successfully used to generate marketed therapeutic antibodies, including ipilimumab (anti-CTLA4), denosumab (anti-Receptor activator of nuclear factor kappa-B ligand [RANKL]) and ofatumumab (anti-CD20) (Brüggemann et al., 2015). For an excellent review of human immune transgenic mice, see Green (2014).

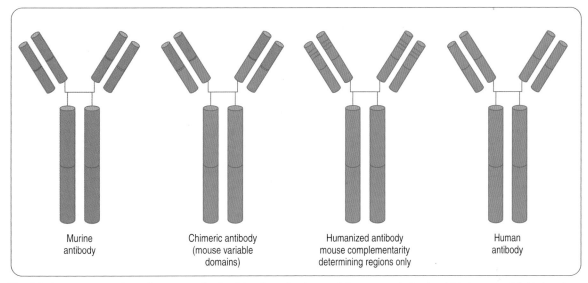

Fig. 8.2 Cartoon comparison of mouse antibody; chimeric antibody containing mouse-derived variable heavy and light domains genetically fused to human constant domains; humanized antibody, where the mouse complementarity-determining regions (CDRs) are grafted into a human antibody; fully human antibody Brown= mouse sequences; Blue= human sequences.

Antibody discovery by *in vitro* technologies

An alternative strategy for creating therapeutic antibodies involves replicating the human immune response *in vitro* in the laboratory. During B-cell development, the naive functional immunoglobulin gene repertoire is generated via the random assembly *in vivo* of variable heavy chain (VH) and variable light chain (VL) gene segments. The naive antibody repertoire is capable of binding to an essentially unlimited diversity of antigen types, with low to moderate affinity. To generate antibodies of higher affinity, when a naive B cell is activated, it undergoes somatic hypermutation, where the amino acid sequence of the CDRs are mutated and improved binding clones enriched.

The power of the *in vivo* immune response can be replicated *in vitro*, where scientists have generated various antibody libraries, including human naive donor libraries, semi-synthetic and fully synthetic libraries. Human naive *in vitro* libraries are generated by cloning the VH and VL (may include both kappa and lambda light chains) antibody gene sequences and replicating the V-D-J and V-J combinations for the variable heavy and light chains, respectively, to create full-length variable heavy and light chains. The cloning can involve using human donor–derived blood samples (typically pooled from multiple donors) to generate a naive library

or generating the VH and VL sequences synthetically by DNA synthesis/polymerase chain reaction (PCR), termed a synthetic library, or a combination of both approaches (semi-synthetic library). Once the antibody library DNA cloning has been performed to replicate the immune repertoire, the genetic information needs to be linked with the physical antibody polypeptide it encodes, referred to as genotype–phenotype linkage. To achieve this genotype–phenotype linkage, phage antibody libraries were developed. This is a powerful technology that enables the identification of a single antibody sequence from a library of 1×10^8 to 1×10^{10} different antibody sequences.

Phage display

To by-pass hybridoma technology and animal immunization, phage display of antibody fragments was developed (Clackson et al., 1991) in which an antibody fragment is typically expressed on the gene III coat protein of nonlytic filamentous bacteriophages (phages), such as M13 or fd. Phages are viruses that infect and replicate in bacteria, such as *Escherichia coli*, generating large numbers of virus particles that are released, and in turn can re-infect more bacteria. Large DNA libraries comprising millions of individual antibody variable genes (VH and VL) are cloned into the phage as either single-chain variable fragment (scFv) or antigen-binding fragment (Fab) fragments and used to transform an *E. coli* culture such that each *E. coli* cell produces only the virus displaying a single antibody specificity on the virus surface (Sheehan & Marasco, 2015). The library of viruses released from the *E. coli* culture provides the critical genotype–phenotype linkage, where the antibody DNA sequence (enabling subsequent cloning of the antibody) is linked with the antigen-binding phenotype of the displayed antibody. The antibody phage library is subjected to multiple rounds of bio-panning against antigens immobilized on a solid surface (i.e., plastic microtitre plate or tube) or in solution (i.e., using biotinylated antigen followed by the addition of streptavidin-coated paramagnetic beads). This enriches for the very rare antigen-binding populations of phage antibody fragments from the vast population (billions) of irrelevant antibody fragments displaying phage. For reviews, see Winter et al. (1994), Frenzel et al. (2017), Sioud (2019) and Hanack et al. (2016).

Phage display technology enabled the generation of naive human libraries (Marks et al., 1991) that can be used to select antibodies against essentially any target antigen, including targets that would not typically elicit an *in vivo* immune response, for example, self-antigens or small chemical haptens. Peripheral blood lymphocytes (PBLs) of unimmunized human donors are isolated and the antibody variable genes recovered by PCR amplification. Genes encoding single-chain Fv fragments or Fab fragments are made by randomly combining heavy and light chain V-genes using PCR and cloned into a phagemid or phage vector that contains the necessary genes and control elements to enable phage virus antibody fragment library production. Synthetic antibody libraries can also be generated (Prassler et al., 2011), where the antibody V-genes for the phage library are synthesized de novo based on antibody gene sequence data. Synthetic libraries can be designed to only use antibody framework sequences that contain desirable properties, such as thermostability, good heterodimer compatibility and frequency found in the natural repertoire, and CDR regions can be engineered to cover diversity observed in natural repertoires determined from hundreds of individuals (Zhai et al., 2011). Semi-synthetic libraries combine approaches of both naive and synthetic library construction, for example, the library framework sequences used may be limited to those possessing desirable biophysical properties, with the CDR3 derived from naive B-cell repertoire and CDR1 and CDR2 derived from memory B repertoire taken from multiple donors. Naive, semi-synthetic and fully synthetic library designs can also be applied to other library display technologies, such as ribosome, yeast or vaccinia display.

Advantages of phage display include the ability to generate fully human therapeutic antibodies without having to immunize animals. The technique can be used to affinity mature antibodies (i.e. to improved the binding of the antibody to its target antigen) and to select antibodies, through deselection, that lack cross-reactivity to closely related proteins. There are disadvantages observed with some antibodies derived from phage systems, including off-target binding resulting in unwanted clinical side-effects and undesirable biophysical properties (e.g., reduced solubility limiting the concentration of mAb that can be formulated for administration, poor expression yields that impact commercial viability when expressing at large scale, immunogenicity in the clinic; Igawa et al., 2011).

Other display technologies

Following the development of phage display, various other display systems have been developed or exploited for antibody discovery. Yeast display, where a yeast cell displays multiple copies of a single antibody specificity in a library of over 100 million yeast cells, with each yeast cell displaying a unique antibody sequence (Sheehan & Marasco, 2015), is a powerful technology enabling more exquisite affinity control of naive selections and affinity maturation, compared with phage selection. It employs flow cytometry to select the desired yeast-binding population (Sivasubramanian et al., 2017). Selections and enrichment of antibodies can be achieved using a combination of phage and yeast display to exploit the strengths of both platforms. For example, using a large phage antibody library for the first rounds of selections, followed by cloning the output into a yeast display platform enables more exquisite affinity pressuring and control of selection conditions during FACS selections. Yeast-displayed antibodies (IgG, scFv or Fab) tend to be more comparable to those produced by mammalian cells, as compared with Fab or scFv produced by *E. coli* libraries. This is because yeast cells use eukaryotic protein expression pathways and incorporate posttranslational modifications (although yeast and mammalian glycosylation profiles are different). A disadvantage of yeast libraries is that they are typically several orders of magnitude smaller than phage-based libraries.

Alternatives to yeast display technologies include mammalian/virus and ribosome display. Vaccinia virus–mediated mammalian cell display has been used to display full-length functional IgG on the surface of mammalian cells (Smith & Zauderer, 2014). Ribosome display (Hanes & Plückthun, 1997; He & Taussig, 1997; Li et al., 2019) utilizes a cell-free system to enable the display of very large DNA libraries (1×10^{12} to 1×10^{14} unique variants). The DNA library is transcribed into mRNA, which is then used as a template for *in vitro* translation. Genotype–phenotype linkage is achieved due to the ribosome stalling on the mRNA (which lacks a stop codon at the 3′ end) thus preventing the ribosome from releasing the newly synthesized scFv polypeptide chain, thereby maintaining a physical link between the mRNA and newly translated protein. Complexes expressing antibody scFv specific for a given target antigen can be selected for a process analogous to phage display, where unbound complexes are washed away, and the remaining complexes eluted, recovered and the antibody sequences amplified by reverse transcription (RT)-PCR.

Hybrid approaches combining both *in vivo* immunization and *in vitro* antibody repertoire screening are also employed by researchers to select lead antibody sequences.

Antibody fragments, bispecific and alternative formats

The focus so far of this chapter has been on the selection of full-length antibody therapeutic molecules; however, academic and industrial antibody engineering laboratories have over the years generated a menagerie of different antibody formats ranging from single-domain antibodies (Enever, 2009) to multivariant constructs (Fig. 8.3) and bispecific antibody formats (Fig. 8.4; for a review, see Spiess et al., 2015) to address specific applications. Some formats have been successful in the clinic, some are still in development and some have failed to make viable therapeutics, usually as a result of poor expression and/or biophysical properties.

The location of the therapeutic target and clinical application are factors that determine which antibody format is most suitable. Antibody single variable domains are around one-tenth the size of IgG_1 (12–15 vs ~150 kDa, respectively), and their small size can confer beneficial or deleterious properties depending on the application. For example, they can modulate both the intracellular and extracellular sides of G-protein-coupled receptors (GPCRs) (Heukers et al., 2019). They have short serum half-lives that are beneficial when being used as imaging reagents (Holliger & Hudson, 2005), where a rapid systemic clearance greatly reduces the nonspecific background signal. A short serum half-life will, however, be unfavourable if the intended mechanism of action is the sustained disruption of a receptor–ligand interaction. The systemic half-life can be extended by genetically fusing the therapeutic variable domain to an albumin-binding peptide or domain (Holt et al., 2008), genetically fusing to an Fc domain or chemically conjugating to polyethylene glycol (PEG) to increase the hydrodynamic radius and apparent molecular weight.

Antibody Fc engineering

The Fc region of an IgG can bind to various activatory FcγR (FcγRI/CD64; FcγRII/CD32; FcγRIII/CD16) or the unique inhibitory FcγR (FcγRIIb/CD32b) (Bruhns, 2012; Takai, 2005) located on the surface of immune cells, acting as a bridge between the adaptive and innate immune responses. Engagement of FcγRs mediates several biological effects, ranging from the induction of antibody-dependent cellular cytotoxicity (ADCC) and antibody-dependent cellular phagocytosis (ADCP), and transcriptional activation of cytokine genes, leading to inflammatory cascades. In addition to engagement of FcγR, antibody Fc can initiate complement activation through binding C1q, resulting in complement-dependent cytotoxicity (CDC), and can bind the FcRn that prolongs the serum half-life of the antibody through endosomal rescue and recycling (Sockolosky and Szoka, 2015).

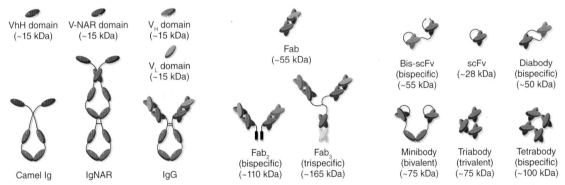

Fig. 8.3 Schematic representation of different antibody formats, showing intact 'classic' immunoglobulin G (IgG) molecules alongside camelid VHH-Ig and shark Ig-NAR immunoglobulins. Camelid VHH-Ig and shark Ig-NARs are unusual immunoglobulin-like structures comprising a homodimeric pair of two chains of V-like and C-like domains (neither has a light chain), in which the displayed V domains bind target independently. Shark Ig-NARs comprise a homodimer of one variable domain (V-NAR) and five C-like constant domains (C-NAR). A variety of antibody fragments are depicted, including Fab, scFv, single-domain VH, VHH and V-NAR and multimeric formats, such as minibodies, bis-scFv, diabodies, triabodies, tetrabodies and chemically conjugated Fab' multimers (sizes given in kilodaltons are approximate). (From Holliger, P., & Hudson, P. J. [2005]. Engineered antibody fragments and the rise of single domains. *Nature Biotechnology*, 23[9], 1126–1136.)

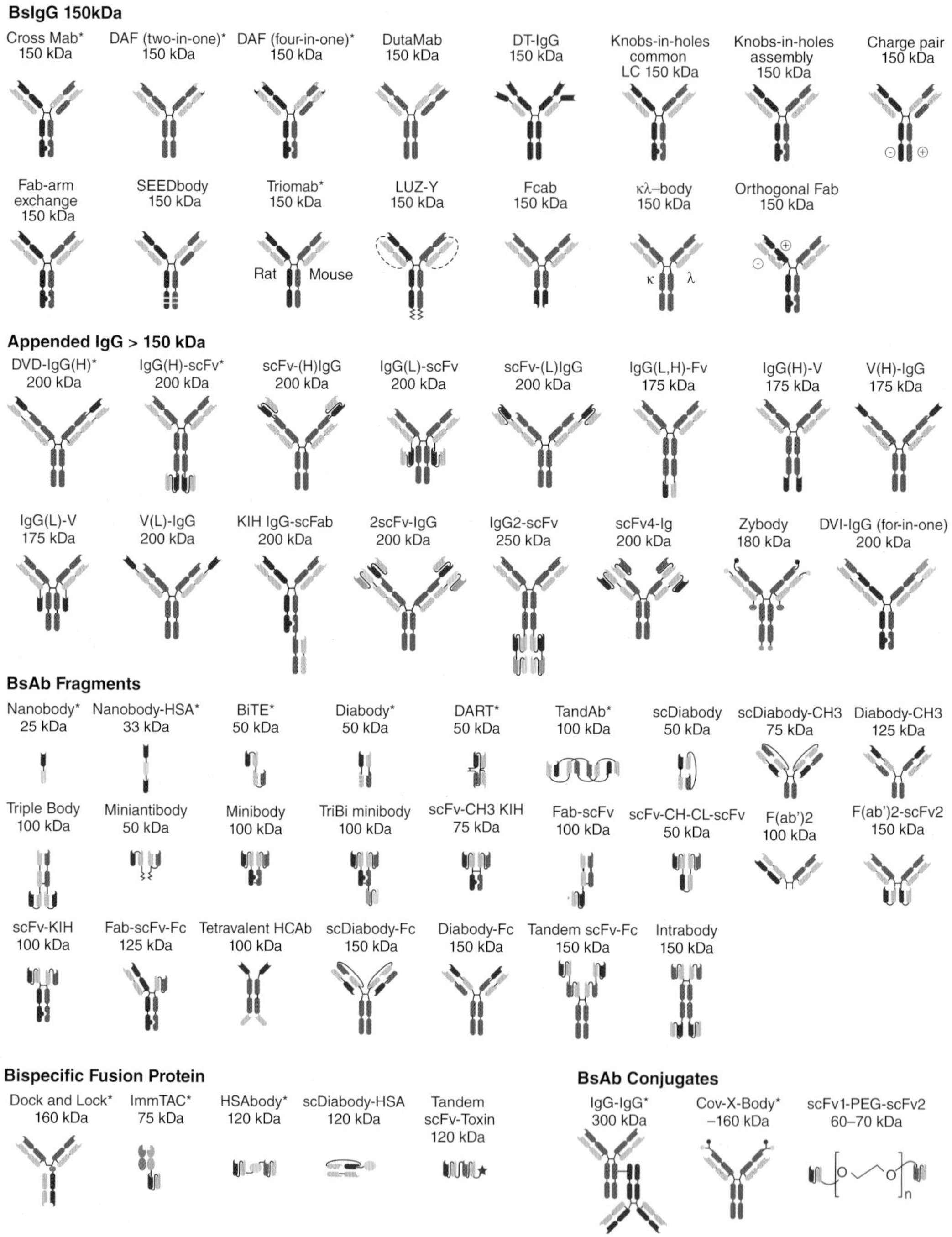

BsIgG 150kDa

Cross Mab* 150 kDa · DAF (two-in-one)* 150 kDa · DAF (four-in-one)* 150 kDa · DutaMab 150 kDa · DT-IgG 150 kDa · Knobs-in-holes common LC 150 kDa · Knobs-in-holes assembly 150 kDa · Charge pair 150 kDa

Fab-arm exchange 150 kDa · SEEDbody 150 kDa · Triomab* 150 kDa (Rat Mouse) · LUZ-Y 150 kDa · Fcab 150 kDa · κλ–body 150 kDa (κ λ) · Orthogonal Fab 150 kDa

Appended IgG > 150 kDa

DVD-IgG(H)* 200 kDa · IgG(H)-scFv* 200 kDa · scFv-(H)IgG 200 kDa · IgG(L)-scFv 200 kDa · scFv-(L)IgG 200 kDa · IgG(L,H)-Fv 175 kDa · IgG(H)-V 175 kDa · V(H)-IgG 175 kDa

IgG(L)-V 175 kDa · V(L)-IgG 200 kDa · KIH IgG-scFab 200 kDa · 2scFv-IgG 200 kDa · IgG2-scFv 250 kDa · scFv4-Ig 200 kDa · Zybody 180 kDa · DVI-IgG (for-in-one) 200 kDa

BsAb Fragments

Nanobody* 25 kDa · Nanobody-HSA* 33 kDa · BiTE* 50 kDa · Diabody* 50 kDa · DART* 50 kDa · TandAb* 100 kDa · scDiabody 50 kDa · scDiabody-CH3 75 kDa · Diabody-CH3 125 kDa

Triple Body 100 kDa · Miniantibody 50 kDa · Minibody 100 kDa · TriBi minibody 100 kDa · scFv-CH3 KIH 75 kDa · Fab-scFv 100 kDa · scFv-CH-CL-scFv 50 kDa · F(ab')2 100 kDa · F(ab')2-scFv2 150 kDa

scFv-KIH 100 kDa · Fab-scFv-Fc 125 kDa · Tetravalent HCAb 100 kDa · scDiabody-Fc 150 kDa · Diabody-Fc 150 kDa · Tandem scFv-Fc 150 kDa · Intrabody 150 kDa

Bispecific Fusion Protein

Dock and Lock* 160 kDa · ImmTAC* 75 kDa · HSAbody* 120 kDa · scDiabody-HSA 120 kDa · Tandem scFv-Toxin 120 kDa

BsAb Conjugates

IgG-IgG* 300 kDa · Cov-X-Body* ~160 kDa · scFv1-PEG-scFv2 60–70 kDa

Fig. 8.4 Alternative formats for bispecific antibodies and other bispecific immunotherapeutics subdivided into five major classes: BsIgG, appended IgG, BsAb fragments, bispecific fusion proteins and BsAb conjugates. Heavy chains are shown in *dark blue, dark pink* and *dark green*, and corresponding light chains are in *lighter shades* of the same colours. Connecting peptide linkers are shown by *thin black lines* and, engineered disulfide bonds by *thin green lines*. Approximate molecular weights are shown assuming ~12.5 kDa per immunoglobulin domain. BsAb formats that have advanced into clinical testing are highlighted (*). *IgG*, immunoglobulin G. (Adapted from Spiess, C., Zhai, Q., & Carter, P. J. [2015]. Alternative molecular formats and therapeutic applications for bispecific antibodies. *Molecular Immunology, 67*, 95–106.)

Analogous to engineering the variable regions of an antibody to improve binding or specificity to a target antigen, the Fc region of the antibody can be engineered to modify how it engages with the FcγR, FcRn and C1q to enhance or silence the biological effects mediated by these receptors or complement molecules. Examples of antibody Fc engineering include:

- The serum half-life of an antibody is extended due to endocytosed antibody binding to the FcRn in a pH-dependent manner. This rescues the antibody from lysosomal degradation and recycles the antibody back into the extracellular environment, thereby extending its half-life (Vaccaro et al., 2005). Further increasing the serum half-life of an antibody is possible through engineering the Fc region to bind with higher affinity to the FcRn (Dall'Acqua et al., 2002), enabling less request dosing of patients (Robbie et al., 2013).

- Mutations can be introduced into the Fc region to dramatically increase C1q binding to the antibody and enhance CDC activity (Idusogie et al., 2001).

- In some circumstances, it is desirable to maintain FcRn-mediated antibody half-life extension but have no functional ADCC activity, for example, for an antagonistic antibody. This can be achieved by introducing L234A and L235A amino acid substitutions into the heavy chain constant region of an IgG1 isotype (Wines et al., 2000). An equivalent effect can be achieved by mutating the IgG4 isotype, where the heavy chain constant region amino acid substitutions S228P and L235E minimize Fab-arm exchange *in vivo* as described by Aalberse (2002), Angal et al. (1993) and Labrijn et al. (2009) and reduce binding to Fc gamma receptors (Reddy et al., 2000).

- Enhanced ADCC activity can be achieved through modifying the glycosylation profile of the antibody (Shields et al., 2002), or alternatively through introducing amino acid mutations into the Fc region (Shields et al., 2001). Modification of the antibody's Fc glycosylation profile by manufacturing in a cell line that does not incorporate fucose into the N-linked carbohydrate (at amino acid position 297) results in improvements of up to 50-fold in the afucosylated antibody's ability to bind human FcγRIIIa (Shields et al., 2002) and improved ADCC activity ex vivo (Iida et al., 2006).

Manufacture, biological and biophysical assessment of therapeutic antibodies

The previous sections have focused on the characteristics of an antibody that make it optimally adapted to its function whether through binding or effector function. To be a viable therapeutic, an antibody must also have suitable biophysical properties that allow manufacturing at scale. The process of identifying a lead antibody sequence and backup molecule(s) to advance into cell line development (cell line used for clinical drug manufacture) is complex and involves extensive *in vitro* and ex vivo biological assessment and preliminary biophysical analysis (Mould & Meibohm, 2016). During cell line development, extensive assessment of the developability properties of the lead antibody is performed, which contributes to a critical data set informing whether the lead antibody candidate can advance into clinical development. Developability assessment involves the evaluation of various drug properties associated with the manufacturability and safety profile of the antibody (Matthews & Friis, 2017), with the aim of producing safe and efficacious therapeutics for patients and to reduce expensive late-stage clinical drug failures. Increasingly, the pharmaceutical industry is performing these assessments earlier during preclinical development to eliminate clones with undesirable biophysical properties (Jarasch et al., 2015).

Following the expiry of patent protection for an innovator antibody drug, biosimilar antibody products from competitor companies can enter the market (after successful clinical trials and marketing approval). Biosimilar drugs can offer alternative lower priced treatment options for patients and healthcare organizations. Unlike small molecules, where generic versions are considered identical to the innovator drug, antibody therapeutics are large complex molecules to manufacture, and a biosimilar version will not be identical to the innovator drug. Biosimilar drugs will possess different ratios of posttranslationally modified products and purity, even though the same genetic sequence is used. This disparity is due to different cell lines, manufacturing and purification processes employed.

Research-grade antibody protein is mainly produced using transiently transfected human embryonic kidney (HEK) cells, and this material is subjected to extensive *in vitro* and ex vivo biological assessment, in silico evaluation (of the amino acid sequence) and preliminary biophysical assessment to generate a data set to guide selection of the lead antibody molecule for cell line development. The *in vitro* and ex vivo biological assessment will vary depending on the therapeutic target and can involve some or all of the following approaches:

- *ELISA binding assay*—where the antibody is titrated against target protein or related proteins to determine cross-reactivity.
- *ELISA receptor binding assay (RBA)*—to determine how effectively the antibody inhibits ligand–receptor interactions (and related receptors/ligands).
- *Kinetic determination*—using surface plasmon resonance (SPR) or similar approach to determine on-rate (k_a)

and off-rate (k_d) and overall equilibrium dissociation constant (K_D) of the antibody for the therapeutic target. For high-affinity interactions (low picomolar [pM] K_D), an orthogonal method may be required.

- *Flow cytometry/FACS*—screening of cells transfected with the target protein and/or primary cells isolated from human donors or tissue biopsy to demonstrate binding specificity of the antibody and lack of cross-reactivity against related or homologous proteins.
- *Functional cell assay*—to determine the activity of antibody by assessing how it modulates the activity of a target cell population (e.g., cytokine readout, cell surface receptor expression, cell viability, cell morphology change).
- *Off-target binding*—determination of binding to related and unrelated targets using, for example, recombinant proteins expressed on an array (Sjöberg et al., 2018).
- *In vivo pharmacokinetic (PK) assays*—where appropriate, assessment of *in vivo* clearance properties of the antibody (typically using mice [wild type or transgenic], occasionally cynomolgus monkey [*Macaca fascicularis*]) by measuring systemic drug concentration over time.
- *In vivo pharmacodynamic (PD) assays*—determination of efficacy, typically performed in either a wild-type or transgenic mouse. When no suitable transgenic mouse model is available, or the lead antibody does not cross-react with the mouse orthologous protein, a mouse target specific 'surrogate' antibody can be created to help demonstrate mechanistic activity. On occasions when the mouse is an inappropriate species, alternative species may be considered. Ideally, *in vivo* studies should be performed using antibody purified from the cell line expression host.

Once a lead (and backup) antibody sequence has been identified, a stable cell line is generated that will eventually be used for clinical manufacture of the drug. Currently, CHO cell lines are commonly used for clinical antibody drug manufacture. Other cell lines less frequently used for antibody manufacture (Kunert & Reinhart, 2016) include NS0 (murine myeloma) and PER. C6 (derived from human embryonic retinal cells). Other non-mammalian expression hosts, such a yeast (Chiba & Akeboshi, 2009) and plants (Holtz et al., 2015; Yusibov & Kushnir, 2016) are also being developed for clinical manufacture of antibodies.

Biophysical assessment of the antibody involves both in silico and physical experimental assessments of how resistant to degradation or modification the antibody sequence/protein is. Preliminary biophysical assessment is typically performed using HEK cell–generated research-grade antibody protein preparations. Later, once the antibody has been expressed in a suitable clinical manufacturing cell line (e.g., CHO), more extensive biophysical assessments are performed. The list below covers a range of biophysical and biological assessments typically performed (not all of these will be performed during the preliminary assessment of HEK-derived antibody material):

- *In silico assessment*—identification of amino acid sequence liabilities such as asparagine deamidation (which can be a major cause of chemical degradation of proteins [Chelius et al., 2005]); methionine residue oxidation propensity (Davies, 2016); identification of amino acid motifs sensitive to protease cleavage; unpaired cysteines; rare or nongermline amino acids; codon optimization for CHO cell expression; immunogenicity prediction; predicted isoelectric point (p*I*); systemic drug availability prediction following subcutaneous administration (Kagan, 2014).
- *Antibody protein purity and fragmentation*—the levels of impurities and fragmentation products can be caused by several of the factors described below in this section and can impact the manufacturing yield.
- *Aggregation*—can impact manufacturing yield, drug shelf-life and storage, and potentially immunogenicity, which can impact patient safety. Chemical or physical changes to the antibody protein can result in protein aggregation.
- *Thermal stability*—assessment of how the antibody protein structure denatures over a temperature range, providing a surrogate for how stable the antibody may be *in vivo*.
- *Charge heterogeneity*—impacted by post-translational modification of charged amino acids creating acidic and basic isoforms. Modifications can include deamidation, oxidation, C-terminal lysine clipping, N-terminal pyroglutamic acid clipping, isomerization, succinimide formation, sialylation.
- *Glycosylation profile*—post-translational glycosylation can influence the stability and the biological activity of an antibody (through Fc engagement with FcγR on immune cells, discussed earlier). Glycosylation is also a source of product heterogeneity.
- *Nonspecific protein–protein interactions*—can adversely impact antibody solubility, aggregation, PK and viscosity at high drug concentrations.
- *Solubility and viscosity*—solubility affects how concentrated the drug formulation can be and therefore what volume of drug can be administered. For subcutaneous administration, concentrations of 100 mg/mL or greater are typically required. The desired drug concentration is impacted by the drug's biological potency, the amount of drug required to achieve the desired concentration *in vivo* and the dosing frequency required to achieve therapeutic efficacy. For intravenous delivery, concentrations can be lower, as administration volumes are larger. Increasing

the protein concentration can increase the viscosity (Tomar et al., 2016) of the solution, which will impact the injection force required to administer the drug and can cause discomfort for the patient.

- *Serum stability*—assessment of antibody stability following ex vivo incubation in serum (i.e., human or mouse), or assessment of samples from *in vivo* studies containing the therapeutic antibody.

- *Accelerated stress studies*—assessment under various conditions, such as elevated temperature, pH range, repeated freeze–thaw cycles, oxidizing agents and physical agitation. These conditions are used to simulate the impact of mechanical and physical stresses the antibody drug product may encounter during manufacture, storage and transport.

- *Nonclinical safety assessment*—assessment of whether there are any unintended toxicological effects of the antibody *in vivo* by observing the behaviour of the test species, testing blood and urine samples and tissue histology. Due to antibodies typically being highly specific for their human target, species cross-reactivity of the antibody may be limited to nonhuman primates (Lansita & Mounho-Zamora, 2015).

- *Tissue cross-reactivity studies*—assessment of whether the antibody binds ex vivo to the expected target tissue or binds unexpectedly (specifically or nonspecifically) to other target tissues (extensively reviewed by Leach et al., 2010).

Optimizing the antibody-producing cell line expression conditions (Li et al., 2010) to provide consistent batch-to-batch supply of purified antibody drug product is critical for marketing approval and supply of drug to the market. Extensive work is undertaken from the late preclinical through to the clinical phase of drug development (Mould & Meibohm, 2016) in the chemistry manufacturing & control (CMC) and late-stage development divisions of pharmaceutical companies. This is a complex aspect of antibody development and is beyond to scope of this chapter. Areas that are evaluated include:

- *Cell line stability over multiple generations*—it is critical to demonstrate that the cell line is stable and monoclonal so that the expression yield and protein quality does not alter over time. Cell culture expression performance may be monitored for 100 to 200 generations to ensure stability.

- *Cell line expression optimization*—identify optimal conditions to enable achievement of high expression yields (>1 g/L and ideally > 5 g/L) with minimal production of heterogeneous contaminants.

- *Downstream antibody purification optimization*—provision of purified antibody, while minimizing yield losses during each step of the purification process. Antibody expression and purification efficiency yield have a major impact on the cost of goods of the antibody drug product. Consistent supply from third-party vendors of filters and reagents required for purifying the antibody from cell culture is essential to ensure an efficient manufacturing process.

- *Drug formulation*—chemical excipients and additives are included in the liquid or lyophilized drug formulation to optimize the stability and storage of the antibody protein.

- *Supply of raw ingredients for clinical manufacture*—critical to ensure a reliable and consistent supply of materials from third-party vendors to enable efficient large-scale expression and purification of the antibody.

Future perspective

The future is of course notoriously difficult to predict as the introduction and application of a disruptive novel technology can completely reset the direction of established processes. However, there are some trends that will undoubtedly have an increasing impact on therapeutic antibody discovery and development.

The development and increasing use of next-generation DNA sequencing (NGS) has enabled the detailed and complete sequence analysis of both synthetic and natural immune repertoire libraries. Applying NGS coupled with powerful bioinformatics software and ingenious experimental selection/screening design can enable the identification of rare antibody sequences that may not be easily identified using traditional binding and screening methodologies. The application of high-throughput miniaturized assays, increased automation and the desire to screen directly for function (rather than identifying antigen binders first, then triaging for function) has the potential to shorten early phase discovery times. However, effort and time will still be required to develop robust functional assays for individual therapeutic targets. For example, if a functional cellular readout is required, a suitable cell line or process to purify primary cells has to be developed, and the associated functional assay must be reproducible to ensure the resulting data are sufficiently robust to enable a definitive decision to be reached as to which antibody clones to advance.

As increasing numbers of antibodies are identified earlier in the screening cascade, there is an increasing desire to assess as early as possible tens to hundreds of clones for indicative favourable developability attributes and other properties, such as immunogenicity. The aim being to generate antibody clones possessing desirable biological and biophysical properties, which bind a diverse range of epitopes on the target protein. This provides researchers with a larger panel of antibody clones from which to select lead molecules to advance into cell line development. The motivation is to reduce project attrition during later stage development due to antibody molecules possessing undesirable properties that cannot be overcome, for example, through formulation. The drive to increase manufacturing cell line productivity and product quality will continue—with the aim of reducing the cost of goods for antibody production. Likewise, there will be continued pressure from insurance companies and national healthcare agencies to scrutinize the cost-effectiveness of drugs and push down the price they are willing to pay.

Administration of antibodies is typically via injection; however, researchers are continually investigating alternative routes of administration, such as pulmonary and oral delivery. Oral, ocular, pulmonary and transdermal routes of administration may become more viable for antibody fragments, or other lower molecular weight binding scaffolds, for some specific indications; however, to achieve the desired systemic concentration of drug, intravenous and subcutaneous delivery will likely remain to be the main routes of delivery. Delivery of antibodies across the BBB and intracellularly remain two challenging applications that, if solved, would broaden the utility of antibody therapeutics.

Antibodies are in essence bispecific molecules due to their ability to engage with antigen and Fc receptors/complement. However, there is a growing trend to develop bispecific (or trispecific) antigen-binding antibodies or related molecular formats to engage multiple therapeutic targets. Particularly in the field of oncology, there may be certain receptor combinations or biparatopic approaches that merit a bispecific or trispecific approach. There is also a case for co-administration of monospecific antibody therapeutics, where clinicians will have greater control over the stoichiometric ratios of drug administered, compared with a bispecific approach, where the ratio is fixed. Another factor that may be critical in determining the efficacy of certain mAbs/target pairs is whether the mAb binds antigens in a monovalent or bivalent manner. If bivalent engagement is necessary for optimum efficacy, some monovalent bispecific antibody formats may struggle to demonstrate superior efficacy compared with co-administration of two monospecific mAbs. Clearly, considerations regarding the antibody molecular format and selecting appropriate therapeutic targets are critical for bispecific antibody design. It will be interesting to see how clinical data from various bispecific approaches read out over the next few years.

The explosion in computational power and development of machine learning, or even the promise of artificial intelligence, will have a dramatic impact on antibody drug discovery. With large and increasingly complex data sets available for computers to analyse, machine learning algorithms will be able to identify trends in large data sets to potentially inform on which clones should be advanced based on lessons learned from legacy data. It may become possible to design, by first intent, high-affinity antibody sequences with low immunogenicity and low developability risk scores. Such de novo antibody design will most likely require a high-resolution crystal structure or homology model of the target protein/molecule to design the corresponding antibody paratope against. Such an approach would negate the requirement to generate and screen physical antibody libraries.

Therapeutic antibodies have already established themselves as one of the most successful classes of therapeutics. Progress to date in the field has been fascinating, and the pace of development is accelerating and holds great promise in delivering many novel therapeutic approaches or potential cures to help patients live longer and improve their quality of life.

References

Aalberse, R. C., & Schuurman, J. (2002). IgG4 breaking the rules. *Immunology, 105*, 9–19.

Angal, S., King, D. J., Bodmer, M. W., Turner, A., Lawson, A. D., Roberts, G., et al. (1993). A single amino acid substitution abolishes the heterogeneity of chimeric mouse/human (IgG4) antibody. *Molecular Immunology, 30*, 105–108.

Beigel, J. H., Tebas, P., Elie-Turenne, M. C., Bajwa, E., Bell, T. E., Cairns, C. B., et al. (2017). Immune plasma for the treatment of severe influenza: An open-label, multicentre, phase 2 randomised study. *Lancet. Respiratory Medicine, 5*(6), 500–511.

Boado, R. J., Zhou, Q. H., Lu, J. Z., Hui, E. K., & Pardridge, W. M. (2010). Pharmacokinetics and brain uptake of a genetically engineered bifunctional fusion antibody targeting the mouse transferrin receptor. *Molecular Pharmaceutics, 7*(1), 237–244.

Brüggemann, M., Osborn, M. J., Ma, B., Hayre, J., Avis, S., Lundstrom, B., et al. (2015). Human antibody production in transgenic animals. *Archivum Immunologiae et Therapiae Experimentalis, 63*(2), 101–108.

Bruhns, P. (2012). Properties of mouse and human IgG receptors and their contribution to disease models. *Blood, 119*(24), 5640–5649.

Carbonetti, S., Oliver, B. G., Vigdorovich, V., Dambrauskas, N., Sack, B., Bergl, E., et al. (2017). A method for the isolation and characterization of functional murine monoclonal antibodies by single B cell cloning. *Journal of Immunological Methods, 448*, 66–73.

Chelius, D., Rehder, D. S., & Bondarenko, P. V. (2005). Identification and characterization of deamidation sites in the conserved regions of human immunoglobulin gamma antibodies. *Analytical Chemistry, 77*(18), 6004–6011.

Chiba, Y., & Akeboshi, H. (2009). Glycan engineering and production of 'humanized' glycoprotein in yeast cells. *Biological & Pharmaceutical Bulletin, 32*(5), 786–795.

Choi, D. K., Bae, J., Shin, S. M., Shin, J. Y., Kim, S., & Kim, Y. S. (2014). A general strategy for generating intact, full-length IgG antibodies that penetrate into the cytosol of living cells. *mAbs, 6*(6), 1402–1414.

Clackson, T., Hoogenboom, H. R., Griffiths, A. D., & Winter, G. (1991). Making antibody fragments using phage display libraries. *Nature, 352*(6336), 624–628.

Dall'Acqua, W. F., Woods, R. M., Ward, E. S., Palaszynski, S. R., Patel, N. K., Brewah, Y. A., et al. (2002). Increasing the affinity of a human IgG1 for the neonatal Fc receptor: Biological consequences. *Journal of Immunology, 169*(9), 5171–5180.

Davies, M. J. (2016). Protein oxidation and peroxidation. *Biochemical Journal, 473*(7), 805–825.

DiMasi, J. A., Grabowski, H. G., & Hansen, R. W. (2016). Innovation in the pharmaceutical industry: New estimates of R&D costs. *Journal of Health Economics, 47*, 20–33.

Enever, C., Batuwangala, T., Plummer, C., & Sepp, A. (2009). Next generation immunotherapeutics—honing the magic bullet. *Current Opinion in Biotechnology, 20*(4), 405–411.

Eyer, K., Doineau, R. C. L., Castrillon, C. E., Briseño-Roa, L., Menrath, V., Mottet, G., et al. (2017). Single-cell deep phenotyping of IgG-secreting cells for high-resolution immune monitoring. *Nature Biotechnology, 35*(10), 977–982.

Frenzel, A., Kügler, J., Helmsing, S., Meier, D., Schirrmann, T., Hust, M., et al. (2017). Designing human antibodies by phage display. *Transfusion Medicine and Hemotherapy, 44*(5), 312–318.

Global Monoclonal Antibodies Market—by Type, Application, Region—Market Size, Demand Forecasts, Company Profiles, Industry Trends and Updates (2017-2023). 2018. Retrieved from www.researchandmarkets.com.

Green, L. L. (2014). Transgenic mouse strains as platforms for the successful discovery and development of human therapeutic monoclonal antibodies. *Current Drug Discovery Technologies, 11*(1), 74–84.

Hanack, K., Messerschmidt, K., & Listek, M. (2016). Antibodies and selection of monoclonal antibodies. In T. Böldicke (Ed.), *From protein targeting compounds, advances in experimental medicine and biology* (Vol. 917). Switzerland: Springer International Publishing. Retrieved from https://doi.org/10.1007/978-3-319-32805-8_2.

Hanes, J., & Plückthun, A. (1997). *In vitro* selection and evolution of functional proteins by using ribosome display. *Proceedings of the National Academy of Sciences of the United States of America, 94*(10), 4937–4942.

He, M., & Taussig, M. J. (1997). Antibody-ribosome-mRNA (ARM) complexes as efficient selection particles for *in vitro* display and evolution of antibody combining sites. *Nucleic Acids Research, 25*(24), 5132–5134.

Heukers, R., De Groof, T. W. M., & Smit, M. J. (2019). Nanobodies detecting and modulating GPCRs outside in and inside out. *Current Opinion in Cell Biology, 57*, 115–122.

Holliger, P., & Hudson, P. J. (2005). Engineered antibody fragments and the rise of single domains. *Nature Biotechnology, 23*(9), 1126–1136.

Holt, L. J., Basran, A., Jones, K., Chorlton, J., Jespers, L. S., Brewis, N. D., et al. (2008). Anti-serum albumin domain antibodies for extending the half-lives of short lived drugs. *Protein Engineering, Design & Selection, 21*(5), 283–288.

Holtz, B. R., Berquist, B. R., Bennett, L. D., Kommineni, V. J., Munigunti, R. K., White, E. L., et al. (2015). Commercial-scale biotherapeutics manufacturing facility for plant-made pharmaceuticals. *Plant Biotechnology Journal, 13*(8), 1180–1190.

Idusogie, E. E., Wong, P. Y., Presta, L. G., Gazzano-Santoro, H., Totpal, K., Ultsch, M., et al. (2001). Engineered antibodies with increased activity to recruit complement. *Journal of Immunology, 166*(4), 2571–2575.

Igawa, T., Tsunoda, H., Kuramochi, T., Sampei, Z., Ishii, S., & Hattori, K. (2011). Engineering the variable region of therapeutic IgG antibodies. *mAbs, 3*(3), 243–252.

Iida, S., Misaka, H., Inoue, M., Shibata, M., Nakano, R., Yamane-Ohnuki, N., et al. (2006). Nonfucosylated therapeutic IgG1 antibody can evade the inhibitory effect of serum immunoglobulin G on antibody-dependent cellular cytotoxicity through its high binding to FcgammaRIIIa. *Clinical Cancer Research, 12*(9), 2879–2887.

Jarasch, A., Koll, H., Regula, J. T., Bader, M., Papadimitriou, A., & Kettenberger, H. (2015). Developability assessment during the selection of novel therapeutic antibodies. *Journal of Pharmaceutical Sciences, 104*(6), 1885–1898.

Jones, P. T., Dear, P. H., Foote, J., Neuberger, M. S., & Winter, G. (1986). Replacing the complementarity-determining regions in a human antibody with those from a mouse. *Nature, 321*(6069), 522–525.

Kagan, L. (2014). Pharmacokinetic modeling of the subcutaneous absorption of therapeutic proteins. *Drug Metabolism and Disposition, 42*(11), 1890–1905.

Köhler, G., & Milstein, C. (1975). Continuous cultures of fused cells secreting antibody of predefined specificity. *Nature, 256*(5517), 495–497.

Köster, S., Angilè, F. E., Duan, H., Agresti, J. J., Wintner, A., Schmitz, C., et al. (2008). Drop-based microfluidic devices for encapsulation of single cells. *Lab on a Chip, 8*(7), 1110–1115.

Kunert, R., & Reinhart, D. (2016). Advances in recombinant antibody manufacturing. *Applied Microbiology and Biotechnology, 100*(8), 3451–3461.

Labrijn, A. F., Buijsse, A. O., van den Bremer, E. T., Verwilligen, A. Y., Bleeker, W. K., Thorpe, S. J., et al. (2009). Therapeutic IgG4 antibodies engage in Fab-arm exchange with endogenous human IgG4 *in vivo*. *Nature Biotechnology, 27*, 767–771.

Lansita, J. A., & Mounho-Zamora, B. (2015). The development of therapeutic monoclonal antibodies: Overview of the nonclinical safety assessment. *Current Pain and Headache Reports, 19*(2) 2.

Leach, M. W., Halpern, W. G., Johnson, C. W., Rojko, J. L., MacLachlan, T. K., Chan, C. M., et al. (2010). Use of tissue cross-reactivity studies in the development of antibody-based biopharmaceuticals: History, experience, methodology, and future directions. *Toxicologic Pathology, 38*(7), 1138–1166.

Leenaars, M., & Hendriksen, C. F. (2005). Critical steps in the production of polyclonal and monoclonal antibodies: Evaluation and recommendations. *ILAR Journal, 46*(3), 269–279.

Li, F., Vijayasankaran, N., Shen, A. Y., Kiss, R., & Amanullah, A. (2010). Cell culture processes for monoclonal antibody production. *mAbs, 2*(5), 466–479.

Li, R., Kang, G., Hu, M., & Huang, H. (2019). Ribosome display: A potent display technology used for selecting and evolving specific binders with desired properties. *Molecular Biotechnology, 61*(1), 60–71.

Male, D., Brostoff, J., Roth, D., & Roitt, I. (Eds.). (2012). *Immunology* (8th ed.). New York: Elsevier.

Marks, J. D., Hoogenboom, H. R., Bonnert, T. P., McCafferty, J., Griffiths, A. D., & Winter, G. (1991). By-passing immunization. Human antibodies from V-gene libraries displayed on phage. *Journal of Molecular Biology, 222*(3), 581–597.

Matthews, D., & Friis, L. (2017). Developability assessment of therapeutic antibodies. *Drug Target Review,* (1). Retrieved from https://www.drugtarget review.com/article/32916/developability-assessment-of-therapeutic-antibodies/.

Mazutis, L., Gilbert, J., Ung, W. L., Weitz, D. A., Griffiths, A. D., & Heyman, J. A. (2013). Single-cell analysis and sorting using droplet-based microfluidics. *Nature Protocols, 8*(5), 870–891.

Morrison, S. L., Johnson, M. J., Herzenberg, L. A., & Oi, V. T. (1984). Chimeric human antibody molecules: Mouse antigen-binding domains with human constant region domains. *Proceedings of the National Academy of Sciences of the United States of America, 81*(21), 6851–6855.

Mould, D. R., & Meibohm, B. (2016). Drug development of therapeutic monoclonal antibodies. *BioDrugs, 30*(4), 275–293.

Prassler, J., Thiel, S., Pracht, C., Polzer, A., Peters, S., Bauer, M., et al. (2011). HuCAL PLATINUM, a synthetic Fab library optimized for sequence diversity and superior performance in mammalian expression systems. *Journal of Molecular Biology, 413*(1), 261–278.

Reddy, M. P., Kinney, C. A., Chaikin, M. A., Payne, A., Fishman-Lobell, J., Tsui, P., Dal Monte, P. R., et al. (2000). Elimination of Fc receptor-dependent effector functions of a modified IgG4 monoclonal antibody to human CD4. *Journal of Immunology, 164*(4), 1925–1933.

Robbie, G. J., Criste, R., Dall'acqua, W. F., Jensen, K., Patel, N. K., Losonsky, G. A., et al. (2013). A novel investigational Fc-modified humanized monoclonal antibody, motavizumab-YTE, has an extended half-life in healthy adults. *Antimicrobial Agents and Chemotherapy, 57*(12), 6147–6153.

Sheehan, J., Marasco, W. A. (2015). Phage and yeast display. *Microbiology Spectrum, 3*(1), 1–17.

Shields, R. L., Lai, J., Keck, R., O'Connell, L. Y., Hong, K., Meng, Y. G., et al. (2002). Lack of fucose on human IgG1 N-linked oligosaccharide improves binding to human Fcgamma RIII and antibody-dependent cellular toxicity. *Journal of Biological Chemistry, 277*(30), 26733–26740.

Shields, R. L., Namenuk, A. K., Hong, K., Meng, Y. G., Rae, J., Briggs, J., et al. (2001). High resolution mapping of the binding site on human IgG1 for Fc gamma RI, Fc gamma RII, Fc gamma RIII, and FcRn and design of IgG1 variants with improved binding to the Fc gamma R. *Journal of Biological Chemistry, 276*(9), 6591–6604.

Simon, J. (2007). Emil Behring's medical culture: From disinfection to serotherapy. *Medical History, 51,* 201–218.

Sioud, M. (2019). Phage display libraries: From binders to targeted drug delivery and human therapeutics. *Molecular Biotechnology, 61*(4), 286–303.

Sivasubramanian, A., Estep, P., Lynaugh, H., Yu, Y., Miles, A., Eckman, J., et al. (2017). Broad epitope coverage of a human *in vitro* antibody library. *mAbs, 9*(1), 29–42.

Sjöberg, R., Andersson, E., Hellström, C., Mattsson, C., Schwenk, J. M., Nilsson, P., et al. (2018). High-density antigen microarrays for the assessment of antibody selectivity and off-target binding. *Methods in Molecular Biology, 1785,* 231–238.

Smith, E. S., & Zauderer, M. (2014). Antibody library display on a mammalian virus vector: Combining the advantages of both phage and yeast display into one technology. *Current Drug Discovery Technologies, 11*(1), 48–55.

Smith, S. (1996). Ten years of Orthoclone OKT3 (muromonab-CD3): A review. *Journal of Transplant Coordination, 6*(3), 109–119.

Sockolosky, J. T., & Szoka, F. C. (2015). The neonatal Fc receptor, FcRn, as a target for drug delivery and therapy. *Advanced Drug Delivery Reviews, 91,* 109–124.

Spiess, C., Zhai, Q., & Carter, P. J. (2015). Alternative molecular formats and therapeutic applications for bispecific antibodies. *Molecular Immunology, 67,* 95–106.

Starkie, D. O., Compson, J. E., Rapecki, S., & Lightwood, D. J. (2016). Generation of recombinant monoclonal antibodies from immunised mice and rabbits via flow cytometry and sorting of antigen-specific IgG+ memory B cells. *PLoS One, 11*(3), e0152282.

Takai, T. (2005). Fc receptors and their role in immune regulation and autoimmunity. *Journal of Clinical Immunology, 25*(1), 1–18.

Tjandra, J. J., Ramadi, L., & McKenzie, I. F. (1990). Development of human anti-murine antibody (HAMA) response in patients. *Immunology and Cell Biology, 68*(6), 367–376.

Tomar, D. S., Kumar, S., Singh, S. K., Goswami, S., & Li, L. (2016). Molecular basis of high viscosity in concentrated antibody solutions: Strategies for high concentration drug product development. *mAbs, 8*(2), 216–228.

Vaccaro, C., Zhou, J., Ober, R. J., & Ward, E. S. (2005). Engineering the Fc region of immunoglobulin G to modulate *in vivo* antibody levels. *Nature Biotechnology, 23*(10), 1283–1288.

Wines, B. D., Powell, M. S., Parren, P. W., Barnes, N., & Hogarth, P. M. (2000). The IgG Fc contains distinct Fc receptor (FcR) binding sites: The leukocyte receptors Fc gamma RI and Fc gamma RIIa bind to a region in the Fc distinct from that recognized by neonatal FcR and protein A. *Journal of Immunology, 164*(10), 5313–5318.

Winter, G., Griffiths, A. D., Hawkins, R. E., & Hoogenboom, H. R. (1994). Making antibodies by phage display technology. *Annual Review of Immunology, 12,* 433–455.

Yusibov, V., Kushnir, N., & Streatfield, S. J. (2016). Antibody production in plants and green algae. *Annual Review of Plant Biology, 67,* 669–701.

Zhai, W., Glanville, J., Fuhrmann, M., Mei, L., Ni, I., Sundar, P. D., et al. (2011). Synthetic antibodies designed on natural sequence landscapes. *Journal of Molecular Biology, 412*(1), 55–71.

Chapter 9

Emerging modalities: nucleotide-based therapies, cell-based therapies, gene therapy

Helen Carnaghan, Raymond G Hill, Duncan B Richards

Introduction

Until comparatively recently, there were only two major approaches to drug treatment of disease, using either small organic molecules or biological therapies (usually monoclonal antibodies or other proteins). Recently there has been an increase in the number of approaches that have been successful in the clinic, and regulatory bodies have licensed medicines using oligonucleotide, cell and gene therapies for a number of diseases, especially cancer and rare genetic conditions. This chapter deals with these recent advances, but it should be remembered that these approaches are not mutually exclusive and for some diseases that are intractable and disabling, multiple approaches are being used employing our established therapeutic approaches and the emerging modalities, for example, sickle cell disease (see Mullard, 2020a; Tambuyzer et al., 2020). Advances in molecular biology and our understanding of the human genome have increased our ability to address difficult to treat diseases (Alberts et al., 2002). Additionally, the use of antisense oligonucleotides (ASOs), small interfering RNAs (siRNAs), gene and cell therapy have allowed previously inaccessible targets, such as transcription factors and dysfunctional intracellular proteins to be tackled. Indeed, there is at least one example of ASOs being designed and used to treat a specific gene missplicing in a single patient with some clinical success. This raises many issues around medical ethics, design of clinical trials and regulatory approval that are outside the scope of this chapter (Mullard, 2020b).

Antisense oligonucleotides and small interfering RNA

The concept of using a synthetic oligonucleotide to change RNA function is not new and the first publications on this topic appeared before the end of the 1970s, yet it is only recently that the regulatory authorities have approved drugs using this mechanism. The reasons for this delay are many and complex, including the need for better knowledge of genomics, oligonucleotide chemistry, the understanding of mechanism and off-target toxicity and strategies for drug delivery. Hundreds of publications dealing with aspects of the above have appeared in the last 20 years, but three recent reviews are especially helpful in aiding the uninitiated to understand this complex topic (Crooke, 2017; Levin, 2019; Setten, 2019).

The first oligonucleotide therapies to be investigated were ASOs. They are single-stranded molecules that bind to complementary messenger RNA (mRNA) by base pairing and thereby initiate its selective enzymatic breakdown (Dean, 2001; Phillips, 2000) and prevent translation. This allows the expression of specific genes to be inhibited. This technique has also been used as an investigational tool so that the role of specific genes in the development of a disease phenotype could be determined. Although simple in principle, the technology is subject to many pitfalls and artefacts in practice, and attempts to use it, without very careful controls, were found likely to give misleading results. As an alternative to using synthetic oligonucleotides, antisense sequences can be introduced into cells by genetic engineering. Examples where this approach has been used to validate putative drug targets include a range of studies on the novel cell-surface receptor uPAR (urokinase plasminogen-activator receptor; see review by Wang, 2001). This receptor is expressed by certain malignant tumour cells, particularly gliomas, and antisense studies have shown it to be important in controlling the tendency of these tumours to metastasize and therefore make it a potential drug target. In a different field, antisense studies have supported the role of a sodium channel subtype, PN3 (now known to be Nav 1.8) (Porreca et al., 1999) and of the metabotropic glutamate receptor mGluR1 (Fundytus et al., 2001) in the pathogenesis of neuropathic pain in animal models. ASOs have the advantage that their effects on gene expression are acute and reversible, and so mimic drug effects more closely than, for example, the changes seen after gene therapy (see later), where in most cases the genetic disturbance is present permanently or for an extended period of time. The production of chemically stable oligonucleotides has been a major task in making drug candidates rather than just experimental tools. Therapeutic oligonucleotides are usually 15 to 30 nucleotides in length and designed to be complementary to a specific region of an RNA coding a disease-related protein or a regulatory RNA. When designing an ASO it is

necessary to synthesize sequences that are highly specific for the target RNA and to avoid sequences that are found in many genes and that would therefore give rise to unwanted off-target effects. Software is now available that will predict sequences that allow specific targets to be attacked even within closely related gene families. However, in practice this is an iterative process that usually involves screening of libraries of matched sequence ASOs to find the ones that have the best properties. Crookes (2017) has described the multistage process by which ASOs exert their effects and it is now clear that there are prehybridization events during which the oligonucleotides interact with proteins at the cell surface and then travel to their site of action within the cell, hybridization (where there are still many unknowns) and posthybridization mechanisms. In this latter phase, RNase H1 is crucial in causing breakdown of the target RNA and thus much effort has been invested in designing ASOs to interact with designated sites on the target RNAs to serve as optimal substrates for RNase H1. Other posthybridization mechanisms have now been exploited using ASOs and in particular the alteration of splicing has proved to be valuable in therapeutic use for treating spinal muscular atrophy (SMA) (Fig. 9.1; Crookes, 2017; Levin, 2019). It is

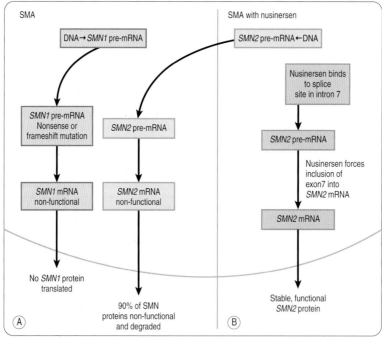

Fig. 9.1 Exon switching induced by nucinersen in spinal muscular atrophy (SMA). In patients with SMA, mutations in *SMN1* (Panel A) lead to nonsense non-functional RNA and hence no functional SMN1 protein is produced. Pre-mRNA for *SMN2* has a natural variant in exon 7 that that results in the exclusion of exon 7 from 90% of *SMN2* mRNA (Panel A). After treatment with nucinersen (Panel B) this oligonucleotide hybridizes to a site on the boundary of exon 7 thus forcing the inclusion of exon 7 into the *SMN2* mRNA. The increased amount of functional SMN2 protein produced compensates for the lack of functional SMN1 protein and means there is no overall SMN protein deficiency (see Levin 2019 for more details).

now possible to design ASOs that bind to upstream open reading frames or translation suppressor elements and thus selectively enhance the translation of specific mRNAs and enhance rather than block specific gene function (Crookes, 2017).

More recently, an alternative approach using double-stranded RNA to produce gene silencing has been developed and is referred to as siRNA (see Setten et al., 2019). This technique depends on the fact that short lengths of double-stranded RNA (siRNAs) activate a sequence-specific RNA-induced silencing complex (RISC), which destroys, by cleavage, the corresponding functional mRNA within the cell (Hannon, 2000; Kim, 2003). Thus specific mRNAs or whole gene families can be inactivated by choosing appropriate siRNA sequences. Gene silencing by this method is highly efficient and is therefore attractive for therapeutic applications. It has also proved to be a rapid and effective tool for discovering new targets, and automated cell assays have allowed the rapid screening of large groups of genes. After initial optimism, in the early 2000s the difficulties inherent in the therapeutic use of this approach became evident and it has not proved to be less problematic than the use of single-stranded ASOs, although it allows a broader range of targets to be addressed and siRNAs may be more potent than ASOs. siRNA interacts with an intrinsic mechanism in which non-coding RNA functions as a central regulator of gene function (Fig. 9.2). The risk of off-target activity is as high with this mechanism as with single-stranded ASOs, but again strategies to ensure specificity are now in place. It is now apparent that in some cases there are commonalities in the way that single-stranded ASO and siRNAs work. As Ago2 has an RNase H domain (see Fig. 9.2), this pathway to RNA degradation could be considered to be an antisense mechanism. Indeed, Crookes and his colleagues have synthesized and stabilized single-stranded RNA-like ASOs that bind to Ago2 and result in cleavage of the target RNA obviating the need for a second strand (Crookes, 2017).

Although the very selective nature of ASO and siRNA therapy reduces body burden of drug and should therefore minimize side effects, there are still a number of issues that introduce unwanted adverse events when this approach is used. This is dealt with in detail in the review by Levin (2019), but briefly, the phosphorothioate single-stranded oligonucleotides (which constitute the most commonly used strategy to produce stable ASOs) can cause injection site reactions, in higher doses fever, chills and other inflammatory reactions and in some cases thrombocytopenia. Toxic effects appear to be dose related and newer ASOs, which use improved chemistry, may have fewer problems but this is an emerging and very complex field (Wan & Seth, 2016). The first clinical trials with unmodified siRNAs produced immune-related toxicity, but improvements in sequence selection and

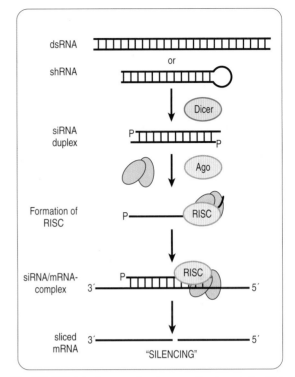

Fig. 9.2 RNA interference—innate gene silencing mechanism. *RISC*, RNA-induced silencing complex.

chemistry have improved tolerability. A wide range of different mechanisms can now be exploited by RNA-based approaches (see Levin, 2020; Table 9.1). Chemical modification within a therapeutic oligonucleotide can determine which antisense mechanism the ASO can interact with within the cell. ASOs that attack the RNA degrading mechanism such as RNase H have more precise design requirements as the modification pattern must be compatible with the specificity of the enzyme, whereas those that function by occupancy-based mechanisms allow a wider variation in ASO sequence and length (Wan & Seth, 2016).

Oligonucleotide therapy has potential in a wide range of diseases but delivering adequate quantities to the desired site of action is still a challenge. Most of the first wave of therapies target the liver, as uptake in the liver is good (a number of mechanisms may be involved depending on the chemistry). Targeting specific organs such as the heart has proven difficult. Topical delivery via intrathecal injection is proving viable for rare severe neurodegenerative conditions.

There are now many alternative ways of using oligonucleotides as drugs including aptamers, immunomodulatory

Table 9.1 Current and potential mechanism of RNA-based therapies

Mechanism	Oligonucleotide
RNase H	Chimeric oligodeoxynucleotides
RNA-induced silencing complex	Double-stranded RNAs or modified single-stranded RNA-like molecules
Exon skipping or splice switching	Single-stranded oligonucleotide
MicroRNA sequestration	Single-stranded or circular oligonucleotide
MicroRNA mimetics	Double-stranded RNA
RNA inducible transcriptional activation	Double-stranded RNA (saRNA)
Transcription-factor decoy	Double-stranded DNA-like oligonucleotide
Synthetic mRNA	Single-stranded RNA
Editing of RNA	Single-stranded oligonucleotide structured to attract adenosine deaminase or RNA co-administered with exogenous Cas enzymes

mRNA, Messenger RNA; *saRNA*, small activating RNA.
From Levin (2019).

oligonucleotides and therapeutic mRNAs will not be considered here (see Wan & Seth, 2016).

Approved oligonucleotide drugs

Nusinersen treatment has led to clinical improvements in motor function in infants and older children suffering from SMA such that the US Food & Drug Administration (FDA) has recently approved its use (Levin, 2019; Fig. 9.1). This ASO induces exon inclusion to increase the production of survival motor neuron (SMN) protein by blocking the splicing signal that causes the exclusion of exon 7 of *SMN-2* and allows the synthesis of more functional SMNs to replace that which is missing because of the defective and nonproductive *SMN-1* gene. The ASO is chemically modified to make it stable to nuclease degradation, so although it must be given by the intrathecal route to be effective it is possible to give maintenance treatment every 4 months after an effect has been achieved with loading doses. Its use has now been expanded to adult patients, with early indication of improved motor function (Hagenacker et al., 2020).

Mipomersen has been shown to reduce low-density lipoprotein (LDL) cholesterol export from the liver and hence reduce circulating LDL cholesterol even in statin-resistant patients. It was approved by the FDA in 2013. It is a single-stranded ASO that produces cleavage of apolipoprotein B mRNA (Levin, 2019).

Patisiran is an siRNA that has recently been approved for the treatment of transthyretin amyloidosis with polyneuropathy (ATTR) when given intravenously once every 3 weeks. Patisiran works by silencing both wild-type and mutant *TTR* mRNAs in hepatocytes and thus reduces circulating TTR protein (Setten et al., 2019). The secret of its success is a lipid nanoparticle formulation optimized for hepatocyte uptake and the siRNA itself is not metabolically stabilized. A single-stranded ASO, inotersen, has also recently been approved for the treatment of ATTR.

A large number of ASOs and siRNA drugs are currently in various stages of clinical evaluation (see Levin, 2019; Setten et al., 2019).

Cell therapy

Cell therapy uses living cells injected, grafted or implanted into a patient to produce a therapeutic effect. The simplest cell therapy is a blood transfusion, which has been used successfully ever since the discovery of blood groups and more recently has been followed by the use of stem cells from bone marrow for stem cell transplantation, but these uses of naturally untransformed cells are outside the scope of this chapter. As always there is overlap and next-generation stem cell therapies are emerging using stem cells that have been transformed using some of the techniques described later (see Kimbrel & Lanza, 2020). Cell therapies for cancer (the most advanced indication at the present time) utilize the adaptive immune system to treat disease, achieve remission and prevent relapse. Adaptive cell therapy involves the infusion of autologous or nonautologous lymphocytes following ex vivo expansion. Lymphocyte infusions include naturally occurring tumour-infiltrating lymphocytes or genetically engineered T cells using chimeric antigen receptor (CAR T, see Fig. 9.3) or T-cell receptor (TCR) technology. CAR T cells are genetically engineered T cells that provide the ability for T cells to recognize specific cancer surface antigens

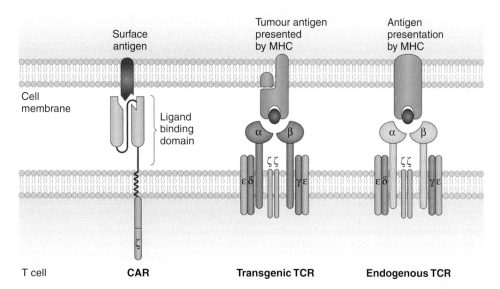

Fig 9.3 Principle of chimeric antigen receptor (CAR) T-cell therapy. *MHC*, Major histocompatibility complex; *TCR*, T-cell receptor. (From Kingswell, 2017).

Table 9.2 Cell therapy is now a reality

Drug (company)	Target	Indications	Status	Key feature
Tisagenlecleucel-t (Novartis)	CD19	Relapsed or refractory B cell ALL	BLA	First-in-modality candidate
Axicabtagene ciloleucel (Kite Pharma)	CD19	Relapsed or refractory aggressive NHL	BLA	First-in-modality candidate
CAR T-meso (Novartis)	Mesothelin	Various solid tumours	Phase I	Targets an antigen upregulated in solid tumours
MB-101 (Fortress Biotech)	IL13Rα2	Glioblastoma	Phase I	Targets an antigen upregulated in solid tumours
JCAR020 (Juno Therapeutics)	MUC16	Fallopian tube and primary peritoneal cancer	Phase I	Co-expresses IL-12
BPX-601 (Bellicum Pharmaceuticals)	PSCA	Various solid tumours	Phase I	Co-expresses rimiducid-activated 'on-switch'
UCART19 (Laboratoires Servier/Pfizer/Cellectis)	CD19	ALL and CLL	Phase I	Potential 'universal' CAR T product
EGFRvIII CAR T (NCI)	EGFRvIII	Glioblastoma or gliosarcoma	Phase I/II	Targets a tumour-specific antigen

ALL, Acute lymphoblastic leukaemia; *BLA*, biologics license application; *CAR*, chimeric antigen receptor; *CLL*, chronic lymphocytic leukaemia; *NHL*, non-Hodgkin's lymphoma.
From Kingswell (2017).

circumventing the need for T-cell activation via the TCR. CAR T cells are therefore not restricted by cancer cell presentation of intracellular antigens, nor matching of T-cell human leukocyte antigens with that of the patient, providing an alternative adaptive cell therapy approach. This currently constitutes the gold standard for cell therapy and provides the first example of late development and licensed products (see Table 9.2). Although dealt with separately here some authorities class CAR T as gene therapy (see later) as the T cells are being genetically modified.

The CAR T-cell receptors are referred to as chimeric because they combine an extracellular domain that enables antigen recognition with an intracellular signalling domain providing T-cell activation. These two domains are connected via a transmembrane region. The extracellular domain is usually derived from an antibody single-chain variable fragment while the intracellular domains are derived from the endogenous TCR CD3ζ signalling domain and costimulatory signals (see Fig. 9.3; June & Sadelain, 2018). The structure of the intracellular domain has evolved from the first-generation composition of only having a CD3ζ signalling domain, to more complex costimulatory intracellular domains leading to second-generation CARs with CD3ζ plus one co-stimulation domain (e.g., 4-1BB or CD28) and third-generation CARs with CD3ζ plus two co-stimulation domains (e.g., CD27, CD28, ICOS, 4-1BB and OX40) enabling augmentation of T-cell persistence, proliferation and survival (Newick et al., 2017; Fig. 9.3). Fourth generation CARs also known as TRUCKs include an additional transgenic product called nuclear factor of the activated T cell (NFAT)-responsive expression cassette, which on engagement of target-initiated CAR CD3ζ signalling stimulates release of transgenic cytokines such as interleukin (IL)-12. IL-12 that improves T-cell activation recruits additional immune cells and modulates the immunological and vascular microenvironment of the tumour, providing a local anti-tumour effect without systemic side effects (Chmielewski & Abken, 2015).

TCR-T and CAR T-cell manufacture

Engineered T-cell receptor (TCR-T) and CAR T cells are manufactured in a similar way involving T-cell source collection, cryopreservation for shipping to a manufacture facility, T-cell selection and/or activation, genetic modification, large-scale expansion and cryopreservation for shipping back to the treatment centre (Levine et al., 2017). Currently, both TCR-T and CAR T cells are autologous cell-based therapies, therefore the process starts with collection of cells from the patient, usually from the peripheral blood, using leukapheresis, which separates the leukocytes and returns the remainder of the blood to the circulation (Smith, 1997). The leukapheresis product is then cryopreserved and shipped to a centre that is capable of TCR-T and CAR T-cell manufacture. The next stage involves separation and enrichment of lymphocytes from other leukapheresis components and isolation of CD4/CD8 T-cell subsets (Powell et al., 2009). At this stage T cells can either be used straight away or cryopreserved for future use providing flexibility with treatment planning (Wang & Rivière, 2016). T cells are activated using a variety of methods such as T-cell culture, with IL-2, beads coated with anti-CD3/anti-CD28 monoclonal antibodies, or APCs (Levine et al., 2017). During this process T cells are incubated with a viral vector, usually retroviral or lentiviral containing the genetic code for TCR alpha and beta chains or CARs. The viral vector attaches to and enters the T cells introducing genetic material in the form of RNA, which is reverse transcribed into DNA therefore permanently integrating with the patient cells and being maintained during cell division (Vannucci et al., 2013). After several days the viral vector is washed out of the culture by dilution and/or medium exchange, following which cells are expanded using bioreactor culture systems designed to provide optimal gas exchange requirements and mixing of the T cells and culture medium enabling large-scale growth of cells. The process may reach a culture volume of 5 L, and it is therefore concentrated before being cryopreserved in an infusible medium and frozen before release. The clinical product is finally transported to the treatment centre where it is thawed and infused into the patient (Levine et al., 2017).

The manufacture of these autologous treatments is, of necessity, on a small scale, using manual processing that is labour intensive, prone to high failure rates, time expensive and costly (Vormittag et al., 2018). The time from leukapheresis to infusion into the patient can be between 2 and 3 weeks, which means there is a risk the treatment may arrive too late for the patient to receive full therapeutic benefit. The financial cost is currently estimated to be in the region of $150,000–$475,000 per treatment with no obvious fixed pricing structure provided by any one company (Walker & Johnson, 2016). Much research is now being invested in finding a safe and effective way of delivering allogenic TCR-T or CAR T cells allowing scaling up of production, improved automation, reduced manufacturing costs and resulting in a true off-the-shelf medicinal product ready and available to be thawed for infusion into patients when needed.

TCR-T and CAR T-cell clinical trial outcomes

Adaptive cell therapy with TCR-T and CAR T cells has been hailed as optimal treatment for some cancers with a huge expansion in clinical trials (Mikkilineni & Kochenderfer, 2017). The fundamental difference between TCR-Ts, which target intracellular antigens presented on major histocompatibility complex (MHC) molecules and CAR T cells that target cell-surface antigens, means they have different applications based on the identified potential cancer antigen target. It could be argued that TCR-Ts have the most potential as they could target almost any cellular protein as long as it is presented on the MHC, whereas only 10% of cellular proteins are expressed on the cell's surface limiting the number of targets available for CAR T cells to act on (Garber, 2018). However, CAR T cells have shown remarkable clinical efficacy due to highly successful targeting of the CD19 cell-surface component of the B-cell receptor complex involved in B-cell activation resulting in impressive rates of complete and durable remission for the treatment of chemorefractory and relapsed leukaemia and lymphoma (Lee et al., 2015; Maude et al., 2014a). To date, two CD19–CAR T-cell therapies (Kymriah and Yescarta) have received FDA approval for clinical use. Kymriah received approval in August 2017 following results from a multicentre clinical phase II trial. Seventy-one paediatric and young adult patients with CD19+ relapsed or chemorefractory B-cell acute lymphoblastic leukaemia (B-ALL) received an infusion with reported overall remission rate in 3 months of 81%, event-free survival and overall survival of 73% and 90%, respectively, at 6 months and 50% and 76% at 12 months (Maude et al., 2018). Shortly afterwards in October 2017 Yescarta was also approved following a multicentre clinical trial including 101 infused adult patients with refractory large B-cell lymphoma in which 54% showed complete remission and an overall survival rate of 52% at 18 months (Neelapu et al., 2017). Adverse events including cytokine release syndrome (CRS), neurological events and haematological side effects were seen with both the licensed therapies. In total five patients died across the studies and Maude et al. (2018) reported 47% of patients were admitted to the intensive care unit for management of CRS, resulting in high circulating levels of inflammatory cytokines secondary to T-cell expansion and activation in response to tumour antigen binding. CRS has been observed in the majority of CD19–CAR T-cell therapies and ranges in severity from flulike symptoms to pyrexia, hypotension, hypoxia, tachycardia and organ failure requiring admission to intensive care for ventilatory and circulatory support. The condition is associated with high levels of inflammatory cytokines (tumour necrosis factor [TNF]-α and IL-6) and markers (C-reactive protein and ferritin). Treatment with anti-IL-6 receptor antibody (tocilizumab) achieves control in the majority of patients, but the impact on the newly infused antitumour cells is unknown. Additionally, corticosteroids may be used but their immunosuppressive action may block T-cell activation and remove clinical benefit. In most cases CRS is reversible and resolves by 2 to 3 weeks postinfusion but can be fatal (Maude et al., 2014b). CD19–CAR T-cell therapy is also associated with neurotoxicity that may occur at the same time as CRS or shortly afterwards but is not controlled by tocilizumab. Symptoms include delirium, confusion, dysphasia, encephalopathy, seizures and cerebral oedema. Usually the condition is self-limiting and resolves but can leave residual symptoms and in severe cases can cause death from cerebral oedema.

TCR-Ts have experienced significant issues with severe toxicity resulting in patient deaths due to cross reactivity with similar antigen MHC complexes and therefore clinical development is continuing cautiously. Currently, three main cancer-associated antigen target categories are being investigated including cancer germline mutations (MAGE-A10, MAGE-A4, PRAME and NY-ESO-1), overexpressed self-antigens (WT1) and tumour somatic mutations/neoantigens. All these approaches have advantages and disadvantages and to date there have been no clear clinical successes. However, TCR-Ts are currently receiving significant interest from pharmaceutical companies and are thought to hold the most promise for successful treatment of solid tumours (Garber, 2018).

Little is known regarding the appropriate dosing levels for adaptive cell therapies. The current dosing strategy follows a principle to deliver as many cells as possible to provide the best chance of success. The main driver is that relapses may not respond to a second infusion of the same T-cell therapy due to escape cell variants no longer expressing the target antigen and the patient's immune system may reject the CAR T cells given a second time around (Fry et al., 2018). As such, to date no optimal target number of cells per infusion has been established. Neelapu et al. (2017) reported a target dose for delivery of 2×10^6 Yescarta anti-CD19 CAR T cells/kg of body weight, while Maude et al. (2018) reported a median dose of 3.1×10^6 Kymriah anti-CD19 CAR T cells/kg of body weight with a range of 0.2×10^6 to 5.4×10^6 cells/kg. Post-infusion cell expansion and cell persistence are important indicators of efficacy but also more severe adverse events (Maude et al., 2018; Neelapu et al., 2017).

Gene therapy

The objective of gene therapy is to produce long-lasting expression of a therapeutic gene at a level that has a significant effect in relieving disease symptoms or even curing the disease. The field has been active for more than 20 years, but recently many of the problems associated with its clinical use have been solved such that there are (since the first in 2016) a number of licensed products available (see High & Roncarolo, 2019). There are different approaches to gene therapy, each with its own advantages and disadvantages.

Autologous ex vivo gene therapy (Fig. 9.4) uses stem cells, derived from the patient, and has similar issues around obtaining cells, modifying them using in vitro cell culture and then injecting them back into the patient to the other cell therapies mentioned above. The long-term objective (as with other cell therapies) is to be able to use allogenic therapy based around cells obtained from

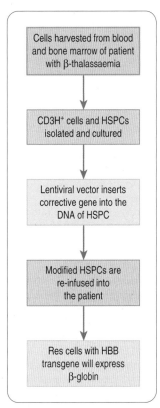

Fig. 9.4 *Ex-vivo* delivery of gene therapy. Block diagram showing the process of *ex-vivo* gene delivery using the example of treatment of β-thalassaemia (see High and Roncarolo 2019 for more details). Hemopoetic stem and progenitor cells (HPSCs) are harvested from the bone marrow or blood of a patient. CD34 +ve HPSCs are isolated using affinity columns and cultured ex vivo in the presence of growth factors to produce and expand a population of self-renewing stem cells. Gene transfer is then achieved using an integrating lentiviral vector containing β-globin cDNA. The patient is then treated to deplete endogenous (faulty) HPSCs from the bone marrow. The gene-corrected HPSCs are then infused back into the patient and engraft in bone marrow where they self-renew and differentiate into hemopoetic cells.

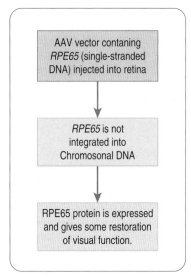

Fig. 9.5 *In vivo* delivery of gene therapy. Block diagram to illustrate the *in vivo* delivery of gene therapy using treatment of vision loss due to a loss of function mutation in *RPE65* (see High and Roncarolo 2019 for more details). The corrective gene is delivered by way of an adeno-associated virus (AAV) vector by injection beneath the retina in an operative procedure. The vector tranduces retinal pigment epithelial (RPE) cells to produce functional enzyme and restore some visual function. The transgene does not integrate into the DNA of the RPE cell.

a donor then expanding and genetically modifying them in a way that allows use in all patients with the relevant gene defect. There are many issues around immunological compatibility of allogenic cells with the recipient that are not yet solved. For some targets it is possible to use suitable vectors to allow in vivo modification of a missing or faulty gene. Although the manufacturing and supply chain is simpler and more scalable for the in vivo approach,

there are still many problems around vector yield and quality control in the manufacturing process that have not been completely solved. It is no accident that those in vivo gene therapies that are currently in use are administered to restricted spaces, such as the eye, so that large amounts of vector are not required (Fig. 9.5). There is much optimism around the use of adeno-associated virus (AAV) as a vector for in vivo gene therapy as this is the only human virus that has been claimed not to cause a disease. Members of this virus family have been engineered to deliver a payload of therapeutic genetic material by swapping viral genes for human genes within the viral capsid. The different crystal structures of the AAV serotypes have been used to design new capsids that can target particular tissues or organs resulting in, for example, AAV8 (whole body transduction), AAV2 (liver, CNS, muscle) and AAV6 (CNS, lung, heart and muscle) (see Li & Samulski, 2020). Two AAV-based drugs (Luxturna and Zolgensma) have been approved by the FDA, and clinical trials using AAV-based therapies are in progress in patients with a number of disorders. Given downstream problems seen in early gene therapy patients it will need long-term follow-up (5–10 years) of approved therapies before it is certain that this approach is beneficial without serious side effects.

The future of gene therapy probably depends upon gene-editing technology. It has been possible to edit genes for many years but only by using complex and time-consuming techniques. In the last 10 years the clustered regularly interspaced palindromic repeats (CRISPR)–Cas methodology has been developed and has transformed this field allowing gene editing to be simple, scalable and effective. CRISPR were discovered as part of a bacterial defence mechanism against viruses, guiding the DNA-cutting enzyme Cas towards the virus sequence to be cleaved. This bacterial mechanism has now been adopted to provide a precise tool to edit the genome. Cas is used as 'molecular scissors' to cut DNA at any point within the genome dictated by a guide RNA. DNA sequences can be removed or inserted to make precise changes (see Jinek et al., 2012). In order to use gene editing to treat a disease, it should be a condition that is chronic and may be progressive such that reversal will have a positive outcome for the patient; there needs to be an identified causative gene and an accessible target tissue in which the gene is expressed such as the brain or liver. If the defective gene is widely expressed throughout the body then the editing therapy is much less likely to be effective. There are three main approaches that have been used: (1) inactivation or deletion of the disease causing gene, (2) repair of the defective sequence to allow coding of normal wild-type protein or (3) insertion of a new DNA sequence to the genome to produce a missing or therapeutic protein. The liver has become the target for the first therapies aimed at human clinical evaluation as a number of genetic diseases are known to originate there. The liver is also among the easiest target organs to reach, with a potential treatment being deliverable in lipid nanoparticles via the bloodstream. For example, a new treatment for ATTR (see ASO section mentioned earlier) is being evaluated by Intellia Therapeutics in collaboration with Regeneron (see https://www.intelliatx.com/pipeline-2/). NTLA-2001 has been tested in nonhuman primates and it has been found that a single dose of a CRISPR–Cas construct, delivered in a lipid nanoparticle formulation, will knock out the *TTR* gene resulting in a 95% reduction in expression of TTR protein that is maintained for up to 12 months. They plan to apply for regulatory approval to proceed to clinical trials in mid-2020. Intellia is also working on approaches where the function of cells is reprogrammed in vitro before the cells are re-administered to the patient (again showing an overlap between cellular and gene therapies). In a project targeting acute myeloid leukaemia (AML) they are replacing the TCR in a patient's T cells with one that expresses the Wilms' tumour antigen (often overexpressed in AML) and

therefore allows the T cells to recognize the AML tumour cells and attack them. They have shown that modified T cells were able to kill patient-derived AML cells in vitro and plan to move into clinical studies in 2021.

CRISPR–Cas is also proving to be a useful tool in drug discovery especially in the field of oncology. For example, Behan et al. (2019) have sequentially knocked out every single gene in cancer cell lines and studied the effect on cancer cell survival. This has uncovered a number of hitherto undiscovered targets. Lin et al. (2019) studied the effects of a range of known anticancer drugs on cancer cells with specific genes deleted. In a number of cases they found that the drug still exerted its cell killing activity even when the gene on which it supposedly worked had been knocked out, revealing that the supposed mode of action was incorrect. This technique allows for the validation of drug target engagement before any patients are exposed to a new drug for the first time. It should lead to drugs that are safer and more effective.

Conclusions

The field of emerging therapies is moving at a rapid pace and many of the approaches that are being used are not covered here. For example, there has been a resurgence in the use of peptides as drugs (Davenport et al., 2020), and some of the delivery problems that prevented their use by the oral route have been overcome (Drucker, 2020) such that this field will almost certainly expand. There is no doubt that the use of cell-based therapies will become more important (see Gottlieb & Marks, 2019), and the FDA has seen a surge in cell- and gene-based therapy products entering early development. It is putting new policies in place to ensure this process is as safe as possible. They estimate that by the end of 2020 they will be receiving more than 200 investigational New Drugs (INDs) per year and in 2019 had more than 800 active cell-based or directly administered gene therapy INDs on file. They estimate that by 2025 they will be approving 10 to 20 cell or gene therapy products a year (Gottlieb & Marks, 2019). The global pipeline of cell-based therapies for cancer is increasing rapidly (see Yu et al., 2019). This trend is illustrated very well in a recent review of the gene-editing pipeline (Mullard 2020c; Fig. 9.6). In a review of novel drug approvals in 2019 Avram et al. (2020) found five classical small molecule drugs, a degrading ASO, an exon-skipping ASO, an siRNA, a peptide, two monoclonal antibodies and two antibody/drug conjugates. This divergence of approach is likely to maximize the chance of success in the treatment of previously intractable diseases.

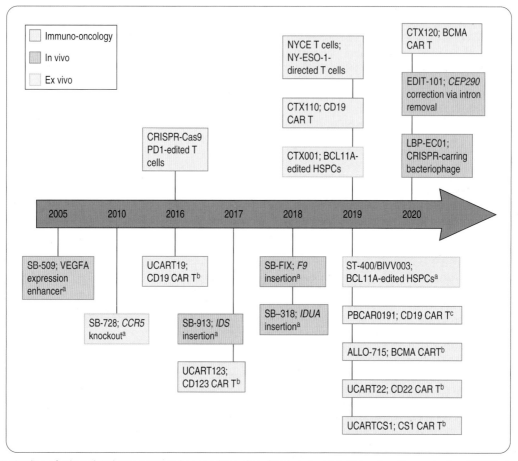

Fig. 9.6 Timeline of selected, industry-supported gene-editing clinical trial starts. *CAR*, Chimeric antigen receptor; *CRISPR*, clustered regularly interspaced palindromic repeats. (From Mullard, 2020c). [a]Zinc-finger proteins [b]Transcription activator-like effector nuclease (TALEN) [c]Meganuclease HPSCs haemopoetic stem and progenitor cells.

References

Alberts, B., Johnson, A., Lewis, J., Raff, M., Roberts, K., & Walter, P. (2002). *Molecular biology of the cell* (4th ed., p. 1463). New York: Taylor and Francis.

Avram, S., Curpan, R., Halip, L., Bora, A., & Oprea, T. I. (2020). Novel drug targets in 2019. *Nature Reviews. Drug Discovery, 19*, 300.

Behan, F. M., Iorio, F., Picco, G., Gon√ßalves, E., Beaver, C. M., Migliardi, G., et al. (2019). Prioritization of cancer therapeutic targets using CRISPR-Cas9 screens. *Nature, 568*, 511–516.

Chmielewski, M., & Abken, H. (2015). TRUCKs: The fourth generation of CARs.

Expert Opinion on Biological Therapy, 15(8), 1145–1154.

Crookes, S. T. (2017). Molecular mechanisms of antisense oligonucleotides. *Nucleic Acid Therapeutics, 27*, 70–77.

Davenport, A. P., Scully, C. C. G., de Graaf, C., Brown, A. J. H., & Maguire, J. J. (2020). Advances in therapeutic peptides targeting G protein coupled receptors. *Nature Reviews. Drug Discovery, 19*, 389–413.

Dean, N. M. (2001). Functional genomics and target validation approaches using antisense oligonucleotide technology.

Current Opinion in Biotechnology, 12, 622–625.

Drucker, D. J. (2020). Advances in oral peptide therapeutics. *Nature Reviews. Drug Discovery, 19*, 277–289.

Fry, T. J., Shah, N. N., Orentas, R. J., Stetler-Stevenson, M., Yuan, C. M., Ramakrishna, S., et al. (2018). CD22-targeted CAR T cells induce remission in B-ALL that is naive or resistant to CD19-targeted CAR immunotherapy. *Nature Medicine, 24*, 20–28.

Fundytus, M. E., Yashpal, K., Chabot, J. G., Osborne, M. G., Lefebvre, C. D., Dray, A., et al. (2001). Knockdown of spinal metabotropic receptor 1 (mGluR1) alleviates pain and restores opioid efficacy after nerve injury in rats. *British Journal of Pharmacology, 132*, 354–367.

Garber, K. (2018). Driving T-cell immunotherapy to solid tumors. *Nature Biotechnology, 36*, 215.

Gottlieb, S., & Marks, P. (2019). *Statement from FDA commissioner Scott Gottlieb MD and Peter Marks MD PhD Director of the Center for Biologics Evaluation and Research on new policies to advance development of safe and effective cell and gene therapies.* FDA. Retrieved from https://www.fda.gov/news-events/press-announcements/statement-fda-commissioner-scott-gottlieb-md-and-peter-marks-md-phd-director-center-biologics.

Hagenacker, T., Wurster, C. D., Günther, R., Schreiber-Katz, O., Osmanovic, A., Petri, S., et al. (2020). Nusinersen in adults with 5q spinal muscular atrophy: A non-interventional, multicentre, observational cohort study. *Lancet Neurology, 19*, 317–325.

Hannon, G. J. (2000). RNA interference. *Nature, 418*, 244–251.

High, K. A., & Roncarolo, M. G. (2019). Gene therapy. *New England Journal of Medicine, 381*, 455–464.

Jinek, M., Chylinski, K., Fonfara, I., Hauer, M., Doudna, J. A., & Charpentier, E. (2012). A programmable dual RNA-guided endonuclease in adaptive bacterial immunity. *Science, 337*, 816–821.

June, C. H., & Sadelain, M. (2018). Chimeric antigen receptor therapy. *New England Journal of Medicine, 379*(1), 64–73.

Lin, A., Giuliano, C. J., Palladino, A., John, K. M., Abramowicz, C., Yuan, M. L., et al. (2019). Off-target toxicity is a common mechanism of action of cancer drugs undergoing clinical trials. *Science Translational Medicine, 11*, eaaw8412.

Kim, V. N. (2003). RNA interference in functional genomics and medicine. *Journal of Korean Medical Science, 18*, 309–318.

Kingswell, K. (2017). CAR – T therapies drive into new terrain. *Nature Reviews. Drug Discovery, 16*, 301–304.

Kimbrel, E. A., & Lanza, R. (2020). Next-generation stem cells – ushering in a new generation of cell-based therapies. *Nature Reviews. Drug Discovery, 19*, 463–479.

Lee, D. W., Kochenderfer, J. N., Stetler-Stevenson, M., Cui, Y. K., Delbrook, C., Feldman, S. A., et al. (2015). T cells expressing CD19 chimeric antigen receptors for acute lymphoblastic leukaemia in children and young adults: A phase 1 dose-escalation trial. *Lancet, 385*, 517–528.

Levin, A. A. (2019). Treating disease at the RNA level with oligonucleotides. *New England Journal of Medicine, 380*, 57–70.

Levine, B. L., Miskin, J., Wonnacott, K., Keir, C. (2017). Global manufacturing of CAR T cell therapy. *Molecular Therapy. Methods & Clinical Development, 4*, 92–101.

Li, C., Samulski, R. J. (2020). Engineering adeno-associated virus vectors for gene therapy. *Nature Reviews. Genetics, 21*, 255–272.

Maude, S. L., Frey, N., Shaw, P. A., Aplenc, R., Barrett, D. M., Bunin, N. J., et al. (2014a). Chimeric antigen receptor T cells for sustained remissions in leukemia. *New England Journal of Medicine, 371*, 1507–1517.

Maude, S. L., Barrett, D., Teachey, D. T., & Grupp, S. A. (2014b). Managing cytokine release syndrome associated with novel T cell-engaging therapies. *Cancer Journal, 20*, 119–122.

Maude, S. L., Laetsch, T. W., Buechner, J., Rives, S., Boyer, M., Bittencourt, H., et al. (2018). Tisagenlecleucel in children and young adults with B-cell lymphoblastic leukemia. *New England Journal of Medicine, 378*, 439–448.

Mikkilineni, L., & Kochenderfer, J. N. (2017). Chimeric antigen receptor T-cell therapies for multiple myeloma. *Blood, 130*, 2594–2602.

Mullard, A. (2020a). Sickle cell disease celebration. *Nature Reviews. Drug Discovery, 19*, 21.

Mullard, A. (2020b). N-of-1 drugs push biopharma frontiers. *Nature Reviews. Drug Discovery, 19*, 151–153.

Mullard, A. (2020c). Gene-editing pipeline takes off, *Nature Reviews. Drug Discovery, 19*, 367–372.

Neelapu, S. S., Locke, F. L., Bartlett, N. L., Lekakis, L. J., Miklos, D. B., Jacobson, C. A., et al. (2017). Axicabtagene ciloleucel CAR T-cell therapy in refractory large B-cell lymphoma. *New England Journal of Medicine, 377*, 2531–2544.

Newick, K., O'Brien, S., Moon, E., Albelda, S. M. (2017). CAR T cell therapy for solid tumors. *Annual Review of Medicine, 68*, 139–152.

Phillips, M. I. (2000). *Antisense technology, Parts A and B.* San Diego: Academic Press.

Porreca, F., Lai, J., Bian, D., Wegert, S., Ossipov, M. H., Eglen, R. M., et al. (1999). A comparison of the potential role of the tetrodotoxin-insensitive sodium channels, PN3/SNS and NaN/SNS2, in rat models of chronic pain. *Proceedings of the National Academy of Sciences of the United States of America, 96*, 7640–7644.

Powell, D. J., Brennan, A. L., Zheng, Z., Huynh, H., Cotte, J., & Levine, B. L. (2009). Efficient clinical-scale enrichment of lymphocytes for use in adoptive immunotherapy using a modified counter-flow centrifugal elutriation program. *Cytotherapy, 11*, 923–935.

Setten, R. L. (2019). The current state and future directions of RNA-based therapeutics. *Nature Reviews. Drug Discovery, 18*, 421–446.

Smith, J. W. (1997). Apheresis techniques and cellular immunomodulation. *Therapeutic Apheresis, 1*, 203–206.

Tambuyzer, E., Vandendriessche, B., Austin, C. P., Brooks, P. J., Larsson, K., Miller Needleman, K. I., et al. (2020). Therapies for rare diseases: Therapeutic modalities, progress and challenges ahead. *Nature Reviews. Drug Discovery, 19*, 93–111.

Vannucci, L., Lai, M., Chiuppesi, F., Ceccherini-Nelli, L., & Pistello, M. (2013). Viral vectors: A look back and ahead on gene transfer technology. *New Microbiologica, 36*, 1–22.

Vormittag, P., Gunn, R., Ghorashian, S., & Veraitch, F. S. (2018). A guide to manufacturing CAR T cell therapies. *Current Opinion in Biotechnology, 53*, 164–181.

Walker, A., & Johnson, R. (2016). Commercialization of cellular immunotherapies for cancer. *Biochemical Society Transactions, 44*, 329–332.

Wan, W. B., & Seth, P. P. (2016). The medicinal chemistry of therapeutic oligonucleotides. *Journal of Medicinal Chemistry, 59*, 9645–9667.

Wang, Y. (2001). The role and regulation of urokinase-type plasminogen activator receptor gene expression in cancer invasion and metastasis. *Medicinal Research Reviews, 21*, 146–170.

Wang, X., & Rivière, I. (2016). Clinical manufacturing of CAR T cells: Foundation of a promising therapy. *Molecular Therapy Oncolytics, 3*, 16015.

Yu, J. X., Hubbard-Lucey, V. M., & Tang, J. (2019). The global pipeline of cell therapies for cancer. *Nature Reviews. Drug Discovery, 18*, 821–822.

Chapter | 10 |

Metabolism and pharmacokinetic optimization strategies in drug discovery

Beth Williamson, Britta Bonn, Bo Lindmark, Nicola Colclough, Stephanie Harlfinger, Antonio Llinas, Constanze Hilgendorf

Introduction

Optimization of drug absorption, distribution, metabolism and excretion (ADME) properties is an integral component of the modern drug discovery process. The objective of the drug metabolism and pharmacokinetics (DMPK) discipline in drug discovery is to aid design and selection of candidate drugs with properties that yield the required efficacy and safety profile in patients. The role of DMPKs at the various stages of drug discovery is summarized in Table 10.1. In vitro and in vivo ADME information is used throughout the drug discovery process to facilitate target validation and safety assessment, and to guide optimization of early screening hits and leads into drug candidates. Indeed, the frontloading of DMPK in drug discovery has resulted in a reduction of the drug attrition rate due to undesirable DMPK properties from approximately 40% in 1990 to 10% in 2000 (Kola & Landis, 2004).

Applying 'quality' over 'quantity' on candidates and therefore shifting attrition to earlier phases has shown that cycle times and costs can be reduced (Paul et al., 2010). In 2011, AstraZeneca started a major revision of its R&D strategy to improve success rates from candidate nomination to phase III completion. The outcome was the implementation of the '5Rs framework' that significantly improved project success rates, decreased the cost per candidate and the cost to reach clinical proof of concept, while dramatically increasing the number of positive proof of mechanisms (PoMs) achieved (Cook et al., 2014; Morgan et al., 2018). This improvement in successful PoMs is mainly due to an increased understanding of human pharmacokinetic (PK), PK/pharmacodynamic (PD) and ADME properties of leads and candidates. A more thorough understanding of drug metabolism and PK is being incorporated into the design of new molecules, and greater focus is applied to quantitative PK scaling and human dose prediction. This strategy has improved the accuracy of human PK predictions for candidates with 76% of compounds predicted within twofold of the observed value, an improvement of ~20% (Morgan et al., 2018).

To help drug hunting project teams focus on the key issues and goals, rather than initiate a multitude of screening assays, it is important to define, as early as possible, a candidate drug target profile (CDTP) in terms of efficacy, ADME, safety and convenience (Bergström & Lindmark, 2019). DMPK plays a central role in defining this target profile. For instance, a commercially attractive best-in-class compound has to be orally active, have a convenient dosing regimen and be able to be administered with or without food and low risk of interactions with other medications. The physicochemical and DMPK attributes that will allow a compound to meet this target profile would be good solubility and permeability, high oral bioavailability, low clearance and reasonable half-life (assuming PD half-life is not the driving parameter) and absence of 'drug–drug interaction' (DDI) potential.

In this chapter, strategies to optimize key DMPK challenges using appropriate in silico, in vitro and in vivo DMPK tools during drug discovery are presented. The rational use of these strategies will help 'drug hunting' projects to advance drug candidates with an attractive DMPK profile and with low risk of failure in development due to DMPK issues. In addition, as prediction of human PK and safe and effective dose is probably the most important activity in drug discovery to ensure that the candidate drug has the attributes required to test the

Table 10.1 Roles of drug metabolism and pharmacokinetics (DMPK) in various phases of drug discovery

Discovery phase	DMPK roles
Target identification	Selection and characterization of tool compounds
	Partner with in vivo pharmacology and toxicology in target validation and safety assessment activities
Hit identification	In silico and in vitro DMPK profiling to help prioritize hit series
Lead identification	Identify DMPK liabilities of lead series
	Determine whether DMPK properties in lead series are optimizable (DMPK liabilities not linked to pharmacophore)
	Develop structure (DMPK) property relationship (SPR)
	Develop 'in vitro in vivo' correlation (IVIVC)
	Guide selection of lead series
	Contribute to development of pharmacodynamic (PD) assay and develop early PK/PD understanding
Lead optimization	Guide optimization of DMPK properties towards target profile
	Comprehensive DMPK characterization of candidate compounds
	Develop biomarker based and/or efficacy/disease-related PK/PD models
	Prediction of human PK
	Prediction of efficacious human dose
	Integration of predicted profile to calculate key margins against side effects

biological hypothesis in patients, strategies to integrate information in discovery to holistically predict PK properties in humans will be discussed.

Optimization of DMPK properties

Optimization principles are described for six key DMPK areas:

- Absorption and bioavailability
- Avoiding PK-based DDIs
- Achieving/avoiding CNS exposure
- Clearance
- Role of metabolite identification:
  - Active metabolites
  - Minimizing risk for reactive metabolites

The following sections summarize current understanding and available tools and suggest best practice for each of the above. Each section introduces the challenges, outlines tactics for dealing with them and identifies areas requiring caution.

Absorption and oral bioavailability

Introduction

As the preferred route of administration for most indications is oral, it is important to characterize oral bioavailability (F) of a compound during drug discovery. Low F must be optimized, as it is often associated with poor and variable exposure and lack of efficacy. F is defined as the percentage of dosed drug that reaches the systemic circulation compared to the intravenous (i.v.) route. F is determined by three serial steps: the fraction of dosed drug absorbed (f_a), the fraction escaping intestinal metabolism (f_g) and the fraction escaping hepatic clearance as it passes from the portal vein to the systemic circulation (f_h) (see Rowland & Tozer, 1989):

$$F = f_a \times f_g \times f_h.$$

The step f_a is influenced by a number of factors including the gastrointestinal (GI) solubility (dose, particle size, pH, solubility profile and formulation), the effective permeability (both passive permeability and active transport processes) and GI stability. The steps f_g and f_h are affected by metabolic enzymes in the intestinal wall and liver, respectively. In addition, f_h can be influenced by transporters if a drug is excreted unchanged into the bile. Both metabolic and active transport processes are saturable and generally obey Michaelis–Menten kinetics. Hence, f_a, f_g and f_h can all display nonlinear effects if compound concentrations are above the Michaelis–Menten constant (K_m) for the particular enzyme– or transporter–drug interaction.

In humans, the combinations of high to low solubility and permeability have led compounds to be categorized according to the biopharmaceutical classification system (BCS) (Amidon et al., 1995). Class 1 compounds, with high solubility and permeability, generally have good absorption properties, while those in class 4 have poor solubility and permeability and are likely to present significant formulation challenges and/or variable and poor exposure. The BCS must be contrasted to the BDDCS (biopharmaceutics drug disposition classification system) introduced by Benet et al. (2016), where high and low clearance complements the permeability range and compounds are classified in terms of their likelihood for high or low extraction and their putative active transport and potential DDI risks.

It is important to estimate the maximum absorbable dose (MAD) of a compound relative to its predicted therapeutic dose, as this will determine the risk of being able to deliver an efficacious dose to humans and guide whether high exposure in safety studies is achievable.

Table 10.2 provides guidance on acceptable pharmaceutical properties for typical oral drug candidates.

Tactics

In theory, it should be relatively simple to obtain good absorption and to ensure that solubility and permeability fall within the optimal ranges. However, the reality is more complex. From an in vivo perspective, the product of absorption and intestinal metabolism can be assessed by accounting for first-pass hepatic clearance in bioavailability estimations:

$$f_a \times f_g = F/f_h.$$

If $f_a \times f_g$ is low, it is important to understand the relative contribution of both f_a and f_g to F so that this can be designed out of the project. Poor absorption can be a result of slow dissolution rate, low solubility in the GI tract, poor effective permeability (passive or active efflux) or instability in GI fluids or in the wall of the GI tract. If absorption is adequate, but F is poor, hepatic clearance (metabolic or biliary elimination) and/or intestinal metabolism may need to be optimized.

To maximize the chances of good absorption, the compound's physicochemical properties must be in an optimal space, as described by Lipinski (rule of 5, Ro5) and others (Johnson et al., 2009; Lipinski et al., 1997; Waring, 2009; Wenlock et al., 2003). Generally, this requires minimizing the number of H-bond donors and acceptors, restricting lipophilicity in the range $\log D_{7.4}$ 0 to 3 and limiting molecular weight to <500. Emerging modalities such as proteolysis targeting chimeras (PROTACs) or compounds (including peptides) targeting protein–protein

---

Table 10.2 Pharmaceutical development candidate drug target profile (CDTP)

Property	CDTP	Impact on pivotal safety studies and initial clinical evaluations if not met	Impact of not meeting on later drug development timelines
Crystallinity Thermal property Hygroscopicity	Crystalline No melt or other event <80°C <2% uptake at 25°C/80% relative humidity	Significant risk of non-robustness of manufacture and performance of drug substance, with the potential for variable exposure in safety and clinical studies due to physical instability Crystalline material required for assessment of formulation approaches and exposure	Significant issues with robustness of manufacture, performance and ease of handling of both drug substance and drug product Potential of compromising clinical studies due to physical instability as drug substance and in drug product requiring additional time and resources
Chemical stability	>90% (in solution formulation after at least 1 day at room temperature)	Insufficient stability for safety assessment (SA) studies. More time and resources needed to understand degradation and mitigate in line with the formulation strategy (storage, pack or formulation) for safety and first time in humans studies	Consideration of the learning in phase I and assess impact and options in line with the formulation strategy. Risk of short shelf-life of the product
Maximum absorbable dose (MAD) Predicted fraction absorbed (f_a) at predicted dose to humans	MAD ≥ predicted dose to humans $f_a \geq 50\%$	Significant risk for not reaching required exposures in early clinical and safety studies. More time and resources needed to develop enhancing formulations as well as a risk of failure	High risk for not reaching clinically relevant exposures using conventional formulations. Strategy with non-conventional formulations will require more time and resources in development. Obvious risk of development failure

interactions (PPIs) often sit beyond the rule of 5 (bRo5) space. Typically, these compounds have molecular weight >800 and $\log D_{7.4} > 4$. In contrast, amino acid–like molecules with molecular weight <250 and negative $\log D_{7.4}$ generally have poor oral absorption and often require a pro-drug or transporter-targeting approach to overcome these issues. These strategies often recruit uptake transporters on the intestinal membrane to improve oral absorption.

Maximizing the absorption of oral drugs is one of the key objectives of any discovery programme. Optimizing the solubility and permeability of the lead compounds becomes therefore of paramount importance. Drug designers know very well that both parameters, crystalline solubility and intrinsic permeability, must be concomi-tantly optimized since a good absorption might be still achieved even if one of these parameters is low, as long as the other one is sufficiently increased (Fig. 10.1).

Both the solubility and passive (or intrinsic) permeabil-ity of a compound should be assessed prior to any in vivo study. Predictive models such as multivariate analysis for these parameters should be assessed for suitability in each project and considered in compound design if either is an issue for a chemical series (Winiwarter et al., 1998). Meas-uring the true thermodynamic solubility of a compound (especially if it is poorly soluble) is not an easy task; many factors, both solution and solid-state aspects, influence the outcome of the measurements (Avdeef et al., 2016). In the Pharma industry, we use different assays depending on

the phase the project is at that moment. For projects in the early phases, when hundreds of compounds need to be measured every week, a high-throughput screening assay is used, typically starting from a dimethylsulfoxide (DMSO) stock solution in a 96-well plate. After an equilibration period (incubation followed by sedimentation), the solid is removed by centrifugation or filtration, and the solution concentration is measured, providing a rough estimation of the kinetic solubility. These solubility measurements will have to be used with caution since the solution often remains supersaturated and the solid is not crystalline, but amorphous. As the project progresses, equilibrium thermo-dynamic solubilities from solid crystalline material will be used to optimize compounds, and ultimately solubility (and dissolution rate) measurements of well-characterized crys-talline material will be performed in relevant GI fluids, that is, FaSSIF and FeSSIF. Fasted State Simulated Intestinal Fluid (FaSSIF) and Fed State Simulated Intestinal Fluid (FeSSIF).

The primary in vitro tools for assessing passive perme-ability are the cell-based Caco-2 permeability assay, where compounds are co-incubated with a cocktail of inhibi-tors of transporters expressed in the Caco-2 cell mem-brane, PAMPA (parallel artificial membrane permeability assay) and in silico predictions. To assess the involvement of transporters (efflux or uptake), bidirectional perme-ability assays can be used, for example, Caco-2 cells or MDCK-MDR1, to flag possible absorption limitations in vivo. However, these transported data cannot be directly

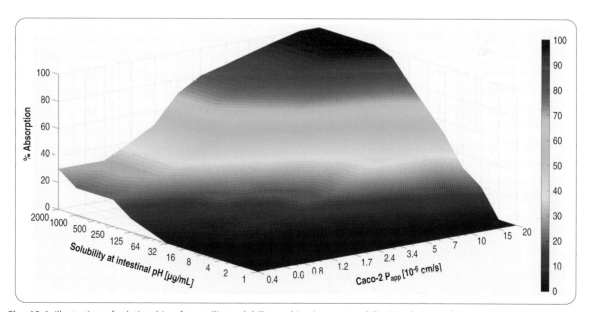

Fig. 10.1 Illustration of relationship of crystalline solubility and in vitro permeability in relation to human absorption. The plot shows that a drug with low crystalline solubility might still have a good fraction absorbed (>50%) if the permeability is sufficiently high, and that for a moderate permeable drug, a solubility of around 120 µg/mL would be required to reach a fraction absorbed about 50%.

extrapolated to quantitative effects in vivo. Modelling tools integrating such in vitro permeability assessment with a relevant solubility measurement (ideally in GI fluids and using crystalline material) are used to estimate human f_a (e.g., GastroPlus (https://www.simulations-plus.com) or Simcyp (Margolskee et al., 2017). Because of its reasonable throughput, the Caco-2 assay can be positioned as an early screen if permeability or efflux is found to be an issue in the project (Fredlund et al., 2017). As a project progresses, these data can also be utilized to predict whether concentration dependence is expected within the likely human dose range or efflux may be saturated. If further evaluation of absorption or efflux is warranted, it is possible to use more physiological models such as sections of fresh intestinal tissue in an Ussing chamber (Sjöberg et al., 2013; Ungell et al., 1998). The Ussing chamber technique can help in understanding regional absorption and cross-species differences and, because the tissue used is enzymatically competent

(metabolic and transporters), the output represents the product of f_a and f_g.

The high lipophilicity of PROTACs and PPIs hinders the use of standard in vitro permeability assays due to the high degree of nonspecific binding, ultimately presenting challenges for in vitro in vivo correlation. For these modalities, in vivo studies are often required to understand the absorption and efflux potential. This approach is similar for peptide prodrugs targeting a specific intestinal transporter, for example, peptide transporter (PepT1). There is currently no enhanced throughput assay available for PepT1, hence in vivo animal PK studies are utilized to understand oral absorption.

Compounds with low hepatic clearance in the rat, good solubility and high effective permeability should exhibit good oral absorption and bioavailability in that species. However, if this is not the case, the troubleshooting decision tree in Fig. 10.2 illustrates the concepts that can be applied to determine the cause(s) of poor absorption,

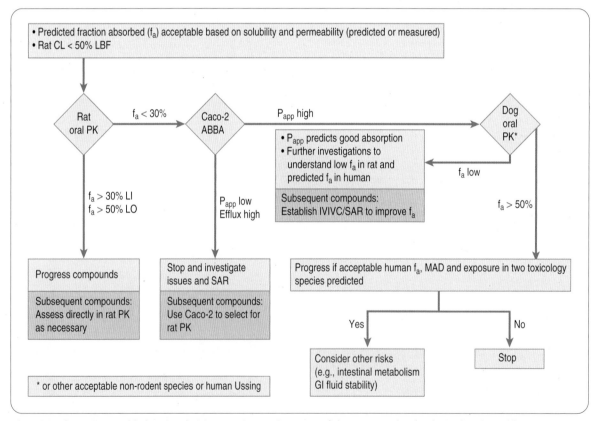

Fig. 10.2 Absorption troubleshooting decision tree, integrating some of the assays and technologies listed in Table 10.3. *Caco-2 ABBA*, Bidirectional transport assay; *CL*, clearance; f_a, fraction of dose absorbed; *GI*, gastrointestinal; *IVIVC*, in vitro to in vivo correlation; *LBF*, liver blood flow; *LI*, lead identification; *LO*, lead optimization; *MAD*, maximum absorbable dose; P_{app}, apparent permeability; *SAR*, structure–activity relationship.

Table 10.3 Assays and techniques used when troubleshooting absorption

Assay/technique	Potential issue/risk addressed	Impacted
PAMPA	Passive permeability	f_a
Absorption profiling on Caco-2 cells	Varying apical to basolateral pH gradient	f_a
	Concentration dependency	
	Use of proteins (e.g., BSA) at various percentages in apical chamber	
	Use of efflux transporter inhibitors	
Transfected cell lines; vesicles expressing specific transporters; Caco-2 efflux assay with and without specific transporter inhibitors	Determine involvement of specific efflux transporters	f_a
GI stability test	Degradation of drug in stomach or intestinal lumen is possible explanation (typical case if predicted F much greater than measured F)	f_a
Intestinal microsomes or S9 fraction	Assess cross-species differences in intestinal metabolism. Nature and source of metabolites can give key information about potential for gut metabolism, as CYP3A and UGTs account for most gut metabolites	f_g
Human metabolic reaction phenotyping	Identify enzymes contributing to gut metabolism	f_g, f_h
Ussing chamber technique	Effective permeability (including transporters) and intestinal metabolism	f_a, f_g
In situ/in vivo portal vein cannulation preparation	Determine amount of drug and metabolites passing through intestine	f_a, f_g
High dose PK studies	Saturation of efflux or metabolism	f_a, f_g, f_h
Simcyp; GastroPlus; or GI-Sim (Sjögren et al., 2013)	Predict absorption rate and extent (software methods)	f_a, f_g

BSA, bovine serum albumin; *fa*, fraction absorbed; *F*, bioavailability; f_a, Fraction absorbed; f_g, fraction escaping intestinal metabolism; f_h, fraction escaping intestinal hepatic clearance; *GI*, gastrointestinal; *PAMPA*, parallel artificial membrane permeability assay; *PK*, pharmacokinetic; *UGTs*, UDP-glucuronosyltransferases.

identify assays to aid in optimizing compound design and understand if the compound is of sufficient quality to progress in the value chain, despite its non-optimal absorption properties.

Table 10.3 lists the assays and techniques that can be used to investigate potential absorption issues and risks, and which parameter (f_a, f_g and/or f_h) the assays impact on.

Cautions

- In contrast to hepatic metabolism, scaling factors for in vitro intestinal metabolism (intestinal microsomes or other subcellular intestinal fractions) are scarce, and it remains difficult to quantitatively assess the contribution of intestinal metabolism to in vivo f_a × f_g. However, physiologically based pharmacokinetic (PBPK)-modelling attempts have been made to use intrinsic Clearance (CLint) CL_{int} from human liver microsomes or S9 fraction to estimate the relative contributions of f_a and f_g to F (Gertz et al., 2010).

- Instead of treating absorption characteristics as a design issue per se, it is often wise to start a multiparameter optimization based on an early predicted human dose, rather than just base the progression of isolated properties of compounds (Page, 2016).

- It is often very difficult to pinpoint why compounds have poor absorption characteristics and, therefore, to resolve this design issue. Thus it is often reasonable to prioritize series with good f_a × f_g, in early discovery even if other properties (e.g., potency, clearance) are less attractive.

- Typically, in preclinical research, oral doses are formulated as suspensions that, on many occasions, may be derived from amorphous material. However, it is important to assess absorption periodically using crystalline material, as physical form may have substantial effects on absorption profiles.

- Particularly for compounds likely to proceed into development, it is important to determine the effect of the polymorphic solid states on absorption. It is also important to ensure that the formulations used are discussed with pharmaceutical development (see Chapter 16) and are appropriate for safety and early clinical development studies.

- If in vitro and in vivo (rat and dog) assessments of f_a do not agree, the risk of an inaccurate estimate of absorption in humans will increase. Sometimes other species have been investigated to mitigate this risk, but it is important to note that there can, for example, be marked discrepancies in $f_a \times f_g$ between cynomolgus monkeys and humans (Takahashi et al., 2009). Evaluation of absorption and pre-systemic metabolism in human intestinal segments in Ussing chambers is a valuable complement to predict human oral absorption.

Avoidance of PK-based drug–drug interactions

Introduction

The design and selection of candidate drugs with a low potential for PK-based DDIs is a key role of discovery DMPK. There are four main forms of PK-based DDI, in which the compound may be a perpetrator or a victim of DDI:

- Competitive (reversible) cytochrome P450 (CYP) inhibition
- Mechanism-based/time-dependent CYP inhibition
- Uptake and efflux transporter inhibition
- CYP induction.

CYP-based DDI is the most frequently observed DDI and mainly occurs in the liver or intestine. Transporter-based DDI generally results in a less than fivefold change of exposure if mediated by a single transporter. More frequently, a multitude of transporters and enzymes are contributing to the overall disposition of a compound. Transporter-mediated DDIs can encompass various processes including intestinal efflux, renal or biliary clearance, and specific issues arising with CNS compounds and hepatic uptake of statins (Tornio et al., 2019). The science and regulatory guidance to support risk assessment of CYP-based DDI are well established and have also significantly advanced for transporter-related issues in recent years (Rekić et al., 2017; US Food and Drug Administration, 2020; Yoshida et al., 2017; International Transporter Consortium, 2018; EMA, 2012).

Tactics

Competitive (reversible) CYP inhibition

Two main types of CYP inhibition assays with different capabilities are currently utilized in drug discovery. Fluorescence-based assays are relatively cheap and have historically enhanced throughput, though in a small but significant number of cases can misrepresent DDI risk due to the occurrence of false positive or negatives (Bell et al., 2008). These assays may still be used for initial profiling of large numbers of compounds, with the data providing guidance of DDI risk in early drug discovery. While LCMS-based assays using specific substrates are more expensive, they provide more representative results and in more recent times have generally replaced the fluorescence-based assays. This assay format is routinely used in lead generation, optimization cycles and for generating compound profiles during more advanced project phases.

Inhibition of the five major CYP isoforms, 1A2, 2C9, 2C19, 2D6 and 3A4, should be evaluated in the earlier phases, while later it would be prudent to also assess potential interactions with isoforms 2A6, 2B6, 2C8, 2E1 and 3A5.

Reduction of CYP inhibition potential is facilitated by the fact that strong quantitative structure–activity relationships (QSARs) are often obtained. It is well established that lipophilicity, aromaticity and charge type are major drivers for inhibiting various CYP enzymes (Gleeson et al., 2007).

Integration of in silico strategies for compound design is becoming complementary to traditional in vitro assays in drug discovery. The availability of large data sets derived from high-throughput screens or clinical databases and bioinformatic algorithms to mine and correlate the data have enabled in silico models for ADME properties including DDI risks (Ferdousi et al., 2017; Zhang et al., 2018).

The risk of DDIs based on phase 2 metabolism (e.g., glucuronidation and sulfation) is usually small, resulting in less than a twofold increase in exposure, and they are rarely observed, possibly due in part to the nature of the enzymatic reaction (high V_{max} [maximum rate] and moderate-to-high K_m values). Such DDIs are not generally evaluated in lead optimization (Williams et al., 2004).

The decision tree in Fig. 10.3 can be used to assess the potential DDI risk of a competitive CYP inhibitor. If still employed, hits identified in a fluorescence-based assay should be confirmed with an LCMS-based assay using drug-like substrates as probes for the different CYP isoforms. Although the ratio $C_{max,u}/K_{i,u}$ can be used to obtain a preliminary estimate of the DDI risk, more accurate evaluation should be conducted using static or PBPK modelling to predict the potential clinical risk (expanded below in the Prediction of DDI risk section).

Mechanism-based/time-dependent CYP inhibition

The inhibition of CYP enzymes may be irreversible (due to covalent binding to the prosthetic haem or the enzyme) or quasi-irreversible (due to the formation of transient complexes with the iron of the haem prosthetic group). Time-dependent inhibition (TDI) methods, using sequential

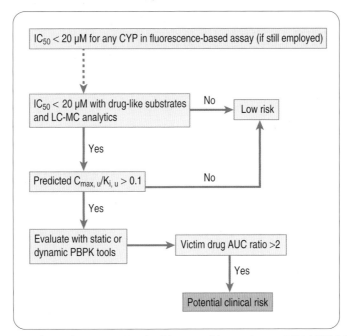

Fig. 10.3 Decision tree to assess drug—drug interaction (DDI) by reversible cytochrome P450 (CYP) inhibition. *AUC*, Area under the concentration-time curve; $C_{max,u}$, unbound maximum concentration; *IC$_{50}$*, concentration producing 50% inhibition; $K_{i,u}$, unbound dissociation constant; *LC-MS*, liquid chromatography - mass spectrometry; *PBPK*, physiologically based pharmacokinetic modelling;.

incubation with test compound and subsequent enzyme activity assessment in recombinant enzymes or microsomes, can be used to determine this (Riley & Wilson, 2015; Stresser et al., 2014). During early phases of drug discovery, a medium throughput screening assay can be used to screen for TDI (Kosaka et al., 2017; Zimmerlin et al., 2011). However, for selecting candidates at later phases, the method employed should provide accurate determination of inactivation rate constant (kinact) k_{inact} and dissociation rate constant (Ki) K_i to properly evaluate the DDI risks of compounds in which preliminary screening indicated the potential for TDI. A positive TDI finding also suggests that the compound or its metabolites may be reactive, and further evaluation should be conducted as specified by reactive metabolite strategies.

A decision tree to help evaluate the potential DDI risk of a TDI CYP inhibitor is shown in Fig. 10.4. If a compound is found to have potential TDI risk based on screening data, K_i and k_{inact} values should be generated to help accurately predict the risk using static equations (Yoshida et al., 2017) or dynamic PBPK prediction tools.

Uptake and efflux transporter inhibition

Compounds that inhibit uptake or efflux transporters may influence absorption, clearance and distribution of drugs that are substrates to those transporters. Unless project specifics warrant it, inhibition potential for efflux of uptake transporters is rarely an early compound design driver, but clearly part of candidate compound characterization. Uptake transporter inhibition assays using human transporter overexpressing cells have proven to be of value (Ward, 2008), but they are highly dependent on chemotype, for example, acids being primarily transported by organic anion transporters (OATs) and likely co-medications, for example, organic cation transporter type 2 (OCT2) and metformin. Acids and zwitterions should be assessed for inhibition of OATP1B1 during drug discovery; this transporter is relevant for hepatic clearance of statins, a widely prescribed cholesterol lowering medication (Kalliokoski & Niemi, 2009). Other uptake inhibition assays (OAT1, OAT3, OATP1B3, OCT1 and OCT2) should be used on a case-by-case basis.

Efflux transporters are believed to serve a protective function and prevent molecules perceived as foreign from gaining entry in cells or tissues. Of the various efflux transporters, P-glycoprotein (Pgp) is the most prevalent and well understood. As specific locations of the Pgp transporter include small intestine enterocytes, hepatocytes, the kidney and the blood–brain barrier (BBB), inhibition of Pgp can affect oral bioavailability, biliary and renal clearance, and brain uptake of compounds that are substrates of Pgp. The bidirectional transport assay using

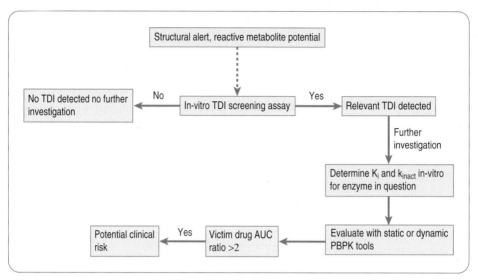

Fig. 10.4 Decision tree to assess time-dependent inhibition (TDI) risk. *AUC*, Area under the curve; K_i, dissociation rate constant; k_{inact}, inactivation rate constant; *PBPK*, physiology-based pharmacokinetic modelling.

either Caco-2 (Pgp, BCRP and MRP2) or MDCK–MDRI cells (specifically for Pgp) is widely available. Inhibition of Pgp can be studied using probe substrates like digoxin. Comparable to Pgp, the importance of BCRP inhibition has developed more recently, in particular in the light of the frequent prescription of statin drugs that involve this transporter (Elsby et al., 2012). If a compound is found to be a transporter inhibitor, the impact of this inhibition in the kidney, liver or gut on co-administered drugs can be assessed based on estimated local concentrations and the IC_{50} (concentration producing 50% inhibition) employing static models (Yoshida et al., 2017) or PBPK tools that allow for dynamic concentration input (e.g., Simcyp).

Determination of clearance mechanism and CYP phenotyping

The potential for a compound to be a victim of a DDI with a co-medication is greatly reduced if there are multiple clearance mechanisms, particularly involving metabolism by multiple CYP enzymes. This should be a consideration if the therapeutic window is low or if the clinical/marketing disadvantage of the interaction would be significant. Quantitative assessment of multiple clearance mechanisms and phenotyping of CYP metabolism should be established for any candidate drug. At nomination, human phenotyping work should include all eight major CYPs (1A2, 2B6, 2C8, 2C9, 2C19, 2D6, 3A4/3A5) and be followed by other enzymes if necessary. Methods for phenotyping the CYP enzymes responsible for a drug's metabolism include the use of individual human

recombinant CYPs (Chen et al., 2011). For a more robust quantitative assessment of individual P450's contribution to clearance, the rate of parent compound disappearance is determined in human hepatocytes in the presence and absence of a specific enzyme inhibitor. For example, the potent CYP3A inhibitor ketoconazole can be used to assess the fraction of total hepatic metabolism mediated by CYP3A4. The remaining rate of metabolism in such an assay can be attributed to non-CYP3A4 pathways like phase 2 enzymes, other CYPs or any other possible mechanism. For compounds with low intrinsic clearance, inhibition of metabolite formation can be monitored instead of loss of parent (Lindmark et al., 2018).

CYP induction-mediated risk for drug–drug interaction

Induction of specific CYP enzymes may not only change a drug's metabolic profile but also have toxicological consequences as CYP enzymes are also involved in the metabolism and synthesis of important endogenous compounds. Although close collaboration with safety functions (see Chapter 15) is needed to evaluate the full impact of CYP induction, it is DMPK's primary responsibility to predict the DDI potential caused by CYP induction in humans. This should be done during optimization with the use of HepaRG cells that are a good surrogate of primary human hepatocytes (gold standard) for AhR-mediated CYP1A induction and PXR- and CAR-mediated CYP3A4 and CYP2B6 induction (Kanebratt & Andersson, 2008). If higher throughput is needed during the optimization phase, the PXR reporter gene assay may be used to minimize PXR-dependent CYP3A4 induction liability. 4-Beta-hydroxycholestrol has also emerged as a promising clinical biomarker for CYP3A induction (Jones et al., 2017).

Prediction of drug–drug interaction risk

Once inhibition potential (of CYP enzymes and/or transporters) has been assessed in vitro, a risk assessment is made by examining the data in relation to the predicted clinical exposures. Predicted free C_{max} is used for a basic assessment for CYPs and for systemically expressed transporters correction of K_i for free values should be considered (US Food and Drug Administration, 2020; EMA, 2013). At candidate drug nomination, a thorough evaluation of CYP and transporter-based DDI risk should be conducted using static equations or dynamic PBPK modelling (e.g., Simcyp). If a potential risk has been identified in the basic assessment, PBPK modelling can be used to estimate relevant concentration of inhibitors at the inlet to the liver or in the gut and to assess DDI risks in various patient populations, particularly in those at most risk.

During early drug discovery, a simple criterion can be used to determine if CYP inhibition presents a risk or not. For this purpose, an IC_{50} of >20 μM provides a reasonable cutoff. Should the predicted therapeutic exposures be very low, then a lower cutoff might be rationally adopted.

To assess CYP induction potential, the E_{max} (maximum response achievable) and EC_{50} (drug concentration giving half maximal effect) obtained from human hepatocytes or HepaRG cells induction assays can be used in conjunction with predicted human exposure (free C_{max} or free liver inlet concentration) to calculate a relative induction score. This is then compared against the relative induction scores of known inducers to estimate the percent human area under the curve (AUC) change of a sensitive CYP substrate.

A compound is likely to be a victim of clinically relevant DDI with co-medication of inhibitors if it has a narrow therapeutic window and is a sensitive substrate to an inhibited enzyme/transporter, as indicated by high values of fraction of the dose eliminated via metabolism (f_m) and high fraction of metabolism via a single CYP ($f_{m,CYP}$). This risk can be reduced by ensuring that the clearance mechanism in question represents <50% of total clearance (resulting in less than a two-fold change in the AUC of the victim compound). At candidate drug nomination, Excel-based DDI templates utilizing static models or software tools such as Simcyp can be used to evaluate the impact of known inhibitors or inducers on the relevant candidate compounds if their clearance is driven mainly by a single enzyme or transporter. If the CYP enzyme involved is polymorphic, the impact of polymorphism should be evaluated to identify high-risk populations. Fig. 10.5 is a decision tree to help in assessing the potential risk that a compound will be a DDI victim.

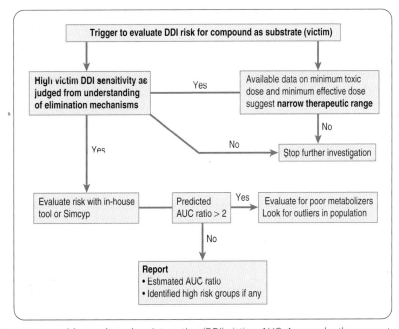

Fig. 10.5 Decision tree to assess risk as a drug–drug interaction (DDI) victim. *AUC*, Area under the concentration-time curve; *CYP*, cytochrome P450; *Simcyp*, software platform.

Cautions

- DDI risk assessment may become complex due to inhibition and induction mechanisms overlaying for a drug molecule; such dynamics can only be assessed by PBPK modelling, for example, with software tools such as Simcyp (Pilla Reddy et al., 2019).
- DDI risk is best assessed by relating IC_{50} to free drug concentrations at the sites of action.

Central nervous system

Introduction

The CNS is protected from the entry of xenobiotics by two barriers, the BBB that separates the brain from the systemic circulation and the blood CSF barrier (BCSFB) that separates the CSF from the systemic circulation. These barriers are formed of cells that have tight junctions ensuring that transport into the brain and CSF can only occur via a transcellular route. Both barriers are rich in efflux transporters particularly Pgp and BCRP. In the BBB, these transporters serve to pump molecules from the brain into the blood.

For CNS therapies where the target resides in the brain, good brain exposure is required. However, for many peripherally targeted therapies, avoidance of CNS exposure is important to avoid unwanted side effects. In both cases, it is important to be able to predict the likely CNS exposure in the clinic. To this end, a cascade of in silico, in vitro and in vivo tools can be employed as outlined below.

Tactics for assessing CNS exposure

In vitro efflux transporter assays are keys in the CNS test cascade and will generally form the front-line assays (Colclough et al., 2019). Typically, these are MDCK cell lines overexpressing either the human Pgp or BCRP transporters or both and serve to readily identify compounds that are transporter substrates. In addition, Caco2 cells in the presence of transporter inhibitors are used to measure the passive permeability of a molecule.

Restricted CNS exposure can be achieved either by efflux of molecules via transporters or from very low passive permeability. However, for oral drugs, passive permeability is generally good, and so the efflux transporters are often the main focus in achieving or restricting CNS exposure in discovery projects.

In silico models trained on in vitro efflux and passive permeability data help discovery projects to design molecules that will give brain exposure (Fredlund et al., 2017). In addition, the physicochemical properties of CNS drug molecules, for example, molecular weight, lipophilicity,

hydrogen bonding, rotatable bonds and polar surface area, have been extensively characterized in the literature and can also serve as a useful guide for design (Rankovic, 2015).

For molecules with the required in vitro efflux properties and passive permeability, for example, for molecules seeking brain exposure, this would be an absence of efflux and good passive permeability, the next step in the cascade would be an assessment of CNS exposure in vivo in the rodent (Colclough et al., 2019). Brain distribution studies may be performed with single or cassettes of compounds using oral or subcutaneous administration with brain and plasma levels sampled over time. The brain AUC to plasma AUC ratio or K_p is then determined. Alternatively, i.v. infusion for several hours can be used to generate a brain/plasma ratio, K_p, at close to steady state.

Unbound concentration in the brain is considered to be the relevant exposure measure for both desired and undesired pharmacological effects. Measurement of total concentration can be very misleading, being to a large extent driven by nonspecific binding to brain tissue and thus strongly correlated with physicochemical properties (e.g., lipophilicity and charge). The fraction unbound in the brain (fu_b) may be determined ex vivo using brain-binding assays, such as the brain homogenate or brain slice (Fridén et al., 2009a; Wan et al., 2007) methods and, together with determined total brain concentration in vivo, enables the calculation of $C_{u,br}$, that is, $C_{total} \times fu_b$. It should be noted, however, that for basic compounds, the brain slice binding method should be used rather than the homogenate method, as the latter, with loss of cellular integrity, gives artifactually higher free levels due to the inability to capture the lysosomal trapping effect (Fridén et al., 2011).

Another key measure of brain exposure is the ratio of free brain to free plasma levels or K_{puu}. This is calculated from the ratio of total brain to total plasma levels, K_p, using fraction unbound in brain fu_b and the fraction unbound in plasma fu_p as shown in the following equation:

$$Kpuu = Kp \times \frac{fub}{fup}$$

Compounds readily able to cross the BBB and giving good brain exposure will typically have $K_{puu} \geq 0.3$, while those compounds with poor BBB penetration typically have $K_{puu} \leq 0.05$. In discovery projects, these cutoffs can serve as useful targets for drug design, where brain exposure or exclusion is sort. In practical terms, discovery projects where the biological target resides in the brain will require a K_{puu} value that delivers unbound drug levels in the brain for the necessary duration to drive clinical efficacy.

For further confirmation of likely brain exposure in the clinic using low dose positron emission tomography (PET), imaging studies can also be undertaken in healthy macaques, which represent the closest BBB model to human. The PET studies, as well as generating images of compound distribution in the brain, enable the percentage of injected radioactivity at C_{max}, K_p and K_{puu} to be determined (Schou et al., 2015).

Beyond the main CNS test cascade, additional problem-solving CNS tools available to enhance understanding of BBB properties include:

1. In vitro efflux studies in alternative cell lines and in cell lines overexpressing animal efflux transporters, for example, mouse, rat and monkey.
2. In vivo distribution studies in rodents in the presence/absence of efflux inhibitors, for example, elacridar. Alternatively, in vivo distribution studies in rodent knockouts (KOs).
3. Mass spectroscopy imaging assessing unlabelled compound distribution in healthy or disease model rodent brains.
4. Rodent quantitative whole-body autoradiography (QWBA) studies.
5. In vivo intracerebral microdialysis. Note, the utility of this technique is limited by the physicochemical properties of the compounds studied.

Cautions

- It is important to note that a relevant brain-to-plasma ratio will only be generated at steady state–like conditions, so the K_{puu} may be very different in steady state and non–steady state conditions. For CNS acting compounds, it is therefore critical to appreciate any acute/steady state differences in CNS distribution. Measurement of K_{puu} at multiple time points can be undertaken to enable understanding of whether a steady state has been achieved.
- There are indications that levels in CSF overestimate free levels in the brain, especially for efflux substrates (Fridén et al., 2009b), although the latter has been challenged (Doran et al., 2005). The Pgp efflux transporter in the BCSFB is reported to pump substrates from the blood into the CSF, in contrast to the BBB, where the transporter pumps substrates from the brain into the blood.
- It may be difficult to assess free levels of acidic compounds in the CNS with standard methodologies (Fridén et al., 2010), because the high plasma protein binding and low tissue binding of such compounds result in inaccurate data due to blood contamination of the brain tissue.
- The brain homogenate binding method has limited use for drugs that reside predominantly in the interstitial space or compounds that are accumulated intracellularly. In such cases, the brain slice method, which retains cell integrity, may provide a better alternative (Fridén et al., 2011).

Clearance optimization

Introduction

Clearance must be suitably low in order to achieve an acceptable half-life and oral bioavailability to ensure appropriate target coverage profile. However, human in vivo clearance cannot be optimized directly in drug discovery, which presents two key challenges. First, there is the need to identify the key elimination processes that determine clearance, and second, those processes must be optimized through appropriate use of human in vitro systems and animal data.

Identification of the likely key human clearance mechanism(s) is supported by a detailed understanding of elimination kinetics in animals. Animal in vitro to in vivo translation increases the confidence in human predictions. This puts emphasis on animal kinetics in all phases of drug discovery to select the appropriate tools and models for both compound optimization and human PK prediction.

Progressing a compound that undergoes numerous routes of elimination can be advantageous, as variability in compound exposure due to single nucleotide polymorphisms of the drug metabolizing enzymes/transporters or DDIs can be minimized. For example, a compound that is eliminated by metabolism via a single drug metabolizing enzyme mainly is vulnerable for DDIs when administered together with an inhibitor or inducer of that enzyme. Furthermore, multiple routes of elimination help to mitigate against exposure variability due to highly variable enzyme activity across populations (i.e., CYP3A4 [see Rawden et al., 2005]) and against polymorphic enzyme metabolism (e.g., CYP2D6 [see Zhou, 2009a, 2009b] and CYP2C19 [see Damle et al., 2009]). The severity of variability in human PK depends on the therapeutic range of the compound as well as safety margins. Further, low variability in human exposure is generally regarded as an advantage for clinical dose escalation studies.

Tactics for optimizing clearance are highly dependent on the nature of the clearance mechanism, as outlined in the following sections dealing with metabolic, renal and biliary clearance, respectively.

Optimization of metabolic clearance

Introduction

Drug metabolizing enzymes are mainly expressed in the liver, but also in other organs at lower levels, for example, the intestine (Gundert-Remy et al., 2014). Optimizing metabolic clearance is one of the most common and challenging activities in drug discovery projects, primarily because high metabolic clearance can be associated with various metabolic pathways and the involvement of numerous enzymes. These include CYP-mediated Nicotinamide adenine dinucleotide phosphate (NADPH-dependent) oxidation or reduction of the compound. CYPs are involved in the metabolic clearance of more than 90% of all drugs (Rendic & Guengerich, 2015). Two CYP isoforms, CYP3A4 and CYP2D6, are involved in the metabolism of more than 50% of all drugs (Zanger & Schwab, 2013; Rendic & Guengerich, 2015). Even though CYPs are responsible for the majority of drug metabolism, non-CYP enzymes contribute to approximately 30% of drug metabolism and should not be ignored (Cerny, 2016; Foti & Deepak, 2016). Examples of other drug-oxidizing enzymes include flavin-containing monooxygenases (FMOs), monoamine oxidase (MAO), aldehyde oxidase (AO) and xanthine oxidase (XO). High metabolic clearance can also be associated with direct or phase 2 conjugation via Uridine 5′-diphospho-glucuronosyltransferase (UDP) UDP-glucuronosyltransferases (UGTs), sulfotransferases, N-acetyltransferases, methyltransferases or glutathione-S-transferases (Jancova et al., 2010). Although less common, whole blood and tissue amidases, esterases, various amine oxidases (diamine oxidase, semi-carbazide sensitive amine oxidase), adenosine deaminase, alcohol and aldehyde dehydrogenase may come into play, depending on the chemotype in question (Cossum, 1988).

During project work, hepatic metabolic clearance can be efficiently screened with available front-line metabolic tools (i.e., microsomes and hepatocytes). Liver microsomes are fragments of the endoplasmic reticulum isolated from hepatocytes. In contrast to hepatocytes, microsomes require co-factors for the catalytic activity of CYPs or UGTs to be activated. In metabolic stability experiments, liver microsomes are often co-incubated with NADPH to activate CYP enzymes only. Lower intrinsic clearance in microsomes compared to hepatocytes can highlight the involvement of phase 2 processes, cytosolic enzymes not associated with the microsomal fraction or the involvement of uptake transporters (Soars et al., 2009). An emerging field of new liver technologies with 2 dimensional (2D) and 3D models and dynamic flow systems are available, for example, co-cultures, spheroids, microphysiological systems, providing a more physiological relevant tool (Bale et al., 2016). However, the complexity of these systems prevents their use in a high-throughput setting, limiting their application to bespoke experiments. When chemotype dictates, for example, esters and amides, whole blood and plasma stability can be used for clearance optimization.

Over the past few decades, small molecules have dominated the oral drug-like space. This paradigm is successively expanding into other drug modalities to access targets that are not druggable with small molecules. Modalities include peptides, small amino acid–like molecules, PROTACs and oligonucleotides (ONs), hence the variety of assays and technologies are adapting accordingly. Peptides are known to be readily metabolized by proteolytic enzymes such as peptidases and proteases, which are expressed mainly in the blood, liver and kidney. Numerous proteolytic enzymes are present in humans, hence it is important to identify which proteolytic enzymes are involved in degradation of a certain peptide due to different cleavage specificity (Werle & Bernkop-Schnürch, 2006). ONs' primary fate of metabolism is via nuclease-mediated hydrolysis of the phosphate backbone to smaller fragments. Nucleases are ubiquitously expressed in the human body. The plasma half-life of natural ONs is in the range of seconds to minutes. Their stability can be substantially increased by chemical modifications of the ribose sugar moiety like 2′-MOE (methoxyethyl) substitution and locked nucleic acids (LNAs) (Andersson et al., 2018). Conversely, small amino acid–like molecules do not undergo hepatic metabolic clearance.

Failure to clarify and control metabolic clearance is a major issue in drug discovery because it can:

- Result in very high total body clearance, low oral bioavailability and short half-life
- Result in an inability to deliver an oral therapeutic drug level
- Lead to excessively long design-make-test-analyse cycles in drug discovery
- Lead to the demise of a project that cannot find an alternative chemotype.

Tactics

Assessment of a compound's metabolic stability in liver microsomes or hepatocytes can be utilized to predict hepatic metabolic clearance. The obtained in vitro intrinsic clearance values can be scaled up to liver proportions, arriving at an in vivo intrinsic clearance value, from which a hepatic metabolic clearance value can be derived utilizing prediction models of variable complexity limited by hepatic blood flow (Hallifax & Houston, 2019; Sohlenius-Sternbeck et al., 2012; Poulin et al., 2012). For in vitro to in vivo extrapolation (IVIVE) of hepatic metabolic clearance, recent analyses have confirmed a standard (CYP/UGT-based) regression correction is suitable for FMO substrates as well (Jones et al., 2017). If the predicted data from animal in vitro systems and the observed total clearance in animal correlate, and there are no obvious features in the structure or physicochemical properties that alert for extrametabolic clearance, project teams can be confident that the compounds' major clearance mechanism is via hepatic metabolism. In a situation where the predicted hepatic metabolic clearance underestimates the observed clearance in animals, or there are obvious structural and/ or physicochemical properties alerting for extrametabolic elimination, a quantitative assessment of renal and biliary clearance is required to fully quantify and understand metabolic clearance in vivo. Underprediction of the observed metabolic clearance may indicate an extrahepatic metabolic clearance mechanism. While not always warranted, if the compound contains esters, amide linkages, aldehydes or ketones, this can be investigated with a simple plasma or blood stability assay.

Addressing high rates of metabolism can be facilitated by understanding the metabolic soft spots of the compound. Reducing the electronic density of the metabolic soft spot and blocking or replacing the metabolically labile functional groups are successful strategies to reduce CYP-mediated clearance. The crystallization and subsequent elucidation of the major CYP isoform structures has enabled structure-based design and in silico methods facilitating the understanding of the metabolic interactions with CYPs 3A4, 2D6 and 2C9. Sun and Scott (2010) provide a review of the 'state of the art' in structure-based design to modify clearance. Combined with knowledge about where in the compound structure the location of catalysis takes place, and knowledge about which CYP enzyme turns over the compound, docking to the CYP enzyme can provide information about how the compound is oriented in the active site of the CYP. As a result, alternative parts of the molecule could be modified to reduce the affinity between substrate and CYP. Such knowledge should, therefore, be used to assist in the rational design to increase metabolic stability of novel compounds. There are types of software available to predict both sites of metabolism and orientation in the CYP enzyme that can be utilized in compound design. Advances in computational approaches provide drug discovery scientists with the ability to review in silico predictions for compounds at the design stage to further refine and ultimately make compounds of the highest quality. Global multivariable models fitted using chemical descriptors are trained on in-house data and utilized to categorize compounds based on their predicted human liver microsome intrinsic clearance. However, with advances in machine learning methods and artificial intelligence, it is hoped these in silico models can be further refined to allow actual intrinsic clearance values to be utilized. Nonetheless, as a compound progresses in silico, models should be complemented with in vitro measurements to allow validation of the models and conduct appropriate risk assessment before significant further investment.

Metabolic stability in terms of unbound clearance is known to correlate with lipophilicity (Broccatelli et al., 2019). Less lipophilic compounds are, in general, more metabolically stable compared with more lipophilic compounds. For more lipophilic compounds, CYP3A4 is usually the main CYP isoform responsible for the metabolism. The rate of such metabolism is sometimes difficult to reduce with specific modifications of soft spots because the catalytic site is large and promiscuous. Commonly, the overall lipophilicity of the molecules needs to be reduced. The correlation between lipophilicity and metabolic stability in vitro should be explored within a compound series, and in turn, used in early screening phases to improve metabolic stability and to influence compound design. For molecules with a low molecular weight and negative $\log D_{7.4}$, for example, amino acid–like drugs, metabolism is generally not the main route of elimination, hence bespoke investigation is required. To optimize metabolic clearance of small molecules, it is essential to understand the enzymatic source of the instability. It is also necessary to have an in vivo assessment of clearance of selected compounds to establish that the in vitro system is predictive of the in vivo metabolic clearance.

Cautions

- Where common in vitro models (e.g., hepatocytes) significantly underestimate in vivo hepatic metabolic clearance and where the chemotype is either a carboxylic acid or a low $\log D_{7.4}$ base, poor scaling may be due to the compound being a substrate for hepatic uptake transporters (e.g., OATPs) that can significantly influence hepatic metabolic clearance. The rate limiting step for poor permeable OATP substrates is the intrinsic uptake clearance that is underpredicted in standard hepatic metabolic in vitro assays (Webborn et al., 2007). Thus, a hepatic uptake experiment will be needed to predict the in vivo hepatic metabolic clearance (see Soars et al., 2007 for methodologies).

- In other instances, carbonyl-containing compounds metabolized by carbonyl reductases in microsomes have been shown to significantly underestimate clearance when in vitro reactions are driven by direct addition of NADPH versus the addition of an NADPH regenerating system (Mazur et al., 2009). Aza-containing heterocycles are potential substrates of AO, which is an NADPH-independent enzyme mainly expressed in the hepatic cytosolic fraction. Similarly, for substrates of carbonyl reductases, hepatic metabolic clearance will be significantly underpredicted in vitro. For compounds carrying a structural alert for AO, any +16Da metabolites detected in a hepatic cytosolic fraction is an alert for AO-mediated metabolism (Hutzler et al., 2012; Zientek et al., 2010).

- By contrast, if hepatic metabolic clearance is overpredicted in vitro, the PK profile should be scrutinized in detail. Possible pitfalls include inaccurate characterization of the elimination phase, enterohepatic circulation or if the compound exposure is well above

K_m and the metabolizing enzymes are saturated (Tse et al., 1982; Williamson et al., 2020).

Optimization of renal clearance

Introduction

For renally cleared drugs, processes including passive glomerular filtration, active tubular secretion and reabsorption can be involved. Renal clearance is most commonly a feature of polar, low $\log D_{7.4}$ ($<\sim 1$) compounds due to their low plasma protein binding, lack of passive permeability (and inability to facilitate re-absorption in the distal tubule), or a compound is a substrate for the renal transporter proteins, for example, OATs and OCTs. Amino acid–like compounds typically possess these physicochemical properties, resulting in renal clearance as the major route of elimination. Similarly, once cleaved by endo- and exo-nucleases, antisense ONs display renal clearance. Passively cleared compounds are generally well predicted from animal data because $CL_r \leq GFR \times f_u$ (where CL_r is renal clearance, GFR is glomerular filtration rate, f_u is the fraction unbound). Hence, simple, related, allometric relationships can be readily established (Paine et al., 2011).

Transporters significantly complicate the prediction of human renal clearance by introducing the potential for large interspecies differences. While there are in vitro assays for animal and human transporters (e.g., OATs) that can be useful for generation of QSAR; their utility for human PK prediction is yet to be fully established.

Tactics

Reducing renal clearance to reduce total body clearance is generally achieved by increasing lipophilicity through modulation of logP or pK_a. All data are amenable to QSAR analysis, and particularly those from cell lines expressing individual transporter proteins.

Based on a few descriptors, a relatively simple diagram (Fig. 10.6) can be used to classify drugs as having high (>1 mL/min/kg), medium (>0.1 to <1 mL/min/kg) or low (≤0.1 mL/min/kg) renal clearance (Paine et al., 2010).

For acids and zwitterions, early determination of renal clearance in rat and dog is recommended as part of establishing the primary clearance mechanism of a compound. Once these data are available, two possible scenarios exist: firstly, a simple allometric relationship can be used to predict human renal clearance or secondly, if such a relationship is not apparent, this prediction should be based on f_u and kidney blood flow–corrected rat or dog data. On balance, there are enough examples to suggest that for acids

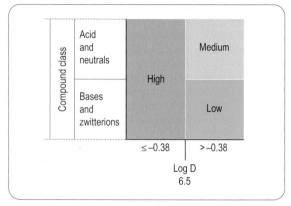

Fig. 10.6 Simple diagram to classify compounds for risk of renal clearance. Low renal clearance is defined as ≤0.1 mL/min/kg, moderate as >0.1 to <1 mL/min/kg and high as >1 mL/min/kg.

and zwitterions, human renal clearance is best predicted from the dog (McGinnity et al., 2007).

Cautions

Accurately predicting renal clearance of acids and zwitterions (i.e., within threefold) is important, as volumes of distribution tend to be low and acceptable half-lives are at risk.

The potential for renal DDI of renal transporter substrates should be considered.

Optimization of biliary clearance

Introduction

The biliary clearance of compounds involves active secretion from hepatocytes by adenosine tri-phosphate (ATP)-dependent transporter proteins (primarily Pgp, MRP2 and BCRP) into the biliary canaliculus, and drainage into the small intestine. It is commonly a feature of acidic and zwitterionic compounds and can be very efficient, resulting in hepatic blood flow limited clearances. This efficiency is partly a consequence of many biliary transporter substrates also being substrates of sinusoidal uptake transporters (e.g., OATPs).

Biliary clearance is a major issue in discovery because it:
- Can result in very high drug clearance and low bioavailability
- Can result in low systemic exposure and small safety margins
- Is difficult to optimize chemically and predict across species

- Is often the synergistic product of two transporter systems in series (uptake and efflux).

Tactics

An overlap between the structure–activity relationship for OATP substrates and biliary-cleared compounds has been shown, depicted by physicochemical descriptors like high molecular weight, large polar surface area, high number of rotatable bonds and hydrogen bonding groups, low lipophilicity and passive permeability (Varma et al., 2012). BDDCS class 3 and 4 drugs, poorly permeable and metabolically stable compounds, are in general primarily excreted into the bile or urine rather than being eliminated via the metabolism (Hosey et al., 2014). In an extensive evaluation of biliary clearance, Yang et al. (2009) showed molecular weight to be a good predictor of biliary clearance in anionic (but not cationic or neutral) compounds, with a threshold of 400 Da in rat and 475 Da in humans.

If total hepatic clearance is underpredicted in vitro metabolic systems or the physicochemical properties alert for biliary clearance, a biliary elimination study in the rat should be considered. For compounds shown to be biliary-cleared in rat, an assessment of efflux by Pgp, BCRP and MRP2 and hepatic uptake by OATP1B1/3 should be considered. For compounds shown to be substrates of efflux but not influx transporters, the biliary clearance is expected to be similar across species when normalized for body weight and corrected for plasma protein binding. For biliary-cleared compounds that are substrates of both efflux and influx transporters, biliary clearance in humans is expected to be at least 10-fold lower compared with that in rat (Grime & Paine, 2013). This can be rationalized by the fact that rat hepatic uptake transporters are more efficient compared with their human counterparts. PK in dog or monkey should be considered for compounds shown to be substrates of hepatic uptake transporters in order to increase confidence in scaling of human biliary clearance.

Tactics for optimization and prediction of biliary clearance include the following:

- Consider physicochemical properties like molecular weight and ionic charge as determinants of biliary CL
- Track progress in rat and dog using i.v. PK studies without bile collection
- Make use of in vitro efflux and hepatic uptake in vitro experiments
- If rat and dog provide ambiguous data, dog is considered a more reliable species for scaling of human biliary clearance if compounds are shown to be substrates of hepatic uptake transporters
- Consider assessing efflux in sandwiched cultured rat and human hepatocytes. An emerging body of literature supports this approach, although quantification is challenging (Li et al., 2009; Kimoto et al., 2017).

Cautions

High biliary clearance in the rat presents a hurdle to a discovery project for two reasons. First, it can be challenging to optimize, and it will be resource-demanding with need for many in vivo PK experiments to track the progress in compound optimization. Second, prediction of human biliary clearance is more uncertain compared with prediction of human metabolic and renal clearance because of species differences in both expression levels and specific activities of hepatic transporters. Hence, high biliary clearance is considered a risk at candidate drug nomination (unless animal specific transporters are the cause). Biliary secretion does not necessarily result in the elimination of compounds from the body, as there is the potential for re-absorption from the GI tract, which can lead to overestimation of volume of distribution at steady state (Vss) V_{ss}.

Role of metabolite identification studies in optimization

Introduction

Knowledge of the metabolites formed from a compound/compound series is often highly beneficial or even essential during drug discovery, because knowing the sites of metabolism facilitates rational optimization of clearance and aids in understanding DDI, particularly time-dependent DDI. As these issues are considered elsewhere (sections on clearance optimization and avoidance of PK-based DDIs), they are not discussed further here. However, two other major areas of drug discovery that are dependent on metabolite identification and on understanding metabolite properties are considered below.

- Assessment of pharmacologically active metabolites
- Avoiding/assessing risk from reactive metabolites.

Active metabolites

Introduction

Active metabolites can influence PD and PK/PD relationships (Gabrielsson & Green, 2009), one example being their major effect on the action of many statins (Garcia et al., 2003). Knowledge about the (structure–activity relationship) SAR for potency should be kept in mind during drug optimization when evaluating pathways of biotransformation since active metabolites with equal or better potency, more favourable distribution or longer half-lives than the parent can have profound effects on PK/PD relationships. Time–response studies will indicate the presence of such metabolites, provided an appropriate PD model is available. Failure to discover the influence of such metabolites may lead to erroneous dose predictions. Assuming similar potency, metabolites with shorter half-lives than the parent will have less effect on dose predictions and are often difficult to elucidate by PKPD modelling. The presence of circulating active metabolites of candidate drugs can be beneficial for the properties of a candidate but also adds significant risk, complexity and cost in development.

Prodrugs are special cases where an inactive compound is designed in such a way as to give rise to pharmacologically active metabolite(s) with suitable properties (Abet et al., 2017). The rationale for design of oral prodrugs is usually that the active molecule is not sufficiently soluble and/or permeable, but a prodrug approach can also be applied for improved organ/tissue selectivity and improved time profile. Examples of successful prodrugs are omeprazole, which requires only one single chemical conversion to activate the molecule (Lindberg et al., 1986), and clopidogrel (Testa, 2009), which is activated through CYP3A4-mediated metabolism.

Tactics

In vitro metabolite identification studies, combined with knowledge about SAR, may suggest the presence of an active metabolite. Studies of plasma metabolite profiles from PKPD animal studies may support their hypothesized presence and relevance. Disconnect between the parent compound's plasma profile and its PD in PKPD studies may be a trigger for in vivo metabolite identification studies.

If active metabolites cannot be avoided during compound optimization, or are considered beneficial for efficacy, their ADME properties should be determined. Advancing the metabolite rather than the parent compound is an option that should be considered. If a prodrug strategy is utilized, the predicted human elimination profile of the prodrug will be of importance to optimize to achieve adequate exposures of the active metabolite.

The decision tree in Fig. 10.7 highlights ways to become alerted to the potential presence of active metabolites, and suitable actions to take.

Cautions

Using preclinical data to predict exposure to an active metabolite in humans is usually accompanied by considerable uncertainty (Anderson et al., 2009). Plasma

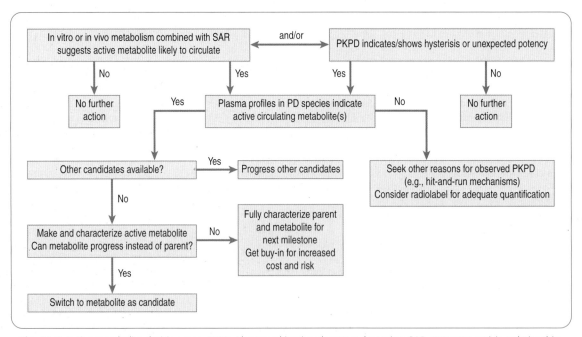

Fig. 10.7 Active metabolite decision tree. *PKPD*, Pharmacokinetics-pharmacodynamics; *SAR*, structure–activity relationship.

and tissue concentrations of metabolites in humans are dependent on a number of factors. Species differences in formation, distribution and elimination need to be included in any assessment.

Minimizing risk for reactive metabolites during drug discovery

Introduction

Many xenobiotics are converted by drug-metabolizing enzymes to chemically reactive metabolites that may react with cellular macromolecules. The interactions may be noncovalent (e.g., redox processes) or covalent and can result in organ toxicity (liver being the most common organ-affected), various immune-mediated hypersensitivity reactions, mutagenesis and tumour formation. Mutagenesis and carcinogenesis arise as a consequence of DNA damage, while other adverse events are linked to chemical modification of proteins and in some instances lipids. Avoiding, as far as possible, chemistry giving rise to such reactive metabolites is, therefore, a key part of optimization in drug discovery.

Tactics

Minimizing the reactive metabolite liability in drug discovery is based on integrating DMPK and safety screening into the design-make-test-analyse process. A number of tools are available to assist projects in this work (Kalgutkar, 2020; Thompson et al., 2011, 2016):

- **Search tools/databases**: this includes in silico tools to: (1) identify substructures associated with potential reactive metabolite formation, (2) identify potential bacterial mutagenicity and (3) learn how to avoid/design away from reactive metabolite formation
- **Trapping studies** in human liver microsomes to enable the detection of reactive metabolites. Agents used to trap unstable reactive intermediates are glutathione (for soft electrophiles) and potassium cyanide (KCN) (for iminium ions) as first-line assays. Structural information can be obtained from further analysis of glutathione and cyanide adduct mass spectrometry data. For very reactive aldehydes, that is, α,β-unsaturated aldehyde, methoxylamine can be used as trapping reagent.
- **Metabolite identification** in human liver microsomes or hepatocytes. Interpretation of the metabolite patterns may give information about existence of putative short-lived intermediates preceding the observed stable metabolites (e.g., dihydrodiols are likely to be result of hydration of epoxides).

- **TDI** studies in human liver microsomes to flag the likelihood of a mechanism-based inhibitor (mainly inhibition of CYPs)
- **Formation and degradation of acyl glucuronides** from carboxylic acids in activated human liver microsomes. This gives an overall estimate of the acylating capability of acyl glucuronides.

If it proves difficult or impossible to optimize away from reactive metabolite signals using the screen assays listed above, yet compounds in the series for other reasons are regarded as sufficiently promising, then a reactive metabolite risk assessment will have to be undertaken. Such assessment could include covalent binding to human hepatocytes in vitro. Predicted dose to humans, C_{max} and fraction of the dose being predicted to be metabolized over the reactive metabolite pathway will have to be taken into account. Other experimental systems that might be used for assaying metabolite-mediated cytotoxicity are cell systems devoid of, or overexpressing, various CYPs and integrated in vitro models for hepatic safety and metabolism, such as human liver spheroids (Foster et al., 2019). Details of such an assessment are beyond the scope of this review but are discussed by Thompson et al. (2012) and Kenna and Utrecht (2018).

Caution

Although reactive metabolites, beyond reasonable doubt, constitute a risk worthwhile to screen away from, the underlying science of potential toxicity is complex; for example, overall covalent binding to proteins is a crude measure indeed. It is possible that covalent binding to some proteins might give rise to antigenic conjugates and consequently pose a toxicity risk; however, the toxicity risk associated with covalent binding to proteins is also highly influenced by the daily dose given, as indicated by Thompson et al. (2012) and Nakayama et al. (2009). Formation of glutathione adducts as such is not alarming, particularly when catalysed by glutathione transferases. The relevance of trapping with an unphysiological agent like cyanide could be even more challenging.

Despite these and other fundamental shortcomings in the reactive metabolite science, most pharmaceutical companies invest significant resources into screening away from chemistry, giving rise to such molecular species. Taking a compound with such liabilities into humans will require complex, and probably even more costly and time-consuming risk assessment efforts.

Human pharmacokinetics and dose prediction

The overriding goal of in silico, in vitro and in vivo DMPK methods conducted at all stages of drug discovery is to help design and select compounds with acceptable human PK. Hence the prediction of human PK is an important component of modern drug discovery and is employed throughout the drug discovery process. In the early stages, it is used to estimate how far project chemistry is from its target profile and to identify the most critical parameters for optimization. At candidate selection, accurate PK and dose prediction is required to determine not only whether the drug candidate meets the CDTP criteria but also to estimate safety margins, compound requirements for early development phases and potential DDI risk.

The prediction of human PK involves two distinct stages—first, the estimation of individual kinetic parameters, and second, the integration of these processes into a model to simulate a concentration–time profile (see Fig. 10.8).

To predict the human PK profile following oral administration, the following fundamental PK parameters must be determined: (1) absorption rate (k_a) and bioavailability (F), (2) volume of distribution (V_{ss}) and (3) clearance (CL, total, hepatic, renal and other routes). Methods used to predict individual PK parameters can be classified into two approaches: empirical or mechanistic. Mechanistic methods are based on knowledge of the underlying mechanisms or processes that define the PK parameters, while empirical methods rely on little or no a priori knowledge. Data required for these methods can be in silico, in vitro or in vivo data, and in general, methods that integrate and use both in vitro and in vivo data. PBPK models utilizing measured parameters (in vivo or in vitro) tend to be more accurate than methods that rely on in silico predictions.

Prediction of absorption rate and oral bioavailability

Although frequently ignored in scaling, accurate prediction of oral absorption rates (k_a) is required to predict C_{max} and to project the potential for DDIs. Oral absorption rate is heavily dependent on the final physical form of the compound, and the prediction of this parameter in the early phase of discovery may be of limited value. The rate of k_a can be scaled empirically using k_a values determined from preclinical species; k_a values are usually obtained from rat or dog, i.v. and p.o. PK studies via deconvolution analysis. Oral absorption determined in the rat was usually found to be in good agreement with that in humans. However, in the dog, oral absorption rates for hydrophilic compounds were usually much faster than in humans (Chiou et al., 2000). Hence, if there is discrepancy in the absorption rate between the two species, the value from the rat should be used for the prediction.

Using various variations of a physiologically based transit model originally developed by Amidon et al. (Yu & Amidon, 1999), k_a can also be predicted mechanistically. The model is termed the compartment absorption and transit (CAT) model and characterizes the fraction of compound absorbed per unit time (based on its dissolution rate, pH solubility profile, effective

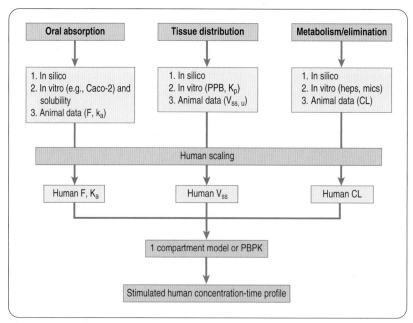

Fig. 10.8 Process for predicting human pharmacokinetics. *PBPK*, Physiologically based pharmacokinetic.

permeability, intestinal metabolism, efflux, etc.) as the compound moves through the different compartments of the GI tract. This approach is used in a number of commercially available tools such as GastroPlus and Simcyp, and can be used to estimate the fraction of the dose absorbed (f_a) and the fraction escaping intestinal metabolism (f_g), in addition to k_a.

As mentioned earlier in the optimizing oral bioavailability section, oral bioavailability is a composite product of (f_a), (f_g) and hepatic 'first-pass' extraction (f_h). Hepatic extraction is a function of hepatic clearance and hepatic blood flow and can be estimated using the following equation:

$$f_h = 1 - CL_h/Q$$

where CL_h is the hepatic clearance and Q is the hepatic blood flow.

Prediction of clearance

Clearance is a primary PK parameter that is used to characterize drug disposition. Total or systemic clearance, the sum of all individual organ clearance responsible for overall elimination of a drug, can be predicted empirically using allometry. Allometric scaling is based on the empirical observations that organ sizes and physiological processes in the mammalian body are proportional to body weight by the following equation:

$$Y = aW^b$$

where Y is the parameter of interest, W is the body weight, and a and b are the coefficient and exponent of the allometric equation, respectively (Mahmood, 2007). Several adaptations to allometric CL predictions have been brought forward in an attempt to improve prediction accuracy of the method (Lombardo et al., 2013).

For individual organ clearance, allometry is useful for flow-dependent clearance processes, for example, renal and high hepatic CL. However, for low CL compounds that exhibit large species differences in metabolism, hepatic clearance and hence total clearance cannot be reliably predicted by allometry. Hepatic clearance can be mechanistically scaled using an in vitro and in vivo correlation (IVIVC) approach. With this approach, intrinsic in vitro clearance is measured using in vitro metabolic stability assays (microsomes or hepatocytes). The measured in vitro clearance values are scaled to an intrinsic in vivo clearance for the whole liver, and then converted to a hepatic clearance using a model that is limited by hepatic blood flow (Hallifax & Houston, 2019; Poulin et al., 2012; Sohlenius-Sternbeck et al., 2012). If IVIVC predicts clearance in animal species, the project team can be confident that the method is applicable for human predictions (albeit due diligence on additional routes must be completed for each chemical series).

Prediction of volume of distribution

Volume of distribution (V) is a primary PK parameter that relates drug concentration measured in plasma or blood to the amount of drug in the body and is used to characterize drug distribution. It is a key parameter, as it is a primary determinant (together with clearance) of drug half-life. Higher volume compounds will have longer half-lives. In a simple system:

$$T1/2 = \ln(2) * V/CL$$

Volume of distribution is a measure of the relative affinity of the compound for plasma/blood constituents and tissue constituents. In general, for moderately lipophilic compounds, acids have a high affinity for albumin and, therefore, have a low volume of distribution (0.1–0.5 L/kg), bases have a high affinity for tissues and, therefore, have high volumes (>3 L/kg), while neutral compounds have volumes around 1 L/kg. Correcting V for plasma protein binding yields a very useful parameter 'unbound volume' (V_u):

$$Vu = V/fu$$

Unbound volume is a measure of the average tissue affinity of a compound, but more importantly should be relatively constant across species. If this consistency is observed in preclinical species, human predictions are relatively straightforward, and a sound basis for the use of more sophisticated tools (e.g., PBPK models, see later) to predict complex distribution profiles is established.

In PBPK modelling, the body is portrayed as a series of compartments that represent tissues and organs. The compartments are arranged to reflect anatomical layout and are connected by arterial and venous pathways. Each tissue has an associated blood flow rate (Q), volume (V_t) and a tissue partition coefficient (K_p), and the rate of change of the drug in each tissue is mathematically described by a differential equation.

The total volume of distribution is the sum of the volume of distribution of all the organs. The volume of distribution in each organ is simply the actual volume of the organ multiplied by its corresponding tissue distribution coefficient (K_p). K_p can be determined experimentally in animals for each organ; however, this is very resource-intensive and impractical. There are two approaches for estimating K_p in various organs. In silico estimation of K_p can be done using various tissue composition methods. This is the approach used in commercial software packages such as GastroPlus and Simcyp. The other approach was developed by Arundel (1997) using rat V_{ss} data and is based on the observation that K_p values are constant for a given V_{ss}, and that they can be predicted from V_{ss} (Arundel, 1997). With the tissue composition methods, partitions to various components in the tissue (neutral lipid, acidic phospholipids, lipoproteins, tissue albumin) are estimated by log$D$ and pK_a of the compound (Poulin

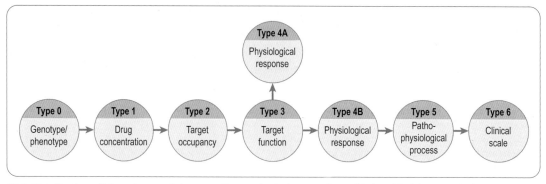

Fig. 10.9 Classification of biomarkers useful to quantify a project's therapeutic model. (Modified from Danhof, M., Alvan, G., Dahl, S. G., Kuhlmann, J., & Paintaud, G. (2005). Mechanism-based pharmacokinetic-pharmacodynamic modeling—a new classification of biomarkers. *Pharmaceutical Research*, 22, 1432–1437.)

& Theil, 2000; Rodgers et al., 2005; Rodgers & Rowland, 2006). A key assumption is that unbound tissue K_p values are constant across species. This underpins the assumption described above, that the unbound volume of distribution is constant across species.

Prediction of plasma concentration-time profile

To accurately estimate C_{max} and C_{min}, which are important exposure parameters for assessing safety and efficacy, the plasma concentration-time profile has to be accurately predicted.

For compounds displaying monoexponential decreases in plasma concentrations over time, the concentration-time profile in humans can be predicted using the following equation:

$$C(t) = \frac{FDk_a}{V\left(ka - \frac{CL}{V}\right)\left(e^{-\frac{CL}{V} \cdot t} - e^{-ka \cdot t}\right)},$$

where C is the concentration at time t, F is bioavailability, D is the dose, k_a is the absorption rate, CL is the clearance and V is the volume of distribution.

For compounds displaying biphasic or multiexponential concentration–time profiles in animals, PBPK modelling is the recommended approach to simulate the profile in humans.

Prediction of human efficacious dose

Estimation of the likely therapeutic dose and dosing frequency in patients requires not only the prediction of the human PK, but also a robust understanding of the concentration–time-response relationship. The quality of the prediction depends on how well the PD effect scales from animals to humans and the linkage between the effect and the clinical outcome. The linkage between the effect

and the clinical outcome is based on a series of translational biomarkers. The different types of biomarkers are classified (Fig. 10.9). The classification is based on the mechanism of drug action and the relationship to the disease process. In general, the closer the relationship of the biomarker is to the disease process, the more relevant and predictive is the biomarker.

Summary

To be a successful drug candidate, a compound, in addition to having good efficacy and safety profile, has to have acceptable DMPK properties. This chapter highlights the roles of DMPK in drug discovery and provides strategies to resolve key DMPK challenges such as improving oral bioavailability, optimizing clearance, avoiding DDI, achieving or avoiding CNS exposure and avoiding risks from metabolites. In addition, approaches used to scale individual PK parameters and strategy to integrate these parameters to predict human PK and dose are discussed in the chapter. The proposed strategy is based on best practices within AstraZeneca, as well as current science, technology and understanding of DMPK. It is our hope that the proposed integrated strategy, which focus DMPK efforts towards the optimization and prediction of DMPK properties in humans, will provide a sound basis to efficiently progress drug discovery projects.

Acknowledgements

The authors wish to thank Pete Ballard, Patrik Brassil, Khan H Bui, Hugues Dolgos, Carl Petersson, Anders Tunek and Peter J H Webborn for their foundational work to layout the strategy, and Ulrik Jurva and Teodor Erngren for their input to this book chapter.

References

Abet, V., Filace, F., Recio, J., Alvarez-Builla, J., & Burgos, C. (2017). Prodrug approach: An overview of recent cases. *European Journal of Medicinal Chemistry, 127*, 810–827.

Arundel, P. (March 23rd–26th, 1997). *A multi-compartment model generally applicable to physiologically based pharmacokinetics. 3rd IFAC Symposium: Modelling and control in biological systems.* Warwick, UK.

Amidon, G. L., Lennernäs, H., Shah, V. P., & Crison, J. R. (1995). A theoretical basis for a biopharmaceutic drug classification: The correlation of in vitro drug product dissolution and in vivo bioavailability. *Pharmaceutical Research, 12*, 413–420.

Anderson, S., Luffer-Atlas, D., & Knadle, M. P. (2009). Predicting circulating human metabolites: How good are we? *Chemical Research in Toxicology, 22*, 243–256.

Andersson, S., Antonsson, M., Elebring, M., Jansson-Löfmark, R., & Weidolf, L. (2018). Drug metabolism and pharmacokinetic strategies for oligonucleotide- and mRNA-based drug development. *Drug Discovery Today, 23*, 1733–1745.

Avdeef, A., Fuguet, E., Llinàs, A., Clara Ràfols, C., Bosch, E., Völgyi, G., et al. (2016). Equilibrium solubility measurement of ionizable drugs–consensus recommendations for improving data quality. *ADMET & DMPK, 4*, 117–178.

Bale, S. S., Moore, L., Yarmush, M., & Jindal, R. (2016). Emerging in vitro liver technologies for drug metabolism and inter-organ interactions. *Tissue Engineering. Part B, Reviews, 22*, 383–394.

Bell, L., Bickford, S., Nguyen, P. H., Wang, J., He, T., Zhang, B., et al. (2008). Evaluation of fluorescence- and mass spectrometry-based CYP inhibition assays for use in drug discovery. *Journal of Biomolecular Screening, 13*, 343–353.

Benet, L. Z., Hosey, C. M., Ursu, O., & Oprea, T. I. (2016). BDDCS, the Rule of 5 and druggability. *Advanced Drug Delivery Reviews, 101*, 89–98.

Bergström, F., & Lindmark, B. (2019). Accelerated drug discovery by rapid candidate drug identification. *Drug Discovery Today, 6*, 1237–1241.

Broccatelli, F., Hop, M., & Wright, M. (2019). Strategies to optimize drug half-life in lead candidate identification.

Expert Opinion on Drug Discovery, 14, 221–230.

Cerny, M. A. (2016). Prevalence of non–cytochrome P450–mediated metabolism in Food and Drug Administration–approved oral and intravenous drugs: 2006–2015. *Drug Metabolism and Disposition, 44*, 1246–1252.

Chen, Y., Liu, L., Nguyen, K., & Fretland, A. J. (2011). Utility of intersystem extrapolation factors in early reaction phenotyping and the quantitative extrapolation of human liver microsomal intrinsic clearance using recombinant cytochromes P450. *Drug Metabolism and Disposition, 39*, 373–382.

Chiou, W., Jeong, Y., Chung, S., & Wu, T. C. (2000). Evaluation of dog as an animal model to study the fraction of oral dose absorbed for 43 drugs in humans. *Pharmaceutical Research, 17*, 135–140.

Colclough, N., Chen, K., Johnström, P., Fridén, M., & McGinnity, D. F. (2019). Building on the success of osimertinib: Achieving CNS exposure in oncology drug discovery. *Drug Discovery Today, 24*, 1067–1073.

Cook, D., Brown, D., Alexander, R., March, R., Morgan, P., Satterthwaite, G., et al. (2014). Lessons learned from the fate of AstraZeneca's drug pipeline: A five-dimensional framework. *Nature Reviews. Drug Discovery, 13*, 419–431.

Cossum, P. A. (1988). Role of the red blood cell in drug metabolism. *Biopharmaceutics & Drug Disposition, 9*, 321–336.

Damle, B. D., Uderman, H., Biswas, P., Crownover, P., Lin, C., & Glue, P. (2009). Influence of CYP2C19 polymorphism on the pharmacokinetics of nelfinavir and its active metabolite. *British Journal of Clinical Pharmacology, 68*, 682–689.

Danhof, M., Alvan, G., Dahl, S. G., Kuhlmann, J., & Paintaud, G. (2005). Mechanism-based pharmacokinetic-pharmacodynamic modeling—a new classification of biomarkers. *Pharmaceutical Research, 22* 1432–1437.

Doran, A., Obach, R. S., Smith, B. J., Hosea, N. A., Becker, S., Callegari, E., et al., (2005). The impact of P-glycoprotein on the disposition of drugs targeted for indications of the central nervous system: Evaluation using the MDR1A/1B knockout mouse model. *Drug Metabolism and Disposition, 33* 165–174.

Elsby, R., Hilgendorf, C., & Fenner, K. (2012). Understanding the critical disposition pathways of statins to assess drug–drug interaction risk during drug development: It's not just about OATP1B1. *Clinical Pharmacology and Therapeutics, 92*, 584–598.

European Medicines Agency. (2012). Guideline on the investigation of drug interactions; web. https://www.ema.europa.eu/en/documents/scientific-guideline/guideline-investigation-drug-interactions-revision-1_en.pdf.

Ferdousi, R., Safdari, R., & Omidi, Y. (2017). Computational prediction of drug–drug interactions based on drugs functional similarities. *Journal of Biomedical Informatics, 70*, 54–64.

Foster, A. J., Chouhan, B., Regan, S. L., Rollison, H., Amberntsson, S., Andersson, L. C., et al. (2019). Integrated in vitro models for hepatic safety and metabolism: Evaluation of a human liver-chip and liver spheroid. *Archives of Toxicology, 93*, 1021–1037.

Foti, R. S., & Deepak, D. K. (2016). Cytochrome P450 and non–cytochrome P450 oxidative metabolism: Contributions to the pharmacokinetics, safety, and efficacy of xenobiotics. *Drug Metabolism and Disposition, 44*, 1229–1245.

Fredlund, L., Winiwarter, S., & Hilgendorf, C. (2017). In vitro intrinsic permeability: A transporter-independent measure of Caco-2 cell permeability in drug design and development. *Molecular Pharmaceutics, 14*, 1601–1609.

Fridén, M., Ducrozet, F., Middleton, B., Antonsson, M., Bredberg, U., & Hammarlund-Udenaes, M. (2009a). Development of a high-throughput brain slice method for studying drug distribution in the central nervous system. *Drug Metabolism and Disposition, 37*, 1226–1233.

Fridén, M., Ljungqvist, H., Middleton, B., Bredberg, U., & Hammarlund-Udenaes, M. (2010). Improved measurement of drug exposure in brain using drug-specific correction for residual blood. *Journal of Cerebral Blood Flow and Metabolism, 30*, 150–161.

Fridén, M., Winiwarter, S., Jerndal, G., Bengtsson, O., Wan, H., Bredberg, U., et al. (2009b). Structure-brain exposure relationships in rat and human using a novel data set of unbound drug concentrations in brain interstitial and cerebrospinal fluids.

Journal of Medicinal Chemistry, 52, 6233–6243.

Fridén, M., Bergström, F., Wan, H., Rehngren, M., Ahlin, G., Hammarlund-Udenaes, M., et al. (2011). Measurement of unbound drug exposure in brain: Modeling of pH partitioning explains diverging results between the brain slice and brain homogenate methods. *Drug Metabolism and Disposition*, 39, 353–362.

Gabrielsson, J., & Green, A. R. (2009). Quantitative pharmacology or pharmacokinetic pharmacodynamic integration should be a vital component in integrative pharmacology. *Journal of Pharmacology and Experimental Therapeutics*, 331, 767–774.

Garcia, M. J., Reinoso, R. F., Sanchez Navarro, A., & Prous, J. R. (2003). Clinical pharmacokinetics of statins. *Methods and Findings in Experimental and Clinical Pharmacology*, 25, 457–481.

Gertz, M., Harrison, A., Houston, J. B., & Galetin, A. (2010). Prediction of human intestinal first-pass metabolism of 25 CYP3A substrates from in vitro clearance and permeability data. *Drug Metabolism and Disposition*, 38, 1147–1158.

Giacomini, K. M., Galetin, A., & Huang, S. M. (2018). International Transporter Consortium, summarizing advances of the role of transporters in drug development. *Clinical Pharmacology and Therapeutics*, 104, 766–771.

Gleeson, P., Davis, A., Chohan, K., Paine, S. W., Boyer, S., Gavaghan, C. L., et al. (2007). Generation of in silico cytochrome P450 1A2, 2C9, 2C19, 2D6, 3A4 inhibition QSAR models. *Journal of Computer-Aided Molecular Design*, 21, 559–573.

Grime, K., & Paine, S. W. (2013). Species differences in biliary clearance and possible relevance of hepatic uptake and efflux transporters involvement. *Drug Metabolism and Disposition*, 41, 372–378.

Gundert-Remy, U., Bernauer, U., Blömeke, B., Döring, B., Fabian, E., Goebel, C., et al. (2014). Extrahepatic metabolism at the body's internal–external interfaces. *Drug Metabolism Reviews*, 46, 291–324.

Hallifax, D., & Houston, J. B. (2019). Use of segregated hepatocyte scaling factors and cross-species relationships to resolve clearance dependence in the prediction of human hepatic clearance. *Drug Metabolism and Disposition*, 47, 320–327.

Hosey, C. M., Broccatelli, F., Benet, L. Z. (2014). Predicting when biliary excretion of parent drug is a major route of elimination in humans. *AAPS Journal*, 16 1085–1096.

Hutzler, J. M., Yang, Y., Albaugh, D., Fullenwider, C. L., Schmenk, J., & Fisher, M. B. (2012). Characterization of aldehyde oxidase enzyme activity in cryopreserved human hepatocytes. *Drug Metabolism and Disposition*, 40, 267–275.

Jancova, P., Anzenbacher, P., & Anzenbacherova, E. (2010). Phase II drug metabolizing enzymes. *Biomedical papers of the Medical Faculty of the University Palacky, Olomouc, Czechoslovakia*, 154, 103–116.

Johnson, T. W., Dress, K. R., & Edwards, M. (2009). Using the golden triangle to optimise clearance and oral absorption. *Bioorganic & Medicinal Chemistry Letters*, 19, 5560–5564.

Jones, B. C., Srivastava, A., Colclough, N., Wilson, J., Reddy, V. P., Amberntsson, S., et al. (2017). An investigation into the prediction of in vivo clearance for a range of flavin-containing monooxygenase substrates. *Drug Metabolism and Disposition*, 45, 1060–1067.

Kalgutkar, A. S. (2020). Designing around structural alerts in drug discovery. *Journal of Medicinal Chemistry*, 63, 6276–6302.

Kalliokoski, A., & Niemi, M. (2009). Impact of OATP transporters on pharmacokinetics. *British Journal of Pharmacology*, 158, 693–705.

Kanebratt, K. P., & Andersson, T. B. (2008). HepaRG cells as an in vitro model for evaluation of cytochrome P450 induction in humans. *Drug Metabolism and Disposition*, 36, 137–145.

Kenna, J. G., & Uetrecht, J. (2018). Do in vitro assays predict drug candidate idiosyncratic drug-induced liver injury risk? *Drug Metabolism and Disposition*, 46, 1658–1669.

Kimoto, E., Bi, Y., Kosa, R. E., Tremaine, L. M., & Varma, M. V. S. (2017). Hepatobiliary clearance prediction: species scaling from monkey, dog, and rat, and in vitro—in vivo extrapolation of sandwich-cultured human hepatocytes using 17 drugs. *Journal of Pharmaceutical Sciences*, 106, 2795–2804.

Kola, I., & Landis, J. (2004). Can the pharmaceutical industry reduce attrition rates? *Nature Reviews. Drug Discovery*, 3, 711–715.

Kosaka, M., Kosugi, Y., & Hirabayashi, H. (2017). Risk assessment using cytochrome P450 time-dependent inhibition assays at single time and concentration in the early stage of drug discovery. *Journal of Pharmaceutical Sciences*, 106, 2839–2846.

Li, N., Bi, Y. A., Duignan, D. B., & Lai, Y. (2009). Quantitative expression profile of hepatobiliary transporters in sandwich cultured rat and human hepatocytes. *Molecular Pharmacology*, 6, 1180–1189.

Lindberg, P., Nordberg, P., Alminger, T., Brändström, A., & Wallmark, B. (1986). The mechanism of action of the gastric acid secretion inhibitor omeprazole. *Journal of Medicinal Chemistry*, 29, 1327–1329.

Lindmark, B., Lundahl, A., Kanebratt, K. P., Andersson, T. B., & Isin, E. M. (2018). Human hepatocytes and cytochrome P450-selective inhibitors predict variability in human drug exposure more accurately than human recombinant P450s. *British Journal of Pharmacology*, 175, 2116–2129.

Lipinski, C. A., Lombardo, F., Dominy, B. W., & Feeney, P. J. (1997). Experimental and computational approaches to estimate solubility and permeability in drug discovery and development settings. *Advanced Drug Delivery Reviews*, 23, 3–25.

Lombardo, F., Waters, N., Argikar, U. A., Dennehy, M. K., Zhan, J., Gunduz, M., et al. (2013). Comprehensive assessment of human pharmacokinetic prediction based on in-vivo animal pharmacokinetic data, part 2: Clearance. *Journal of Clinical Pharmacology*, 53, 178–191.

Mahmood, I. (2007). Application of allometric principles for the prediction of pharmacokinetics in human and veterinary drug development. *Advanced Drug Delivery Reviews*, 59, 1177–1192.

Margolskee, A., Darwich, A. S., Pepin, X., Aarons, L., Galetin, A., Rostami-Hodjegan, A., et al. (2017). IMI—oral biopharmaceutics tools project—evaluation of bottom-up PBPK prediction success part 2: An introduction to the simulation exercise and overview of results. *European Journal of Pharmaceutical Sciences*, 96, 610–625.

Mazur, C. S., Kenneke, J. F., Goldsmith, M. R., & Brown, C. (2009). Contrasting influence of NADPH and a NADPH-regenerating system on the metabolism of carbonyl-containing compounds in hepatic microsomes. *Drug Metabolism and Disposition*, 37, 1801–1805.

McGinnity, D. F., Collington, J., Austin, R. P., & Riley, R. J. (2007). Evaluation of human pharmacokinetics, therapeutic dose and exposure predictions using marketed oral drugs. *Current Drug Metabolism*, 8, 463–479.

Morgan, P., Brown, D. G., Lennard, S., Anderton, M. J., Barrett, J. C., Eriksson, U., et al. (2018). Impact of five-dimensional framework on R&D productivity at AstraZeneca. *Nature Reviews. Drug Discovery, 17*, 167–181.

Nakayama, S., Atsumi, R., Takakusa, H., Kobayashi, Y., Kurihara, A., Nagai, Y., et al. (2009). A zone classification system for risk assessment of idiosyncratic drug toxicity using daily dose and covalent binding. *Drug Metabolism and Disposition, 37*, 1970–1977.

Page, K. M. (2016). Validation of early human dose prediction: A key metric for compound progression in drug discovery. *Molecular Pharmaceutics, 13*, 609−620.

Paine, S. W., Menochet, K., Denton, R., McGinnity, D. F., & Riley, R. J. (2011). Prediction of human renal clearance from preclinical species for a diverse set of drugs that exhibit both active secretion and net reabsorption. *Drug Metabolism and Disposition, 39*, 1008–1013.

Paine, S. W., Barton, P., Bird, J., Denton, R., Menochet, K., Smith, A., et al. (2010). A rapid computational filter for predicting the rate of human renal clearance. *Journal of Molecular Graphics & Modelling, 29*, 529–537.

Pilla Reddy, V., Bui, K., Scarfe, G., Zhou, D., & Learoyd, M. (2019). Physiologically based pharmacokinetic modeling for olaparib dosing recommendations: Bridging formulations, drug interactions, and patient populations. *Clinical Pharmacology and Therapeutics, 105*, 229–241.

Paul, S. M., Mytelka, D. S., Dunwiddie, C. T., Persinger, C. C., Munos, B. H., Lindborg, S. R., et al. (2010). How to improve R&D productivity: The pharmaceutical industry's grand challenge. *Nature Reviews. Drug Discovery, 9*, 203–214.

Poulin, P., & Theil, F. P. (2000). A priori prediction of tissue: plasma partition coefficients of drugs to facilitate the use of physiologically-based pharmacokinetic models in drug discovery. *Journal of Pharmaceutical Sciences, 89*, 16–35.

Poulin, P., Kenny, J. R., Hop, C. E. C., & Haddad, S. (2012). In-vitro-in-vivo extrapolation of clearance: Modeling hepatic metabolic clearance of highly bound drugs and comparative assessment with existing calculation methods. *Journal of Pharmaceutical Sciences, 101*, 838–851.

Rankovic, Z. (2015). CNS drug design: Balancing physicochemical properties for optimal brain exposure. *Journal of Medicinal Chemistry, 58*, 2584−2608.

Rawden, H. C., Carlile, D. J., Tindall, A., Hallifax, D., Galetin, A., Ito, K., et al.

(2005). Microsomal prediction of in vivo clearance and associated interindividual variability of six benzodiazepines in humans. *Xenobiotica, 35*, 603–625.

Rekić, D., Reynolds, K. S., Zhao, P., Zhang, L., Yoshida, K., Sachar, M., et al. (2017). Clinical drug-drug interaction evaluations to inform drug use and enable drug access. *Journal of Pharmaceutical Sciences, 106*, 2214–2218.

Rendic, S., & Guengerich, P. F. (2015). Survey of human oxidoreductases and cytochrome P450 enzymes involved in the metabolism of xenobiotic and natural chemicals. *Chemical Research in Toxicology, 28*, 38–42.

Riley, R. J., & Wilson, C. E. (2015). Cytochrome P450 time-dependent inhibition and induction: Advances in assays, risk analysis and modelling. *Expert Opinion on Drug Metabolism & Toxicology, 11*, 557–572.

Rodgers, T., Leahy, D., & Rowland, M. (2005). Physiologically based pharmacokinetic modeling 1: Predicting the tissue distribution of moderate-to-strong bases. *Journal of Pharmaceutical Sciences, 94*, 1259–1276.

Rodgers, T., & Rowland, M. (2006). Physiologically based pharmacokinetic modelling 2: Predicting the tissue distribution of acids, very weak bases, neutrals and zwitterions. *Journal of Pharmaceutical Sciences, 95*, 1238–1257.

Rowland, M., & Tozer, T. N. (1989). *Clinical pharmacokinetics—concepts and applications* (2nd ed.). London: Lea and Febiger.

Schiou, M., Varnäs, K., Lundquist, S., Nakao, R., Amini, N., Takano, A., et al. (2015). Large variation in brain exposure of reference CNS drugs: A PET study in nonhuman primates. *International Journal of Neuropsychopharmacology, 18*, pyv036

Sjöberg, Å., Lutz, M., Tannergren, C., Wingolf, C., Borde, A., & Ungell, A. L. (2013). Comprehensive study on regional human intestinal permeability and prediction of fraction absorbed of drugs using the Ussing chamber technique. *European Journal of Pharmaceutical Sciences, 48*, 166–180.

Sjögren, E., Westergren, J., Grant, I., Hanisch, G., Lindfors, L., Lennernäs, H., et al. (2013). In silico predictions of gastrointestinal drug absorption in pharmaceutical product development: Application of the mechanistic absorption model GI-Sim. *European Journal of Pharmaceutical Sciences, 49*, 679–698.

Soars, M. G., Grime, K., Sproston, J. L., Webborn, P. J., & Riley, R. J. (2007). Use

of hepatocytes to assess the contribution of hepatic uptake to clearance in vivo. *Drug Metabolism and Disposition, 35*, 859–865.

Soars, M. G., Webborn, P. J., & Riley, R. J. (2009). Impact of hepatic uptake transporters on pharmacokinetics and drug-drug interactions: Use of assays and models for decision making in the pharmaceutical industry. *Molecular Pharmacology, 6*, 1662–1677.

Sohlenius-Sternbeck, A., Jones, C., Ferguson, D., Middleton, B. J., Projean, D., Floby, E., et al. (2012). Practical use of the regression offset approach for the prediction of in vivo intrinsic clearance from hepatocytes. *Xenobiotica, 42*, 841–853.

Stresser, D. M., Mao, J., Kenny, J. R., Jones, B. C., & Grime, K. (2014). Exploring concepts of in vitro time-dependent CYP inhibition assays. *Expert Opinion on Drug Metabolism & Toxicology, 10*, 157–174.

Sun, H., & Scott, D. O. (2010). Structure-based drug metabolism predictions for drug design. *Chemical Biology & Drug Design, 75*, 3–17.

Takahashi, M., Washio, T., Suzuki, N., Igeta, K., & Yamashita, S. (2009). The species differences of intestinal drug absorption and first-pass metabolism between cynomolgus monkeys and humans. *Journal of Pharmaceutical Sciences, 98*, 4343–4353.

Testa, B. (2009). Drug metabolism for the perplexed medicinal chemist. *Chemistry & Biodiversity, 6*, 2055–2070.

Thompson, R. A., Isin, E. M., Yan, L., Weaver, R., Weidolf, L., Wilson, I., et al. (2011). Risk assessment and mitigation strategies for reactive metabolites in drug discovery and development. *Chemico-Biological Interactions, 192*, 65–71.

Thompson, R. A., Isin, E. M., Yan, L., Weidolf, L., Page, K., Wilson, I., et al. (2012). In vitro approach to assess the potential for risk of idiosyncratic adverse reactions caused by candidate drugs. *Chemical Research in Toxicology, 25* 1616–1632.

Thompson, R. A., Isin, E. M., Ogese, M. O., Mettetal, J. T., & Williams, D. (2016). Reactive metabolites: Current and emerging risk and hazard assessments. *Chemical Research in Toxicology, 29*, 505–533.

Tornio, A., Filppula, A. M., Niemi, M., & Backman, J. T. (2019). Clinical studies on drug-drug interactions involving metabolism and transport: Methodology, pitfalls, and interpretation. *Clinical Pharmacology and Therapeutics, 105*, 1345–1361.

Tse, F. L., Ballard, F., & Skinn, J. (1982). Estimating the fraction reabsorbed in drugs undergoing enterohepatic circulation. *Journal of Pharmacokinetics and Biopharmaceutics, 10,* 455–461.

Ungell, A. L., Nylander, S., Bergstrand, S., Sjöberg, A., & Lennernäs, H. (1998). Membrane transport of drugs in different regions of the intestinal tract of the rat. *Journal of Pharmaceutical Sciences, 87,* 360–366.

US Food and Drug Administration. (2020). In vitro drug interaction studies—cytochrome P450 enzyme- and transporter-mediated drug interactions guidance for industry. Retrieved from https://www.fda.gov/regulatory-information/search-fda-guidance-documents/vitro-drug-interaction-studies-cytochrome-p450-enzyme-and-transporter-mediated-drug-interactions.

Varma, M. V. S., Chang, G., Lai, Y., Feng, B., El-Kattan, A. F., Litchfield, J., et al. (2012). Physicochemical property space of hepatobiliary transport and computational models for predicting rat biliary excretion. *Drug Metabolism and Disposition, 40,* 1527–1537.

Wan, H., Rehngren, M., Giordanetto, F., Bergström, F., & Tunek, A. (2007). High-throughput screening of drug-brain tissue binding and in silico prediction for assessment of central nervous system drug delivery. *Journal of Medicinal Chemistry, 50,* 4606–4615.

Ward, P. (2008). Importance of drug transporters in pharmacokinetics and drug safety. *Toxicology Mechanisms and Methods, 18,* 1–10.

Waring, M. J. (2009). Defining optimum lipophilicity and molecular weight ranges for drug candidates—molecular weight dependent lower logD limits based on permeability. *Bioorganic &*

Medicinal Chemistry Letters, 19, 2844–2851.

Webborn, P. J. H., Parker, R. L., Dento, R. L., & Riley, R. J. (2007). In vitro-in vivo extrapolation of hepatic clearance involving active uptake: Theoretical and experimental aspects. *Xenobiotica, 37,* 1090–1109.

Wenlock, M. C., Austin, R. P., Barton, P., Davis, A. M., & Leeson, P. D. (2003). A comparison of physiochemical property profiles of development and marketed oral drugs. *Journal of Medicinal Chemistry, 46,* 1250–1256.

Werle, M., & Bernkop-Schnürch, A. (2006). Strategies to improve plasma half life time of peptide and protein drugs. *Amino Acids, 30,* 351–367.

Williams, J., Hyland, R., Jones, B., Smith, D. A., Hurst, S., Goosen, T. C., et al. (2004). Drug-drug interactions for UDP-glucuronosyltransferase substrates; a pharmacokinetic explanation for typically observed low exposure (AUCi/AUC) ratios. *Drug Metabolism and Disposition, 32,* 1201–1208.

Williamson, B., Colclough, N., Fretland, A. J., Jones, B. C., Jones, R. D. O., & McGinnity, D. F. (2020). Further considerations towards an effective and efficient oncology drug discovery DMPK strategy. *Current Drug Metabolism, 21,* 145–162.

Winiwarter, S., Bonham N. M., Ax, F., Hallberg, A., Lennernäs, H., Karlén, A. (1998). Correlation of human jejunal permeability (in vivo) of drugs with experimentally and theoretically derived parameters. *A multivariate data analysis approach. J Med Chem, 41*(25):4939–49.

Yang, X., Gandhi, Y. A., Duignan, D. B., & Morris, M. E. (2009). Prediction of biliary excretion in rats and humans using molecular weight and quantitative

structure-pharmacokinetic relationships. *AAPS Journal, 11,* 511–525.

Yoshida, K., Zhao, P., Zhang, L., Abernethy, D. R., Rekić, D., Reynolds, K. S., et al. (2017). In vitro-in vivo extrapolation of metabolism- and transporter-mediated drug-drug interactions-overview of basic prediction methods. *Journal of Pharmaceutical Sciences, 106,* 2209–2213.

Yu, L. X., & Amidon, G. L. (1999). A compartmental absorption and transit model for estimating oral absorption. *International Journal of Pharmaceutics, 186,* 119–125.

Zanger, U. M., & Schwab, M. (2013). Cytochrome P450 enzymes in drug metabolism: Regulation of gene expression, enzyme activities, and impact of genetic variation. *Pharmacology & Therapeutics, 138,* 103–141.

Zhang, W., Chen, Y., Li, D., & Yue, X. (2018). Manifold regularized matrix factorization for drug-drug interaction prediction. *Journal of Biomedical Informatics, 88,* 90–97.

Zhou, S. F. (2009a). Polymorphism of human cytochrome P450 2D6 and its clinical significance: Part I. *Clinical Pharmacokinetics, 48,* 689–723.

Zhou, S. F. (2009b). Polymorphism of human cytochrome P450 2D6 and its clinical significance: Part II. *Clinical Pharmacokinetics, 48,* 761–804.

Zientek, M., Jiang, Y., Youdim, K., & Obach, R. S. (2010). In vitro-in vivo correlation for intrinsic clearance for drugs metabolized by human aldehyde oxidase. *Drug Metabolism and Disposition, 38,* 1322–1327.

Zimmerlin, A., Trunzer, M., & Faller, B. (2011). CYP3A time-dependent inhibition risk assessment validated with 400 reference drugs. *Drug Metabolism and Disposition, 39,* 1039–1046.

Chapter | 11 |

Pharmacology

Duncan B Richards

Introduction

Pharmacology as an academic discipline, loosely defined as the study of the effects of chemical substances on living systems, is broad in its sweep but all too often is associated only with classical small-molecule agonists and antagonists. The pharmacology of biological therapies is often complex and does not easily fit with the traditional pharmacological terms; nonetheless, the principles of understanding the exposure response relationship are as important for small molecules.

In this chapter, we begin with an outline of the fundamental aspects of the physical interaction between a drug molecule and its target, and how that will define many aspects of the behaviour of the drug.

A clear understanding of the in vitro characteristics of a drug is the vital starting point but then it is important to gain a more holistic understanding in vivo. Typically, this has been through the use of animal models, and we will discuss the pros and cons of such models. Safety pharmacology studies form part of the evaluation of drugs at this stage (see Chapter 12).

The single most important development in this field in recent times has been the use of mathematical models to describe and, increasingly, predict aspects of the behaviour of drugs. These models are increasing in sophistication, and regulatory authorities are encouraging their use to improve the quality and rigour of drug development. We will discuss how these models are changing approaches to drug discovery and development.

Overview

Once a target has been selected, then the first decision is whether one wishes to block or activate the system. When a disease is directly caused by an activating mutation, this decision is easy; for many modern targets, however, there is often evidence of a pathological role with both over- and underactivity. It is not uncommon for these types of targets to see parallel development programmes for both agonists and antagonists. For most drugs, the target will be the active site of the protein molecule (e.g., substrate-binding site of an enzyme, ligand-binding site of a transmembrane receptor). Binding at these sites can sometimes be challenging, for example, when there are a range of pathological mutations—finding a molecule that has the desired properties in cases can be difficult. As a result, there has been increasing interest in 'allosteric' pharmacology, where drugs bind to a site distant from the active site but induce a conformational change in the protein that has the desired blocking or activating effect. Agonism and antagonism is a helpful shorthand, but the underlying pharmacology is often more complex and may involve concepts as partial agonism, inverse agonism and biased agonism. These are explained in more detail in the primary pharmacology section.

Location of the drug target is a vital consideration when considering the likely effects of your intervention. Achieving cell-surface receptor subtype selectivity was a major focus of drug development in the 20th century, as this can provide a degree of tissue selectivity. When the drug target is a second messenger system or on an immune cell, effects may be seen in multiple organs. The route of administration can be manipulated to provide a degree of selectivity in some cases—inhaled corticosteroids for asthma have fewer systemic metabolic adverse effects than systemic steroids.

Pharmacological evaluation

Typically, when a molecular target has been selected, and lead compounds have been identified that act on it selectively, and which are judged to have 'drug-like' chemical attributes (including suitable pharmacokinetic properties), the next stage is a detailed pharmacological evaluation. This means investigation of the effects, usually of a small number of compounds, on a range of test systems, up to and including whole animals, to determine which, if any, is the most suitable for further development (i.e., for nomination as a drug candidate).

Our understanding of pharmacological responses has become more sophisticated in recent years. A full agonist is capable of eliciting a maximal response, while a partial agonist elicits a submaximal response for a given degree of receptor occupancy. When a full agonist (often the natural ligand) and partial agonist are present, the partial agonist has the effect of a competitive antagonist (Fig. 11.1). Buprenorphine is a partial agonist at opioid receptors. It may be given to those in pain for its agonist properties to provide analgesia. It is also used in the treatment of opioid misuse, where its partial agonist actions reduce the pharmacological effects if the subject also takes a full agonist. In recent years, it has been recognized that some drugs with antagonist effects are in fact inverse agonists. In this case, the drug binds to the same site as the agonist but has the opposite effect. Examples of drugs that act in this way include most antihistamines, carvedilol (beta adrenoceptors) and naloxone (mu opioid receptors). This type of pharmacology is seen when the receptor has a degree of basal or intrinsic activity. By contrast, a neutral antagonist induces no activity in the receptor—it can block the effect of an agonist (natural ligand) and can also block the effect of inverse agonists. A recent development has been the

concept of biased agonism. In this case, the drug is able to elicit distinct cellular signalling profiles by preferentially stabilizing different active conformational states of the receptor. It has been described in the G-protein-coupled receptors, and the hope is that it will provide a means to optimize treatments and improve therapeutic index.

Although these properties are generally described for traditional drugs, the principles also apply to biological molecules, such as antibodies. TGN1412 was a CD28 agonist antibody administered to healthy volunteers in a commercial clinical trials unit. This was a new type of agonist antibody described by some as a superagonist. In this context, this means the antibody was capable of stimulating T cells in the absence of the usual co-signalling molecules (Fig. 11.2). Within 90 minutes of receipt of a single intravenous dose of the drug, all six volunteers had a systemic inflammatory response characterized by a rapid induction of proinflammatory cytokines requiring critical care. This incident had long-term consequences for the participants and led to substantial changes in the conduct of first-in-human trials (Expert Group on Phase One Clinical Trials 2006).

Pharmacological evaluation typically involves the following:

- **Selectivity screening,** consisting of in vitro tests on a broad range of possible drug targets to determine whether the compound is sufficiently selective for the chosen target to merit further investigation.
- **Pharmacological profiling in vitro,** aimed at evaluating in isolated tissues or normal animals the range of effects of the test compound that might be relevant in

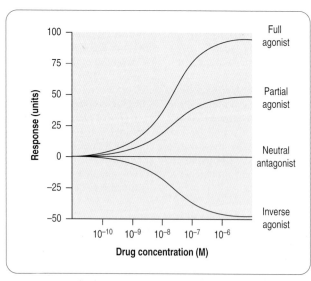

Fig. 11.1 Dose response curves of a full agonist, partial agonist, neutral antagonist, and invverse agonist

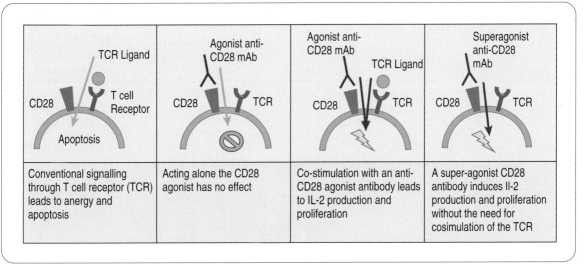

Fig. 11.2 Properties of a 'superagonist' antibody

the clinical situation. Some authorities distinguish between *primary pharmacodynamic studies*, concerning effects related to the selected therapeutic target (i.e., therapeutically relevant effects), and *secondary pharmacodynamic studies*, on effects not related to the target (i.e., side effects). At the laboratory level, the two are often not clearly distinguishable, and the borderline between secondary pharmacodynamic and safety pharmacology studies (see later) is also uncertain. Nevertheless, for the purposes of formal documentation, the distinction may be useful.

- **Pharmacological testing in vivo.** Typically, this will be conducted in using animals and animal models of disease. These investigations should be hypothesis-driven.
- **Safety pharmacology.** This is a form of in vivo profiling but is not entirely hypothesis-driven. It takes a more open-minded approach, consisting of a series of standardized animal tests aimed at revealing undesirable side effects, which may be unrelated to the primary action of the drug. This topic is discussed in Chapter 12.

Some aspects of drug development are highly regimented, but the pharmacological evaluation of lead compounds does not in general follow a clearly defined path. Often, it will vary greatly in its extent, depending on the nature of the compound, the questions that need to be addressed and the inclinations of the project team. How much information is needed to progress is a matter of judgement, and directing this phase of the drug discovery project efficiently, and keeping it focused on the overall objective of putting a compound into development, is highly skilled. The work will likely generate interesting findings; deciding which of these are materially important for the development of the drug, and which although scientifically interesting are potentially a distraction, takes real judgement and experience.

An important principle in pharmacological evaluation is the use of a *hierarchy* of test methods, covering the range from the most reductionist tests on isolated molecular targets to much more elaborate tests of integrated physiological function. Establishing and validating such a series of tests appropriate to the particular target and indication being addressed is one of the most important functions of pharmacologists in the drug discovery team. In general, assays become more complicated, slow and expensive, and more demanding of specialist skills as one moves up this hierarchy.

The strengths and weaknesses of these test systems are summarized in Table 11.1.

Pharmacological characterization of a candidate compound often has to take into account active metabolites, based on information from drug metabolism and pharmacokinetics (DMPK) studies (see Chapter 10). If a major active metabolite is identified, it will be necessary to synthesize and test it in the same way as the parent compound in order to determine which effects (both wanted and unwanted) relate to each. Particular problems may arise if the metabolic fate of the compound shows marked species differences, making it difficult to predict from animal studies what will happen in humans. Some drugs are prodrugs and require metabolic transformation to become active—ensure your test system is evaluating the pharmacologically active molecule.

Table 11.1 Characteristics of pharmacological test systems

Test system attribute	Molecular/cellular assays	In vitro pharmacology	Whole animal pharmacology (normal animals)	Whole animal disease models
Throughput	High (thousands/day)	Moderate (c. 10/day)	Low (<10/day)	Generally low or very low, depending on nature of model
Quantitative precision	Good	Good, but may be subject to environmental and physiological variation	Relatively poor, due to uncontrolled pharmacokinetic and physiological factors	As for whole animal pharmacology, plus added variability of disease model phenotype
Cost	Low	Fairly low depending on number and cost of animals needed	High, depending on number and cost of animals needed	High, depending on number and cost of animals needed
Flexibility of experimental design	Generally inflexible. Washout effects, repeat dose effects, etc., difficult to study	Highly adaptable	Adaptable, but limitations imposed by pharmacokinetics	
Suitability for chronic experiments	Unsuitable	Unsuitable	Depends on model. Suitable if repeated noninvasive readouts are feasible. Possible, but expensive for one-off terminal readouts	As for whole animal, provided disease phenotype remains stable
Species dependence	Often performed on human cell lines or cloned human targets	Rarely possible with human tissues	Animal studies may not be applicable to humans	Animal studies may not be applicable to humans
Usefulness for predicting therapeutic efficacy	OK for me-too drugs. Poor for drugs acting through novel mechanisms	OK for me-too drugs. Poor for drugs acting through novel mechanisms	As above	Variable, depending on characteristics of model
Usefulness for predicting side effects	Useful if broad selectivity screen is performed	Sometimes useful	Generally useful as basis for 'safety pharmacology' screening	Usually not informative

Although most of the work involved in pharmacological characterization of a candidate drug takes place before clinical studies begin, it does not normally end there. Both ongoing toxicological studies and early trials in man may reveal unpredicted effects or novel metabolites that may need to be investigated pharmacologically. The discovery team needs to remain actively involved and be able to perform experiments well into the phase of clinical development.

Screening for selectivity

The selectivity of a compound for the chosen molecular target needs to be assessed at an early stage. Compounds selected for their potency, for example, on a given amine receptor, protease, kinase, transporter or ion channel, are very likely to bind also to related—or even unrelated—molecular targets, and thereby cause unwanted side effects. Selectivity is, therefore, as important as potency in choosing potential development candidates, and a 'selectivity screen' is usually included early in the project. The range of targets included in such a screen depends very much on the type of compound and the intended clinical indication. Ligands for monoamine receptors and transporters form a large and important group of drugs, and several contract research organizations (e.g., CEREP, MDL) offer a battery of assays. In most cases, the initial screen will identify whether the compound binds to the targets. This should be followed up by functional assays to understand whether this physical interaction has pharmacological consequences. Initial screens tend to be conducted at a single (high) concentration; follow-up information will usually involve a range of concentrations. Always consider these data in the context of the likely concentrations of your drug in man. Off-target effects of antibiotics are relatively common because they are typically given in large doses; another type of drug may have a similar potential but because the dose is low these may not manifest in man. Antibody drugs are generally highly specific for their target, and off-target effects are very rare.

Off-target effects on certain types of receptor are known to have a poor safety and/or tolerability profile and will often lead to termination of the compound. Examples include peripheral muscarinic receptors, adrenergic receptors or histamine (particularly H_1) receptors. Blockade of the potassium channel known as the *hERG channel* predisposes to a potentially fatal cardiac arrhythmia called torsade de pointes. Evidence of blockade of hERG should be followed up with electrophysiological measurements on isolated myocardial cells, and then more integrated test systems such as the rabbit ventricular wedge assay. Most drugs shown to have a significant hERG liability would be terminated, but in some cases, where unmet need is high or avoiding this liability proves impossible, the compound may be taken forward but very close cardiac monitoring will be required in clinical trials.

Note on the interpretation of binding assays

Binding assays, generally with membrane preparations made from intact tissues or receptor-expressing cell lines, are widely used in drug discovery projects because of their simplicity and ease of automation. Detailed technical manuals describing the methods used for performing and analysing drug binding experiments are available (Keen, 1999; Vogel, 2002). Generally, the aim of the assay is to determine the dissociation constant, K_D, of the test compound, as a measure of its affinity for the receptor. In most cases, the assay (often called a *displacement assay*) measures the ability of the test compound to inhibit the binding of a high-affinity radioligand that combines selectively with the receptor in question, correction being made for 'nonspecific' binding of the radioligand.

In the simplest theoretical case, where the radioligand and the test compound bind reversibly and competitively to a homogeneous population of binding sites, the effect of the test ligand on the amount of the radioligand specifically bound is described by the simple mass-action equation:

$$B/B_{max} = ([A]/K_A)/([A]/K_A + [L]/K_L + 1) \qquad (1)$$

where B = the amount of radioligand bound, after correcting for nonspecific binding, B_{max} = the maximal amount of radioligand bound, that is, when sites are saturated, $[A]$ = radioligand concentration, K_A = dissociation constant for the radioligand, $[L]$ = test ligand concentration and K_L = dissociation constant for the test ligand.

By testing several concentrations of L at a single concentration of A, the concentration, $[L]_{50}$, needed for 50% inhibition of binding can be estimated. By rearranging Eq. 1, K_L is given by:

$$K_L = [L]_{50}/([A]/K_A + 1) \qquad (2)$$

This is often known as the Cheng–Prusoff equation and is widely used to calculate K_L when $[L]_{50}$, $[A]$ and K_A are known. It is important to realize that the Cheng–Prusoff equation applies only (1) at equilibrium, (2) when the interaction between A and L is strictly competitive and (3) when neither ligand binds cooperatively. However, an $[L]_{50}$ value can be measured for any test compound that inhibits the binding of the radioligand by whatever mechanism, irrespective of whether equilibrium has been reached. Applying the Cheng–Prusoff equation if these conditions are not met can yield estimates of K_L that are quite meaningless, and so it should strictly be used only if the conditions have been shown experimentally to be satisfied—a fairly laborious process. Nevertheless, Cheng–Prusoff estimates of ligand affinity constants are often quoted without such checks having been performed. In most cases, it would be more satisfactory to use the experimentally determined $[L]_{50}$ value as an operational measure of potency. A further important caveat that applies to binding studies is that they are often performed under conditions of low ionic strength, in which the sodium and calcium concentrations are much lower than the physiological range. This is done for technical reasons, as low $[Na^+]$ commonly increases both the affinity and the B_{max} of the radioligand, and omitting $[Ca^{2+}]$ avoids clumping of the membrane fragments. Partly for this reason, ligand affinities estimated from binding studies are often considerably higher than estimates obtained from functional assays, although the effect is not consistent, presumably because ionic bonding, which will be favoured by the low ionic strength medium, contributes unequally to the binding of different ligands. Consequently, the correlation between data from binding assays and functional assays is often rather poor (see later). Fig. 11.3 shows data obtained independently on serotonin 5HT$_3$ and 5HT$_4$ receptors; in both cases, the estimated K_D values for binding are on average about 10 times lower than estimates from functional assays, and the correlation is very poor.

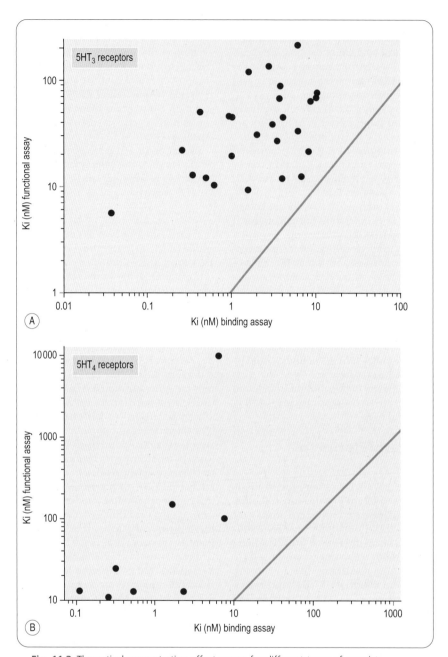

Fig. 11.3 Theoretical concentration effect curves for different types of agonist

Pharmacological profiling in vitro

Pharmacological profiling aims to determine the pharmaco-dynamic effects of the new compound—or more often of a small family of compounds—on in vitro model systems, for example, cell lines or isolated tissues, normal animals and animal models of disease. The last of these is particularly important, as it is intended to give the first real pointer to therapeutic efficacy as distinct from pharmacodynamic activity. It is valuable to assess the activity of the compounds in a series of assays representing increasingly complex levels of

Box 11.1 **Example of a pharmacology package for a novel G-protein-coupled receptor antagonist**

- Ligand-binding assay on membrane fragments from a cell line expressing the cloned receptor
- Inhibition of agonist activity in a cell line, based on a functional readout (e.g., raised intracellular calcium)
- Antagonism of a selective agonist in an isolated tissue (e.g., smooth muscle, cardiac muscle). Such assays will normally be performed with nonhuman tissue, and so interspecies differences in the receptor need to be taken into account. Sometimes, specific questions have to be asked about effects on human tissues for particular compounds, and then collecting viable tissues to use becomes a major challenge
- Antagonism of the response (e.g., bronchoconstriction, vasoconstriction, increased heart rate) to a selective receptor agonist in vivo. Prior knowledge about species specificity of the agonist and antagonist is important at this stage.

organization. The choice of test systems depends, of course, on the nature of the target. For example, characterization of a novel antagonist of a typical G-protein-coupled receptor might involve the following (Box 11.1).

Pharmacological profiling is designed as a hypothesis-driven programme of work, based on the knowledge previously gained about the activity of the compound on its specific target or targets. In this respect, it differs from safety pharmacology (see later), which is an open-minded exercise designed to detect unforeseen effects. The aim of pharmacological profiling is to answer the following questions:

- Do the molecular and cellular effects measured in screening assays actually give rise to the predicted pharmacological effects in intact tissues and whole animals?
- Does the compound produce effects in intact tissues or whole animals not associated with actions on its principal molecular target?
- Is there correspondence between the potency of the compound at the molecular level, the tissue level and the whole animal level?
- Do the in vivo potency and duration of action match up with the pharmacokinetic properties of the compound?
- What happens if the drug is given continuously or repeatedly to an animal over the course of days or weeks? Does it lose its effectiveness, or reveal effects not seen with acute administration? Is there any kind of 'rebound' after effect when it is stopped?

In vitro profiling

Measurements on isolated tissues

Studies on isolated tissues have been a mainstay of pharmacological methodology ever since the introduction of the isolated organ bath by Magnus early in the 20th century. The technique is extremely versatile and applicable to studies on smooth muscle (e.g., gastrointestinal tract, airways, blood vessels, urinary tract, uterus, biliary tract, etc.), as well as cardiac and striated muscle, secretory epithelia, endocrine glands, brain slices, liver slices and many other functional systems. In most cases, the tissue is removed from a freshly killed or anaesthetized animal and suspended in a chamber containing warmed oxygenated physiological salt solution. With smooth muscle preparations, the readout is usually mechanical (i.e., tension, recorded with a simple strain gauge). For other types of preparation, various electrophysiological or biochemical readouts are often used. Vogel (2002) gives details of a comprehensive range of standard pharmacological assay methods, including technical instructions.

Studies of this kind have the advantage that they are performed on intact normal tissues, as distinct from isolated enzymes or other proteins. The recognition molecules, signal transduction machinery and the mechanical or biochemical readout are assumed to be a reasonable approximation to the normal functioning of the tissue. There is abundant evidence to show that tissue responses to G-protein-coupled receptor activation, for example, depend on many factors, including the level of expression of the receptor, the type and abundance of the G proteins present in the cell, the presence of associated proteins such as receptor activity-modifying proteins (RAMPs; see Sexton et al., 2006), the state of phosphorylation of various constituent proteins in the signal transduction cascade and so on. For compounds acting on intracellular targets, functional activity depends on permeation through the membrane, as well as affinity for the target. For these reasons—and probably also for others that are not understood—the results of assays on isolated tissues often differ significantly from results found with primary screening assays. The discrepancy may simply be a quantitative one, such that the potency of the ligand does not agree in the two systems, or it may be more basic. For example, the *pharmacological efficacy* of a receptor ligand, that is, the property that determines whether it is a full agonist, a partial agonist or an antagonist, often depends on the type of assay used, and this may have an important bearing on the selection of possible development compounds. Examples that illustrate the poor correlation that may exist between measurements of target affinity in cell-free assay systems, and functional activity in intact cell systems, are shown in Figs 11.3 and 11.4. Fig. 11.3 shows the relationship between binding and func-

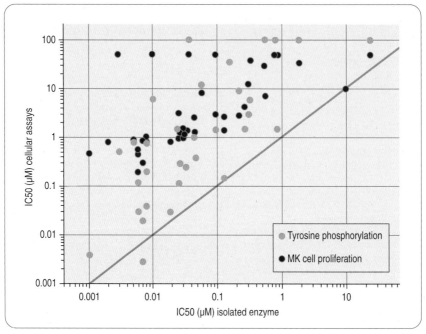

Fig. 11.4 Correlation of cellular activity of Epidermal growth factor receptor (EGFR) receptor kinase inhibitors with enzyme inhibition. (From Traxler et al.,1997.)

tional assay data for $5HT_3$ and $5HT_4$ receptor antagonists. In both cases, binding assays overestimate the potency in functional assays by a factor of about 10 (see earlier), but more importantly, the correlation is poor, despite the fact that the receptors are extracellular, and so membrane penetration is not a factor. Fig. 11.4 shows data on tyrosine kinase inhibitors, in which activity against the isolated enzyme is plotted against inhibition of tyrosine phosphorylation in intact cells, and inhibition of cell proliferation for a large series of compounds. Differences in membrane penetration can account for part of the discrepancy between enzyme and cell-based data, but the correlation between intracellular kinase inhibition and blocking of cell proliferation is also weak, which must reflect other factors.

It is worth noting that these examples come from very successful drug discovery projects. The quantitative discrepancies that we have emphasized, though worrying to pharmacologists, should not therefore be a serious distraction in the context of a drug discovery project.

A very wide range of physiological responses can be addressed by studies on isolated tissues, including measurements of membrane excitability, synaptic function, muscle contraction, cell motility, secretion and release of mediators, transmembrane ion fluxes, vascular resistance and permeability and epithelial

transport and permeability. This versatility and the relative technical simplicity of many such methods are useful attributes for drug discovery. Additional advantages are that concentration–effect relationships can be accurately measured, and the design of the experiments is highly flexible, allowing rates of onset and recovery of drug effects to be determined, as well as measurements of synergy and antagonism by other compounds, desensitization effects and so on.

The main shortcomings of isolated tissue pharmacology are (1) that tissues normally have to be obtained from small laboratory animals, rather than humans or other primates; and (2) that preparations rarely survive for more than a day, so that only short-term experiments are feasible.

In vivo profiling

Valuable though information from isolated tissue is, insight into the integrated response to a drug or intervention is important. For many years, this has meant conducting experiments in animal models of disease. The predictive value of these experiments has been brought into question in recent years, as there has been a long history of drugs that work brilliantly in animal models but show little or no efficacy in humans. This debate has taken place at a time when the need to reduce the numbers of animals used in research has been recognized. The 3Rs are now an embedded part of the approach to in vivo studies (NC3RS National Centre for the Replacement, Refinement and Reduction of Animals in Research, 2020):

- Replacement—methods that replace the use of animals with other approaches
- Reduction—strategies that result in fewer animals being used
- Refinement—modification of husbandry or experimental procedures to minimize pain and distress.

A beneficial outcome of this approach is a much stronger focus on the scientific design of in vivo studies both to improve reproducibility of results and to obtain the maximum information from the smallest number of animals.

An approach to the design of in vivo studies

The key to success in the use of in vivo studies is to be clear about the question to be answered (Table 11.2). Most animal models only model some aspects of the human disease; indeed very few are truly 'disease models'. For example, human allergic asthma involves: (1) an immune response, (2) increased airway resistance, (3) bronchial hyperreactivity, (4) lung inflammation and (5) structural remodelling of the airways. Animal models, mainly

Table 11.2 Epilepsy and epileptogenesis models

Model	Procedure	Face validity	Construct validity	Predictive validity
Acute seizure models				No acute seizure models show 'treatment-resistance' to conventional antiepileptic drugs, though this occurs in ~30% of human cases
Maximal electroshock model	Acute seizures evoked by whole-brain stimulation. Measure: proportion of mice responding with seizures	Weak. No spontaneous seizures. No neuropathological changes	Weak. Production of seizures not related to epileptogenesis	Good. Predictive of activity of drugs against partial seizures and generalized tonic–clonic seizures (with some false positives). Poor prediction of drugs effective in absence seizures
Pentylenetetrazole (PTZ)-induced seizure model	Seizures induced by subcutaneous s.c. injection of the convulsant drug PTZ. Measure: proportion of mice responding with seizures	As above	As above	Quite good as predictor of efficacy in absence seizures. Unreliable for other clinical types
Epileptogenesis models				
Kindling model	Weak electrical stimulation of amygdala repeated over several days. Evoked full-blown seizures develop gradually	Moderate, though spontaneous seizures are rarely produced Histological, electrophysiological and biochemical changes similar to human epilepsy	Uncertain	Moderate, but model is generally more drug-responsive than human epilepsy

continued

Table 11.2 Epilepsy and epileptogenesis models—cont'd

Model	Procedure	Face validity	Construct validity	Predictive validity
Postseizure models	Various procedures (e.g., injection of kainate, lithium or other agents into brain, sustained stimulation of amygdala or other pathways) evoke sustained seizures, with ongoing spontaneous seizures appearing days or weeks later. Can be used to test drug effects on fully kindled seizures, or on the kindling process	Good. Spontaneous seizures, latent period after initial trigger. Replicates histological and other changes, including neurodegeneration	Probably good for some clinical forms of epilepsy	As maximal electroshock (MES) for antiseizure drugs. Uncertain for antiepileptogenic drugs, of which there are no proven clinical examples
Surgical procedures	Cortical undercutting. Isolated region of cortex gradually develops spontaneous seizure activity	Good as model of posttraumatic epilepsy. Replicates histological and other changes	Probably good for post-traumatic epilepsy	As above

based on guinea pigs, whose airways behave similarly to those of humans, can replicate each of these features, but no single model reproduces the whole spectrum. A model of bronchial hyperreactivity is likely to be uninformative for a drug that may reduce the incidence of exacerbations. Studies that interrogate mechanistic aspects that are recapitulated by the animal model are likely to be much more helpful. A specific example is illustrated here. Systemic amyloidosis is a rare (but not very rare) condition in which misfolded protein fibrils accumulate in the extracellular matrix of vital organs causing progressive dysfunction and in many cases, organ failure and death. So far 26 globular proteins have been shown to be capable of forming amyloidogenic fibrils, and the pattern of deposition is variable both between fibril types and between individuals with the same fibril type. This is a considerable challenge for drug discovery and identification of a suitable animal model in which to explore pharmacology. Pepys et al. identified that despite this diversity, a normal plasma protein, serum amyloid P (SAP) component universally decorated amyloid and was thus a drug target. This observation also meant that the well-characterized inflammatory (AA) amyloidosis mouse model could be used to probe mechanisms of drug action. In a series of experiments, they showed that antibodies directed against SAP were capable of triggering amyloid removal through a complement-dependent macrophage giant cell response (Bodin et al., 2010). Each of these experiments focused on a different aspect of the putative mechanism of action and together built a picture of the complete response. Although the

pattern of deposition of AA amyloid in the mouse model is not the same as in humans, and there are important differences between mouse and human immune systems, the fundamental architecture of the response could be characterized in mouse and proved broadly translational to the human setting.

Transgenic models

The ability to knock out specific genes, most commonly in mice, has been proved to be a powerful tool. In many cases, these models have been used to support validation of targets. One disadvantage of the original methods in which the gene is knocked out right from the single-cell stage is that this may be lethal during development or lead to substantial developmental abnormalities. This can limit the ability to define the role in the adult and its role in disease of later onset. Newer methods allow for genes to be knocked out in specific organs and to be 'switched off' in adult life. These approaches have extended the translational value of these models.

Another important use of transgenic (knockout) models is in the interrogation of mechanism of action of drugs. For example, in the amyloidosis example given earlier, mice with knockout of specific components of the complement pathway showed that this was an important contributor to the mechanism of action of anti-SAP antibodies.

Transgenic models that 'knock-in' a (human) gene can also be informative, although careful consideration needs to be given to the context: a human gene expressed in a mouse may behave differently from the same gene in a human context. The same caution should be applied to models in which a receptor or other protein is overexpressed. These models may give some insight into the biological role of a protein, but are unlikely to be an accurate representation of human disease.

Imaging

Studies involving imaging can be particularly informative—these fall into two broad categories: studies that examine the distribution of a drug and/or its target, and those where imaging is used to assess a physiological or physical response to the intervention.

A major advantage of imaging approaches is that they allow assessments over a period of time, whereas traditional (histological) approaches would require a separate cohort of animals for each time point. Radiolabelling of small molecules is well established, and although initial preparation of the radiolabelled molecule can be expensive, its value is usually justified by the value distribution information that can be derived. Radiolabelling biological molecules is more complex, as the radiolabelling process can disrupt the three-dimensional architecture of the molecule and thus its pharmacological properties. Despite the effort and expense, there is increased focus on the use of radiolabelled biological molecules in both animal and human studies. An alternative approach is to use optical techniques. These make use of the fluorescent properties of biological molecules or in the case of bioluminescence imaging, light generated by chemiluminescent enzymatic reactions. The principal limitation of these methods is the depth of penetration that can be achieved; as a result, use in humans is limited, but in small animals, they may be more practical.

Structural methods

Spatial resolution of structural imaging is improving all the time such that methods such as computed tomography (CT) with X-rays and magnetic resonance imaging (MRI) are widely employed as measures of pharmacological response. They can be combined with labelling techniques to provide additional information.

Positron emission tomography (PET) can provide useful functional information. For example, the PET ligand fluorine-18 (^{18}F) fluorodeoxyglucose (FDG) is widely used as a means to assess the metabolic activity of tissues including tumours. It remains, however, an expensive technique owing to the infrastructure requirements for the creation of ligands and imaging facilities.

A particularly important role for in vivo experiments is to evaluate the effects of long-term drug administration on the intact organism. 'Adaptive' and 'rebound' effects (e.g., tolerance, dependence, rebound hypertension, delayed endocrine effects, etc.) are often produced when drugs are given continuously for days or weeks. Generally, such effects, which involve complex physiological interactions, are evident in the intact functioning organism but are not predictable from in vitro experiments.

The programme of in vivo profiling studies for characterization of a candidate drug depends very much on the drug target and therapeutic indication. A comprehensive catalogue of established in vivo assay methods appropriate to different types of pharmacological effect is given by Vogel (2002). Charting the appropriate course through the plethora of possible studies that might be performed to characterize a particular drug can be difficult.

A typical example of pharmacological profiling is summarized in Box 11.2. The studies were carried out as part of the development of a cardiovascular drug, *beraprost* (Melini & Goa, 2002). Beraprost is a stable analogue of prostaglandin I_2 (PGI_2) that acts on PGI_2 receptors of platelets and blood vessels, thereby inhibiting platelet aggregation (and hence thrombosis) and dilating blood vessels. It is directed at two therapeutic targets, namely, occlusive peripheral vascular disease and pulmonary hypertension (a serious complication of various types of cardiovascular disease, drug treatment or infectious diseases), resulting in hypertrophy

---

Box 11.2 Pharmacological profiling of beraprost

In vitro studies

Binding to prostaglandin I_2 (PGI_2) receptors of platelets from various species, including humans

PGI_2 agonist activity (cAMP formation) in platelets

Dilatation of arteries and arterioles in vitro, taken from various species

Increased red cell deformability (hence reduced blood viscosity and increased blood flow) in blood taken from hypercholesterolaemic rabbits

In vivo studies

Increased peripheral blood flow in various vascular regions (dogs)

Cutaneous vasodilatation (rat)

Reduced pulmonary hypertension in rat model of drug-induced pulmonary hypertension (measured by reduction of right ventricular hypertrophy)

Reduced tissue destruction (gangrene) of rat tail induced by ergotamine/epinephrine infusion

Reduction of vascular occlusion resulting from intraarterial sodium laureate infusion in rats

Reduction of vascular occlusion and thrombosis following electrical stimulation of femoral artery in anaesthetized dogs and rabbits

Reduction of vascular damage occurring several weeks after cardiac allografts in immunosuppressed rats

and often contractile failure of the right ventricle. The animal studies were, therefore, directed at measuring changes (reduction in blood flow, histological changes in vessel wall) associated with peripheral vascular disease, and with pulmonary hypertension. As these are progressive chronic conditions, it was important to establish that long-term systemic administration of beraprost was effective in retarding the development of the experimental lesions, as well as monitoring the acute pharmacodynamic effects of the drug.

Species differences

It is important to take species differences into account at all stages of pharmacological profiling. For projects based on a defined molecular target—nowadays the majority—the initial screening assay will normally involve the human isoform. The same target in different species will generally differ in its pharmacological specificity; commonly, there will be fairly small quantitative differences, which can be allowed for interpreting when pharmacological data in experimental animals, but occasionally the differences are large, so that a given class of compounds is active in one species but not in another. An example is shown in Fig. 11.5, which compares the activities of a series of bradykinin receptor antagonists on cloned human and rat receptors. The complete lack of correlation means that, for these compounds, tests of functional activity in the rat cannot be used to predict activity in man.

Species differences are, in fact, a major complicating factor at all stages of drug discovery and preclinical development. The physiology of disease processes such as inflammation, septic shock, obesity, atherosclerosis and so on differs markedly in different species. Most importantly (see Chapter 10), drug metabolism often differs, affecting the duration of action, as well as the pattern of metabolites, which can in turn affect the observed pharmacology and toxicity.

Validity criteria

Obviously, an animal model produced in a laboratory can never replicate exactly a spontaneous human disease state, so on what basis can we assess its 'validity' in the context of drug discovery?

Three types of validity criteria were originally proposed by Willner (1984) in connection with animal models of depression. These are:
- Face validity
- Construct validity
- Predictive validity.

Face validity refers to the accuracy with which the model reproduces the phenomena (symptoms, clinical signs and pathological changes) characterizing the human disease.

Construct validity refers to the theoretical rationale on which the model is based, that is, the extent to which the aetiology of the human disease is reflected in the model.

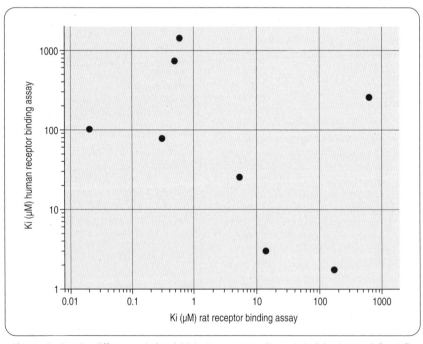

Fig. 11.5. Species differences in bradykinin B_2 receptors. (From Dziadulewicz et al. [2002]).

A transgenic animal model in which a human disease-producing mutation is replicated will have, in general, good construct validity, even if the manifestations of the human disorder are not well reproduced (i.e., it has poor face validity).

Predictive validity refers to the extent to which the effect of manipulations (e.g., drug treatment) in the model is predictive of effects in the human disorder. It is the most pragmatic of the three and the most directly relevant to the issue of predicting therapeutic efficacy but also the most limited in its applicability, for two main reasons. First, data on therapeutic efficacy are often sparse or non-existent, because no truly effective drugs are known (e.g., for Alzheimer's disease, septic shock). Second, the model may focus on a specific pharmacological mechanism, thus successfully predicting the efficacy of drugs that work by that mechanism but failing with drugs that might prove effective through other mechanisms. The knowledge that the first generation of antipsychotic drugs act as dopamine receptor antagonists enabled new drugs to be identified by animal tests reflecting dopamine antagonism, but these tests cannot be relied upon to recognize possible 'breakthrough' compounds that might be effective by other mechanisms. Thus, predictive validity, relying as it does on existing therapeutic knowledge, may not be a good basis for judging animal models where the drug discovery team's aim is to produce a mechanistically novel drug. The basis on which predictive validity is judged carries an inevitable bias, as the drugs that proceed to clinical trials will normally have proved effective in the model, whereas drugs that are ineffective in the model are unlikely to have been developed. As a result, there are many examples of tests giving 'false positive' expectations, but very few false negatives, giving rise to a commonly held view that conclusions from pharmacological tests tend to be overoptimistic.

Good laboratory practice compliance in pharmacological studies

Good laboratory practice (GLP) comprises adherence to a set of formal, internationally agreed guidelines established by regulatory authorities, aimed at ensuring the reliability of results obtained in the laboratory. The rules (Good Laboratory Practice Regulations 1999, amended 2004) cover all stages of an experimental study, from planning and experimental design to documentation, reporting and archiving. They require, among other things, the assignment of specific GLP-compliant laboratories, certification of staff training to agreed standards, certified instrument calibration, written standard operating procedures covering all parts of the work, specified standards of experimental records,

reports, notebooks and archives and much else. Standards are thoroughly and regularly monitored by an official inspectorate, which can halt studies or require changes in laboratory practice if the standards are thought not to be adequately enforced. Adherence to GLP standards carries a substantial administrative overhead and increases both the time and cost of laboratory studies, as well as limiting their flexibility.

The regulations are designed primarily to minimize the risk of errors in studies that relate to safety. They are, therefore, not generally applied to pharmacological profiling as described in this chapter. They are obligatory for toxicological studies that are required in submissions for regulatory approval. Though not formally required for safety pharmacology studies, most companies and contract research organizations choose to do such work under GLP conditions. An important development in recent years has been that pharmacodynamic assays (usually pharmacologically based) that are primary or secondary endpoints in clinical studies, or are used for clinical decision making, should be conducted in a laboratory that is compliant with good clinical practice (GCP). This is not the same as the GLP legislation but many of the principles of good practice are similar.

Pharmacology in the development phase

There has been a tendency to pigeon-hole pharmacology as a preclinical discipline. Pharmacology data were used to make somewhat crude predictions of human dose based on basic exposure response estimates. Many of these estimates proved inaccurate. The impetus for change and greater precision increased after human subjects suffered severe neurological harm, and one subject died while participating in a first-in-human study with a fatty acid amide inhibitor. Subsequent investigation identified a need for in-stream pharmacodynamic markers as the harmful off-target effects in the study were seen at doses higher than needed to achieve the desired pharmacology (EMA, 2017). The discipline of quantitative systems pharmacology (QSP) combines computational modelling and experimental data to examine the relationships between a drug, the biological system and the disease process. These are brought together in a quantitative model. As far as possible, the understanding of biological, physiological and metabolic differences between model systems (e.g., cell cultures, organs on a chip or animal models) should be used to characterize the multifaceted effects of the drug intervention. A critical element of these models is that they should address the concentration of the drug at its site of action. Human physiology is highly complex and to try to model all aspects of the test system would be near impossible. An important aspect of model building is therefore the identification of those processes that have the greatest effect and to obtain good estimates of the parameters that govern them.

QSP is particularly associated with dose prediction in first-in-human studies, but the value of this approach extends well beyond the first-in-human study. Pharmacology and pharmacodynamics are inextricably linked with drug exposure. Further information on the pharmacokinetic aspects is outlined in Chapter 10. In this section, we focus on the pharmacological aspects of these models.

Modelling and simulation and model-based drug development

Pharmacokinetic/pharmacodynamic (PK/PD) models have formed an important part of drug development for some time. The first models linked exposure to the drug with a direct pharmacodynamics effect—for example, time above a certain concentration and effect of heart rate for a beta blocker. These first models had two important limitations: they rely on a direct relationship between the concentration of a drug and the effect of interest, and they are largely retrospective, seeking to explain observations that have been made rather than predicting what might happen. Much of the innovation in this field has been aimed at addressing this latter point. Model-based drug development is actively encouraged by regulatory authorities and forms an increasingly important part of the drug development framework.

Physiologically based pharmacokinetic models and population pharmacokinetic models

As mentioned earlier, the earliest PK/PD models linked exposure (typically time above a certain concentration) with a direct effect of the drug based on data from a single clinical experiment. The next evolution was the population pharmacokinetic modelling (POPPK) that sought to link pharmacodynamic effect or efficacy with population-based PK measures. These measures might include sex, age, ethnic origin, concomitant medication, seeking to establish which of these had a clinically significant impact and thus might require a dose adjustment. Important though this technique is, it does not provide a mechanistic basis for the observations. Our enhanced understanding of the link between genetic variation and drug metabolism and receptor pharmacology provides an opportunity to define a mechanistic basis for variation observed in POPPK models. For example, a POPPK model might identify that overall patients of Southeast-Asian origin

respond to a lower dose of the drug. The mechanistic basis of this may be that 30% of people of this heritage are slow metabolizers of the drug in question. This more granular information allows a more sophisticated and targeted approach to dose adjustment. Those patients who are slow metabolizers may require a 50% dose reduction; this may be 30% of the Southeast-Asian population but 5% of a White population. In this case, ethnic origin has been used as a tag to identify the mechanistic basis of variation but is not in itself the basis for that variation.

A limitation of the POPPK approach is that it relies on population-based parameters to detect variation. An evolution has been the physiologically based pharmacokinetic (PBPK) model. These models seek to describe the behaviour of a drug through mathematical constructs of its absorption, distribution, metabolism and elimination. This has been particularly important for the modelling of biological molecules such as antibodies. For small chemical molecules, variation in response is often driven by variations in metabolism of the drug; by contrast, variation in response to antibodies is often driven by distribution to the tissue of interest and will not be identified by traditional PKPD models or POPPK approaches. The creation of a PBPK model requires different types of data, for example, the penetration of antibodies into tissues varies widely based on blood flow and the nature of the endothelium. These factors may have a much larger effect than the physical characteristics of the molecule itself.

The role of models is evolving from a retrospective means to explain clinical observations to a way to predict what will happen and thus to define the design of clinical studies. Traditional methods of defining the starting dose of a drug for human testing are based on allometric scaling and based on the no observed adverse effect level (NOAEL) in animal studies. The limitations of this approach are widely recognized and regulatory guidance makes clear that dose selection should be based on an understanding of the pharmacology through concepts such as the minimal biologically active level (MABEL). These approaches require the construction of a model that predicts the likely pharmacology of a drug based on the predicted exposure from a putative dose. The construction of such models should now form a routine part of the preclinical workup of a molecule; importantly, these models may dictate different types of preclinical experiments from the traditional package in order to define the key parameters. For example, permeability of the drug into muscle would not be part of a typical preclinical package, but if this is the location of the drug target estimating, it would be a vital component of a PBPK model.

Modelling and simulation should now form an integral part of the drug development process throughout. For example, traditional approaches to dose-ranging studies would seek to test high, optimal and inadequate dose levels. If one picks correctly, this works well, but all too often reality does not align with one's predictions. A model-based approach would seek to test a range of doses (exposures) in phase II with the aim of modelling the optimal dose for formal testing in phase III. These are now several examples of drugs where the dose selected for phase III testing is different from any of the doses tested in phase II but was identified based on a PKPD model.

Models are becoming more and more sophisticated, and the ultimate goal is the in silico clinical trial. This is close to reality in a few areas. Our understanding of cardiac electrophysiology is now sufficiently sophisticated, that is, it is possible to build a model of how a drug that alters that physiology will behave at a whole organ level. This raises the potential of an in silico early clinical development paradigm, where the only clinical trial required will be the definitive phase III registration trials, with doses defined by the in silico models.

References

Bodin, K., Ellmerich, S., Kahan, M. C., Tennent, G. A., Loesch, A., Gilbertson, J. A., et al. (2010). Antibodies to human serum amyloid P component eliminate visceral amyloid deposits. *Nature*, 468(7320), 93–97.

Dziadulewicz EK, Ritchie TJ, Hallett A, et al. Nonpeptide bradykinin B_2 receptor antagonists: conversion of rodent-selective bradyzide analogues into potent orally active human bradykinin B_2 receptor antagonists. *Journal of Medicinal Chemistry* 2002;45:2160–72.

EMA. (2017). Guideline on strategies to identify and mitigate risks for first-in-human and early clinical trials with investigational medicinal products. Retrieved from https://www.ema.europa.eu/en/documents/scientific-guideline/guideline-strategies-identify-mitigate-risks-first-human-early-clinical-trials-investigational_en.pdf.

Expert Group on Phase One Clinical Trials (chairman: Professor Gordon W. Duff) *Expert group on phase one clinical trials: Final report 2006 TSO*. The Stationery Office.

Keen, M. (Ed.). (1999). *Receptor binding techniques*. Totowa, NJ: Humana Press.

Melini, E. B., & Goa, K. L. (2002). Beraprost: a review of its pharmacology and therapeutic efficacy in the treatment of peripheral arterial disease and pulmonary hypertension. *Drugs, 62*, 107–133.

NC3RS National Centre for the Replacement, Refinement and Reduction of Animals in Research. (2020). *The 3Rs*. Retrieved from https://www.nc3rs.org.uk/the-3rs.

Sexton, P. M., Morfis, M., Tilakaratne, N., Hay, D. L., Udawela, M., Christopoulos, G., et al. (2006). Complexing receptor pharmacology: modulation of family B G protein-coupled receptor function by RAMPs. *Annals of the New York Academy of Sciences, 1070*, 90–104.

Traxler P, Bold G, Frei J, et al. Use of a pharmacophore model for the design of EGF-R tyrosine kinase inhibitors: 4-(phenylamino) pyrazolo[3,4-d] pyrimidines. *Journal of Medicinal Chemistry* 1997;40:3601–16.

Vogel, W. H. (Ed.). (2002). *Drug discovery and evaluation: Pharmacological assays*. Heidelberg: Springer-Verlag.

Willner, P. (1984). The validity of animal models of depression. *Psychopharmacology, 83*, 1–16.

Chapter 12

Nonclinical safety assessment

Duncan B Richards

Many of the elements of nonclinical assessment of safety have arisen following clinical disasters in which patients have been harmed by adverse drug reactions that were not predicted. The best known of these was the thalidomide disaster in which a drug given for nausea associated with pregnancy caused life-changing limb defects ('phocomelia') in babies. Following this, nonclinical testing for drugs to be given to women of child bearing potential became mandatory. Not all adverse effects of drugs can be predicted from nonclinical studies, and when they can, the animal model system that predicts them has usually been designed to pick up a specific adverse effect of interest; it does not mean that the model system will be equally good at identifying other potential harms.

Nonclinical package to support first-in-human studies

The nonclinical package to support a drug in development continues to evolve throughout the process but has a particularly important role to support the first human studies. We use the term nonclinical studies rather than preclinical because although these studies are before the clinic, later studies will be running in parallel with human studies (Fig. 12.1).

Toxicity from medicines may arise from the following:

- On-target pharmacology—while short-term effects are often predictable, long-term adaptive responses to the primary pharmacology may be adverse.
- Off-target pharmacology—while every effort is made to make medicines specific for their target, small chemical molecules in particular may also interact with other cell and receptor systems.
- 'Chemical toxicity'—in some cases, the parent molecule but more commonly a metabolite or degradant may cause toxicity through, for example, formation of reactive intermediates.

The schema outlined later has developed over many years based on experience, but the preclinical evaluation of potential medicines should never become a tick-box exercise.

Primary and secondary pharmacology

Understanding the primary pharmacology of a new chemical entity is an essential element of the nonclinical package. This is discussed in detail in Chapter 11, but some features have an impact on safety. Any molecule that has irreversible actions (perhaps through covalent binding) cannot easily be reversed in the event of an excessive pharmacological effect, and therefore this property is generally not favoured. Nonetheless, there are some important medicines that have an irreversible mode of action: aspirin irreversibly blocks cyclooxygenase, and proton pump inhibitors (e.g., omeprazole) irreversibly inhibit the H^+/K^+-adenosine triphosphate (ATPase) enzyme found at the secretory surface of gastric parietal cells. Drugs that are antagonists have traditionally been considered 'safer' than drugs that have an agonist action, usually because they have a wider therapeutic index.

Secondary pharmacology is an important source of unwanted effects of drugs. This may relate to relative lack of specificity leading to actions on other isoforms of the primary target but also includes action on enzymes, receptors and ion channels that are unrelated. A number of screening platforms are available that will identify the potential for a new molecule to bind to a wide range of other targets. These are important screening tools but in most cases only identify the potential for binding; they do not establish whether a molecule has agonist or antagonist properties—further tests are required to provide more detailed information (Lynch et al., 2017). As in all matters of pharmacology, concentration is important.

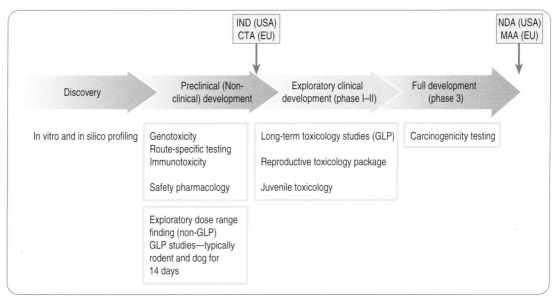

Fig. 12.1 Timing of the main safety assessment studies during drug discovery and development. *GLP*, Good laboratory practice; *IND*, Investigational New Drug; *CTA*, Clinical trial authorisation; *MAA*, Marketing authorisation application; *NDA*, New drug application.

Many molecules will have off-target effects at very high concentrations—whether these are clinically relevant will depend on the primary pharmacology and concentrations needed to achieve the desired effect.

Safety pharmacology

Nonclinical pharmacological studies (see also Chapter 11) are exploratory (i.e., surveying the effects of the compound with respect to selectivity against a wide range of possible targets) or hypothesis driven (checking whether the expected effects of the drug, based on its target selectivity, are actually produced). In contrast, safety pharmacology comprises a series of protocol-driven studies, aimed specifically at detecting possible undesirable or dangerous effects of exposure to the drug in therapeutic doses (see ICH Guideline S7A). The emphasis is on acute effects produced by single-dose administration, as distinct from toxicology studies, which focus mainly on the effects of chronic exposure. Safety pharmacology evaluation forms an important part of the dossier submitted to the regulatory authorities.

ICH Guideline S7A defines a *core battery* of safety pharmacology tests, and a series of *follow-up* and *supplementary* tests (Table 12.1). The core battery is normally performed on all compounds intended for systemic use. Where they are not appropriate (e.g., for preparations given topically), their omission has to be justified on the basis of

information about the extent of systemic exposure that may occur when the drug is given by the intended route. Follow-up studies are required if the core battery of tests reveals effects whose mechanism needs to be determined. Supplementary tests need to be performed if the known chemistry or pharmacology of the compound gives any reason to expect that it may produce side effects (e.g., a compound with a thiazide-like structure should be tested for possible inhibition of insulin secretion, this being a known side effect of thiazide diuretics; similarly, an opioid needs to be tested for dependence liability and effects on gastrointestinal motility). Where there is a likelihood of significant drug interactions, this may also need to be tested as part of the supplementary programme.

The core battery of tests listed in Table 12.1 focuses on acute effects on cardiovascular, respiratory and nervous systems, based on standard physiological measurements.

The follow-up and supplementary tests are less clearly defined, and the list given in Table 12.1 is neither prescriptive nor complete. It is the responsibility of the team to decide what tests are relevant and how the studies should be performed, and to justify these decisions in the submission to the regulatory authority.

Tests for QT interval prolongation

The ability of a number of therapeutically used drugs to cause a potentially fatal ventricular arrhythmia (*torsade de pointes*) has been a cause of major concern to clinicians and regulatory authorities (see Committee for Proprietary

Table 12.1 Safety pharmacology

Type	Physiological system	Tests
Core battery	Central nervous system	Observations on conscious animals Motor activity Behavioural changes Coordination Reflex responses Body temperature
	Cardiovascular system	Measurements on anaesthetized animals Blood pressure Heart rate ECG changes Tests for delayed ventricular repolarization (see text)
	Respiratory system	Measurements on anaesthetized or conscious animals Respiratory rate Tidal volume Arterial oxygen saturation
Follow-up tests (examples)	Central nervous system	Tests on learning and memory More complex test for changes in behaviour and motor function Tests for visual and auditory function
	Cardiovascular system	Cardiac output Ventricular contractility Vascular resistance Regional blood flow
	Respiratory system	Airways resistance and compliance Pulmonary arterial pressure Blood gases
Supplementary tests (examples)	Renal function	Urine volume, osmolality pH Proteinuria Blood urea/creatinine Fluid/electrolyte balance Urine cytology
	Autonomic nervous system	Cardiovascular, gastrointestinal and respiratory system responses to agonists and stimulation of autonomic nerves
	Gastrointestinal system	Gastric secretion Gastric pH Intestinal motility Gastrointestinal transit time
	Other systems (e.g., endocrine, blood coagulation, skeletal muscle function, etc.)	Tests designed to detect likely acute effects

Medicinal Products, 1997; Haverkamp et al., 2000). The arrhythmia is associated with prolongation of the ventricular action potential (delayed ventricular repolarization), reflected in ECG recordings as prolongation of the QT interval. Drugs known to possess this serious risk, many of which have been withdrawn, include several *tricyclic antidepressants*, some antipsychotic drugs (e.g., *thioridazine, droperidol*), antidysrhythmic drugs (e.g., *amiodarone, quinidine, disopyramide*), antihistamines (e.g., *terfenadine, astemizole*) and certain antimalarial drugs (e.g., *halofantrine*). The main mechanism responsible appears to be inhibition of a potassium channel, termed the hERG channel, which plays a major role in terminating the ventricular action potential.

Screening tests have shown that QT interval prolongation is a common property of 'drug-like' small molecules, and the patterns of structure–activity relationships have revealed particular chemical classes associated with this effect. Ideally, these are taken into account and avoided at an early stage in drug design, but the need remains for functional testing of all candidate drug molecules as a prelude to tests in humans.

Proposed standard tests for QT interval prolongation have been formulated as ICH Guideline S7B. They comprise (1) testing for inhibition of hERG-channel currents in cell lines engineered to express the hERG gene; (2) measurements of action potential duration in myocardial cells from different parts of the heart in different species and (3) measurements of QT interval in ECG recordings in conscious animals. These studies are usually carried out on ferrets or guinea pigs, as well as larger mammalian species, such as dog, rabbit, pig or monkey, in which hERG-like channels control ventricular repolarization, rather than in rat and mouse.

Because of the importance of drug-induced QT prolongation in humans, and the fact that many diverse groups of drugs appear to have this property, there is a need for high-throughput screening for hERG-channel inhibition to be incorporated early in a drug discovery project. The above methods are not suitable for high-throughput screening, but alternative methods, such as inhibition of binding of labelled *dofetilide* (a potent hERG-channel blocker), or fluorimetric membrane potential assays on cell lines expressing these channels, can be used in high-throughput formats, as increasingly can automated patch clamp studies. It is important to note that binding and fluorescence assays are not seen as adequately predictive and cannot replace the patch clamp studies under the guidelines (ICH 7B). These assays are now becoming widely used as part of screening before selecting a clinical candidate molecule, though there is still a need to confirm presence or absence of QT prolongation in functional in vivo tests before advancing a compound into clinical development.

Important though QT prolongation is, it is not the only mechanism by which drugs can cause clinically significant arrhythmias, and some have argued that the focus on QT has distracted attention from other mechanisms. Identification of better predictive model systems for arrhythmia is an important area of research in drug development and is discussed later in this chapter.

Toxicology

The principle of toxicology is to administer the study material to a relevant animal species in order to identify potential toxicities. There are several important principles that need to be considered when designing a toxicology package. The animal species chosen must be relevant to humans—if the animal lacks the target receptor or the molecule does not bind the animal form of the target, then only off-target effects can be assessed. This is particularly

relevant for biological and advanced therapies and is discussed in more detail later in the chapter. For small-molecule pharmaceuticals, the usual expectation is that toxicity will be explored in one rodent (usually rat) and one nonrodent (usually dog) species. The absorption, distribution, metabolism and excretion (ADME) characteristics of the molecule must be similar in humans and the chosen animal species. If the molecule undergoes a completely different metabolic pathway in animals from humans, the results may be falsely reassuring or alarming. At this preclinical stage of development, the human ADME characteristics are of course unknown, but in vitro tests (e.g., human hepatocytes) can inform the choice of relevant animal species. Pathology is a complex discipline, and considerable expertise is required in the interpretation of histopathological specimens from toxicology studies. Not every tissue from every animal will be 100% 'normal', even if there is no drug-induced toxicity. Reference data providing information on natural variability are vital to the assessment of toxicology studies, and therefore there is a strong steer to use well-described strains for these studies. There is an expectation from regulatory authorities that at least one dose level will show evidence of toxicity. If one knows the nature of the toxicity and has information at what exposure it occurs, this provides for a more secure basis for setting limits to human exposure. A clean bill of health from toxicology studies may be ostensibly appealing but may induce a request from regulators to explore higher dose levels.

Exploratory (dose range-finding) toxicology studies

Given the importance of dose (exposure) selection, the first stage of toxicological evaluation usually takes the form of a *dose range-finding (DRF) study* in a rodent and/or a nonrodent species. The species commonly used in toxicology are mice, rats, guinea pigs, hamsters, rabbits, dogs, minipigs and nonhuman primates. Usually two species (rat and mouse) are tested initially, but others may be used if there are reasons for thinking that the drug may exert species-specific effects. A single dose is given to each test animal, preferably by the intended route of administration in the clinic, and in a formulation shown by previous pharmacokinetic studies to produce satisfactory absorption and duration of action (see also Chapter 10). Generally, widely spaced doses (e.g., 10, 100, 1000 mg/kg) will be tested first, on groups of three to four rodents, and the animals will be observed over 14 days for obvious signs of toxicity. The regulatory expectation is that the dose range will include a maximum tolerated dose (MTD), or in rare circumstances, the maximum feasible dose (generally 2000 mg/kg in rodents). Alternatively, a *dose escalation* protocol may be used, in which each animal is treated with increasing doses of the drug at intervals (e.g., every 2 days), until signs of toxicity appear, or until a dose of

2000 mg/kg is reached. With either protocol, the animals are killed at the end of the experiment and autopsied to determine if any target organs are grossly affected. The results of such DRF studies provide a rough estimate of the *no observed adverse effect level* (NOAEL, see Toxicity measures, fig. 12.2) in the species tested, and the nature of the gross effects seen is often a useful pointer to the main target tissues and organs. The word 'observed' is important here as the NOAEL tends to lower as drug development proceeds and the drug is administered for longer periods. Doses that show no observed toxicity over 7–14 days may well show adverse effects when given for 3–6 months. Margins of safety that look very generous at the start of a development programme may be much narrower by the end.

The dose range-finding study may be followed by a more detailed single-dose toxicological study in two or more species, the doses tested being chosen to span the estimated NOAEL. Four or five doses may be tested, ranging from a dose in the expected therapeutic range to doses well above the estimated NOAEL. A typical protocol for such an acute toxicity study is shown in Fig. 12.2. The data collected consist of regular systematic assessment of the animals for a range of clinical signs on the basis of a standardized checklist, together with gross autopsy findings of animals dying during a 2-week observation period, or killed at the end. The main signs that are monitored are shown in Table 12.2.

As most drugs are given repeatedly in many cases, the single dose work will be limited, and the focus will shift to a multiple dose-ranging study in which the drug is given daily or twice daily, usually for 2 weeks, with the same observation and autopsy procedure as in the single-dose study, in order to give preliminary information about the toxicity after chronic treatment.

Formal toxicology studies

The information from the dose range-finding studies will be used to design the formal (good laboratory practice [GLP]) studies that will support human studies. Usually

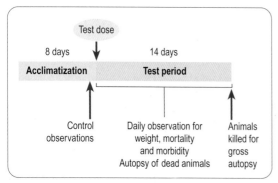

Fig. 12.2 Typical protocol for a single-dose toxicity study.

these are of 14 days duration, as this supports up to 14 days administration in humans. Three dose levels are typically tested. Based on the preliminary findings of the DRF studies, consider whether any special tests should be included or whether a recovery group should be included to see if observed toxicities recover off-treatment. Careful consideration needs to be given to the drug material used in these studies. It must be representative of the material that will be given to humans. At this stage of development, the level of control of impurities and degradants may not be as tight as would be expected for a final drug product. It is important that material used for toxicology studies (and of course human studies) is of high quality, but at this stage it must not be 'purer' than that which will be given to humans.

The three Rs (reduce/refine/replace) are core principles of modern toxicology, and regulators have provided guidance (ICHM3 R2) on alternative approaches to the scheme above which enable human studies with a slimmer toxicology package. These approaches are particularly useful when there are several drug candidates and one wishes to select the best based on its human pharmacokinetics; for this, a microdose may be all that is required. The guidance also allows for administration of small pharmacologically active doses to test target or pharmacological engagement; again, this can be a particularly useful approach for novel mechanisms and when doses can be administered locally, for example, to a segment of the lung.

Chronic toxicology studies

Assuming that initial human studies are encouraging, then additional toxicological information will be required to support longer duration clinical trials and ultimately marketing of the product; the prescribed durations are summarized in Table 12.3. The key point is that these longer studies evaluate toxicity when a steady state is achieved, that is, when the rate of drug administration equals the rate of elimination. There is usually some further refinement of the dose range, typically with a narrowing of the range explored as top doses are not tolerated in the long term. Usually the doses will include one that is clearly toxic, one in the therapeutic range and at least one in between. Ideally, the in-between doses will exceed the expected clinical dose by a factor of 10 for rodents and 5 for nonrodents, yet lack overt toxicity, this being the 'window' normally required by regulatory authorities. At least one recovery group is usually included, that is, animals treated with the drug at a toxic level, and then allowed to recover for 2–4 weeks so that the reversibility of the changes observed can be assessed. The aim of these studies is to determine (1) the cumulative biological effects produced by the compound and (2) at what exposure level

Table 12.2 Clinical observations in acute toxicity tests

System	Observation	Signs of toxicity
Nervous system	Behaviour	Sedation
		Restlessness
		Aggression
	Motor function	Twitch
		Tremor
		Ataxia
		Catatonia
		Convulsions
		Muscle rigidity or flaccidity
	Sensory function	Excessive or diminished response to stimuli
Respiratory	Respiration	Increased or decreased respiratory rate
		Intermittent respiration
		Dyspnoea
Cardiovascular	Cardiac palpation	Increase or decrease in rate or force
	Electrocardiography	Disturbances of rhythm.
		Altered ECG pattern (e.g., QT prolongation)
Gastrointestinal	Faeces	Diarrhoea or constipation
		Abnormal form or colour
		Bleeding
	Abdomen	Spasm or tenderness
Genitourinary	Genitalia	Swelling, inflammation, discharge, bleeding
Skin and fur		Discoloration
		Lesions
		Piloerection
Mouth		Discharge
		Congestion
		Bleeding
Eye	Pupil size	Mydriasis or miosis
	Eyelids	Ptosis, exophthalmos
	Movements	Nystagmus
	Cornea	Opacity
General signs	Body weight	Weight loss

(see later) they appear. The initial repeated dose studies, by revealing the overall pattern of toxic effects produced, also give pointers to particular aspects (e.g., liver toxicity, bone marrow depression) that may need to be addressed later in more detailed toxicological investigations.

Experimental design

Chronic toxicity testing must be performed under GLP conditions, with the formulation and route of administration to be used in humans. Tests are normally carried out on one rodent (usually rat) and one nonrodent species (usually dog), but additional species (such as monkey or pig) may be tested if there are special reasons for suspecting that their responses may predict effects in humans more accurately than those of dogs.

Pharmacokinetic measurements are included, so that extrapolation to humans can be done on the basis of the concentration of the drug in blood and tissues, allowing for differences in pharmacokinetics between laboratory animals and humans (see Chapter 10). Separate male and female test groups are used. The recommended number of animals per test group (see Gad, 2002) is shown in Table 12.4. There are strong reasons for minimizing the number of animals used in such studies, and the figures given take this into account, representing the minimum shown by experience to be needed for statistically reliable conclusions to be drawn. An average study will require 200 or more rats and about 60 dogs, dosed with compound and observed regularly, including blood and urine sampling, for several months before being killed and autopsied, with tissue samples being collected

Table 12.3 Recommended duration of repeated-dose toxicity studies to support clinical trials and marketing

Clinical studies		
Duration of clinical study	Rodent	Nonrodent
Up to 2 weeks	2 weeks	2 weeks
Between 2 weeks and 6 months	Same duration as clinical trial	
>6 months	6 months	9 months
Marketing		
Duration of indicated treatment	Rodent	Nonrodent
Up to 2 weeks	1 month	1 month
>2 weeks to 1 month	3 months	3 months
>1 month to 3 months	6 months	6 months
>3 months	6 months	9 months

See ICH M3 for more details

Table 12.4 Recommended numbers of animals for chronic toxicity studies (Gad, 2002)

Study duration	Rats (per sex)	Dogs (per sex)	Primates (per sex)
4 weeks	5–10	3–4	3
3 months	20	6	5
6 months	30	8	5
12 months	50	10	10
2-year (carcinogenicity)	50–80		

for histological examination. It is a massive and costly experiment requiring large amounts of compound prepared to good manufacturing practice (GMP) standards, the conduct and results of which will receive detailed scrutiny by regulatory authorities, and so careful planning and scrupulous execution are essential.

Evaluation of toxic effects

During the course of the experiment, all animals are inspected regularly for mortality and gross morbidity, severely affected animals being killed and all dead animals subjected to autopsy. Specific signs (e.g., diarrhoea, salivation, respiratory changes, etc.) are assessed against a detailed checklist and specific examinations (e.g., blood pressure, heart rate and ECG, ocular changes, neurological and behavioural changes, etc.) are also conducted regularly. Food intake and body weight changes are monitored, and blood and urine samples collected at intervals for biochemical and haematological analyses.

At the end of the experiment, all animals are killed and examined by autopsy for gross changes, and samples of all major tissues being prepared for histological examination. Tissues from the high-dose group are examined histologically, and any tissues showing pathological changes are also examined in the low-dose groups to enable a dose threshold to be estimated. The reversibility of the adverse effects can be evaluated in these studies by studying animals retained after the end of the dosing period.

As part of the general toxicology screening described earlier, specific evaluation of possible *immunotoxicity* is required by the regulatory authorities, the main concern being immunosuppression. If effects on blood, spleen or thymus cells are observed in the 1-month repeated-dose studies, additional tests are required to evaluate the strength of cellular and humoral responses in immunized animals. A battery of suitable tests is included in the ICH S8 guideline.

The large body of data collected during a typical toxicology study should allow conclusions to be drawn about the main physiological systems and target organs that underlie the toxicity of the compound, and also about the dose levels at which critical effects are produced. In practice, the analysis and interpretation are not always straightforward, for a variety of reasons, including:

- Incorrect choice of doses
- Variability within the groups of animals
- Spontaneous occurrence of 'toxic' effects in control or vehicle-treated animals
- Missing data, owing to operator error, equipment failure, unexpected death of animals and so on
- Problems of statistical analysis (qualitative data, multiple comparisons, etc.).

Overall, it is estimated that correctly performed chronic toxicity tests in animals successfully predict 70% of toxic reactions in humans (Olson et al., 2000); skin reactions in humans are the least well predicted.

Long-term toxicology studies are time-consuming, costly and consistent with the principles of the three Rs and should not be undertaken lightly. Moving directly from 14 days dosing directly to long-term administration (6–9 months depending on species) may be appealing from an efficiency point of view, but it is very unlikely that the 14-day studies provide sufficient scientific information to design the long-term studies properly. A study of intermediate duration is likely to be a prudent approach. Scheduling these studies is complex; one needs sufficient confidence from the clinical programme results to move forward but also suitable drug material and time to collate and submit the results. The reporting of toxicology studies usually takes at least as long as the physical duration of the study; a long-term study will involve tens of thousands of slides that need to be read and peer-reviewed.

Special tests

The standard procedures discussed here are appropriate for the majority of conventional synthetic compounds intended for systemic use. Additional specific testing may be required, often related to the route of administration. Illustrative examples are provided here:

- A drug for intravenous administration will need to be tested to ensure it does not cause haemolysis.
- Drugs for topical use and their excipients (vehicle) will need to be tested to ensure they do not cause unacceptable irritation at the site of delivery.
- Some drugs accumulate in the skin, especially if they bind to melanin. This can cause phototoxicity; guidance on assessment is provided in ICH S10 and ICH M3R2.

The toxicology package forms the core of the nonclinical package for a drug, but there are important additional elements to consider; these are now outlined.

Genotoxicity

Foreign substances can affect gene function in various ways, the two most important types of mechanism in relation to toxicology being:

- *Mutagenicity*, that is, chemical alteration of DNA sufficient to cause abnormal gene expression in the affected cell and its offspring. Most commonly, the mutation arises as a result of covalent modification of individual bases (point mutations). The result may be the production of an abnormal protein if the mutation occurs in the coding region of the gene, or altered expression levels of a normal protein if the mutation affects control sequences. Such mutations occur continuously in everyday life and are counteracted more or less effectively by a variety of DNA repair mechanisms. They are important particularly because certain mutations can interfere with mechanisms controlling cell division and thereby lead to malignancy or, in the immature organism, to adverse effects on growth and development. In practice, most carcinogens are mutagens, though by no means all mutagens are carcinogens. Evidence of mutagenicity therefore sounds a warning of possible carcinogenicity, which must be tested by thorough in vivo tests.

- *Chromosomal damage*, for example, chromosome breakage (clastogenesis), chromosome fusion, translocation of stretches of DNA within or between chromosomes, replication or deletion of chromosomes and so on. Such changes result from alterations in DNA, more extensive than point mutations and less well understood mechanistically; they have a similar propensity to cause cancerous changes and to affect growth and development.

The most important end results of genotoxicity—carcinogenesis and impairment of fetal development (teratogenicity)—can only be detected by long-term animal studies. There is, therefore, every reason to pre-screen compounds by in vitro methods, and such studies are routinely carried out before human studies begin. Because in many cases the genotoxicity is due to reactive metabolites rather than to the parent molecule, the in vitro tests generally include assays carried out in the presence of liver microsomes or other liver-derived preparations, so that metabolites are generated. Often, liver microsomes from rats treated with inducing agents (e.g., a mixture of chlorinated biphenyls known as Arochlor 1254) are used, in order to enhance drug-metabolizing activity.

Selection and interpretation of tests

Many in vitro and in vivo test systems for mutagenicity have been described, based on bacteria, yeast, insect and mammalian cells (see Gad, 2002 for details). The ICH Guideline S2R1 stipulates a preliminary battery of three tests:

- *Ames test: a test of mutagenicity in bacteria.* The basis of the assay is that mutagenic substances increase the rate at which a histidine-dependent strain of *Salmonella typhimurium* reverts to a wild type that can grow in the absence of histidine. An increase in the number of colonies surviving in the absence of histidine therefore denotes significant mutagenic activity. Several histidine-dependent strains of the organism that differ in their susceptibility to particular types of mutagen are normally tested in parallel. Positive controls with known mutagens that act directly or only after metabolic activation are routinely included when such tests are performed.

- *An in vitro test for chromosomal abnormalities in mammalian cells or an in vitro mouse lymphoma tk cell assay.* To test chromosomal damage, Chinese hamster ovary (CHO) cells are grown in culture in the presence of the test substance, with or without liver microsomes. Cell division is arrested in metaphase, and chromosomes are observed microscopically to detect structural aberrations, such as gaps, duplications, fusions or alterations in chromosome number. The mouse lymphoma cell test for mutagenicity involves a heterozygous (tk +/−) cell line that can be killed by the cytotoxic agent bromodeoxyuridine (BrDU). Mutation to the *tk* −/− form causes the cells to become resistant to BrDU, and so counts of surviving cells in cultures treated with the test compound provide an index of mutagenicity. The mouse lymphoma cell mutation assay is more sensitive than the chromosomal assay but can give positive results with noncarcinogenic substances. These tests are not possible with compounds that are inherently toxic to mammalian cells.

- *An in vivo test for chromosomal damage in rodent haemopoietic cells.* The mouse micronucleus test is commonly used. Animals are treated with the test compound for 2 days, after which, immature erythrocytes in bone marrow are examined for micronuclei, representing fragments of damaged chromosomes.

If these three tests prove negative, no further tests of genotoxicity are generally needed before the compound can be tested in humans. If one or more is positive, further in vitro and in vivo genotoxicity testing will usually be carried out to assess more accurately the magnitude of the risk. In a few cases, where the medical need is great and the life expectancy of the patient population is very limited, development of compounds that are clearly genotoxic—and, by inference, possibly carcinogenic—may still be justified, but in most cases, genotoxic compounds will be abandoned without further ado.

Drug products may contain degradants and impurities that have mutagenic properties and so may represent a carcinogenic risk. The approach here is to limit the amount in the material to a level that they represent a negligible risk to patients. One common approach is to set a threshold of toxicological concern; a benchmark is 1.5 µg/day corresponding to a theoretical 10^{-5} excess lifetime risk of cancer, which is generally considered acceptably low. Higher intakes may be acceptable if the duration of exposure is limited (e.g., during early clinical trials). Specific guidance is provided in the ICH M7 Guideline.

Reproductive toxicology

Two incidents led to greatly increased concern about the effects of drugs on the fetus. The first was the thalidomide disaster of the 1960s. The second was the high incidence of cervical and vaginal cancers in young women whose mothers had been treated with diethylstilbestrol (DES) in early pregnancy, with the aim of preventing early abortion. DES was used in this way between 1940 and 1970, and the cancer incidence was reported in 1971. These events led to the introduction of stringent tests for teratogenicity as a prerequisite for the approval of new drugs, and from this flowed concern for other aspects of reproductive toxicology that now must be fully evaluated before a drug is marketed. Current requirements are summarized in ICH Guideline S5R3.

Drugs can affect reproductive performance in three main ways:

- Fertility (both sexes, fertilization and implantation), addressed by *Segment 1* studies
- Embryonic and fetal development or teratology, addressed by *Segment 2* studies
- Peri- and postnatal development, addressed by *Segment 3* studies.

It is usually acceptable for phase I human studies on male volunteers to begin before any reproductive toxicology data are available, so long as the drug shows no evidence of testicular damage in 2- or 4-week repeated-dose studies. The requirement for reproductive toxicology data as a prelude to clinical trials differs from country to country, but, as a general rule, clinical trials involving women of childbearing age should be preceded by relevant reproductive toxicology testing. In all but exceptional cases, such as drugs intended for treating life-threatening diseases, or for use only in the elderly, registration will require comprehensive data from relevant toxicology studies so that the reproductive risk can be assessed.

Segment 1 tests of fertility and implantation involve treating both males (for 28 days) and females (for 14 days) with the drug prior to mating, then measuring sperm count and sperm viability, numbers of implantation sites and live and dead embryos on day 6 of gestation. For drugs that either by design or by accident reduce fertility, tests for reversibility on stopping treatment are necessary.

Segment 2 tests of effects on embryonic and fetal development are usually carried out on two or three species (rat, mouse, rabbit), the drug being given to the female during the initial gestation period (day 6 to day 16 after mating in the rat). Animals are killed just before parturition, and the embryos are counted and assessed for structural abnormalities. In vitro tests involving embryos maintained in culture are also possible. The main stages of early embryogenesis can be observed in this way, and the effects of drugs added to the medium can be monitored. Such in vitro tests are routinely performed in some laboratories but are currently not recognized by regulatory authorities as a reliable measure of possible teratogenicity.

Segment 3 tests on pre- and perinatal development entail dosing female rats with the drug throughout gestation and lactation. The offspring are observed for motility, reflex responses and so on, both during and after the weaning period, and at intervals, some are killed for observations of structural abnormalities. Some are normally allowed to mature and are mated, to check for possible second-generation effects. Mature offspring are also tested for effects on learning and memory.

Reproductive and developmental toxicology is a complex field in which standards in relation to pharmaceuticals have not yet been clearly defined. The experimental studies are demanding, and the results may be complicated by species differences, individual variability and 'spontaneous' events in control animals.

It is obvious that any drug given in sufficient doses to cause overt maternal toxicity is very likely to impair fetal development. Nonspecific effects, most commonly a reduction in birthweight, are commonly found in animal studies, but provided the margin of safety is sufficient—say 10-fold—between the expected therapeutic dose and that affecting the fetus, this will not be a bar to developing the compound. The main aim of reproductive toxicology is to assess the risk of specific effects occurring within the therapeutic dose range in humans. Many familiar drugs and chemicals are teratogenic in certain species at high doses. They include *penicillin, sulfonamides, tolbutamide, diphenylhydantoin, valproate, imipramine, acetazolamide, ACE inhibitors* and *angiotensin antagonists*, as well as many *anticancer drugs* and also *caffeine, cannabis* and *ethanol*. Many of these are known or suspected teratogens in humans, and their use in pregnancy is to be avoided. A classification of drugs based on their safety during pregnancy has been developed by the US Food and Drug Administration (FDA) (A, B, C, D or X). Category A is for drugs considered safe in human pregnancy, that is, adequate and well-controlled studies in pregnant women have failed to demonstrate a risk to the fetus in any trimester of pregnancy. Few drugs belong to this category. Category X is reserved for drugs (e.g., *isotretinoin, warfarin*) that have been proved to cause fetal abnormalities in humans and are therefore contraindicated in pregnancy. Category B covers drugs with no evidence of risk in humans; category C covers drugs in which a risk cannot be ruled out; and category D covers drugs with positive evidence of risk. Requirements for the reproductive safety testing of biologicals are laid out in the Addendum to S6 (2011), and there are specific considerations, for example, the inability of some high-molecular-weight proteins to cross the placenta that do not apply to small molecules.

Carcinogenicity

Drugs that are expected to be given to large numbers of patients and for extended periods will be expected to have carcinogenicity testing before the drug is marketed, although it is not usually required for clinical trials.

It is also required if there are special causes for concern, for example, if:

- The compound belongs to a known class of carcinogens, or has chemical features associated with carcinogenicity; nowadays such compounds will normally have been eliminated at the lead identification stage (see Chapter 7)
- Chronic toxicity studies show evidence of precancerous changes

- The compound or its metabolites are retained in tissues for long periods.

Drugs that are given for short periods or for rare diseases may be exempt from carcinogenicity testing. A carcinogenicity programme will typically take 3 years and many millions of pounds to complete, so it is vital that developers discuss the need for and design of such programmes early in the clinical development process.

If a compound proves positive in tests of mutagenicity (see earlier), it must be *assumed* to be carcinogenic, and its use restricted accordingly, so no purpose is served by in vivo carcinogenicity testing. Only in very exceptional cases will such a compound be chosen for development.

ICH Guidelines S1A, S1B and S1C on carcinogenicity testing stipulate one long-term test in a rodent species (usually rat), plus one other in vivo test, which may be either: (1) a short-term test designed to show high sensitivity to carcinogens (e.g., transgenic mouse models) or to detect early events associated with tumour initiation or promotion; or (2) a long-term carcinogenicity test in a second rodent species (normally mouse). If positive results emerge in either study, the onus is on the pharmaceutical company to provide evidence that carcinogenicity will not be a significant risk to humans in a therapeutic setting. Until recently, the normal requirement was for long-term studies in two rodent species, but advances in the understanding of tumour biology, and the availability of new models that allow quicker evaluation, have brought about a change in the attitude of regulatory authorities such that only one long-term study is required, together with data from a well-validated short-term study.

Long-term rat carcinogenicity studies normally last for 2 years and are run in parallel with phase III clinical trials. (Oral contraceptives require a 3-year test for carcinogenicity in beagles.)

Three or four dose levels are tested, plus controls. Typically, the lowest dose tested is close to the maximum recommended human dose, and the highest is the MTD in rats (i.e., the largest dose that causes no obvious side effects or toxicity in the chronic toxicity tests). Between 50 and 80 animals of each sex are used in each experimental group (see Table 12.4), and so the complete study will require about 600–800 animals. Premature deaths are inevitable in such a large group and can easily ruin the study, so that housing the animals under standard disease-free conditions is essential. At the end of the experiment, samples of about 50 different tissues are prepared for histological examination and rated for benign and malignant tumour formation by experienced pathologists. Carcinogenicity testing is therefore one of the most expensive and time-consuming components of the toxicological evaluation of a new compound. New guidelines for dose selection were adopted from 2008 that allow a more rational approach to the selection of the high dose on the basis of a 25-fold higher exposure of the rodent than that seen in human subjects on the basis of area-under-the-curve (AUC) measurements in plasma rather than MTD.

Several transgenic mouse models have been developed that provide data more quickly (usually about 6 months) than the normal 2-year carcinogenicity study (Gad, 2002). These include animals in which human proto-oncogenes, such as hRas, are expressed, or the tumour suppressor gene P53 is inactivated. These mice show a very high incidence of spontaneous tumours after about 1 year, but at 6 months, spontaneous tumours are rare. Known carcinogens cause tumours to develop in these animals within 6 months.

Advances in this area are occurring rapidly, and as they do so, the methodology for carcinogenicity testing is expected to become more sophisticated and faster than the conventional long-term studies used hitherto (https://www.alttox.org/ttrc/toxicity-tests/carcinogenicity/).

Toxicology studies to support use in children

It is now a regulatory expectation that any medicine in development that has potential utility in children (whether for the adult indication or another paediatric-specific one) will have a paediatric development plan in place. Children are both developing and growing, both of which represent considerable challenges for the assessment of safety. At any given point, there will be a complex interplay between these factors and the impact of the disease process, a child with a chronic disease may well experience reduced growth and delayed puberty. For these reasons, the ICH guidance (S11) recommends a weight of evidence approach rather than relying on single tests.

Specific considerations for biopharmaceuticals and advanced therapies

The emergence of biopharmaceuticals and monoclonal antibodies in particular has necessitated a different approach to the nonclinical assessment of safety. A fundamental feature of monoclonal antibodies is their specificity—in practical terms, they only bind to their target. Much of the focus of the nonclinical assessment of traditional pharmaceuticals is on off-target effects—these are very uncommon with biopharmaceuticals. The targets for many antibodies are complex elements of the immune system, and therefore the most pressing question is to fully understand the biological consequences of hitting that target. The nonclinical package for a biopharmaceutical will therefore typically include a detailed survey of the location of the target within human tissues and a series of in vitro and in vivo studies exploring the biology of the target. In many cases, this will involve studies in nonhuman primates, but transgenic mouse models may be used. Interpretation of data from model systems is complex—a humanized antibody will not interact with the mouse immune system in the same way as a murine one. Indeed, it will usually induce the formation of anti-human immunoglobulin (Ig)G antibodies leading to fatal immunotoxicity if a second dose is administered to a mouse. This illustrates a second key area of focus for the nonclinical package for biopharmaceuticals. Small molecules may cause immunotoxicity, usually through the formation of haptens, but this is uncommon. By contrast, immune responses to monoclonal antibodies are common. In many cases, this will lead to the formation of neutralizing antibodies, which although they may not directly impact safety, they may render the treatment less effective over time. In other cases, interaction with the immune system can fundamentally alter the properties of the drug. For example, naturally occurring antibodies present in 50% of healthy subjects in a first-in-human study were found to bind to the variable heavy (VH) chain framework sequences, resulting in crosslinking of the (domain) antibody molecules. The target of the molecule was the tumour necrosis factor (TNF)-α receptor 1, and the effect of this crosslinking was to induce signalling through the receptor rather than the intended blocking effect (Holland et al., 2013).

The manufacture of biopharmaceuticals relies on biological processes that are inherently more difficult to control than traditional chemical synthetic routes. As development progresses, so the scale of manufacturing increases. It is very important to ensure that these changes in scale do not introduce changes in, for example, the glycosylation pattern of the molecule, as these can have a material impact on the pharmacology and hence safety of the molecule. The release specification for most biopharmaceuticals will include some form of bioassay to ensure that it not only has the same physical properties as previous batches, but also behaves in the same way.

Advanced and cellular therapies present a particular challenge for safety assessment. On the one hand, many of these are derived from the patient's own cells and therefore are not going to be toxic in the same way that an exogenous chemical might be. On the other hand, they raise challenging long-term questions that are difficult to answer: what is the fate of the genetically engineered cells in the body, how long do they last and what are the risks that genetic material is incorporated in a place where it may raise the risk of cancer in the future? There is no standardized approach yet for these therapies, and each has to be considered on its merits. The core principal is to take a question-based approach, and then design appropriate in vitro and in vivo systems to address these questions. In many cases, these programmes may include any traditional toxicology studies.

The future—new approaches in translational toxicology

In this final nonclinical section, we consider some of the current trends and developments in the field of translational toxicology.

In the field of small molecules, there is a particular focus on the use of in silico techniques to predict toxicity and off-target effects based on structural motifs. There is also increasing use of mathematical modelling, illustrated by emerging approaches to predict pro-arrhythmic potential. Detailed assessment in vitro of the potential of a molecule to alter function of specific ion channels is integrated in a mathematical model to predict risk of arrhythmia. In vivo techniques are becoming more sophisticated; monitoring techniques such as a cardiovascular telemetry and EEG are being used to combine safety pharmacology and toxicology assessments in a single animal, providing both a more comprehensive assessment and reduction in number of animals used.

For biologics there is a particular focus on improved techniques to capture the complex biodistribution of these molecules. There is also increased used of sophisticated measures of pharmacology including imaging to link exposure to response in target tissues. Bispecific molecules and combination therapy present a complex challenge—in many cases, the approach is to conduct a detailed combination toxicology study in nonhuman primates coupled with an assessment of the potential for cytokine release in human cell studies. Cytokine release is a feature of many immuno-oncology approaches (biological molecules and cell therapies), and there are ongoing attempts to better characterize this risk in order to guide dose selection. In addition to traditional cytokine concentration assays, there is increased use of flow cytometry to assess cell-surface markers of activation.

For cell-based therapies, especially stem cell therapies, there is a particular need to assess where in the body these cells distribute to, as this is likely to be a critical driver of both efficacy and safety. Because these cells persist, careful assessment of genetic stability over time is a key safety assessment.

At this time, the rapid advance of technology means that many of the novel approaches are considered on a case-by-case basis, but we can expect some regulatory conventions and expectations to emerge in the near future as experience develops.

References

Committee for Proprietary Medicinal Products. (1997). Points to consider for the assessment of the potential QT prolongation by non-cardiovascular medicinal products. *Publication CPMP 986/96.* Human Medicines Evaluation Unit, London.

Gad, S. C. (2002). *Drug safety evaluation.* New York: Wiley Interscience.

Haverkamp, W., Breitlandt, G., Comm A. J., Janse, M. J., Rosen, M. R., Antzelevitch C., et al. (2000). The potential for QT prolongation and proarrhythmias by non-anti-arrhythmic drugs: Clinical and regulatory implications. *European Heart Journal, 21,* 1232–1237.

Holland, M. C., Wurthner, J. U., Morley, P. J., Birchler, M. A., Lambert, J., Albayaty, M., et al. (2013). Autoantibodies to variable heavy (VH) chain Ig sequences in humans impact the safety and clinical pharmacology of a VH domain antibody antagonist of TNF-α receptor 1. *Journal of Clinical Immunology, 33*(7), 1192–1203.

Lynch, J. J., Van Vleet, T. R., Mittelstadt, S. W., & Blomme, E. A. J. (2017). Potential functional and pathological side effects related to off-target pharmacological activity. *Journal of Pharmacological and Toxicological Methods, 87,* 108–126.

Olson, H., Betton, G., Robinson, D., Thomas, K., Monro, A., Kolaja, G., et al. (2000). Concordance of the toxicity of pharmaceuticals in humans and animals. *Regulatory Toxicology and Pharmacology, 32,* 56–67.

Further reading

The international conference on harmonization (ICH) produces comprehensive guidance on safety topics. The following is a list of the current guidances. These undergo regular review, so it is important to check for the most current version when planning a programme. The guidances can be accessed at the ICH website https://www.ich.org/products/guidelines/safety/article/safety-guidelines.html

S1A–S1C Carcinogenicity Studies
S2 Genotoxicity Studies
S3A–S3B Toxicokinetics and Pharmacokinetics
S4 Toxicity Testing
S5 Reproductive Toxicology

S6 Biotechnological Products
S7A–S7B Pharmacology Studies
S8 Immunotoxicology Studies
S9 Nonclinical Evaluation for Anticancer Pharmaceuticals
S10 Photosafety Evaluation
S11 Nonclinical Paediatric Safety

Chapter | **13** |

Therapeutic vaccines

Federica Cappuccini, Jakub Kopycinski, Rachel Tanner

Introduction

Therapeutic vaccines aim to modulate host immune responses after an infection, cancer or other chronic disease is established. This is in contrast to prophylactic vaccines, which act to prevent the initial establishment of infection or disease. Therapeutic vaccines differ from drug therapies in that they focus on reinforcing, broadening, redirecting or curbing the host immune response rather than targeting the cause or result of the condition itself, and therefore fall under the umbrella of 'immunotherapy'. Other, passive, immunotherapy approaches including the direct administration of monoclonal, bi- or tri-specific antibodies; genetic engineering of lymphocyte populations (as in the case of chimeric antigen receptor T and natural killer (NK) cells); or the use of cytokines are beyond the scope of this chapter.

Therapeutic vaccines may be particularly desirable in situations where (1) drugs are not available or efficacious, (2) drugs are available but have adverse side effects or long-term toxicity or (3) drugs are selected for resistance due to inability to clear the pathogen or tumour. They are often designed for use following, or in conjunction with, drug therapies. A prerequisite for the biological feasibility of a therapeutic vaccine is that the immune system has the potential to control the condition, which may be indicated by some degree of natural or prophylactic vaccine–induced immune control in at least a proportion of patients.

There are several challenges to therapeutic vaccine development, including understanding relevant immune correlates, identifying target antigens and potentially contending with an immune system that has reached exhaustion or been subjected to tolerance or polarization mechanisms that help to sustain the disease. Furthermore, in cases where chronic conditions induce immunopathology, boosting specific immunity may be ineffective or even detrimental. Immune correlates associated with success of a therapeutic vaccine generally differ from prophylactic correlates of protection that operate at the time of pathogen entry. For example, humoral immunity is critical in preventing infection with human papillomavirus (HPV), but cell-mediated responses are thought to be more important in regression of resulting precancerous lesions and clearance of infection. Consequently, antigens targeted by prophylactic and therapeutic vaccines also differ, particularly for pathogens that express different proteins at different stages of their lifecycle and/or of disease. An additional challenge is the phenomenon of immune evasion: both pathogens and tumours under selective immune pressure may evolve and adapt to escape, necessitating induction of a broad response.

Vectors, adjuvants and delivery systems

The choice of vector and/or adjuvant (enhances immune response to vaccine) can influence the magnitude and nature of the immune response induced, favouring, for example, humoral over cellular responses or a T-helper cell type 1 (Th1) over Th2 response. Selecting the appropriate formulation and delivery system is therefore a key factor in determining the success of any vaccine (Fig. 13.1).

Whole cell vaccines

Whole cell vaccines consist of either an attenuated (weakened) version of the pathogen of interest/related pathogen in the case of infectious disease, or of whole tumour cells in the case of cancer. They arguably induce immune responses against the widest range of antigens

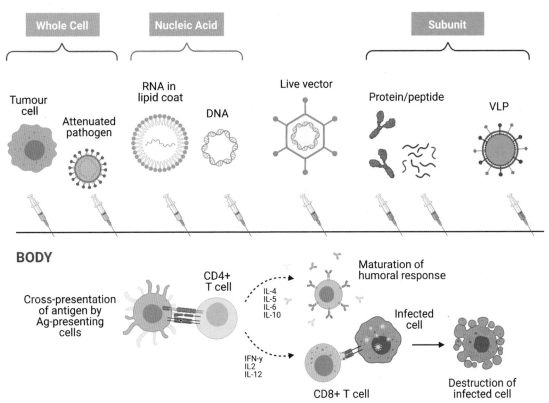

Fig. 13.1 Therapeutic vaccine formulations and delivery systems. The choice of vaccine formulation and delivery system can influence the magnitude and nature of the immune response induced. Whole cell vaccines consist of either an attenuated version of the pathogen of interest/related pathogen in the case of infectious disease, or of whole tumour cells in the case of cancer. Nucleic acid–based vaccines introduce genetic material and exploit the host's cellular machinery to produce the antigen encoded. Certain live attenuated viruses or bacteria have the capacity to be engineered to carry and deliver recombinant heterologous antigens in order to elicit immunity against the pathogen or tumour from which such antigen was derived. Subunit vaccines deliver a single immunogenic antigen, or a combination of antigens, from the pathogen of interest or tumour. In the case of protein or peptide vaccines, purified recombinant antigens or synthetic peptides (8–15 amino acids in length) corresponding to defined epitopes are used to stimulate specific immune responses. VLPs may be applied as carrier molecules or delivery systems for antigenic proteins. *VLPs*, Virus-like particles.

and eliminate the need to identify the most optimal targets. However, the responses elicited are not necessarily the most effective, as illustrated by the underwhelming efficacy of the prophylactic bacillus Calmette-Guérin (BCG) vaccine against pulmonary tuberculosis (TB). Furthermore, certain pathogens are considered too high risk even in their attenuated forms, particularly when vaccinating infants or the immune-compromised/-impaired. The potential for incomplete inactivation or reversion to a more virulent strain also raises concerns. Cancer whole cell vaccines may be either autologous, in which case they will express the same antigens as the tumour, or allogeneic, whereby several cell lines derived from different tumours are combined. Both have potential drawbacks: autologous whole cell cancer vaccines are not always

feasible and are costly and time-consuming to produce, while vaccines made from allogeneic cells raise issues around human leukocyte antigen (HLA) mismatch.

Subunit vaccines

An alternative to whole cell vaccines is to deliver a single immunogenic antigen, or a combination of antigens, from the pathogen of interest or tumour. So-called subunit vaccines do not contain live components of the pathogen/tumour cell; only the parts necessary to elicit a protective immune response. Subunit vaccines offer advantages over whole cell vaccines in terms of safety, ease of manufacture and precise immune targeting. However, effective antigen selection requires detailed understanding of specific responses and the pathways in which they operate. Furthermore, antigens alone are often poorly immunogenic, necessitating the use of additional components, known as adjuvants, to help stimulate protective immunity.

The concept of adjuvants first arose following observations that an abscess at the inoculation site, even one generated by unrelated substances, resulted in higher specific antibody titres. Early adjuvants including aluminium salts (alum) and oil-in-water emulsions are generalized in their mode of action, but as knowledge of immune pathways has increased, compounds better tailored to trigger or prolong certain responses have been developed. Adjuvants may be used to bias or switch the immune system towards Th1 or Th2 immunity, and this 'directing' of the immune response may ultimately determine vaccine efficacy and safety. The benefits of adjuvants must be balanced against the risk of adverse side effects, including local reactions of inflammation, swelling and pain, as well as systemic reactions such as fever, nausea, anaphylaxis and immunotoxicity.

Peptide-/protein-based vaccines

In the case of protein or peptide vaccines, purified recombinant antigens or synthetic peptides (8–15 amino acids in length) corresponding to defined epitopes are used to stimulate specific immune responses. Indeed, once the antigens of interest have been identified, the recognition and targeting of the most antigenic peptides might be a useful approach when designing a therapeutic vaccine, as any potentially competing nonimmunogenic peptides can be excluded. These vaccines are safe and easy to manufacture, although they generally require the use of potent adjuvants or conjugation to Toll-like receptor (TLR) agonists to overcome their generally poor immunogenicity.

While protein-based vaccines include numerous T-cell epitopes and are therefore not restricted by patient HLA type, short peptides require HLA-binding prediction for each individual patient. Furthermore, short peptides do not stimulate CD4+ T-helper cells, which are necessary for a potent cytotoxic response. Finally, the protein/peptide might not be processed or presented by professional antigen-presenting cells (APCs) and induced responses lacking the proper co-stimulatory signals might lead to suboptimal generation of antipathogen or antitumour responses, or even tolerogenic responses and T-cell dysfunction.

Methods to improve the efficacy of peptide vaccines include the use of multivalent synthetic long peptides (SLPs) (28–35 amino acids) containing both major histocompatibility complex (MHC) class I and II epitopes to elicit a balanced induction of antigen-specific CD4+ and CD8+ T-cell responses. SLPs are also preferentially taken up by dendritic cells (DCs), guaranteeing the optimal stimulatory signals for an efficient antipathogen or antitumour response. However, it should be noted that repeated immunizations with SLPs may lead to preferential expansion of T cells recognising a single immunodominant epitope. Antigens and peptides can also be altered to increase binding to the MHC molecule or to the T-cell receptor (TCR), thus increasing their immunogenicity. Other approaches include the encapsulation of peptides in structures such as liposomes or nanoparticles, which might enhance T-cell priming by professional APCs.

Virus-like particles

Virus-like particles (VLPs) self-assemble to mimic the overall structure of a native virus but generally lack the viral genome. They are highly immunogenic, often to a similar extent as the virus from which they derive, due to the presence of key features such as repetitive surfaces, particulate structures and pathogen-associated molecular patterns (PAMPs). VLPs have several advantages over native viruses, including an enhanced safety profile due to their nonreplicative and noninfectious nature, with no risk of reversion or recombination. There is also no requirement for attenuation or inactivation, which limits the risk of epitope modification.

In addition to their utility as direct immunogens, VLPs may also be applied as carrier molecules or delivery systems for other, unrelated antigenic proteins. Such proteins are displayed on the surface of the VLP, resulting in ready uptake by APCs and stimulation of both cellular and humoral immunity. While more efficacious than standard protein/peptide subunit vaccines, VLP-based vaccines are generally still formulated with adjuvants such as alum to optimize activity, enhance potency and, in some cases, increase stability.

Nucleic acid–based vaccines

Rather than introducing antigenic proteins, an alternative vaccine approach is to introduce genetic material and exploit the host's cellular machinery to produce the antigen encoded. DNA vector vaccines consist of a recombinant DNA plasmid encoding the antigen/s of interest under control of an appropriate promoter. Following their uptake into host cells, the plasmids express their recombinant antigens, which are then processed endogenously. Once expressed, the encoded protein will be presented on MHC class I and II molecules for CD8+ and CD4+ T-cell recognition and activation. Innate immune responses are also stimulated, as bacterial unmethylated CpG (5'-C-phosphate-G-3') motifs of the plasmid will be recognized as a danger signal by cytosolic sensors.

DNA vaccines offer a range of advantages over other vectors, including their ability to persistently express antigens that more closely resemble native epitopes, which can elicit both cellular and humoral responses, their potential for rapid and large-scale low-cost production, thermostability and an excellent safety profile. However, cellular uptake of naked DNA in vivo has been found to be somewhat inefficient, and much of the injected DNA remains extracellular. DNA vaccines have been poorly immunogenic in clinical trials and are thus often modified to include genes encoding immunostimulatory molecules or elements that enhance antigen presentation. In addition, codon optimization has been used to increase the antigenicity and immune-cell stimulation of these vaccines. Safety concerns were previously raised regarding the potential for DNA integration into host cellular DNA that could result in insertional mutagenesis and lead to inactivation of tumour suppressor genes or activation of oncogenes. However, there has been little evidence that this occurs in practice.

RNA vaccines make use of messenger RNA (mRNA) transcripts encoding antigens of interest, which are more rapidly translated and processed by the host cell machinery and presented to immune cells compared with DNA vaccines. RNA vaccines can also activate the innate immune system by acting as agonists for the Toll-like receptors TLR7 and TLR8. Unlike DNA vaccines, RNA vaccines do not require nuclear translocation, which increases the probability of successful transfection and circumvents the risk of insertional mutagenesis or genomic alteration. However, RNA vaccines are generally susceptible to degradation because of the ubiquitous presence of ribonucleases (RNases). To overcome this issue, RNA can be encapsulated in nanoparticles or chemically modified, or modified nucleotides can be incorporated into the vaccine. In their simplest form, RNA vaccines consist of a nonreplicating strand of mRNA, but self-replicating RNA vaccines have also been introduced, with the advantage of a longer persistence and a lower required dose.

Live vectors

As cellular uptake of naked nucleic acids is very low, recent research has focussed on methods to improve transfection efficiency. Certain live attenuated viruses or bacteria have the capacity to be engineered to carry and deliver recombinant heterologous antigens in order to elicit immunity against the pathogen or tumour from which such antigen was derived; such vectors are useful in their natural ability to invade host cells and replicate. Furthermore, these vectors may exert adjuvant-like effects by stimulating facets of the innate immune system via PAMPs and other 'danger signals' normally expressed by the native pathogen. Live vectors are thought to be more suitable in circumstances where a cellular rather than humoral response is desirable, as they enable expression of intracellular antigens by MHC molecules on APCs leading to the induction of robust T-cell responses.

However, similar to some whole cell vaccines, live replicating vectors may pose potential safety risks to both the young and the immunocompromised. Certain vectors are capable of integrating their genomes into that of the host, potentially risking cell transformation or other unforeseen pleiotropic effects. Another important issue is the possibility of preexisting immune responses against the vector that can limit the generation of an effective response against the antigen of interest through clearance of the vector. One of the principal reasons for avoiding homologous prime/boost vaccine strategies (where the same vector is used to both prime and boost immune responses) is that the responses induced de novo against the vector following primary vaccination may be amplified with subsequent homologous vaccine boosts and render the boost less effective than a heterologous vector. Such issues are now being overcome by the use of strains that do not circulate in humans and/or different strains for prime and boost immunizations.

Viral vectors. Viral-vectored vaccines consist of viruses in which nonessential genes have been replaced with those encoding the antigen/s of interest from the pathogen or tumour. To ensure safety, viral vectors must be nonpathogenic or genetically engineered to make them attenuated and/or replication-deficient. Viruses are particularly useful in their ability to transduce their genetic information into host cells, resulting in high efficiency expression of the encoded antigen/s. They have several advantages over nucleic acid vaccines, including high efficiency of transduction, highly specific delivery of genes to target cells and induction of robust immune responses with increased cellular immunity, as well as stimulation of innate immunity, without the need for an adjuvant.

Commonly used viral vectors derive from poxviruses such as modified vaccinia ankara (MVA), adenoviruses such as chimpanzee adenovirus (ChAd) and alphaviruses such as Venezuelan equine encephalitis (VEE) virus. These vectors have been shown in their attenuated or replication-defective versions to be well tolerated and immunogenic in numerous clinical trials. For optimal immune stimulation, repeated vaccinations are often required; in such cases, a heterologous prime-boost regimen is recommended to avoid viral neutralization; this is achieved by targeting the same antigen through the engineering of different viral vectors. Preexisting antivector immunity may be circumvented by vaccinating patients with nonhuman-specific viruses. For example, ChAd has been frequently used as priming agent in clinical trials, inducing immune responses of high quality and magnitude against the engineered antigens and a good safety profile. Poxviruses such as MVA have mainly been used as potent boosting agents, as they are less prone to neutralization.

Bacterial and yeast vectors. Live bacteria and yeasts are also attractive therapeutic vaccine vehicles currently under assessment in clinical settings. Attenuated strains of these microorganisms can be easily engineered to deliver DNA or proteins, have a large capacity for foreign DNA and can be produced at very low costs. They are stable, safe and well tolerated, while remaining potent immune stimulators with the capacity to induce mucosal, as well as humoral and/or cell-mediated systemic immunity. Like viral vectors, their immunostimulatory properties circumvent the need for adjuvants. Furthermore, multiple administrations do not elicit neutralization by the host immune system. However, potential concerns include the risk of environmental contamination, lateral gene transfer conferring resistance to antibiotics and reversion to a more virulent form.

Recombinant yeast-based vaccines commonly used in clinical settings derive from the nonpathogenic heat-killed *Saccharomyces cerevisiae* and offer the advantage of a eukaryotic expression system, essential for posttranslational modifications and the secretion of human antigens. Commonly employed bacteria strains include *Salmonella*, *Listeria* and *Lactococcus*. Target antigens can be encoded in the chromosomal genetic material or in plasmids, with the former offering advantages in terms of stability of expression, lack of antibiotic selection and simultaneous expression of multiple antigens. Plasmids, on the other hand, may be present in multiple copies within a single vector and thus express high levels of the target antigen. To maximise antigen expression, potent promoters or inducible systems are used for chromosomal inserted genes, while balanced lethal systems have been introduced to overcome the instability of plasmids. In this approach, the antigen-encoding plasmids also express critical proteins essential for bacterial survival; the loss of the plasmid will therefore result in cell death.

Bacterial spores such as *Bacillus subtilis* have also been explored as potential vaccine vectors. *B. subtilis* is found as a gut commensal in humans, and its spores are known to be both safe and adjuvantic. They also readily bind protein antigens, have a low production cost and demonstrate resistance to adverse conditions for long periods. However, some studies have reported low antigen expression, which may lead to poor immunogenicity, and a short residency time in the gastrointestinal tract following oral administration.

Therapeutic vaccines for infectious diseases

Despite considerable advances in global health, infectious diseases remain a leading cause of human morbidity and mortality. While many prophylactic vaccines have been extremely effective at reducing rates of initial infection or acute disease, they are not designed to deal with established infections. Therapeutic vaccines aim to reinforce host immunity after infection with a pathogen has occurred, which can act to prevent complications of a chronic infection. Such complications include severe immunodeficiency caused by human immunodeficiency virus (HIV), cancer induced by HPV and chronic hepatitis, cirrhosis and hepatocarcinoma caused by hepatitis B virus (HBV). However, often immunopathological events aggravate these disease states, in which case, it may in fact be counterproductive to boost specific immunity.

Therapeutic HIV vaccines

Acquired Immunodeficiency Syndrome (AIDS) caused by HIV continues to be a major global health crisis, with 1.7 million new infections and 770,000 deaths annually attributable to HIV-related causes. Despite the introduction of antiretroviral therapy (ART), which has led to substantial reductions in both morbidity and mortality, HIV has not been eradicated largely due to its ability to establish latency reservoirs inaccessible to antiretroviral drugs. Discontinuation of ART results in viral rebound in the majority of patients, necessitating life-long treatment with significant associated toxicity.

Unlike for HPV and HBV, no successful preventative vaccine has yet been developed for HIV-1, despite the completion of numerous phase III efficacy trials. Of note, VAX003 and 004 trials used alum-adjuvanted AIDSVAX clade BE or BB monomeric envelope glycoproteins gp120, respectively, and despite their ability to induce nonneutralizing antibodies, neither vaccine demonstrated efficacy. STEP HIV Vaccine Trials Network 502 (HVTN 502) and Phambili (HVTN503) trials subsequently used recombinant adenovirus 5 vectors expressing HIV proteins. Although vaccine-specific T-cell responses were successfully induced, the STEP trial was terminated due to the risk of infection being almost doubled in the vaccine group compared with the placebo group, with no difference in the mean viral load set-point (Sekaly et al., 2008).

The RV144 trial gave the first indication that a preventative vaccine strategy could yield promising results. Here, a heterologous ALVAC pox vector, encoding clade B Group Antigens (gag)/protease and clade AE envelope protein (env), prime with an AIDSVAX gp120 protein boost yielded a 31% reduction in the risk of infection. The main correlate associated with its protective effects was unexpected: nonneutralizing immunoglobulin (Ig)G responses to V1 and V2 epitopes on gp120, capable of mediating antibody-dependent cell cytotoxicity (ADCC). This effect was mitigated by the finding that the induction of env-specific IgA responses offset this protective effect. Further investigation using the COMPASS analysis tool identified a further protective effect in polyfunctional env-specific CD4+ T cells; this had previously been missed by other conventional analysis strategies.

Similar to other viral infections, most preventative HIV vaccines have focussed on the induction of humoral responses that neutralize HIV through preventing virus attachment and subsequent infection of CD4+ T cells. Therapeutic vaccine candidates, however, have largely aimed to induce CD8+ T-cell responses, which may eliminate infected cells through priming or boosting the recognition of cognate epitopes derived from virus sequences in the context of class I HLA molecules. CD8+ T-cell responses have been shown to be critical in controlling HIV replication during acute infection (McMichael & Rowland-Jones, 2001). Nonhuman primate models have demonstrated that depletion of CD8+ T-cell populations with monoclonal antibodies (mAbs) results in rebound of simian immunodeficiency virus (SIV) plasma viraemia, and this is only controlled on their reemergence. Similarly, CD8+ T-cell depletion abrogates control of SIV replication despite continuation of ART in monkeys.

In humans, the emergence of HIV-specific CD8+ T cells following acute infection coincides with a reduction of viral load and establishment of virus set-point, which subsequently defines the time to progression. The specificity of such populations, as dictated by the class I HLA background of an individual, has a strong bearing on HIV replication. Protective class I alleles such as HLA B*27 and B*57 are highly enriched in individuals who control virus replication and maintain normal CD4+ T-cell counts in the absence of ART. The loss of control in these individuals often coincides with escape mutations in epitopes being presented by these alleles, allowing variants to escape recognition by CD8+ T-cell. Moreover, CD8+ T-cell responses found to target highly conserved regions of the HIV Gag protein have also been associated with superior viral control—a phenomenon that is largely independent of the individual's HLA background.

Multiple hurdles must be overcome by a successful therapeutic HIV vaccine. First, the vaccine must be safe and not burden an already weakened immune system. Second, it must be capable of eliciting effective immune responses in the context of the immunocompromised environment caused by HIV infection, as initial infection results in massive depletions in CD4+ T-cell populations and broad dysfunction/exhaustion of both innate and adaptive immune populations. Expression of the co-inhibitory receptors cytotoxic T lymphocyte-associated protein-4 (CTLA4), Programmed cell death protein-1 (PD-1), T-cell immunoglobulin and mucin-domain containing-3 (TIM3), T-cell immunoreceptor with Ig and ITIM domains (TIGIT) and Lymphocyte-activation gene-3 (LAG-3) by both CD4+ and CD8+ T cells, which occurs as a result of chronic stimulation by replicating virus, is a characteristic of HIV infection and could hinder the subsequent generation of a functional vaccine-specific response. Indeed, addition of antibodies blocking these co-inhibitory receptors enhances HIV-specific

T-cell proliferation and function; macaque models have demonstrated that anti-PD-1 therapy resulted in improved frequencies of SIV-specific CD8+ T cells, decreased viral loads and improved survival rates (Day et al., 2006).

Furthermore, the extent of sequence variation in the HIV-1 genome may render the majority of infected cells undetectable to T-cell responses already focussed on wild-type or consensus epitopes. The use of ART therapies, which make HIV-1 viral loads undetectable, along with established HIV reservoirs, where the viral genome has integrated into that of the host in a transcriptionally silent manner, both prevent immune responses from recognizing viral antigens. It is unclear how a therapeutic vaccine could successfully clear HIV in the absence of antigen expression. The measurement of efficacy also needs to be addressed in these contexts; it may be necessary to delay restart of ART until after rebound and allow a threshold level of viral replication to be reached that would enable vaccine-induced responses to be effective.

To address safety and immunogenicity issues, several therapeutic vaccine trials have used protein/peptide or DNA vaccines, which exhibit improved safety profiles over recombinant vaccine vectors. The Vacc-4X trial compared the responses of HIV-seropositive individuals vaccinated with conserved domains of the HIV capsid protein p24 to a placebo group. Despite one major adverse event, proliferative responses to the vaccine antigens were induced that coincided with a modest decrease in viral load in vaccinated individuals following combination ART (cART) interruption. In the AIDS Clinical Trials Group (ACTG) A5187 trial, Rosenberg et al. vaccinated 20 ART-experienced HIV-infected subjects with an HIV-1 DNA vaccine encoding a clade B Gag-Pol (reverse transcriptase)-Nef (negative factor) fusion protein and clades A, B and C Env. The vaccine was found to be safe and well tolerated with no serious grade 3 or 4 events; however, it did not induce or boost T-cell responses above baseline and, following discontinuation of therapy, made no difference in time to rebound, viral loads or CD4+ T-cell counts between the treatment and placebo arms.

In a randomized, double-blind trial using recombinant adenovirus 5 expressing gag, Schooley et al. reported that, despite the induction of significant gag-specific CD4+ and CD8+ T-cell responses, there was no impact on viral rebound following treatment interruption. Furthermore, a randomized, placebo-controlled trial vaccinating chronically infected individuals on ART with ALVAC-HIV vCP1452 incorporating Gag and gp120 proteins, along with a segment of Pol and known Nef and Pol cytotoxic T-lymphocyte (CTL) epitopes, found that despite the induction of T-cell responses, vaccination was associated with reduced control of viral replication on treatment interruption and a shorter time to virus rebound. This result could partially be explained by the presence of individuals with controlling HLA alleles B*27 and B*57 in the placebo group, who were absent from the vaccine arm, and conversely, individuals possessing the HLA B*35 allele that exhibited quicker viral rebound were present in the vaccine arm but not the placebo.

Though disappointing, the failure of the STEP trial did highlight that a T-cell-focussed vaccine strategy could induce a 'sieve effect', whereby the 'founder' viruses that established infection carried mutations in epitopes targeted by responses induced following vaccination. That these mutations occurred in regions deemed less critical for virus replication, alongside the existence of defective proviruses, capable of diverting T-cell responses through acting as 'decoys', suggests that future vaccines should focus on targeting only highly conserved regions of the HIV proteome. Consequently, several therapeutic HIV vaccine candidates have sought to induce CD8+ T-cell responses to such regions, aiming to 'educate' the host immune response to better control the virus.

Two such trials have used chimpanzee adenovirus 63 (ChAd63) vector prime, MVA boost regimens expressing an insert containing the 14 most conserved elements of the HIV proteome (HIVconsv). Both found the vaccines to be safe, tolerable and capable of refocussing CD4+ and CD8+ T-cell responses towards conserved elements of the HIV-1 proteome. However, neither trial showed any reduction in viral load or total viral DNA. More recently, vaccine candidates have used polyvalent mosaic inserts. These aim to induce broader immune responses enabling the recognition of multiple versions of HIV epitopes, allowing them to deal with viral escape variants through increasing response breadth and depth.

To address the issue of virus latency several so-called 'Shock or kick and kill' trials have been attempted. Here, HIV-1 infected individuals receiving ART are vaccinated and then treated with latency reversal agents (LRAs), which induce viral reactivation from previously latently infected cells. These cells subsequently express virus antigens, which are recognised and eliminated either by pre-existing or vaccine-induced CTL. The effectiveness of these strategies is assessed through measuring the size of the reservoir or through measuring the time to rebound following treatment interruption.

Two notable examples of this are the REDUC and BCN02 trials. The REDUC single-arm, phase Ib/IIa trial involved administration of Vacc-x4: a gag p24-based vaccine with granulocyte-macrophage colony-stimulating factor (GM-CSF), followed by the LRA histone DeACetylase inhibitor (HDACi) romidepsin, to 17 individuals. Vaccine-induced proliferative CD8+ T-cell responses were associated with decreased levels of total DNA but not integrated DNA compared with baseline. In BCN02, an extension of the BCN01 trial, 15 ART-experienced HIV+ individuals were given a HIVconsv ChAd63 prime MVA, boost regimen followed by romidepsin. Thirteen of these individuals developed HIVconsv-specific CD8+ T-cell responses, although 8/13 rebounded after 4 weeks; the remaining five maintained viral control for >27 weeks following treatment interruption. Furthermore, all of these individuals were found to have lower levels of total virus DNA. The principal caveat to both trials is that neither included a control arm; as such, it is unclear whether delays in virus rebound may be mediated by the vaccine or are examples of spontaneous viral control that can occur as a result of early ART intervention.

To address this, the phase II randomized placebo-controlled RIVER trial (National Clinical Trial number NCT02336074) enrolled individuals who were given ART during acute infection and stratified them into two groups. The first were maintained on ARTs (including raltegravir); the second also stayed on ARTs but were also given the HIVconsv ChAd63 prime, MVA boost vaccine regimen followed by 10 doses of the LRA vorinostat. Although polyfunctional CD4+ and CD8+ T responses were both elevated in the treatment arm and the CD8+ T-cell responses maintained their capacity to inhibit virus replication following randomization compared with the placebo group, there was no significant difference in total virus DNA between the two groups. A large mitigating factor was that vorinostat only had a small and transient effect on viral gene expression, potentially limiting the reservoir that could be eliminated by virus-specific T cells. Another potential drawback to using HDACi (such as romidepsin and vorinostat) as LRAs is that they only act on lymphocytes, not on myeloid subsets, which might serve as another potential reservoir.

Therapeutic vaccines against chronic hepatitis B

HBV causes both acute and chronic infections of the liver. While the acute stage resolves within 6 months, chronic hepatitis B (CHB), characterized by detection of virus proteins for >6 months, may result in cirrhosis and cancer. Despite the existence of a safe and effective prophylactic HPV vaccine, an estimated 240 million people are believed to be chronically infected with HBV; of those that remain untreated, 15%–40% develop cirrhosis (Tang et al., 2018). For individuals with CHB, treatment by pegelated (peg)-interferon (IFN) and nucleoside/nucleotide analogues can suppress viral replication to undetectable levels; but similar to HIV ART, they cannot achieve functional cure.

While individuals with acute, self-limiting HBV infection exhibit potent CD4+ and CD8+ T-cell responses, these are largely absent in CHB. Cellular immune responses have long been associated with clearance of HBV during acute infection, as demonstrated by woodchuck models, and the role played by CD8+ T cells in particular is well established with the detection of intrahepatic HBV-specific CD8+ T-cell populations corresponding to a reduction of HBV DNA. Furthermore, depletion of CD8+ T-cell populations in primate models delays clearance and reduces levels of alanine aminotransferase (ALT), a proxy measurement of liver inflammation or damage. Elimination of HBV-infected cells occurs through lytic and nonlytic means with IFN-γ and tumour necrosis factor (TNF)-α, both playing a critical role. However, the contribution of CD4+ T cells is less clear, with CD4+ T-cell depletions in primate models having no effect on virus clearance or peak virus titre.

CHB largely results from the development of immune tolerance. While this process is critical in reducing immunopathology and maintaining liver function, it also prevents viral clearance. Immune tolerance may result from deletion of antigen-specific T cells, lack of expansion or 'arming' of effector T cells (deletional tolerance), functional adaptation or, similar to HIV, the exhaustion of the immune response that arises from massive persistent antigenic exposure. Therapeutic HBV vaccines aim to overcome immune tolerance and achieve at least a functional (if incomplete) cure. The fact that this can occur naturally, with a small proportion (<1%) of chronically infected patients each year demonstrating anti-HBs seroconversion, lends support to the potential of a therapeutic vaccine.

However, there are two major hurdles that any therapeutic vaccine against HBV must overcome. First, the vast majority of the ~10^{12} hepatocytes in the human liver can be infected and therefore induction of strong cytolytic T-cell responses against infected cells may risk immunopathology; the measurement of ALT levels is thus critical postvaccination. Second, although chronic HBV infection can be characterized by the presence of HBsAg, HBeAg and HBV DNA for more than 6 months, individuals who have been cured functionally, as defined by undetectable HBV DNA and HBsAg in the peripheral blood, still harbour a reservoir of both hepatic and extrahepatic cells where transcriptionally silent HBV genomes exist in a covalently closed circular (ccc) form. HBV can reactivate from this form should infected individuals be exposed to immunosuppressive therapies.

Attempts to apply existing prophylactic vaccines in a therapeutic setting have been largely unsuccessful in resolving CHB and few novel therapeutic HBV vaccine candidates have entered the clinical trials pipeline. Candidates based on subviral particles with alum-based adjuvants showed initial promise but were unable to reduce HBV DNA. Viral vector vaccines, which stimulate a broad range of immune responses, have been more successful—particularly in heterologous prime-boost regimens. One such example is the CpG-adjuvanted hepatitis B surface antigen (HBsAg) protein prime/MVA boost regimen, which was found to induce high frequencies of HBV-specific CD4+ and CD8+ T cells in a mouse model.

HBV transgenic (HBVtg) mice that differed in levels of serum HBeAg prior to vaccination were all found capable of developing vaccine-induced CD8+ and CD4+ T-cell responses, suggesting that high levels of HBV antigen, such as those present during chronic infection, would not preclude the induction of responses by the vaccine. However, vaccine-induced CD8+ T-cell populations in medium or high antigenaemia mice tended to express a reduced functional profile, similar to those found in exhausted CD8+ T-cell populations during chronic infections.

Pancholi et al. demonstrated that a DNA HBsAg prime followed by CanaryPox HBsAg, PreS1+2 boost was sufficient to induce robust T-cell responses in chimpanzees, which coincided with a reduction in levels of HBV DNA in the blood at 1 week postboost that was maintained for > 200 weeks postvaccination. However, HBV ccc genome could still be detected by QC-PCR (quantitative competitive polymerase chain reaction), suggesting that infection was not fully cleared. Interestingly, this control was associated with IFN-γ production and not cytolytic activity. A similar DNA prime/poxvirus boost regimen was attempted in humans by Cavenaugh et al.; unfortunately, no reductions in HBV DNA levels occurred, although this must be caveated with the fact that this was an unblinded study where the schedule using an MVA boost lacked PreS1 and S2 antigens. Mancini-Bourgine et al. trialled an intramuscular DNA vaccine encoding HBV envelop proteins in 10 CHB individuals; low-frequency T-cell responses in all vaccinees, with 2/10 also showing increased transaminase activity, which was associated with a fall in HBV DNA and may have been related to vaccine-induced T-cell responses.

The multicentre phase II GS-4774 trial employed a heat-inactivated, yeast-derived vaccine encoding a fusion protein of HBV surface, core and X antigens (HBsAg, HBcAg and HBXAg, respectively). Immunization-induced T-cell responses are measurable by IFN-γ ELISpot in 30/60 (50%) of individuals across three dose groups, with 90% of vaccines displaying antigen-specific lymphoproliferative responses. A controlled, randomized phase II trial using CHB-infected individuals who were not on antiviral therapy found that GS-4774 predominantly induced polyfunctional CD8+ T-cell responses to the core antigen, either in the presence or absence of the antiviral drug tenofovir. Although vaccination did not result in significant decreases in mean HBsAg levels at weeks 12, 24 or 48, only individuals who had been vaccinated with the highest dose of GS-4774 were found to have reductions in HBsAg levels of >0.5_{log} IU/mL. The failure of the vaccine to induce significant CD4+ T-cell responses was highlighted as a potential explanation for the relative lack of reduction of HBsAg levels, given their ability to help the development of nascent humoral and CD8+ T-cell responses.

Therapeutic EBV vaccines

Epstein–Barr virus (EBV) is a near-ubiquitous gamma-herpes virus that, in the majority of cases, is transmitted orally during childhood, resulting in an asymptomatic infection and life-long persistence. However, when infection is delayed, in a proportion of adolescents and young adults, EBV infection causes infectious mononucleosis (IM). IM is thought to arise from massive cellular responses targeting EBV-infected cells and its incidence increases the risk of several lymphoproliferative and nonlymphoid malignancies in later life; indeed, the relative risk of Hodgkin's lymphoma and multiple sclerosis (MS) in EBV seropositive individuals increases by 4 and 2.2, respectively. Following lytic infection of the oropharynx, EBV establishes latency in naive B cells. Here, the virus is restricted to expressing specific latency genes that enable it to achieve persistence. The capacity of EBV to propagate through the transformation of cells results from its expression of transactivating proteins such as Epstein–Barr nuclear antigens (EBNAs) and latent membrane proteins (LMPs), which simultaneously provide signals for cell survival and proliferation. The differential expression of latency proteins coincides with different stages of EBV latency, and these are, in turn, associated with specific malignancies.

To date, there is no effective prophylactic vaccine against EBV. Development of vaccine candidates has historically focussed on blocking entry of EBV into B cells through induction of antibodies to the envelope protein gp350, which is required for attachment and entry, primarily via the CD21 receptor. A phase II double-blinded placebo-control trial showed that although it reduced the incidence of IM in the intention-to-treat group, an alum-adjuvanted subunit gp350 vaccine was unable to prevent infection despite induction of neutralizing antibody responses. Other preventative strategies have included targeting EBNA3A epitopes, VLPs and antigen–antibody complexes that target T-cell epitopes towards B cells through conjugation with CD19/CD20/CD21-specific antibodies.

Because EBV has the ability to persist in different stages of latency, where the expression of latency stage–specific antigens depends on the state of the cell, the virus poses a unique challenge for any therapeutic vaccine. The main strategy that has been pursued is the incorporation of antigens that are expressed in several different phases of latency and are known to be targeted by T-cell responses. EBNA1 and LMP2 are particularly attractive candidates and have been the focus of several vaccine trials, both being known targets for T-cell responses and expressed during latency stages I–III and II–III, respectively. Therapeutic vaccines incorporating such antigens could potentially enable the elimination of multiple cancers. One potential caveat to this is the persistence of EBV in quiescent B cells; here, virus gene expression is entirely absent (latency 0), rendering it entirely hidden from immune responses. In these circumstances it is unclear whether sterilizing immunity is even possible without reactivation of the virus.

MVA-EL, a poxvirus vector encoding an EBNA1/LMP2 fusion protein, was assessed in a phase I dose-escalation trial in nasopharyngeal carcinoma (NPC) patients. Only the C-terminal half of the EBNA1 gene was included; this contained most of the known EBNA1 T-cell epitopes, while also lacking the N-terminal half previously found to contain the glycine-alanine repeat domain known to interfere with antigen presentation. CD4+ and CD8+ T-cell responses to both antigens were increased in 15/18 individuals, with the individuals in the two highest doses showing the strongest responses. Because NPC is more common in South East Asia and the protein sequences were derived from EBV strains of Chinese origins that contained variations in T-cell epitopes, the trial was repeated using a UK cohort and sequences derived from UK strains. Data from this second trial confirmed the findings of the first, showing the vaccine to be safe with boosting of vaccine-induced polyfunctional CD4+ and CD8+ T-cell responses. A phase II trial is currently ongoing.

In a separate trial, 16 individuals with residual NPC were given four doses of autologous DCs loaded with HLA-A1101-, -A2402-, or B40011-restricted CD8+ T-cell epitopes derived from the LMP2. LMP2-specific CD8+ T-cell responses were induced in 9/16 (56%) of individuals, with two of these nine patients showing tumour regression; these responses were detectable and able to mediate cytolysis for 3 months postvaccination.

Therapeutic HPV vaccines

HPVs asymptomatically infect epithelial cells, with most infections being spontaneously resolved. To date, over 200 types of HPVs have been characterized. A subgroup of types termed high risk (HR)-HPV account for the vast majority of cervical, anogenital and oropharyngeal cancers; within the high-risk types, HPV16 and 18 are the most prevalent. While the prophylactic vaccines Gardasil and Cervarix have been highly effective in preventing infection through induction of neutralizing antibodies against the L1 capsid protein, they have been found to be of little therapeutic benefit to infected individuals (Hildesheim et al., 2007).

HPV infects cells of the basal epithelium or mucosa following abrasions caused by trauma. Once inside the cell, the viral genome migrates to the nucleus and forms extrachromosomal episomes, which are maintained alongside division of keratinocytes by the early proteins E1 and E2. HPV genome copy number rapidly expands upon differentiation of the keratinocyte, where expression of E6 and E7 oncoproteins allows cell-cycle checkpoints to be overridden, enabling the formation of warts. In high-risk types, the viral genome can integrate into that of the host, disrupting or entirely losing other open reading frames, including the L1 protein targeted by prophylactic vaccines and early genes E1 to E5. The loss of L1 proteins abrogates any protective benefit prophylactic vaccines might have. Disruption or loss of the early protein E2, either through epigenetic changes or integration, averts its ability to negatively regulate expression of oncoproteins E6 and E7, which, in turn, allows their overexpression. E6 and E7 oncoproteins of high-risk types have higher affinities for tumour suppressor proteins p53 and Rb, respectively, which they inactivate, thus forcing the cell cycle into S phase (Synthesis Phase). This results in the unchecked proliferation and genomic instability required for malignancies to occur. In the case of cervical cancer, this manifests itself as precancerous lesions to the three stages of cervical intraepithelial neoplasia (CIN).

Despite the fact that all cases of cervical carcinoma develop from CIN stages II/III, approximately 30% of CIN spontaneously regress, and the infiltration of CD8+ T cells into the tissue lesions has long been associated with regression. E6 and E7 proteins of HPV16 and 18 form the basis of most therapeutic vaccine strategies, as they are known targets for CD8+ T-cell responses and are constitutively expressed in the various stages of CIN. However, despite these two genotypes being responsible for most HPV-associated cancers, there are multiple other HR-HPV types that would potentially not be covered by such vaccines. Furthermore, expression of other early antigens is not always lost in precancerous lesions, and their inclusion would increase the number of targets for vaccine-directed immune responses.

Several therapeutic vaccines have progressed to phase II clinical trials, notably VGX3100, which comprises two DNA plasmids encoding E6/E7 proteins of HPV16 and 18 administered through electroporation. In a double-blinded placebo-controlled trial, 49% of vaccinated individuals showed regression in HPV16/18-associated CIN2/3, corresponding to an increase of > 19% over that of the placebo group (Trimble et al., 2015). Elevated HPV-specific CD8+ T-cell responses, as well as an increased proportion of CD137+Perforin+ CD8+ T cells responding to HPV16 and 18 peptide antigens, could be detected in vaccinated individuals; these responses were found to correlate with regression. An earlier uncontrolled single-group phase II study used nine and four SLPs spanning HPV16 E6 and E7, respectively, with incomplete Freund's adjuvant to vaccinate 20 HPV16+ women with grade 3 vulvar intraepithelial neoplasia (VIN3). Lesion regression was seen in 79% of patients, and complete regression was seen in 49% of patients 1 year after the last dose of vaccine, with complete clinical responses being associated with stronger CD4+ and CD8+ T-cell responses.

More recently, Tipapkinogen Sovacivec (TS) vaccine, composed of MVA encoding human interleukin-2 (IL-2) and modified HPV16 E6 and E7 proteins, was administered in a placebo-controlled phase II trial to women

with CIN2/3. The vaccine was administered intradermally, with 24% of vaccines found to have complete resolution of CIN2/3 regardless of HR-HPV type compared with placebo groups (10%). DNA clearance was also significantly elevated in the vaccinated group, and this was maintained for 2.5 years of follow-up. In another phase IIa trial, a similar MVA-vectored E6/E6/IL2 vaccine, TG4001, resulted in regression in 10/21 patients with HPV16-related CIN2/3. Of the 10 individuals with regression, eight had clearance of HPV16 DNA with no recurrence of high-grade lesions in the 24 months following treatment.

The bacteria *Listeria monocytogenes* (Lm) is an attractive vector due to its ability to access both the cytoplasm and endosomal compartments, resulting in presentation of antigen on MHC class I and II to CD8+ and CD4+ T cells, respectively (Zenewicz & Shen, 2007). The therapeutic HPV vaccine candidate ADXS11-001 consists of *L. monocytogenes* expressing HPV-16 E7 antigen fused to a fragment of Lm protein listeriolysin O (LLO) and has shown promise in phase II clinical trials, with intravenous vaccination increasing the 1-year survival rate to 38% in patients with persistent or recurrent metastatic cervical cancer compared with the expected rate of 24%.

Therapeutic TB vaccines

TB, caused by *Mycobacterium tuberculosis* (M.tb), is the leading cause of death due to an infectious agent with 1.6 million deaths in 2018 (WHO, 2018). While 10% of infected individuals develop active disease, the majority mount an effective immune response, leading to successful containment of *M.tb* growth—a condition known as latent *M.tb* infection or LTBI. LTBI, characterized by the formation of caseous granulomas, is asymptomatic but has a 5%–10% lifetime risk of reactivation to overt disease. Antibiotics are available for the treatment of LTBI and active TB disease, but regimens are long and complex with frequent side effects, resulting in poor compliance. The emergence of drug-resistant and multi-drug–resistant strains is a serious and growing global threat, reflecting treatment failure of drug-sensitive disease. The problems with drug toxicity and compliance and the presence of drug-resistant strains, together with the high likelihood of reinfection in endemic countries following treatment, mean that there is an urgent need for therapeutic TB vaccines. Unlike chemotherapy, therapeutic vaccines do not directly target the causative organism and as such are not involved in the development of antimicrobial resistance.

The concept of therapeutic vaccination to enhance the host immune response to *M.tb* was first proposed as early as 1890 by Robert Koch, whose attempts at immunotherapy by repeated injection of 'Old Tuberculin' (*M.tb* culture supernatant) appeared promising. This method exploited the tissue destructive aspect of the immunopathology of TB, with administration of tuberculin increasing necrosis of tuberculous lesions and reducing availability of oxygen to bacteria. However, tuberculin therapy caused severe and sometimes fatal adverse reactions in active TB patients, thought to result from a tissue-damaging 'cytokine storm', with exacerbated release of TNF-α and other downstream proinflammatory cytokines. Friedmann postulated that a less pathogenic species belonging to the same genus as *M.tb* (and therefore sharing many common antigens) might be as effective as Koch's therapy, but less dangerous, and reported some success using live *Mycobacterium chelonae* isolated from a diseased turtle in the Berlin Zoo (Friedmann, 1903).

In the 1970s, heat-killed *Mycobacterium vaccae* (a nonpathogenic species commonly found in soil and water) was proposed as an immunotherapeutic agent following observations that some people in areas where this species was abundant had a degree of natural protection to TB. Unlike Koch's necrosis-inducing tuberculin method, *M. vaccae* acts to convert the existing necrotizing response into a protective one by promoting the Th1 response and suppressing the Th2 response. The safety of *M. vaccae* has been well documented and, in combination with chemotherapy, it has been reported to improve the sputum conversion rate and X-ray appearances of TB patients. However, clinical trials have shown conflicting efficacy outcomes, and while some systematic reviews or meta-analyses find *M. vaccae* to be an effective treatment (Huang & Hsieh, 2017), others disagree. *M. vaccae* is now approved in China as an immunotherapeutic agent to help shorten TB therapy and is currently in phase III trials to assess effectiveness in preventing active disease in LTBI individuals. *Mycobacterium indicus pranii* (MIP; previously *Mw*) is another inactivated whole cell mycobacterium. While preclinical studies showed promising results, it had no immunotherapeutic benefit in patients with TB pericarditis in a phase III clinical trial of 1400 patients. However, the use of MIP in sepsis was associated with improved outcomes in a recent randomized trial, and this vaccine has now progressed to a phase IIb trial in patients with severe sepsis (NCT02330432).

An alternative approach is to increase the surveillance capacity against so-called 'persister' or nonreplicating bacteria. *M.tb* has a unique ability to transform phenotype into a nonreplicative dormant state under stress conditions, allowing it to persist in the face of the host immune response and antimicrobial treatment. Targeting such persister bacilli could improve treatment success rates and shorten treatment duration. The first therapeutic vaccine to be designed with this aim, RUTI, is composed of detoxified fragments derived from *M.tb* that has been cultured under stress to induce expression of latency-associated antigens. Administered following a short period of chemotherapy during which active growing bacilli are killed, RUTI aims to induce an immune response that will kill the remaining persister

bacilli and reduce the probability of them regrowing. Prior chemotherapy also acts to reduce bacillary load and local inflammatory responses so as to avoid the Th2-related exacerbated immune response observed by Koch. Preclinical studies of RUTI have demonstrated induction of a broad polyantigenic response with no toxicity, and efficacy in controlling LTBI. A phase II clinical trial in South Africa demonstrated acceptable tolerability and good immunogenicity in HIV-infected and uninfected subjects, with LTBI following 1 month of isoniazid treatment, and a phase III trial is planned.

The H56 (Statens Serum Institut, SSI) vaccine candidate contains the latency-associated antigen Rv2660 in addition to Ag85B and TB10.4, which are immunodominant in the secreted proteins of active replicating *M.tb*. This vaccine is designed to protect before *M.tb* exposure, as well as to enhance protective immunity in individuals with LTBI, preventing reactivation and facilitating clearance of infection. H56 was well tolerated and immunogenic in non-human primate (NHP) studies and showed protective efficacy against active TB disease and reactivation of latent infection. Phase I/IIa trials in healthy adults without or with LTBI demonstrated safety and immunogenicity. A phase II prevention-of-infection study is planned (NCT03265977). Interestingly, V5 immunitor, an oral therapeutic vaccine originally developed for the management of chronic hepatitis, has been shown to be beneficial when administered to TB patients. V5 is derived from inactivated pooled blood from donors positive for hepatitis B and C virus; it has been hypothesized that immune responses may be stimulated by circulating latency-associated *M.tb* antigens resulting from LTBI in some of the donors.

Conclusions

Despite the relative lack of success of therapeutic vaccines in the context of infectious disease, there are reasons to believe that such an approach could be effective in the future. Numerous therapeutic vaccines have already been shown to be safe and capable of inducing robust immune responses in previously infected individuals, often in spite of immune impairments in vaccine cohorts. Furthermore, several lines of evidence suggest that vaccine-induced responses are able to recognize and eliminate infected cells and improve clinical outcomes. Tumour regression and increased survival rates at 1 year have been observed in CIN patients given therapeutic HPV vaccines. In HIV, delayed virus rebound following treatment interruption has been demonstrated when vaccines have been used with LRA, while increased ALT levels alongside decreases in HBV DNA following therapeutic HBV vaccination suggest the destruction of HBV-infected cells.

Nevertheless, several barriers must be overcome for therapeutic vaccines to be successful (Fig. 13.2). First, the

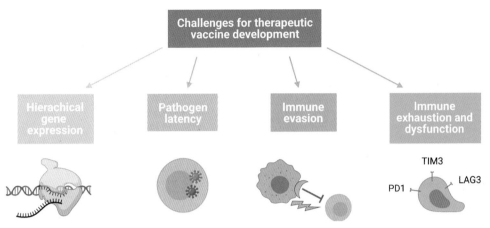

Fig. 13.2 Challenges for therapeutic vaccine development. Several barriers must be overcome for therapeutic vaccines to be successful. These include antigenic variability or alteration of antigen availability, immune evasion strategies and immune exhaustion and dysfunction resulting from prolonged antigenic re-stimulation caused during chronic infections.

antigen availability, or variability, of specific pathogens must dictate a more coherent strategy for vaccine insert design. This will be critical to circumvent pathogen latency (as seen in HIV/EBV/HBV/TB), hierarchical gene expression (EBV/HPV/TB) and immune evasion strategies including sequence variation (HIV/HPV), which are recurrent themes in many infections. To address this, vaccine inserts are being designed to include only the most conserved regions of the antigens most commonly expressed during the replication cycle of the pathogen; thus by refocussing or reeducating immune responses away from sequences that are either hypervariable or rarely expressed, the likelihood of only conserved epitopes being seen increases. Where latency is established following infection, the combined use of epigenetic-targeted therapies such as LRAs alongside vaccination might yield promise. Several of these including HDACs have already been trialled to induce HIV, HBV and EBV reactivation or expression of lytic antigens; although at present their potency may be insufficient to allow the clearance of viral reservoirs, novel agents may well improve this.

Immune exhaustion and dysfunction (as characterized by overexpression of inhibitory receptors such as PD-1, TIGIT, CTLA-4, TIM-3 by lymphocytes) result from prolonged antigenic re-stimulation caused during chronic infections and may also preclude the efficacy of therapeutic vaccination. Vaccines boosting exhausted populations are unlikely to improve functional capacity to react to antigen and mediate destruction of infected cells. Reversing this exhausted phenotype through addition of antibodies blocking inhibitory receptors reinvigorates the ability of previously exhausted cells to target and eliminate infected cells. Together, with recent advances in vaccine insert design, epigenetic modulation and inhibitory

receptor blockage could result in a three-pronged therapeutic approach that would increase the likelihood of successfully eliminating specific infections.

Therapeutic cancer vaccines

The safety, affordability and effectiveness of vaccines to prevent and, in some cases, eradicate bacterial and viral infections make this approach attractive for the treatment of other diseases including cancer. In particular, the application of prophylactic vaccines to control certain viral infections, namely HBV and HPV, has proven effective in the prevention of virus-induced malignancies. With this rationale, the use of vaccines for the treatment of cancer has been extensively investigated in recent decades, although with limited clinical benefits. Nonetheless, improved understanding in the fields of immunology and molecular biology, together with continuous advances in technology, is paving the way for the development of effective therapeutic cancer vaccines.

Tumours originate from normal cells that undergo a complex series of genetic alterations affecting the regulation of the normal cell physiology. The tumorigenic process happens as a progressive transformation through modifications of oncogenes and tumour suppressor genes and leads to the generation of dysregulated cells with aberrant proliferation and homeostasis. During tumour development, cells become self-sufficient in growth signals and acquire limitless replicative potential, can invade other tissues and metastasize. Additional key neoplastic changes include insensitivity to antigrowth signals, evasion of apoptotic cell death and angiogenic ability to sustain oxygen and nutrient supply. These hallmark capabilities, which allow cancer cells to survive, proliferate and disseminate, are shared among almost all cancer types, although the order in which they are acquired seems to be very variable across different cancer types and subtypes.

The identification and study of these hallmarks have helped researchers to understand the pathogenesis of neoplastic diseases. However, tumours are not only composed of proliferating cancer cells; rather, they include multiple diverse cell types that constitute the tumour microenvironment. These nonmalignant cells, such as fibroblasts, stromal cells, endothelial cells and immune cells, are in direct contact and continuously interact with tumour cells, possibly contributing to tumorigenesis. In particular, the role of inflammation and immune escape in cancer development and progression is now widely recognized (Hinshaw and Shevde, 2019). For example, a high regulatory T-cell (Treg) to effector T-cell ratio or high levels of suppressor macrophages within the tumour microenvironment have been associated with a poorer clinical outcome (Coventry, 2019). Understanding these interactions and the immune response to cancer can aid in identifying the best approach to effectively target tumours with cancer vaccine therapies.

Cancer vaccine challenges

Target antigens

A key aspect in cancer vaccine design is the choice of target antigens. The ideal antigen should be (1) unique to the tumour and completely absent in healthy cells, (2) expressed homogeneously in all tumour cells, (3) immunogenic and (4) essential for cancer survival such that it cannot be downregulated. Very few antigens though meet all of these criteria, and it is not common for these to be shared among patients or tumours.

Tumour-associated antigens (TAAs) have been widely used as targets for cancer vaccines. These antigens are self-proteins preferentially or abnormally expressed in tumour cells, but still present at some level in healthy cells. TAAs are usually classified into cancer testis antigens (CTAs) that are mainly expressed in germline cells, tissue-specific differentiation antigens unique to the tumour and the normal tissue of origin, and antigens encoded by overexpressed genes in tumours. There are several considerations when targeting a TAA. First, as a mechanism of defence from potential autoimmune reactions, T and B cells with high affinity receptors to self-antigens are depleted during development in the thymus and the periphery through negative selection. Only cells with absent or low-affinity receptors to presented self-antigens will mature and enter the bloodstream. The final repertoire of receptors will then shape any future responses against not only infections, but also tumours.

Therefore, an insufficient antitumour response following cancer vaccination might be a consequence of these low-affinity interactions between adaptive immune cells and presented TAAs, ordinarily meant to prevent autoimmunity. Second, in such a scenario, a cancer vaccine would need to amplify any remaining low-affinity or rare TAA-reactive cells, breaking the immunological tolerance towards self-antigens, without causing any collateral toxicity to vital organs.

As opposed to TAAs, neoantigens represent immunogenic vaccine targets. These are tumour-specific antigens (TSAs) that arise from mutations in cancer cells and are therefore exclusive to single tumours. The immune system will have retained the necessary specificity to recognize them as foreign antigens and therefore potentially mount an antitumour immune response in favourable conditions. It is indeed well established that tumours with a high mutational rate are more immunogenic and, as a consequence, generally associated with improved survival. A single tumour will encode hundreds of mutated genes and present a fraction of the mutated antigen peptides on their surface. Inevitably, the high variability of point or frameshift mutations and translocations generated within the same tumour mass, together with the even higher variability of mutated peptides presented by the same tumour types among different individuals, make the identification and targeting of neoantigens more challenging. Thus, a personalized therapeutic approach is essential to identify patient-specific mutations as effective vaccine targets, resulting in a relatively slow initiation of the therapeutic treatment, which will necessarily have a very limited application.

Immune evasion mechanisms

Through the process of immune surveillance, the immune system constantly monitors cells and tissues and can recognize new antigens arising from genetic abnormalities during the oncogenic process as a danger signal. As a consequence, incipient cancer cells, and even small tumours early on in their development, can be eliminated by tumour-reactive immune cells. Indeed, spontaneous antitumour immune responses have been described in many studies; moreover, the presence of tumour-infiltrated lymphocytes (TILs) is associated with improved clinical outcome, confirming the key role of the immune system in controlling and eliminating cancer cells. Nevertheless, some tumour cells can survive the elimination phase and escape immune pressure, eventually leading to malignancy. It is now widely recognized that the development of cancer in immunocompetent individuals can be directly influenced by immunologically driven events. Indeed, the elimination of immunogenic tumour cells could lead to a selective survival of less immunogenic variants favouring the formation of tumours that are poorly recognizable by the immune system, or that have an improved ability to suppress immune responses. These events constitute so-called 'cancer immune-editing'—a process characterized by a dynamic interaction between the immune system and cancer cells. Further evidence for the close association between tumour development and the immune system is that immune dysfunction is often linked to an increased incidence of malignancies. Immunocompromised patients with congenital or acquired immunodeficiencies (e.g., HIV infection), as well as immunosuppressed patients (such as transplant recipients), do indeed suffer a higher occurrence of viral and nonviral cancers, respectively.

Tumour cells do not simply rely on immune defects to develop but also actively evolve specific mechanisms to escape immune recognition and attack (Fig. 13.3). Tumour cells are able to evade the immune system through the loss of stimulatory cytokines and co-stimulatory molecules. Furthermore, expression of negative regulators of T-cell activation (e.g., Galectin-1) and the production of cytokines, such as transforming growth factor (TGF)-β, help to maintain an immunosuppressive microenvironment. The downregulation or loss of specific TAAs, as well as dysregulation, or even complete loss, of HLA class I molecules is a further strategy to reduce or eliminate tumour recognition and immunogenicity. A major goal of therapeutic cancer vaccines is therefore to overcome immune escape mechanisms put in place by tumours and thus restore functional antitumour activity of the host immune system.

Therapeutic cancer vaccine platforms

As discussed, therapeutic cancer vaccines aim to efficiently generate or stimulate antitumour responses through empowering activation mechanisms or suppressing inhibitory processes directed towards the immune system. This can be achieved through passive or active immunotherapy strategies. Passive immunotherapy, which does not rely on direct involvement of the host immune system, encompasses the use of cytokines, mAbs, adoptive cell therapy or oncolytic viruses. The effects are immediate but also transient, as these agents do not induce immunological memory, therefore a continuous administration of the agent is necessary to achieve prolonged responses. Active immunotherapy engages directly with the host immune system, so the effects will be deferred, but protracted and durable, as tumour-specific induced responses lead to immunological memory. As a consequence, each patient will respond differently to the same active therapy depending on individual factors that influence their general immunological status. Active immunotherapy agents include tumour cells, DCs, proteins and peptides, genetic vaccines and recombinant viral vectors.

Cell-based cancer vaccines

Whole tumour cell vaccines. The use of autologous tumour cells was one of the first vaccination strategies applied in the field of cancer immunotherapy. Patient-derived tumour cells are irradiated to prevent cell division and readministered to the same patient, typically combined with an adjuvant, such as BCG. The advantage of whole tumour cell vaccines is that the patient immune system will be exposed to the entire spectrum of cancer antigens, inclusive of known or undefined TAAs and mutated antigens, presented by the host MHC class I and II molecules. The display of a complete range of epitopes eliminates the need for prospective identification of target antigens. However, this strategy relies on the availability of tumour biopsies and is therefore not applicable to all cancer types and stages. Allogeneic tumour cell vaccines overcome this issue, as they are formulated as a combination of multiple established cancer cell lines. The disadvantage is the arguable similarity between allogeneic cell and endogenous cancer antigens and their effective presentation to the patient's immune system, although some TAAs might be shared between patients.

Whole tumour cells, both endogenous and allogeneic, can also be engineered to express immunostimulatory cytokines (e.g., GM-CSF and IL-2) aimed at improving immunogenicity. GVAX vaccines are GM-CSF ex vivo transfected tumour cells using viral or nonviral vectors; they have been widely used in clinical settings, showing immunogenicity but limited efficacy. In addition, tumour lysates can be used to load APCs ex vivo, and autologous or allogeneic tumour cells can be fused to autologous APCs in order to enhance the antigen-presenting properties of these vaccines. Similar to whole tumour cells, the advantages of such fusion vaccines are the presentation of a broad spectrum of epitopes and induced immune responses to more than one target antigen, but also the extended duration of the antigen presentation itself due to antigen processing in the APCs.

Dendritic cell cancer vaccines. DCs are specialized APCs that function as potent initiators of adaptive immune responses and therefore represent a powerful alternative approach for cancer immunotherapies. Autologous DCs are isolated from cancer patients by leukapheresis and can be loaded with tumour lysates, cancer peptides or antigens, or transfected with cancer genes and mRNA before readministration to the patient, making DC vaccines a versatile therapeutic strategy. Expression of TAAs in DCs can also be achieved through loading with bacterial or viral vectors, although preexisting immunity against the vectors themselves may limit the immune responses towards the TAAs in vivo. Prestimulation and maturation of APCs ex vivo after isolation is also common, as cells benefit from the optimal ex vivo culture conditions; after reinfusion, they can more efficiently trigger antitumour immune responses. This process helps to overcome the immunosuppressive signals often found in the tumour microenvironment. To further increase migration to the lymph nodes and better

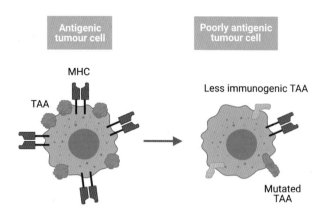

A. Reduction of immune recognition

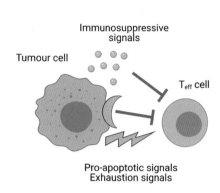

B. Increased resistance/ reduction of immune stimulation

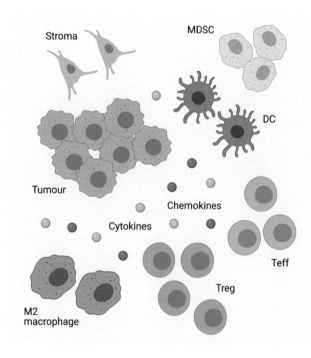

C. Establishment of immunosuppressive microenvironment

Fig. 13.3 Immune evasion mechanisms in cancer. The dynamic interaction between the immune system and cancer cells constitutes the so-called 'cancer immune-editing'. During carcinogenesis, the immune system can recognize and eliminate incipient cancer cells. However, the immune pressure could favour the selective proliferation of less immunogenic variants of tumour cells surviving this elimination phase. Tumour cells also evolve specific mechanisms to actively escape immune-mediated elimination. (A) Loss of antigenicity. Reduction of immune recognition might happen via downregulation or loss of specific tumour-associated antigens (TAAs), as well as dysregulation, or even complete loss, of major histocompatibility (MHC) expression. In addition the expression of mutated TAAs might increase the chances of escaping antitumour immune cells. (B) Loss of immunogenicity. Tumour cells could gain additional immunosuppressive properties upregulating or secreting molecules directly suppressing or inactivating tumour-reactive lymphocytes. (C) Induction of an immunosuppressive microenvironment. Tumours may also establish and orchestrate an immunosuppressive microenvironment, recruiting suppressor cells or negatively influencing the activation of antitumour immunity, thus promoting immune evasion and tumour progression. *DC*, Dendritic cells; *MDSC*, (myeloid-derived suppressor cells); *Teff*, (effector T cells); *Treg*, regulatory T cell.

induce antitumour responses, TLR agonists are commonly administered together with DC vaccines.

DC vaccines have been extensively assessed in clinical trials for the treatment of a variety of cancer types, showing only mild toxicity while inducing antigen-specific T-cell responses, irrespective of the route of administration. The DC vaccine sipuleucel-T was the very first cancer vaccine to be licensed by the US Food and Drug Administration (FDA) for cancer treatment, specifically of hormone-refractory prostate cancer. Sipuleucel-T is composed of patient-derived and enriched DCs incubated in vitro with a recombinant fusion protein, namely the TAA prostatic acid phosphatase (PAP) protein, linked to GM-CSF. This vaccine has resulted in an average of 4 months increase in overall survival (OS) in metastatic castration-resistant prostate cancer (mCRPC) patients over the placebo control in a phase III clinical trial. Despite the modest clinical effects, the production of sipuleucel-T and other DC vaccines is very complex and costly, which currently limits the widespread use of such vaccines.

Protein/peptide cancer vaccines

Protein and peptide vaccines have been shown to be immunogenic in many cancer trials, but no significant clinical benefit has been achieved to date. The various disadvantages of protein/peptide vaccines are discussed in the earlier section on peptide-/protein-based vaccines, but an explanation for the disappointing results may also be found in the failure to account for tumour heterogeneity when stimulating immune responses towards a single TAA or one or a few epitopes of a TAA. The loss of antigen expression by tumours may also contribute to the failure of protein/peptide vaccines. Targeted patient-specific use of mutated antigens is an effective strategy to improve the efficacy of such vaccines, although considerable additional labour and cost is associated with identification of the mutations, with the further disadvantage that the resulting vaccine is exclusive to an individual patient.

Genetic cancer vaccines

DNA and RNA vaccines have been widely investigated in the field of cancer immunotherapy with the benefits of low cost of production and the ability to deliver multiple antigens in the same construct. Another important characteristic is the good tolerability of these vaccines, which have very few side effects. In addition, the target antigen will be expressed/translated, processed and presented by the host cell machinery, allowing these vaccines to be used irrespective of the HLA haplotype of the patient.

Cancer DNA vaccines are able to induce systemic immune responses, beneficial in metastatic patients and also to generate immunological memory, providing a long-lasting antitumour response. Despite their huge potential, the clinical benefits of DNA vaccines have been disappointing so far, although encouraging results have been observed using DNA-encoding tumour antigens from different species that share significant homology with the target species. Additional vaccination with the xenogeneic form has been shown to generate a cross-reactive response to the self-antigen and to induce a protective antitumour immune response in both preclinical and clinical settings. A xenogeneic DNA vaccine encoding the human version

of tyrosinase has been licensed for the treatment of canine melanoma, offering hope for this strategy as a potentially efficacious treatment for human cancers.

Clinical trials of RNA vaccines in cancer patients have mainly used mRNA, although self-replicating RNA vaccines have also been introduced, with the advantage of a longer persistence and a lower dose required. To increase the stability and cellular uptake, many delivery vehicles have been formulated, such as nanoliposomes. To date, there have been a number of RNA-based cancer vaccines clinically tested in phase I/II trials, including the enrolment of advanced castration-resistant prostate cancer, melanoma, renal cell carcinoma (RCC) or non–small cell lung cancer (NSCLC) patients.

Viral-vectored cancer vaccines

Viral vectors are potent inducers of antigen expression and presentation and, in addition, the immune system will also respond to the viral infection itself. Many viruses allow the insertion of large fragments of foreign DNA and can be engineered to target multiple TAAs, thus decreasing chances of treatment failure due to antigen loss in the tumour. For optimal immune cell stimulation, repeated vaccinations are often required. In such cases, a heterologous prime-boost regimen is the recommended strategy to avoid viral neutralization; this is achieved targeting the same antigen through the engineering of, and vaccination with, different viral vectors. A classic example of this approach is represented by the use of PROSTVAC-VF/TRICOM in prostate cancer patients. Genes encoding the tumour target antigen PSA (prostate specific antigen) and co-stimulatory molecules CD54 (Intracellular Adhesion Molecule 1, ICAM-1), CD58 (lymphocyte function-associated antigen 3, LFA3) and CD80 (B7.1) (TRIad of COstimulatory Molecules, TRICOM) are delivered via a prime vaccination using a recombinant replication-competent vaccinia virus (PROSTVAC-V) and subsequent boost vaccinations using a replication-incompetent fowlpox virus (PROSTVAC-F). Despite early encouraging results and activation of PSA-specific T-cell responses, this strategy has failed to significantly increase OS in a phase III clinical trial in prostate cancer metastatic patients.

Poxviruses, such as MVA, are potent boosting agents, and they have been successfully used in heterologous prime-boost regimens, not only in cancer patients. In particular, the prime-boost vaccination strategy using ChAd and MVA vectors has induced the most potent and durable T-cell response ever described in healthy volunteers (Sheehy et al., 2011). The use of such vector combinations has already demonstrated promising results in preclinical studies of cancer immunotherapy and is currently being evaluated in phase I/II trials enrolling prostate cancer patients. As a single agent, TroVax has been used in several trials to treat metastatic colorectal cancer (CRC), metastatic renal cancer and hormone-refractory prostate cancer. This vaccine is a recombinant MVA virus encoding the oncofoetal antigen 5T4, a TAA highly expressed in many tumour types. Despite inducing potent and sustained immune responses in cancer patients, TroVax failed to significantly increase OS in a phase III trial in metastatic renal cancer patients. However, data collected from TroVax trials have been extensively analysed to identify potential biomarkers predictive of clinical benefit.

Bacterial-/yeast-vectored cancer vaccines

Bacteria- and yeast-based cancer vaccines have been, or are currently being, tested in phase I/II trials in a variety of cancer types, where they are used as single agents or in combination with different therapeutic interventions.

Combination immunotherapy for the treatment of cancer

Despite antitumour immune responses being detected in many cancer vaccine clinical trials, none of the various platforms discussed has translated into appreciable success in terms of clinical benefit when used as monotherapies. One possible explanation is that vaccination-induced activation and expansion of TAA-specific cytotoxic cells might be too weak to achieve any significant efficacy. It is also important to remember that many of the strategies described have limitations and, in addition, tumours themselves have diverse mechanisms to evade or suppress the immune system. To improve the efficacy of cancer immunotherapy, much effort is focussed not only on the optimization of the distinct platforms, but also on exploring combinatorial approaches to achieve a synergistic antitumour effect. The rationale behind a combination strategy is to stimulate a more sustained and potent antitumour immune response, achievable not only through the optimal activation of new or weak preexisting antitumour immune responses, but also through the release of the intrinsic immunological breaks that control autoimmune reactions. At the same time, combination therapies aim to maximize the clinical efficacy of cancer vaccines in overcoming the immunosuppressive and evasive mechanisms of tumours. For this purpose, multiple cancer vaccines have been combined with adoptive T-cell transfer therapy, therapeutic antibodies and cytokines.

Most recently, immune modulators such as co-stimulatory molecules and checkpoint inhibitors have been extensively investigated. Among these, antibodies blocking CTLA-4 and programmed death-1 (PD-1) receptor have been approved as antitumour therapeutics in several cancer types, such as metastatic melanoma, NSCLC and RCC. Under normal conditions, these inhibitory co-receptors play an important role in limiting the generation of self-reactive T cells that could lead to autoimmune responses. The suppressive role of CTLA-4 specifically is exerted in the early activation phase of T cells within the lymphatic tissue. CTLA-4 binds to the B7 ligand of CD28 with higher affinity than CD28 itself, thus preventing the prolonged activation of T cells. PD-1 regulates adaptive immune responses and has a role in the effector phase of T-cell activation mainly in peripheral tissues, where once bound to its ligands PD-L1 and PD-L2, it down-regulates signalling from the T cell receptor (TCR). In the context of tumour vaccination, this checkpoint blockade helps release the full potential of tumour-reactive T cells, facilitating their generation and/or effector functions.

The development of new immunotherapies and combination therapies will necessarily overlap with and integrate into the standard of care, namely chemotherapy and radiotherapy, for most tumours. Local tumour radiation and certain chemotherapeutic agents can act in synergy with immunotherapy by generating an inflammatory microenvironment, facilitating the release of TAAs due to induced cell death, depletion of Tregs, and by favouring immune responses via effects on the tumour microenvironment. An understanding of the interactions and benefits of combining certain vaccines with available treatments is crucial to achieve synergistic or additive effects and ultimately improve clinical benefit. Importantly, the timing and schedule of the different combination therapies must be optimized in order to take advantage of the single component effects on the different levels and stages of the immune response. For example, an initial treatment could aim to reduce immunosuppressive cells in the tumour, providing a favourable microenvironment in which the vaccine can act. Therapies administered close to, or in combination with, vaccination will have an impact on T-cell activation preventing immune regulation, thus improving the quality and efficacy of vaccine-induced T-cell responses. Therapies administered postvaccination will maintain optimal conditions for tumour elimination and generally boost vaccine-induced antitumour responses.

Clinical trials

Despite the multitude of clinical trials employing a wide range of cancer vaccine therapies, as single agents or in combination with conventional cancer treatments or other immunotherapeutic interventions, only modest successes have been obtained so far in the field of therapeutic cancer vaccines. Nevertheless, clinical trials have been, and still are, essential to improve our understanding of cancer immunoregulation. An in-depth analysis of clinical studies is necessary to unveil crucial regulatory mechanisms, to identify prognostic factors and to determine surrogate and predictive biomarkers of clinical benefit. Only through the development of optimized and personalized therapeutic strategies will it be possible to fully unleash the potential of active immunotherapy and significantly improve clinical benefit in cancer patients. In the next paragraphs, a brief overview of past and current clinical trials in a number of major solid tumours will be provided.

Melanoma

Incidence rates of melanoma have dramatically increased in recent decades. Early detection of this skin cancer permits surgical resection and complete cure in the majority of cases, but advanced melanoma is associated with poor prognosis. Melanoma has a very high mutational load that increases the risk of neoantigen formation; moreover, it is an immunogenic tumour and therefore represents a suitable cancer type for immunotherapy. In 2011 and 2014, the FDA approved the use of CTLA-4 and PD-1 antibodies, respectively, for the treatment of metastatic melanoma patients. Despite a drastic increase in OS, approximately half of patients do not benefit from these treatments. Furthermore, associated adverse events often necessitate the termination of antibody therapy (Weiss et al., 2019).

In the study that led to the approval of anti-CTLA-4 (ipilimumab), 676 patients with unresectable stage III or IV melanoma were randomly assigned to receive antibody therapy plus gp100 peptide vaccine, anti-CTLA-4 alone or gp100 peptide vaccine alone. The median OS was 10.1 months with ipilimumab alone and 10.0 months among patients receiving ipilimumab plus gp100, while patients receiving gp100 alone showed an OS of 6.4 months. The gp100 antigen has been frequently used in clinical trials, as adoptive transfer with gp100-specific TILs is associated with tumour regression in patients with melanoma.

Other therapeutic cancer vaccines assessed in clinical trials for metastatic melanoma target tumour antigens such as tyrosinase, melan-A (MART-1), melanoma-associated antigen 3 (MAGE-A3) and New York esophageal squamous cell carcinoma-1 (NY-ESO-1). A cocktail of peptides derived from these melanoma antigens has been used to pulse autologous DCs in a phase II clinical trial against metastatic melanoma. OS was significantly improved in patients receiving the DC-pulsed vaccine and further prolonged in patients who demonstrated a positive CTL response after vaccination. Peptide cocktail–pulsed DC vaccines proved safe and effective in metastatic melanoma and as adjuvant treatment, and a phase III trial is currently ongoing to confirm clinical efficacy of DC vaccines in a larger cohort of patients (NCT02993315).

A prime-boost regimen using vaccinia and fowlpox viruses expressing NY-ESO-1 also showed preliminary evidence of clinical benefit in patients with melanoma at high risk of recurrence or progression. In this phase II clinical trial (LUD00-014), median progression-free survival (PFS) (9 months) and median OS (48 months) were significantly extended in patients with detectable NY-ESO-1-specific immune responses and more pronounced in patients with a preexisting immunity to the vaccine antigen.

Taking advantage of the recent advances in whole exome and RNA sequencing, a personalized approach is also showing promising results. Carreno et al. reported results of a phase I clinical trial on three melanoma patients using neoantigen-pulsed DCs. T cells specific for the personalized neoantigens expanded after vaccination and subdominant neoantigens were also identified. Later, Ott et al. demonstrated efficacy of SLPs encoding up to 20 personalized neoantigens in four out of six patients receiving vaccination. The remaining two patients had disease recurrence but complete tumour regression after anti-PD-1 therapy.

Lung cancer

Therapeutic cancer vaccines are a promising alternative for the treatment of lung cancer, an aggressive tumour with the highest cancer mortality rate worldwide. NSCLC accounts for approximately 85% of all cases, and less than 5% of patients survive for more than 5 years after cytotoxic chemotherapy or targeted therapy. Lung cancer is among cancers with the highest mutation burden, particularly in the case of tumours found in smokers, as somatic mutations are generally higher after exposure to carcinogens. As seen for melanoma, NSCLC also benefits from treatment with checkpoint inhibitors, and since 2017, anti-PD-1 therapy has been approved for advanced/metastatic NSCLC. Results from the study leading to the licensing of nivolumab were reported by Brahmer et al. In their phase III clinical trial, 272 patients with disease recurrence were enrolled and randomized to nivolumab or docetaxel, a second-line treatment chemotherapeutic. The median OS was 9.2 months in the nivolumab group against the 6.0 months in the docetaxel group, and the rate of PFS at 1 year was 21% in the nivolumab group versus 6% in the docetaxel group.

Many cancer vaccines have been tested in NSCLC patients in recent years, but promising results obtained in phase I clinical trials have not been replicated in late-phase development. To illustrate, TG4010, a recombinant MVA encoding Mucin 1 (MUC1) and IL-2 was combined with first-line chemotherapy in a phase IIb trial in patients with advanced NSCLC. The vaccine increased the median OS in the experimental group, and the objective response was associated with longer survival in this group. However, in a subsequent double-blind, placebo-controlled, randomized phase IIb/III clinical trial of 222 patients with advanced NSCLC, the OS was 10.9 months in the control group and 15.5 months in patients receiving TG4010. Importantly, the development of a MUC1-specific response after treatment with TG4010 was strongly associated with an improved clinical outcome, with a median OS of 32.1 months for patients with antigen-specific responses, versus 12.7 months in nonresponders. TG4010-treated patients also showed a broadened response to other TAAs, a phenomenon that could contribute to improved tumour control.

A further example is CIMAvax-EGF, a protein vaccine designed to induce a humoral immune response towards the epidermal growth factor (EGF), an antigen involved in carcinogenesis and associated with poor prognosis in many cancer types. In a phase III clinical trial, patients receiving at least four doses of CIMAvax-EGF had a survival advantage over the control arm (median OS was 12.43 months versus 9.43 months), with vaccination mainly benefitting patients who had high EGF concentration after front-line chemotherapy. CIMAvax is licensed in Cuba for stage IIIB–IV NSCLC.

Overall, cancer vaccines to treat advanced NSCLC have failed to significantly improve survival over available second-line treatments, although they have proven safe and immunogenic. Combination therapies with other immunotherapeutic agents might be the way forward to significantly improve the clinical outcome of these malignancies.

Breast cancer

The clinical benefits observed in other cancer types such as melanoma and lung cancer after the introduction of checkpoint inhibitors have yet to be replicated in breast cancer. Breast cancer is a heterogeneous disease with limited innate immunogenicity. Nevertheless, the presence of TILs has been shown to be associated with better prognosis in early stage breast cancer, particularly in triple-negative breast cancer (TNBC) and human epidermal growth factor receptor 2 (HER2)-positive breast cancer. Therefore, there is a potential for immunotherapy to improve therapy outcome for advanced breast cancer cases. Targets evaluated in therapeutic cancer vaccines include HER2, MUC1, carcinoembryonic antigen (CEA), p53, survivin and others.

NeuVax is a peptide vaccine given in combination with GM-CSF. The synthesized peptide E75 belongs to the extracellular domain of HER2. Data from a phase III clinical trial in 182 evaluable patients showed a 57% reduction in relative risk of recurrence at 24 months postvaccination. Interestingly, low HER2 tumour expression was associated with a statistically significant improvement in disease-free survival (DFS) rates. Similarly, patients with HER2 low-expressing tumours mounted a more robust and sustained CTL response after vaccination as compared to patients with overexpressed HER2, as described in previous reports from the same group.

In a phase I/II trial, DCs infected with an adenoviral vector expressing p53 (Ad.53) were used in combination with indoximod, an inhibitor of the indoleamine 2,3-dioxygenase pathway. CD8+ T-cell responses were detected in 30% of the evaluable patients. Median PFS was 13.3 weeks, and median OS was 20.71 weeks, with no significant differences between immunological responders and nonresponders. Nine patients had either stable disease (SD) (one patient), partial response (PR) (seven patients) or complete response (CR) (one patient) on imaging. An autologous DC vaccine loaded with Wilms' tumour protein 1 (WT1) peptides has also been tested in a phase I/II clinical trial that enrolled 10 patients. The vaccine was well tolerated. Four patients had a significant immunological response postvaccination; in two of these, tomography scans revealed a regression of metastatic tumours and tumour shrinkage following DC vaccination. In general, after the initial vaccination, seven patients had an SD, but at follow-up time point, six patients had died.

A DNA vaccine, INVAC-1, encoding a modified human telomerase reverse transcriptase (hTERT) protein was well tolerated in a phase 1 clinical trial. Vaccination-induced hTERT-specific CD4+ and CD8+ T-cell responses and, although no CR or PR could be observed, disease stabilization was observed in 58% of patients. PFS was 2.7 months, median OS was 15 months and estimated 1-year survival rate reached 65.4%. A number of phase I clinical trials are currently exploring personalized vaccines in TNBC patients. Among these, one study is administering a personalized polyepitope DNA vaccine (NCT02348320), a second trial is using a personalized SLP vaccine strategy (NCT02427581) and a third one is recruiting patients to receive a neoantigen-pulsed DC vaccine (NCT04105582).

Prostate cancer

Prostate cancer is the second most common malignancy in men worldwide and the fifth in terms of mortality. Although early diagnosis effectively reduces prostate cancer–specific mortality, therapeutic options for advanced stages of the disease are still palliative. The FDA approval in 2010 of sipuleucel-T for the treatment of asymptomatic and minimally symptomatic mCRPC represents a turning point in the field of cancer vaccines. The licensing resulted from observations obtained in a double-blind, placebo-controlled, phase III trial (IMPACT). In this study, 512 patients were randomly assigned to receive either sipuleucel-T (341 patients) or placebo (171 patients). As already mentioned, sipuleucel-T consists of autologous peripheral-blood mononuclear cells (PBMCs), including APCs, loaded with PAP protein fused to GM-CSF. Kantoff et al. observed a relative reduction of 22% in the risk of death, as compared with the placebo group. Median survival improved from 21.7 months in the placebo group to 25.8 months in the sipuleucel-T group. Furthermore, probability of 3-year survival was 31.7% in the sipuleucel-T group versus 23.0% in the placebo group. Subsequent analysis of the IMPACT trial showed that sipuleucel-T treatment was more beneficial (greater OS) in patients with lower baseline PSA levels. In the PROCEED trial, almost 2000 patients with mCRPC have been enrolled from 2011 to 2017 and treated with sipuleucel-T. Follow-up was for 3 years or more. The median OS was 30.7 months, and the median time from the first infusion to death for prostate cancer progression was 42.7 months. Interestingly, patients enrolled in the PROCEED trial had lower median baseline levels of PSA, as compared to patients in the IMPACT trial, although a survival benefit could not be determined, as there was no control group in this trial.

The GVAX approach has also been used extensively for the immunotherapy of prostate cancer. The prostate GVAX vaccine consists of the allogeneic prostate cancer cell lines LNCaP (Lymph Node Carcinoma of the Prostate) and PC-3 secreting GM-CSF. Despite encouraging results from a phase I/II study, where a statistically significant decrease in PSA velocity was reported in 16 of 21 patients at 20 weeks after first therapy (Simons et al., 2006), subsequent phase III clinical trials were terminated early and GVAX has not been investigated further in prostate cancer trials.

The PROSTVAC vaccine has also failed to demonstrate survival benefit to date. As described, PROSTVAC consists of a heterologous prime-boost strategy employing vaccinia and fowlpox viral vectors encoding PSA and TRICOM. In a phase II randomized, double-blind, placebo-controlled study, PROSTVAC treatment failed to prolong PFS, although an association with OS was suggested. In a phase III trial, asymptomatic or minimally symptomatic mCRPC patients were randomized 1:1:1 to PROSTVAC plus GM-CSF, PROSTVAC plus placebo GM-CSF or vaccine placebo plus placebo GM-CSF. The primary endpoint was not met in this trial, as median OS was 34.4 months in the PROSTVAC arm, 33.2 months in the PROSTVAC+GM-CSF arm and 34.3 months in the placebo arm.

TroVax is an engineered MVA expressing the tumour antigen 5T4. In a phase II study assessing clinical benefit of TroVax alone and in combination with GM-CSF, the median time to progression (TTP; number of days from treatment to disease progression) was longer in patients who mounted a positive 5T4-specific T-cell response. Patients in the TroVax alone arm had a significantly greater median TTP (4.05 months) compared with TroVax + GM-CSF (2.1 months). Nevertheless, all patients had disease progression and no objective clinical response was reported. A phase II trial assessing efficacy of TroVax and docetaxel was terminated early, despite encouraging results on PFS in the combination group. MVA.5T4 is currently being tested as a boosting agent in a heterologous regime together with ChAdOx1.5T4 as the priming vector, and in association with cyclophosphamide (phase I trial; NCT02390063) in early stage prostate cancer patients, as well as with anti-PD-1 therapy in early and advanced prostate cancer patients (phase I/II trial; NCT03815942).

Other therapeutic vaccines are currently being tested in combination with checkpoint inhibitors (anti-CTLA-4, anti-PD-1 and anti-PD-L1) in clinical trials on advanced prostate cancer patients. CPIs as single agents have not been as clinically efficacious as seen for other malignancies to date.

Renal cancer

RCC is a heterogeneous disease that accounts for 90% of all renal malignancies. Similar to prostate cancer, surgical resection can be curative when the disease is localized, but patients with recurrent disease have limited therapeutic options. Advances in the field of immunotherapy led to the FDA approval of anti-PD-1 therapy for the treatment of metastatic RCC (mRCC). Initially, in a phase II clinical trial, nivolumab treatment of clear cell mRCC (ccmRCC) patients resulted in a median PFS ranging from 2.7 to 4.2 months, an objective response rate (ORR) of 20%–22% and a median OS of 18.2–25.5 months. Subsequently, nivolumab was compared with everolimus, an mTOR (Mechanistic Target of Rapamycin) inhibitor, in a phase III clinical trial on 821 ccmRCC patients. The trial met the primary endpoint, in that the median OS was 25.0 months in patients receiving PD-1 therapy and 19.6 months in the everolimus-treated group. PR and CR were observed in 24% and 1% of patients, respectively, in the nivolumab group, versus 5% and <1% of patients in the everolimus group. PFS was similar in the two groups, but the ORR favoured the nivolumab group, with a benefit observed irrespective of PD-L1 expression. Nivolumab was then established as a new standard of care as the second-line treatment for ccmRCC.

Several other therapeutic vaccines have reached phase III clinical trials. For example, IMA-901, a multipeptide vaccine consisting of several tumour-associated peptides (TUMAPs), was identified through an antigen discovery platform. In a retrospective analysis of a phase I clinical trial, immunogenicity to more than one TUMAP was found to be significantly associated to the frequency of SD or PR; moreover, responses to multiple TUMAPs were associated with low percentages of Treg cells before vaccination. In a phase II trial, IMA-901 was co-administered with cyclophosphamide in order to reduce Tregs and improve immunogenicity and efficacy of the vaccine. Among immune responders, survival was prolonged in the case of cyclophosphamide pretreatment, whereas there was no difference in survival in nonresponders independent of cyclophosphamide conditioning. As seen in the phase I trial, responses to multiple TUMAPs were associated with extended OS. When taken to phase III, IMA 901 failed to improve OS when co-administered with sunitinib, and it was not possible to infer any associations between immune response and clinical outcomes.

TroVax has also been investigated in RCC. In a phase II trial, it was used in combination with IL-2 treatment, known to be associated with durable objective responses in less than 20% of patients. No objective responses were observed in vaccinated patients; however, 3/25 patients were disease-free after additional surgery and 12/25 had SD, which was associated with an increase in the effector T cell to regulatory T-cell ratio (NCT00083941). When tested in phase III, TroVax in combination with IFN-α, IL-2 or sunitinib as standard-of-care mRCC therapy failed to meet the primary end-point of improved OS. The study reported a median OS of 20.1 and 19.2 months for MVA-5T4 and placebo-treated patients, respectively.

Other vaccines investigated include WT1-peptide-pulsed autologous DCs, autologous tumour lysate-loaded DCs and vascular endothelial growth factor receptor 1 (VEGFR1) peptide vaccination, with others currently being tested as monotherapies or combination therapies.

Colorectal cancer

CRC is the fourth deadliest cancer worldwide. It originates from precancerous polyps evolving to cancerous tissue. The availability of screening tests and general advances in therapeutic interventions have contributed to reduce mortality rates in recent years, but the occurrence of distant metastasis still affects around one in four patients. Surgery, chemotherapy and radiation therapy are the recommended treatments; however, the 5-year survival rate in metastatic patients still only reaches c. 12%. The CEA and MUC1 are the most commonly targeted TAAs in CRC vaccine candidates. An adenoviral vector (Ad5) expressing CEA was tested in a phase I/II clinical trial in 32 patients with metastatic CRC. Following vaccination, the majority of patients had specific cell-mediated immunity and experienced a 1-year survival probability of 48%, with no association with preexisting immunity to the viral vector. All but three patients had progressive disease after treatment.

OncoVAX is an autologous tumour cell vaccine combined with BCG as an adjuvant that has demonstrated promising results in a phase III clinical trial. A total of 254 patients with stage II or III colon cancer were randomly assigned to OncoVAX therapy or no treatment after curative surgery of primary tumours. Patients treated with OncoVAX had a lower incidence of disease progression (30.5% versus 38.9% in the control group). Stage II cancer patients showed a 5-year survival rate of 37.7% versus 21.3% of control group, a 41.4% relative risk reduction of disease progression. Stage III cancer patient did not experience any significant benefit. A phase IIIb trial recruiting 550 patients with stage II colon cancer is underway (NCT02448173).

In a randomized phase II clinical trial, disease-free CRC patients who had undergone metastasectomy received autologous DCs modified with PANVAC-V/PANVAC-F, vaccinia and fowlpox viruses encoding modified MUC1 and CEA, and TRICOM, or were treated with prime-boost PANVAC-V/PANVAC-F with GM-CSF adjuvant. The magnitude of the specific T-cell response was similar in the two arms, as was the proportion of patients with no recurrence of disease within 2 years of resections (47% for the DC/PANVAC arm versus 55% for the PANVAC plus GM-CSF arm). Vaccinated patients from the two arms combined had a significant OS advantage when compared to a contemporary group of patients with similar characteristics who had not received vaccination.

TroVax has also been assessed in CRC patients in a phase II trial. A total of 55 patients with inoperable mCRC were randomized to receive cyclophosphamide, TroVax, cyclophosphamide plus TroVax or no treatment. Patients receiving TroVax vaccination with or without cyclophosphamide showed a significant association between immune responses and PFS or OS, although there was no significant difference in terms of survival benefits between the treated groups. Moreover, all treated patients showed improved PFS, but no significant OS benefit compared with the control group.

Pancreatic cancer

Pancreatic cancer is an aggressive tumour with a very poor prognosis. Incidence of this malignancy is rapidly increasing with data suggesting that it will become the second leading cause of cancer deaths in the next 20 years. Tumour resection is a curative option in only 10%–20% of patients, although complications after surgery are frequent and patients with recurrent disease experience a median survival of less than 2 years. Among the treatment options for locally advanced or metastatic disease, immunotherapy and therapeutic vaccination are a promising approach for the management of recurrent or unresectable disease.

GV1001 is an hTERT peptide vaccine shown to be immunogenic in more than 60% of patients in a phase I/II clinical trial. The study inferred a possible association of vaccination with survival benefit and demonstrated a significant advantage in immune responders (7.2 months) over nonresponders (2.9 months). In a phase III clinical trial, GV1001 was administered concurrently or after chemotherapy and compared with chemotherapy alone. Unfortunately, the trial failed to meet the primary end-point, as there was no difference in median OS between the chemotherapy-only treated arm and the vaccine arms, either concurrent or delayed. Furthermore, no differences were found in median PFS or PR/CR in the three groups.

GVAX vaccine has also been investigated for the treatment of metastatic pancreatic adenocarcinoma. In a phase IIb clinical trial, GVAX (allogeneic pancreatic tumour cells secreting GM-CSF) was administered with cyclophosphamide and live, attenuated *L. monocytogenes* expressing mesothelin (CRS-207), in comparison to CRS-207 monotherapy or standard chemotherapy. The primary efficacy endpoint was not met in the trial, as the cyclophospha-mide/vaccines combination did not improve survival over standard chemotherapy.

A personalized peptide vaccine (PPV) has also been tested in phase II clinical trials in advanced pancreatic cancer patients who had failed at least first-line chemotherapy. Two to four personalized peptides per patient were chosen among some of the most frequently expressed antigens in tumour cell lines and selected through screening of preexisting peptide-specific IgG responses. PPV vaccine was combined with chemotherapeutic agents or used as a stand-alone therapy. The study reported no CR or PR during PPV, with the majority of patients experiencing an SD (28 of 41). Median survival time was 9.6 months when PPV was administered with chemotherapies and 3.1 months when PPV was used as single agent.

Clinical trials with checkpoint inhibitors as second-line treatment have reported no significant clinical benefit to date, perhaps unsurprisingly, since pancreatic cancer is not well infiltrated by immune cells and is not an immunogenic tumour. Several combination treatment studies are currently ongoing using anti-CTLA-4 and anti-PD-1 therapies in addition to GVAX, with some encouraging results.

Conclusions

In the last century, the field of cancer therapy has evolved from the exclusive use of radiotherapy and surgery to chemotherapeutic agents, with cancer research mainly focussing on genomic mutations and generation of oncogenes, and discovery of new, more effective and less toxic anticancer drugs, targeting biochemical and molecular pathways. Only in the last decade has the importance of the immune system in cancer research emerged as one of the hallmarks of cancer, with cancer immunotherapy recognized as a scientific breakthrough of the year in 2013. Since then, even more intensive effort has been invested in the development and optimization of new and old cancer vaccine platforms and into combinatorial therapies, which have resulted in exceptional progress in the fight against tumours. There is now a better understanding of tumour evasion mechanisms and tumour–host interactions, but the challenges are still many, and success of immunotherapy is far from satisfactory. In particular, several aspects need to be addressed in order to achieve effective cancer vaccines.

Because of tumour heterogeneity, vaccination against a single cancer antigen needs to be revisited. Targeting multiple antigens, and where possible mutated antigens, would not only improve immune responses, but may also help to overcome the dynamic changes within tumours (e.g., antigen loss). Furthermore, the phenomenon of antigen spread following treatment might be a helpful resource for the identification of new immunogenic TAAs. Indeed, cancer vaccines have been shown to trigger immune responses to additional antigens expressed within the tumours; in fact, the initial tumour cell death releases secondary antigens that are cross-presented to the host immune system, inducing responses to nonvaccine targets. Importantly, recent advances in exome and RNA sequencing analysis, mass spectrometry and bioinformatics can now lead to an accelerated identification of cancer antigens and consequently expedited production of personalized cancer vaccines.

Only a minority of cancer patients respond to immunotherapy, and this may be partly due to some tumours being nonimmunogenic, or 'cold'. Selecting the most appropriate vaccine strategy to transform 'cold' tumours into 'hot' tumours, for example, through targeting the immunosuppressive tumour microenvironment, is essential to increase the number of responders. Likewise, the identification of the most appropriate cohort of patients is key to the success of immunotherapy. It is well established that cancer patients with preexisting antitumour immunity at diagnosis and patients with more tumour infiltrating T cells show improved clinical outcome, highlighting the potential to harness immune cells within tumours and the general immunological fitness of cancer patients to further develop cancer therapy. In addition, the presence of validated biomarkers may be of great help in prospectively identifying patients who are more likely to benefit from immunotherapy. Therapeutic cancer vaccines require time to induce a clinically relevant immune response and do not have an immediate impact on tumour burden; because of the slower kinetics, cancer vaccination is more beneficial when patients are treated at earlier stages of the disease, as these patients are also generally less immunosuppressed.

Cancer vaccines need to be safe, and therefore optimization of the different platforms (or development of more sophisticated vaccines) and their doses, routes of administration and combinations is of utmost importance to minimize adverse effects and maximize clinical benefit. Furthermore, the interplay of conventional treatments and immunotherapy needs to be investigated further in clinical settings. The development of safe and effective combinatorial approaches requires a more extensive knowledge of how standard-of-care therapies influence the clinical efficacy of immunotherapy. As discussed, integrated approaches must be timed appropriately in order to maximize the synergistic effect at the level of intensity of antitumour responses, as well as in terms of reduction/elimination of immunosuppressive mechanisms.

Despite the enormity of the challenges ahead, the successes obtained to date in clinical settings are very encouraging, and together with the increasing knowledge on cancer–host dynamics and advances in available technologies, the development of effective anticancer therapies no longer seems the daunting mission it once was. Optimism is growing about the potentialities of therapeutic cancer vaccines, and they could soon become an integral part of routine antitumour therapies.

Therapeutic vaccines for other chronic diseases

Autoimmune disease

The rates of autoimmune diseases, including MS, type 1 diabetes (T1D), Crohn's disease and rheumatoid arthritis (RA), are rapidly rising. These conditions result from immunological hypersensitivity, whereby mechanisms that ordinarily regulate responses to endogenous host proteins break down, and the immune system destroys or disrupts the body's own tissues. Susceptibility is influenced by complex interactions between environmental and genetic factors. The identification of many associations with genes encoding MHC class I and II suggests a central role for autoreactive T cells. Autoreactive T cells may be activated by cross-presentation of viral epitopes homologous to self-antigens ('molecular mimicry'), microbial superantigens or nonspecific proinflammatory antigenic factors of the innate immune system. Disturbances in Treg function have also been reported in several autoimmune diseases, and likely also contribute to loss of self-tolerance.

Current treatment strategies are palliative rather than curative, and compliance is often poor due to toxicity and serious side effects. Furthermore, many therapies induce generalized immunosuppression, leading to increased susceptibility to opportunistic infections and risk of malignancy. The fact that autoimmune disease can be naturally reversible (e.g., RA can transiently resolve during pregnancy), offers hope for the biological feasibility of therapeutic vaccines in this context. Therapeutic vaccines for autoimmune disease aim to reestablish tolerance to autoantigens or induce antigen-specific immunoregulatory responses, for example, through eliciting Tregs (Fig. 13.4). This unique challenge of inducing a safe and effective immune response against 'self' is not trivial.

Multiple sclerosis

MS is a chronic neuroinflammatory disease of the brain and spinal cord that affects approximately 2.5 million people worldwide. It is caused by autoreactive lymphocytes that mount responses against self-antigens of the central nervous system, and by a weakening of immunoregulatory mechanisms. This leads to inflammation and break down of the myelin sheath around nerve cells, resulting in the formation of hallmark lesions and the disruption of neuronal signalling (Dendrou et al., 2015). Several disease-modifying drugs have been marketed for MS, but they generally act to delay rather than prevent disease progression, and side effects are common and sometimes life-threatening. Furthermore, currently-available drugs attenuate the global function of the immune system without antigen-specific discrimination. Therapeutic vaccine candidates for MS aim to restore self-tolerance to specific antigens while leaving the healthy immune system intact, causing minimal side effects. As for many autoimmune diseases, the primary target antigen/s are not yet known, although myelin basic protein (MBP), myelin oligodendrocyte glycoprotein (MOG) and proteolipid protein (PLP) within the myelin sheath are thought to represent important targets (Willekens & Cools, 2018).

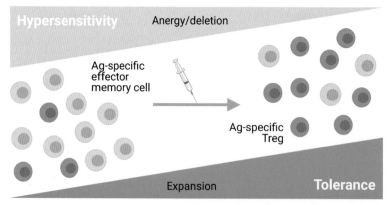

Fig. 13.4 Therapeutic vaccines for autoimmune diseases. Many therapeutic vaccine candidates for autoimmune diseases aim to suppress undesired immune activation and/or expand antigen-specific immunoregulatory responses, for example, through eliciting regulatory T cells (Tregs).

Following the success of peptide-based therapies for allergies, similar approaches to inducing antigen-specific tolerance are being explored in MS. The transdermal application of peptides derived from MBP, MOG and PLP has been reported to induce immunological tolerance via activation of Langerhans cells and induction of IL-10 secreting T cells. This was associated with reduced disease activity in patients with relapsing-remitting MS. However, administration of an altered peptide ligand of MBP in a proinflammatory environment induced hypersensitivity reactions in 9% of patients in a phase II trial, resulting in suspension of the trial. An alternative approach is the use of apitopes: soluble synthetic peptides designed to mimic naturally processed epitopes and to induce antigen-specific expansion of Tregs. ATX-MS-1467 comprises a mixture of four short peptides derived from MBP and has shown a favourable safety profile. In a phase IIa trial, ATX-MS-1467 treatment was associated with reduction in lesion number in patients with relapsing MS, although it should be noted that there was no placebo arm. An alternative approach is the use of amino acid sequences derived from the TCR of autoreactive T-cell clones to induce immune responses directed at those clones. Clinical trials of such vaccines have reported the induction of TCR peptide-specific T cells, reduction of MBP-specific T cells and concomitant clinical improvement.

Other approaches include the use of DNA vaccines or cell-based vaccines. The leading DNA vaccine candidate for MS is BHT-3009 (Bayhill Therapeutics), which encodes a modified full-length human MBP driven by a cytomegalovirus (CMV) promoter. BHT-3009 has been shown to be safe and effective in inducing antigen-specific tolerance to myelin proteins with positive brain MRI improvements, but did not significantly impact lesion reduction or risk or rate of relapse in phase II clinical trials. In the case of autologous T-cell vaccination, myelin-reactive T cells (MRTCs) are isolated from the patient's own peripheral blood and inactivated before being readministered, with the aim of inducing a specific immune response against other circulating autoreactive T cells. This approach has been shown to be safe and immunogenic and was associated with a 40% reduction in relapse rate over the following 1–2 years with stabilization of progression, although additional repetitive injections were required to ensure durability. The combination of T-cell vaccine, Tcelna, consisting of attenuated MRTCs with multiple peptides derived from MBP, PLP and MOG, showed promise in a placebo-controlled trial in 26 patients with relapsing-progressive MS but did not demonstrate efficacy in a phase IIb trial of 183 patients with secondary-progressive MS. A phase I trial of a tolerization regimen using a single infusion of autologous PBMCs chemically coupled with seven myelin peptides from MOG, MBP and PLP demonstrated

safety and tolerability, with decreased antigen-specific T-cell responses in the high-dose group.

Due to the key role of DCs in maintaining the balance between immunity and tolerance, tolerance-inducing DC (tolDC)-based therapies have been developed with the aim of restoring immunological balance in MS and other autoimmune disorders. tolDC therapy has shown promise in in vitro and preclinical models and three phase I clinical trials are in progress to evaluate the safety and tolerability of myelin-derived, peptide-pulsed tolDCs administered intradermally, intranodally or intravenously (NCT02618902, NCT02903537 and NCT02283671). Other next-generation approaches include the use of nanoparticles as a delivery system for self-antigens. As described, EBV infection is a primary risk factor for MS, and therefore a vaccine that prevents or treats EBV might also reduce the rate of MS (Cohen, 2018).

Diabetes

Diabetes is a metabolic disease characterized by chronic hyperglycaemia, which can lead to blindness, kidney failure, heart attacks, stroke and lower limb amputations. Insulin usually acts to move glucose from the bloodstream into the cells, where it can be used for energy. There are two main types of diabetes: type 1—when the immune system attacks and destroys insulin-producing cells; and type 2—failure to produce or react to insulin. In both cases, glucose consequently remains in the blood stream at high levels. Treatment success is limited by poor adherence and the economic burden associated with life-long treatment.

Type 1 diabetes. T1D is a chronic autoimmune disease in which the immune system destroys the insulin-producing β cells of the pancreatic islets. Both a T-cell–mediated inflammatory response within the islets (known as insulitis) and a humoral response with production of autoantibodies specific to β-cell antigens have been described. There is evidence for genetic variants associated with susceptibility or protection, and environmental factors such as viruses, toxins or foods may also play a role in triggering the onset of disease.

The BCG vaccine, originally developed over 100 years ago as a prophylactic vaccine against TB, is a known inducer of TNF and was therefore hypothesized to have some therapeutic benefit in T1D. In phase I trials conducted in 2012, BCG vaccination was associated with reduced insulin-autoreactive T cells and increased Tregs. Long-term follow-up showed normalization of blood sugars from 3 years later that persisted for the next 5 years. The mechanism is thought to be due to a systemic shift in metabolism from oxidative phosphorylation to aerobic glycolysis (a state of high glucose utilization), as well as the epigenetic resetting of central Treg genes restored tolerance. Phase II trials are currently underway.

An alternative approach is the use of antigen-specific immunomodulation, which may be more likely to restore immunological tolerance to β cells. Proinsulin, islet antigen 2 (IA-2), zinc transporter 8 (ZnT8) and the 65-kDa isoform of glutamic acid decarboxylase (GAD) are major autoantigens in T1D patients that represent attractive vaccine targets. Administration of GAD with the aluminium hydroxide adjuvant (GAD-alum) has shown promise in murine models, but human trials have given conflicting results. NBI-6024 is an altered peptide ligand corresponding to an amino acid region of the insulin B chain, an epitope recognized by IFN-γ producing Th1 cells in T1D patients. A phase I clinical trial suggested that NBI-6024 resulted in a shift from a Th1 to Th2 regulatory phenotype. However, a subsequent study found no effect on improving or maintaining β-cell function. A natural peptide sequence derived from proinsulin (MonoPepT1De) has also been evaluated and shown to be safe and well tolerated, with some evidence of both antigen-specific and nonspecific immune modulation. A plasmid DNA vaccine encoding proinsulin (BHT-3021) was associated with reduced insulin-specific CD8+ T cells and temporarily maintained β-cell function, but the effect diminished after discontinuation of therapy. The DiaPep277 vaccine (p277 peptide derived from the heat shock protein HSP60 in oil) reached phase III trials but the publication was retracted amid allegations of serious misconduct.

In addition to single peptides or multiple peptides from the same antigen, multiple peptides from different antigens may be used. Chimeric vaccines such as Dipeptidyl Peptidase 41-Insulinoma antigen-2, D41-IA2(5)-P2-1 and U-IA-2(5)-P2-1 (UIP-1) have been shown to increase insulin levels and reduce blood glucose levels in mice. A phase I trial of MultiPepT1De (comprising a mixture of peptides from islet autoantigens) has recently completed, and results are expected soon. Next-generation approaches include the modification of peptides to improve affinity (known as Imotopes), the targeting of peptides to the erythrocyte and encapsulation of peptides into nanoparticles or liposomes.

Type 2 diabetes. Type 2 diabetes (T2D; also referred to as noninsulin-dependent diabetes mellitus or adult-onset diabetes) affects over 400 million adults globally, with rapidly increasing rates associated with the rise in obesity and population ageing. The mechanism differs from T1D, with patients showing insulin resistance and/or insulin deficiency, resulting in hyperglycaemia. While it has traditionally been considered a metabolic disease, emerging evidence indicates an altered function of specific T-cell populations including Tregs, suggesting that T2D may be at least partially attributable to an autoimmune phenomenon.

Proinflammatory cytokines, including IL-1β, are produced in fat tissues and may contribute to the pathogenesis of insulin resistance and β-cell dysfunction in T2D. The hIL1bQb vaccine (Cytos) consists of full-length recombinant IL-1β coupled to Qβ bacteriophage VLP and aims to induce neutralizing antibodies against IL-1β. In a phase I/II clinical trial, neutralizing specific antibody responses were detectable only after six high-dose injections but were long-lived and associated with improvement in glycaemia and inflammatory levels. As obesity is a significant risk factor for T2D, obesity management is being explored as a therapeutic approach, including the use of obesity vaccines. The CYT009-GhrQb vaccine (Cytos) was designed to induce neutralizing antibodies to ghrelin, an endogenous peptide that enhances appetite and food intake. However, despite mounting a strong specific antibody response, patients did not lose weight, and this vaccine has been discontinued. Other potential targets for obesity vaccines include adipose tissue antigens, somatostatin and glucose-dependent insulinotropic polypeptide (GIP). A DNA vaccine that induces antibodies against dipeptidyl peptidase 4 (DPP4) aims to increase levels of the glucagon-like peptide 1 hormone (GLP-1) and thus improve insulin sensitivity. Although promising in preclinical murine studies, DPP4 vaccines have not yet progressed to clinical trials.

Hypertension

Hypertension, affecting approximately one-third of the global population, is the most important risk factor for potentially fatal cardiovascular diseases including stroke, heart failure and coronary artery disease. The renin-angiotensin system (RAS) plays a key role in the regulation of blood pressure and thus represents an important target for pharmacological treatments including angiotensin converting enzyme (ACE) inhibitors and angiotensin II type I receptor blockers. While these therapies are effective in lowering blood pressure and reducing incidence of disease, side effects and long-term requirements in the absence of symptoms result in poor compliance. Patients may also suffer from morning pressure surges when drug levels are at their lowest.

Active therapeutic vaccination aims to induce long-lived specific antibody responses that target key regulators of blood pressure, thus addressing the issues associated with drug treatments. Renin is the initial and rate-limiting enzyme of the RAS cascade, generating the angiotensin peptides and was the first therapeutic vaccine target to be tested in the 1940s. However, while inducing a significant decrease in blood pressure in a primate model, active immunization against renin-induced lethal autoimmune disease of the kidney, where renin levels are abundant. More recently, the antigenic peptide hR32, which mimics a catalytic site of human renin, has demonstrated low cross-reactivity in rats and may thus represent a safer approach to a renin-based vaccine.

Angiotensin I and II, which are too small to permit the formation of immune complexes, do not pose such risks and have been the focus of more recent vaccine development. The antiangiotensin I vaccine PMD3117 (Protherics) consists of angiotensin I peptides coupled to keyhole limpet haemocyanin carrier protein with aluminium hydroxide adjuvant. This vaccine showed promising efficacy in a rat model and was associated with increased specific antibody titres in phase I and II clinical trials, but blood pressure was not significantly reduced in these patients. The antiangiotensin II vaccine AngQb-Cyt006, comprising angiotensin II peptides coupled to Qβ VLPs, is the first therapeutic vaccine for hypertension to demonstrate a successful reduction in blood pressure in clinical trials (Tissot et al., 2008). Interestingly, a second study involving an increased number and frequency of injections induced higher levels of antiangiotensin II antibodies but a considerably smaller reduction in blood pressure. This reduced efficacy correlated with reduced antibody affinity (strength of binding to angiotensin II), which may have resulted from impairment of affinity maturation due to the frequency of antigen administration. Development of AngQb-Cyt006 has consequently been discontinued. Future vaccine assessment should consider quality, as well as quantity, of antibodies induced.

Next-generation approaches including the use of DNA vaccination and nanoparticles for vaccine development are also being explored. The DNA vaccine pcDNA3.1-HBc-Ang II consists of a plasmid vector encoding a fusion protein between Ang II and a hepatitis B core. Having induced a decrease in blood pressure that correlated with antigen-specific antibody titre in rats while avoiding the activation of self-reactive T cells, this vaccine is currently in ongoing phase I/II clinical trials. A nanoparticle-based nasal vaccine against the angiotensin II type I receptor, AT1R, aims to avoid localized adverse reactions associated with systemic injection and has shown promise in the rat model.

Allergic disorders

Similarly to autoimmune disease, allergies arise due to inappropriate immune responses—in this case, directed against innocuous environmental antigens rather than self-antigens. Allergic disorders include allergic rhinitis, atopic dermatitis, asthma and anaphylaxis and may be life-threatening. Globally, more than 30% of children are estimated to have allergies, and prevalence is increasing—particularly in low- and middle-income countries.

T cells play an important role in the pathogenesis of allergy. As CD4+ T cells develop, they can become polarized and restricted to producing either Th1 or Th2 patterns of cytokines, a process dependent on genetic factors and environmental stimuli including the cytokine milieu surrounding the differentiating cells. Microbial activation of APCs under the influence of IL-12 leads to the differentiation of Th1 cells that primarily secrete IFN-γ, while the Th2 response is dependent on co-stimulation mediated via CD28/B7 interactions and is dominated by cells producing IL-4, IL-5 and IL-10. Allergy is broadly considered the result of a Th2-driven hypersensitivity due to polarization of the allergen-specific T-cell memory response towards Th2. Th2 cells and group 2 innate lymphoid cells (ILC2s) drive IgE synthesis by B cells, tissue eosinophilia, mucous overproduction and smooth muscle contraction via the production of cytokines such as IL-4, IL-13 and IL-5. The increased incidence of allergic disorders has been widely, albeit controversially, attributed to reduced exposure to microbes during childhood, as a result of the sanitized Western lifestyle, known as the 'hygiene hypothesis'. The loss of infectious pressure is thought to lead to a reduction in Th1 cells and IFN-γ and a consequent increase in Th2 immunity, as each response counter-regulates the other. This theory has been extensively supported by mouse models of allergy and studies showing lower incidence of allergic disorders in children with a higher frequency of infections.

However, several important lines of evidence suggest that the dysregulation of the immune system observed in allergy cannot be explained simply by the Th1/Th2 dichotomy: (1) allergen-specific Th1 cells are not a predominant feature of allergen-specific T-cell repertoires in healthy individuals, (2) helminth infections, which are accompanied by Th2 responses, eosinophilia and IgE responses to the parasite, are protective against allergy and (3) there has been a concomitant increase in autoimmune disorders, which are associated with increased Th1 responses. Thinking has now shifted towards a loss of Tregs or IL-10 producing regulatory B cells being responsible for increased Th2 responses in those living a Western lifestyle. This revised hypothesis is known as the 'Old Friends' hypothesis, in which humans need exposure to chronic infections such as intestinal parasites, mycobacteria or *Helicobacter* (which may be lacking in those living Western lifestyles) to drive the development of Tregs. While allergen-specific Tregs dominate the response in healthy individuals, allergic individuals show the co-existance of Tregs and memory/effector Th2 cells. Therefore it is the balance of T-cell effectors and T-cell regulators that is the determining factor in allergy development.

Current treatments for allergic disorders, such as antihistamines, are largely palliative and of varying efficacy; they are also nonspecific and effects are short-lived. That children can 'grow out of' food allergies suggests that allergic disorders may be reversible; furthermore, natural exposure to allergens has been shown to alter risk of allergic disorders, offering hope for immunotherapeutic approaches. Allergen-specific immunotherapy (AIT) aims to induce immune tolerance through repetitive administration of the disease-causing allergen and may be considered a form of therapeutic vaccination. The first attempt at AIT was made by Noon in 1911, who injected increasing doses of pollen extract into hay fever patients, resulting in some degree of clinical improvement. AIT has since become accepted clinical practice for the treatment of allergy to many aeroallergens and insect venoms. Mechanistically, AIT is thought to function through a shift in T-cell function from a Th2 profile towards a Th0/Th1 profile with increased production of IFN-γ, induction of Tregs and/or induction of allergen-specific IgG antibodies that interfere with the allergen–IgE interaction. While treatment has been successful in certain individuals and may prevent the progression of mild forms of allergy to severe forms, AIT remains underused; in part due to adherence issues and safety concerns including instances of fatal adverse reactions due to intact allergens with retained IgE activity. Consequently, there has been a move towards different routes of administration, improved standardization of allergen extracts and exploring novel approaches such as use of recombinant antigen, allergen-derived peptides, VLPs or potent adjuvants.

Initial attempts to improve the safety and efficacy of AIT included the introduction of allergoids—allergenic proteins that have been chemically modified using formaldehyde or glutaraldehyde to destroy IgE epitopes and reduce allergenic activity. In the 1980s, new technologies permitted the determination of the immune function of allergens and their constituent epitopes, as well as their protein molecular structure, paving the way for the cloning of allergen proteins using recombinant DNA technology. Unlike crude allergen extracts, recombinant allergen can be formulated with a reproducible and precise quantity of relevant, high quality allergen. A vaccine consisting of a mixture of five recombinant grass pollen allergens was found to ameliorate symptoms of allergic rhinitis associated with promotion of IgG and reduction of IgE antibodies, consistent with the induction of IL-10 producing Tregs. The rBet v 1a vaccine using recombinant birch pollen allergen derivatives also induced a highly specific immune response and was safe and effective.

While clinical trials of recombinant allergen vaccines have demonstrated good efficacy profiles with strong modulation of specific T- and B-cell responses, many retain the allergenic properties of natural allergen extracts, necessitating long and inconvenient up-dosing schedules. Genetically engineered modifications to the protein structure can result in reduced allergenicity and increased immunogenicity. Such modifications aim to reduce IgE reactivity while retaining T-cell epitopes and have demonstrated safety and promise in eliminating IgE-mediated side effects and efficacy against birch pollen or cat allergy; they are also in clinical trials for fish allergy. These hypoallergenic allergen derivatives allow injection of higher doses compared with wild-type allergens. However, it is not clear whether it will be possible to produce immunogenic and nonallergenic derivatives for all allergen sources using this technology; to date, there is only one report describing an IgG-inducing hypoallergenic derivative of the major house dust mite allergen Der p 1.

Peptide vaccines, containing synthetic immunodominant T-cell epitopes, are designed to reduce the adverse effects of conventional AIT (through avoidance of IgE-mediated activation) and increase efficacy by inducing T-cell tolerance. Vaccination with ALLERVAX CAT, which uses synthetic peptides of the major cat allergen Fel d 1, has been shown to improve tolerance to cat dander and pulmonary function in patients who failed previous conventional immunotherapy. Reduced allergen-specific skin reactivity was accompanied by decreased Th1 and Th2 responses and increased IL-10 production. A mixture of three peptides of the major honeybee venom allergen phospholipase A2 (PLA) was safe and well tolerated in a trial of 10 patients allergic to bee stings. The vaccine induced epitope-specific anergy in peripheral T cells and partial protection from bee sting challenge. However, such vaccines do pose challenges, such as the large number of peptides required to address MHC diversity among patients, and manufacture-related issues with solubility and aggregation of certain peptides. The peptides must also mimic the conformation of the naturally processed epitope of the allergen to ensure MHC binding and effector cell recognition. Evidence from mouse models suggests that tolerance may be a peripheral phenomenon and therefore duration of responses poor, necessitating repeated dosing.

A more recent, alternative approach is the use of B-cell epitope–based vaccines that contain non-IgE reactive peptides derived from the IgE-binding sites of major allergens. Such vaccines aim to induce an IgG antibody response that blocks IgE from binding to the allergen and make use of unrelated carrier proteins to boost immunogenicity by inducing helper T-cell responses. This strategy has been found to be safer and more effective at reducing allergenic activity than vaccines based on recombinant or synthetic hypoallergens, as they show reduced induction of late-phase T-cell-mediated side effects. This permits the use of higher doses and more convenient schedules. New routes of administration are also being explored amid safety concerns associated with subcutaneous administration of allergens (SCIT). There has been increasing use of sublingual administration, which has several advantages including the ability to self-administer and reduced risk of anaphylaxis (Valenta et al., 2016).

Therapeutic vaccines for dementia

Alzheimer's disease

Alzheimer's disease is the most common form of dementia, estimated to affect over 44 million people globally. It is characterized by the accumulation of aggregated amyloid β (Aβ) and tau proteins, leading to the formation of amyloid plaques, neurofibrillary tangles and neuronal loss. Although drug treatments may temporarily lessen symptoms, there are no currently available disease-modifying therapeutics. Active therapeutic vaccine strategies to date have predominantly targeted pathological forms of Aβ through induction of antibodies thought to function via (1) peripheral clearance of Aβ species, thus increasing efflux of these proteins from the brain via passive diffusion; (2) binding fibrillar Aβ in plaques, leading to disassembly of large aggregates; (3) sequestering monomeric Aβ in the brain thus preventing oligomerization into larger aggregates and (4) binding to fibrillar Aβ, leading to phagocytosis-mediated clearance via Fc (fragment crystallizable) receptors on microglia (Herline et al., 2018).

The first Aβ-targeted therapeutic vaccine for Alzheimer's disease to enter clinical trials was AN1792, composed of aggregated human Aβ42 peptides and the QS-21 adjuvant. While showing promise in phase I trials with over half of patients mounting a positive anti-Aβ antibody response, there was no evidence of clinical improvement, and a larger phase IIa trial was terminated when 6% of vaccinated patients developed T-cell-mediated meningoencephalitis. Consequently, next-generation approaches have predominantly utilized N-terminus Aβ fragments that contain the B-cell epitope while avoiding the T-cell epitope. Two such candidates (ACC-001 and AD02) have been discontinued following phase II trials, but several remain in active clinical development. The GlaxoSmithKline/Novartis candidate CAD106 comprises Aβ1-6 conjugated to a bacteriophage coat protein. A 450-μg dose elicited strong anti-Aβ IgG responses in over 80% of patients, with no induction of specific T-cell responses and no occurrences of meningoencephalitis.

ABvac40 (Araclon Biotech) is composed of the C-terminal fragment of Aβ40 conjugated to a cyanine carrier protein, with aluminium hydroxide as an adjuvant. It was well tolerated in phase I trials, and 92% of individuals receiving three doses developed anti-Aβ40 antibodies, and phase II trials are underway. UB-311 (United Neuroscience) comprises a novel Aβ synthetic peptide with an alum adjuvant. In phase I trials, a high anti-Aβ40 antibody response was induced, and rate of cognitive decline slowed significantly in a subset of patients with mild disease. Results are also expected from early clinical trials of ACI-24 (AC Immune

SA) and Lu AF20513 (Otsuka Pharmaceutical Co. Ltd.), following promising preclinical findings.

Unlike amyloid or plaque burden, the presence of neocortical neurofibrillary tangles correlates with disease progression, and hyperphosphorylated tau (the main component of neurofibrillary tangles) may therefore be a more attractive immunotherapeutic target. Anti-tau antibodies are thought to cross the blood–brain barrier and interact with intra- and extraneuronal tau proteins. Targeting of extracellular pathological tau species may prevent them from infecting naive neurones and thus reduce the spread of tau pathology that otherwise propagates with a prion-like mechanism, inducing misfolding of intracellular tau. Anti-tau antibodies are also found in the endosomal–autophagosome–lysosome system associated with tau aggregates, suggesting that they disassemble multimers of pathological tau. The candidate ACI-35 (AC Immune SA, Janssen) consists of 16 copies of a tau fragment that is phosphorylated at sites known to be pathological phosphorylation sites, anchored to a liposome and combined with the adjuvant MPLA. Preclinical testing was promising, and results are expected from a phase I dose-escalation trial. ADDvac1 (Axon Neuroscience SE) consists of tau294-305 coupled to haemocyanin with the aluminium hydroxide adjuvant. In a phase I trial, three doses were well tolerated and induced a specific IgG response in 29 out of 30 patients, and phase II trials are underway.

Synucleinopathies

Synucleinopathies are a group of neurodegenerative diseases characterized by the abnormal accumulation of the α-synuclein protein in neurones and glia, leading to a progressive decline in motor, cognitive, behavioural and autonomic functions. These disorders include Parkinson's disease (PD), dementia with Lewy bodies (DLB), pure autonomic failure (PAF) and multiple system atrophy (MSA). To date, there are no disease-modifying treatments for synucleinopathies; available therapies focus on managing early symptoms but become less effective as disease progresses. Active immunization strategies predominantly target α-syn due to its central role in synucleinopathies, although a limited number have proceeded to clinical development. The AFFITOPE PD01A vaccine (AFFiRiS) for PD comprises a pool of peptides that mimic α-syn, conjugated to KLH and adjuvanted with aluminium oxyhydroxide. PD01A was found to be safe and induced an antibody response against α-syn in phase I clinical trials. A second α-syn targeting vaccine from AFFiRiS, PD03A, has also been found to be safe and immunogenic in phase I trials in PD. Both vaccines are also being assessed in MSA as the rapid progression of this disease allows for shorter trial duration.

A number of additional novel approaches are under preclinical development, including the use of short α-syn peptides expressed by VLPs that have an inherent adjuvant effect without inducing T cells against the target. DNA vaccines such as an α-syn gene–based nucleic acid for PD and the multivalent vaccine pVAX1-IL-4/SYN-B have shown promise in preclinical mouse models. Heat shock proteins have previously been used as carriers to enhance the antibody response to bound antigen, and Hsp70 is known to bind to α-syn aggregates and monomers. Administration of an α-syn/Hsp70 complex resulted in a shift towards an immunomodulatory phenotype in mice but did not enhance the antibody response to α-syn. Vaccines targeting DCs or Tregs are also in active development.

Therapeutic vaccines for addiction

Use of addictive drugs is a growing medical, social, economic and political problem, and for many drugs such as cocaine and methamphetamine, there are no approved pharmacological options. For those seeking treatments for heroin and morphine, access is often problematic, side effects are common and relapse rates high. While medications against dependence-inducing drugs generally interact with brain receptors, therapeutic vaccines aim to stimulate the immune system to recognize addictive substances and produce specific antibodies against them, thus avoiding any adverse effects on the central nervous system. As the molecules of addictive substances are ordinarily nonimmunogenic, efforts have been made to modify them so as to elicit an immune response, beginning with work on morphine in the late 1960s. Current therapeutic vaccine strategies for addiction make use of carrier proteins or VLPs including tetanus toxoid, cholera toxin B and haemocyanin, to stimulate antibody production (Fig. 13.5). Vaccines for nicotine, opioid, cocaine, methamphetamine and phencyclidine (PCP) are in various stages of development, though no candidates have yet been licenced for clinical use. The development of vaccines for addiction may prove more challenging than other applications, in part due to the associated stigma and consequent lack of funding, but also difficulties recruiting motivated trial participants, and the complex nature of addiction that likely requires a combination of pharmacological and psychosocial management strategies.

Nicotine addiction

Approximately 1.1 billion people worldwide smoke tobacco, resulting in over 7 million deaths per year. Pharmacotherapies for nicotine abuse, which focus on reducing symptoms of withdrawal and craving, have had limited success with poor adherence and high rates of relapse; less than 5% of individuals who try to quit smoking are successful. Nicotine stimulates the rapid release of dopamine from the brain, thus 'rewarding' the smoker and positively reinforcing the behaviour. Therapeutic vaccines aim to stimulate the immune system to generate nicotine-specific antibodies. When nicotine molecules enter the bloodstream via the lungs, antibody binding results in the formation of an antigen–antibody complex that is too large to cross the blood–brain barrier, preventing nicotine from reaching the central nervous system and reducing the 'rewarding' effect of smoking.

To date, five nicotine vaccines have been tested in clinical trials: NIC002, Niccine, NicVAX, NicQb and TA-NIC. Despite promising outcomes from preclinical animal studies, results in humans have been disappointing, with weak and variable induction of specific antibody responses. While NicVAX (Nabi Biopharmaceuticals/GSK), consisting of a nicotine derivative conjugated to detoxified *Pseudomonas* exoprotein A, reached phase III clinical trials, vaccine recipients were no more likely to cease smoking than those given a placebo. A Cochrane Review concluded that there is currently no evidence that nicotine vaccines enhance long-term smoking cessation (Hartmann-Boyce et al. 2012), and the need for investment in nicotine vaccine development has been questioned. Nonetheless, next-generation vaccines including synthetic nicotine-like haptens conjugated with diphtheria toxin, and other novel approaches such as using a nanoparticle surface to replace the conventional protein, or conjugating nicotine to a liposome complex, are in preclinical development.

Opioid addiction

Opioid vaccines are not yet in clinical trials but have been shown to reduce behavioural and/or psychoactive effects of heroin intake in preclinical animal models. A bivalent vaccine using the tetanus toxoid as a protein conjugate induced high levels of antibodies that recognized both heroin and morphine and prevented relapse to heroin addiction in rodents. One challenge in opioid vaccine development is that addicted individuals frequently switch or transition between different opioids, and thus strategies include the co-administration of two or more vaccines concurrently to target multiple abusable opioids such as the morphine and oxycodone bivalent vaccine candidates OXY-KLH and M-KLH. Furthermore, within seconds of injection, heroin undergoes rapid deacetylation to the active metabolites 6-acetylmorphine and morphine. Vaccines that elicit nonselective opiate antibodies are easily overcome by increasing the dose, and thus a 'dynamic' vaccine has recently been proposed that presents a multihaptenic structure to the immune system, eliciting antibodies against both heroin and its metabolites.

Cocaine and methamphetamine addiction

Following promising preclinical studies of vaccines based on the succinyl norcocaine hapten, human studies began

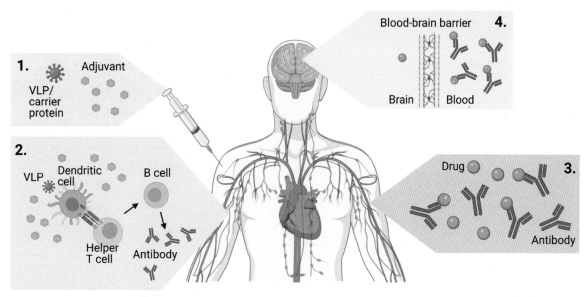

Fig. 13.5 Therapeutic vaccines for addiction. Current therapeutic vaccine strategies for addiction make use of carrier proteins or virus-like particles to stimulate the production of antibodies against the drug or addictive substance. When the drug enters the bloodstream, antibody binding results in the formation of an antigen–antibody complex that is too large to cross the blood–brain barrier, preventing it from reaching the central nervous system and generating a 'rewarding' effect. *VLPs*, Virus-like particles. "Adapted from Yang H. Ku/C&EN/Shutterstock"

in 2014 using TA-CD (succinyl norcocaine conjugated to a cholera toxin with an aluminium hydroxide adjuvant). In a phase II trial, subjects developed high anticocaine antibody titres initially, but these fell rapidly, and after 6 months, there was a high relapse rate (Martell et al., 2005). In a larger phase III trial of 300 subjects given five doses of TA-CD, outcomes were mixed, and even when high antibody titres were induced, they did not correspond to a significant reduction in cocaine use. The candidate vaccine dAd5GNE, which links a cocaine-like molecule (GNE) to a disrupted protein on an inactive adenovirus adjuvant, is currently in phase I clinical trials. Second-generation vaccines are exploring conjugation to nanofibres or the bacterial protein flagellin to boost the immune response, or co-administration of the vaccine with cocaine-degrading enzymes. Methamphetamines are cleared much more slowly than cocaine, and immunotherapy has thus focussed on mAbs, although active conjugated vaccines (such as succinyl methamphetamine conjugated to tetanus toxoid with the E6020 adjuvant) are in preclinical development.

Conclusions

The global burden of chronic diseases continues to grow alongside an ageing population and risk factors such as smoking, obesity and hypertension. With recent advances in our understanding of the immunological basis of chronic diseases and molecular biology technologies, the potential to adapt the vaccine concept to novel situations has become more feasible. Numerous preclinical and clinical proof-of-concept studies have demonstrated that autoimmune or allergen-directed responses are to some extent reversible, and that antibodies can be induced against key molecules identified as risk factors for dementia, hypertension or addiction. However, to date, no vaccines have been licenced for these diseases and many challenges remain. Suitable target antigens must be identified, bearing in mind safety issues and often high patient-to-patient variability in antigen reactivity. Antibodies induced must be of appropriate quality and quantity, and the dose, route and frequency of administration, as well as selection of carriers or adjuvants must be carefully optimized. The safe and effective targeting of self-antigens is particularly challenging in the context of an immune system that has evolved to avoid autoreactive responses; also, the quantity and affinity of antibody necessary for neutralization is considerably higher than required to protect against disease-causing pathogens. Given the growing financial burden noncommunicable chronic diseases place on healthcare systems, therapeutic vaccines offer a promising, affordable alternative to disease-modifying drugs. Acknowledgements: Figures were created with BioRender.com.

References

Brahmer, J., et al., *Nivolumab versus Docetaxel in Advanced Squamous-Cell Non-Small-Cell Lung Cancer.* N Engl J Med, 2015. 373(2): p. 123–35.

Carreno, B. M., et al., *Cancer immunotherapy. A dendritic cell vaccine increases the breadth and diversity of melanoma neoantigen-specific T cells.* Science, 2015. 348(6236): p. 803–8.

Cavenaugh, J. S., Awi, D., Mendy, M., Hill, A. V., Whittle, H., McConkey, S.J. Partially randomized, non-blinded trial of DNA and MVA therapeutic vaccines based on hepatitis B virus surface protein for chronic HBV infection. PLoS One. 2011 Feb 15;6(2):e14626. doi: 10.1371/journal.pone.0014626. PMID: 21347224; PMCID: PMC3039644.

Cohen, J. I. (2018). Vaccine development for Epstein–Barr virus. *Advances in Experimental Medicine and Biology*, 1045, 477–493.

Coventry, B. J. (2019). Therapeutic vaccination immunomodulation: Forming the basis of all cancer immunotherapy. *Therapeutic Advances in Vaccines and Immunotherapy*, 7, 2515135519862234.

Day, C. L., Kaufmann, D. E., Kiepiela, P., Brown, J. A., Moodley, E. S., Reddy, S., et al. (2006). PD-1 expression on HIV-specific T cells is associated with T-cell exhaustion and disease progression. *Nature*, 443(7109), 350–354.

Dendrou, C. A., Fugger, L., & Friese, M. A. (2015). Immunopathology of multiple sclerosis. *Nature Reviews Immunology*, 15, 545.

Friedmann, F. F., 1903, "Der Schildkrötentuberkelbacillus, seine Züchtung, Biologie und Pathogenität," DMW-Deutsche Medizinische Wochenschrift, 29(26), pp. 464–466.

Hartmann-Boyce, J., Cahill, K., Hatsukami. D., Cornuz. J. Nicotine vaccines for smoking cessation. Cochrane Database of Systematic Reviews 2012, Issue 8. Art. No.: CD007072. DOI: 10.1002/14651858.CD007072.pub2.

Herline, K., Drummond, E., & Wisniewski, T. (2018). Recent advancements toward therapeutic vaccines against Alzheimer's disease. *Expert Review of Vaccines*, 17(8), 707–721.

Hildesheim, A., Herrero, R., Wacholder, S., Rodriguez, A. C., Solomon, D., Bratti, M. C., et al. (2007). Effect of human papillomavirus 16/18 L1 virus-like particle vaccine among young women with preexisting infection: A randomized trial. *Journal of the American Medical Association*, 298(7), 743–753.

Hinshaw, D. C., & Shevde, L. A. (2019). The tumor microenvironment innately modulates cancer progression. *Cancer Research*, 79(18), 4557.

Huang, C. Y., & Hsieh, W. Y. (2017). Efficacy of *Mycobacterium vaccae* immunotherapy for patients with tuberculosis: A systematic review and meta-analysis. *Human Vaccines & Immunotherapeutics*, 13(9), 1960–1971.

Kantoff, P.W., et al., *Sipuleucel-T immunotherapy for castration-resistant prostate cancer.* N Engl J Med, 2010. 363(5): p. 411–22.

Kaufman, H.L., et al., *Phase II trial of Modified Vaccinia Ankara (MVA) virus expressing 5T4 and high dose Interleukin-2 (IL-2) in patients with metastatic renal cell carcinoma.* J Transl Med, 2009. 7: p. 2.

Koch R (1891) A further communication on a remedy for tuberculosis. BMJ 1(1568):125–127.

Mancini-Bourgine, M., Fontaine, H., Scott-Algara, D., Pol, S., Bréchot, C., Michel, M. L. Induction or expansion of T-cell responses by a hepatitis B DNA vaccine administered to chronic HBV carriers. Hepatology. 2004 Oct;40(4):874–82. doi: 10.1002/hep.20408. PMID: 15382173.

Martell, B. A., Mitchell, E., Poling, J., Gonsai, K., & Kosten, T. R. (2005). Vaccine pharmacotherapy for the treatment of cocaine dependence. *Biological Psychiatry*, 58(2), 158–164.

McMichael, A. J., & Rowland-Jones, S. L. (2001). Cellular immune responses to HIV. *Nature*, 410, 980.

Noon, L., 1911, "Prophylactic inoculation against hay fever," Lancet, pp. 1572–1573.

Ott, P.A., et al., *An immunogenic personal neoantigen vaccine for patients with melanoma.* Nature, 2017. 547(7662): p. 217–221.

Pancholi, P., Lee, D. H., Liu, Q., Tackney, C., Taylor, P., Perkus, M., Andrus, L., Brotman, B., Prince, A. M. (2001) DNA prime/canarypox boost-based immunotherapy of chronic hepatitis B virus infection in a chimpanzee. Hepatology 33:448–454.

Rosenberg, E.S., et al., Safety and immuno-genicity of therapeutic DNA vaccination in individuals treated with antiretroviral therapy during acute/early HIV-1 infection. PLoS One, 2010. 5(5): p. e10555

Schooley, R.T., et al., AIDS clinical trials group 5197: a placebo-controlled trial of immunization of HIV-1-infected persons with a replication-deficient adenovirus type 5 vaccine expressing the HIV-1 core protein. The Journal of infectious diseases, 2010. 202(5): p. 705–716.

Sekaly, R. P. (2008). The failed HIV Merck vaccine study: A step back or a launching point for future vaccine development? *Journal of Experimental Medicine*, 205(1), 7–12.

Sheehy, S. H., Duncan, C. J., Elias, S. C., Collins, K. A., Ewer, K. J., Spencer, A. J., et al. (2011). Phase Ia clinical evaluation of the *Plasmodium falciparum* blood-stage antigen MSP1 in ChAd63 and MVA vaccine vectors. *Molecular Therapy*, 19(12), 2269–2276.

Simons, J.W., et al., *Phase I/II trial of an allogeneic cellular immunotherapy in hormone-naive prostate cancer.* Clin Cancer Res, 2006. 12(11 Pt 1): p. 3394–401.

Tang, L. S. Y., Covert, E., Wilson, E., & Kottilil, S. (2018). Chronic Hepatitis B infection: A review. *Journal of the American Medical Association*, 319(17), 1802–1813.

Tissot, A. C., Maurer, P., Nussberger, J., Sabat, R., Pfister, T., Ignatenko, S., et al. (2008). Effect of immunisation against angiotensin II with CYT006-AngQb on ambulatory blood pressure: A double-blind, randomised, placebo-controlled phase IIa study. *The Lancet*, 371(9615), 821–827.

Trimble, C. L., Morrow, M. P., Kraynyak, K. A., Shen, X., Dallas, M., Yan, J., et al. (2015). Safety, efficacy, and immunogenicity of VGX-3100, a therapeutic synthetic DNA vaccine targeting human papillomavirus 16 and 18 E6 and E7 proteins for cervical intraepithelial neoplasia 2/3: A randomised, double-blind, placebo-controlled phase 2b trial. *The Lancet*, 386(10008), 2078–2088.

Valenta, R., Campana, R., Focke-Tejkl, M., & Niederberger, V. (2016). Vaccine development for allergen-specific immunotherapy based on recombinant allergens and synthetic allergen peptides: Lessons from the past and novel mechanisms of action for the future. *Journal of Allergy and Clinical Immunology*, 137(2), 351–357.

Weiss, S. A., Wolchok, J. D., & Sznol, M. (2019). Immunotherapy of melanoma: Facts and hopes. *Clinical Cancer Research*, 25(17), 5191–5201.

WHO. (2018). *Global tuberculosis report 2018*. Geneva: World Health Organization.

Willekens, B., & Cools, N. (2018). Beyond the magic bullet: Current progress of therapeutic vaccination in multiple sclerosis. *CNS Drugs*, 32(5), 401–410.

Zenewicz, L. A., & Shen, H. (2007). Innate and adaptive immune responses to *Listeria monocytogenes*: A short overview. *Microbes and Infection*, 9 (10), 1208–1215.

Chapter | **14** |

An introduction to drug development

Duncan B Richards, Raymond G Hill

Introduction

The development of a new medicine is a highly complex integrated process involving many disciplines. Within this complexity, however, there are four key decisions that are critical to success (Fig. 14.1). The first two are outlined in the preceding sections: the selection of the target and the identification of the molecule with which to prosecute against the target.

Drug development comprises all the activities involved in transforming a compound from drug candidate (the end-product of the discovery phase) to a product approved for marketing by the appropriate regulatory authorities. Traditional representations of the development process give the impression that this is a linear process like building a car, but this is false (Fig. 14.2). The risks of failure at all stages of development remain high. Only about 20% of drugs are successful in phase II—the most common reason for failure being a lack of or inadequate efficacy. A better way of thinking about development is to consider it in terms of a learning phase and a confirming phase. In simplest terms, phases I and II are learning and phase III should be confirming. For a traditional drug receptor target (e.g., beta blocker, H_2 antagonist), the endpoint in the phase II proof-of-concept study will be very similar to the registrational endpoint for phase III. In this setting, the distinction between learning and confirming is clear, and the translational risk between phase II and III is low—if it worked in phase II, it is likely to work in the larger study with the same endpoint in phase III. For many modern drug targets, however, the phase II endpoint is a surrogate clinical endpoint, and the link to the registrational endpoint is sometimes distant. For example, we have observed that inhibition of Lipoprotein-associated phospholipase A2 (Lp-PLA(2)) results in a reduction of interleukin (IL)-6 and hs-CRP- high sensitivity C-reactive protein

(hs-CRP) after 12 weeks, suggesting a possible reduction in inflammatory burden. Large-scale phase III studies, however, did not show a reduction in cardiovascular events. In these circumstances, we are 'learning' throughout the development process, and as a result, the probability of success is low.

The concept of learning and confirming is also helpful because is drives towards a question-based approach to development. The linear process model implies that the process is about generating larger and larger datasets until one has enough to seek registration. A traditional development plan with two replicate placebo-controlled phase III studies may look like this, but these types of plans are now the exception rather than the rule. Novel treatments for cancer and rare diseases may be approved on much smaller datasets, providing they adequately answer the questions that need to be addressed. An illustrative example of how these approaches differ is given in Table 14.1. The question-based approach directly influences the design of studies, ensuring that the data collected are relevant to the important questions. Every data point collected in the clinic is costly; if you do not know what you need to collect, the study will cost a fortune, and you may still not be able to answer critical development questions.

The nature of drug development

The development of novel medicines is one of the most complex tasks that we undertake, requiring a truly multidisciplinary approach to be successful. When someone mentions drug development, for many this means a series of clinical trials. The clinical components of the process are core but equally as important is the development of

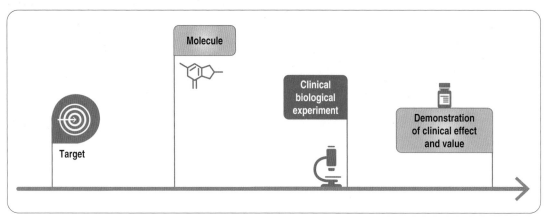

Fig. 14.1 Four key decisions in the development of a medicine.

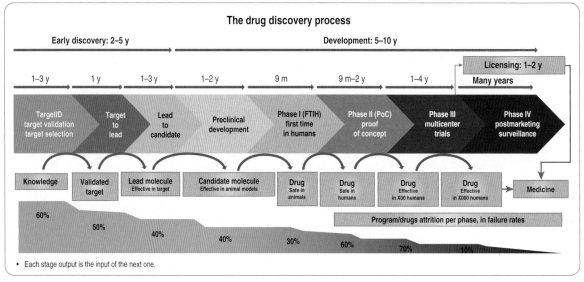

Fig. 14.2 A process-driven view of drug development.

Table 14.1 A data vs question-based approach to early drug development	
Data-driven approach	**Question-based approach**
• I have tested six doses at single dose and three doses on repeat dosing • I can describe the pharmacokinetics characteristics of the drug • The drug was 'safe and well tolerated' at the doses tested • The drug reduced cytokine concentrations in a challenge model	• I understand the exposure response relationship and can select a dose for further development • I have not observed any of the adverse events I was most concerned about based on the mechanism of action

the physical drug product. Success will only come when these two very different elements interdigitate effectively.

The heart of the drug development process is the project team. A multidisciplinary group comes together with the clear objective of developing a medicine for patients. Although this sounds obvious, it is fundamental to success. If individual departments within companies are left to prioritize work on their own, it is very unlikely these will line up in the best interests of the project. The project representative has a vital role as both champion but also as stern dispassionate critic when a molecule does not look like it will deliver. The costs associated with drug development are huge, and while a problem-solving approach is vital, it is also important that team members recognize when the profile is no longer viable and investment must stop.

In such a complex process, leadership is essential. No one in this complex process can be the content area expert on all aspects of the development process. Leadership in this setting is marked by an ability to set a clear vision for the project, and then align the multidisciplinary team around it to deliver. Many of these projects will have a budget of several hundred million pounds, and so there are many aspects of the role akin to that of a CEO of a medium-sized company.

While drug development is a journey of scientific exploration, it cannot be approached in a haphazard fashion. Effective and detailed project management is a vital skill. This is not simply a matter of setting out a good plan and ensuring everyone delivers their component. Every drug development project encounters the unexpected—a drug batch fails its specification, a new competitor enters the race, a new clinical safety signal; project management in this setting requires the anticipation of problems and the development of options to address emergent issues.

The work of the project team is multidisciplinary, but in terms of skills, there are three broad categories: *technical*, *investigative* and *managerial*:

- Technical skills—medicinal products must be of the highest quality. Delivering this requires the team to solve a wide range of technical issues. These include synthesis and formulation of the drug substance, developing appropriate packaging, developing a companion diagnostic to identify the target patient population and development of a novel imaging technique to measure the effect of the drug.
  - Main functions involved: chemical development, pharmaceutical development.
- Investigative skills—it is an inherent feature of the development of a novel therapeutic that efficacy and safety of the product is unknown. Establishing these requires investigative skills through a learning and confirming process to establish the profile of a new medicine and its place in the therapeutic pathway.
  - Main functions involved: safety pharmacology, toxicology, pharmacokinetics, clinical development.

- Managerial skills:
  - Coordination—drug development projects are large, multidisciplinary and complex. Progress depends on managing quality control, logistics, communication and decision-making.
  - Main function involved: project management.
  - Drug development is a highly regulated and expensive process involving treatments given to humans. A high standard of documentation of decision-making and risk management is mandatory. The ability to summarize and present information to oversight bodies, both internal and external (e.g., regulatory authorities) is essential.
  - Main function involved: regulatory affairs.

A critical element drawing these skills together is the vision for the medicine. This is a succinct description of the potential for the new medicine, the minimally acceptable profile, the base case and what an upside profile might look like. This should be a holistic view, not just the safety and efficacy profile but also the requirements for the drug product such as its presentation and shelf life. This is a vital document because the project team must continually refer to it as development progresses. There are numerous examples of projects that by the end of development are so far from the original expectation of the medicine that they are not commercially viable. For a commercial company this is the worst possible outcome— all the money for development has been spent, but there is little expectation of revenue.

At each stage of development, it is important to set clear go/no-go criteria. An approach based on 'show me the data and then I will decide' is open to unacceptable levels of bias. Time and again, it has been shown that in this situation, the 'believers' will always find the good in the data, and the 'detractors' will always find problems. Effective decision-making is much better done on the basis of pre-agreed criteria than the zeitgeist of the meeting on the day.

Components of drug development

Fig. 14.3 summarizes the main activities involved in developing a typical synthetic compound. It shows the main tasks that have to be completed before the compound can be submitted for regulatory approval, but needs to be translated into an operational plan (Fig. 14.4) that will allow the project to proceed as quickly and efficiently as possible. It is obvious that certain tasks have to be completed in a particular order. For example, a supply of pure compound, prepared in an acceptable formulation, has to be available before phase I clinical studies can begin. Animal toxicity data must also be available before the compound can be given to

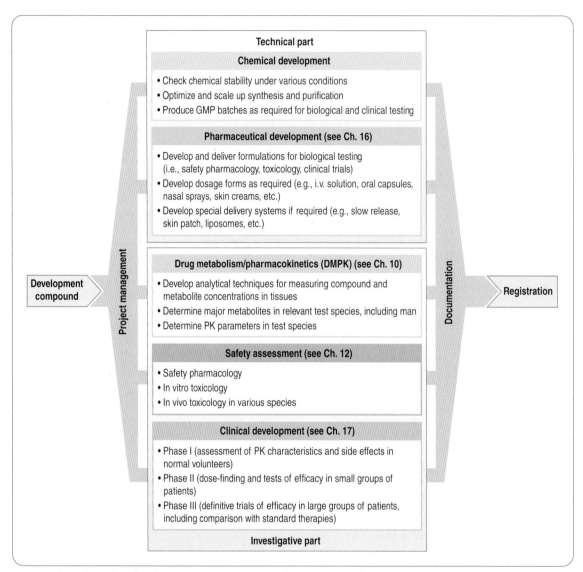

Fig. 14.3 The main technical and investigative components of a typical drug development project. *GMP*, Good manufacturing practice; *i.v.*, intravenous; *PK*, pharmacokinetics.

humans. Deciding on the dosage schedule to be used in efficacy trials requires knowledge of the pharmacokinetics and metabolism of the compound in humans. Because the data generated will be included in the final registration proposal, it is essential that each part of the work should be formally reported and 'signed off' by the group responsible and archived for future reference. It is important to recognize the difference between collection of sufficient data to make an internal decision to progress or not, and the standard required for

regulatory review. Regulators have a statutory obligation to ensure that their reviews are based on secure data, and the time required to quality check and report data should be incorporated into timelines. It is also naive to assume that all reviewing bodies will approve plans when first presented, time for discussion and debate should be incorporated into a realistic timeline. Most development plans are overoptimistic about the time taken to undertake development. Small companies with a fixed budget that do not plan for this may fail because

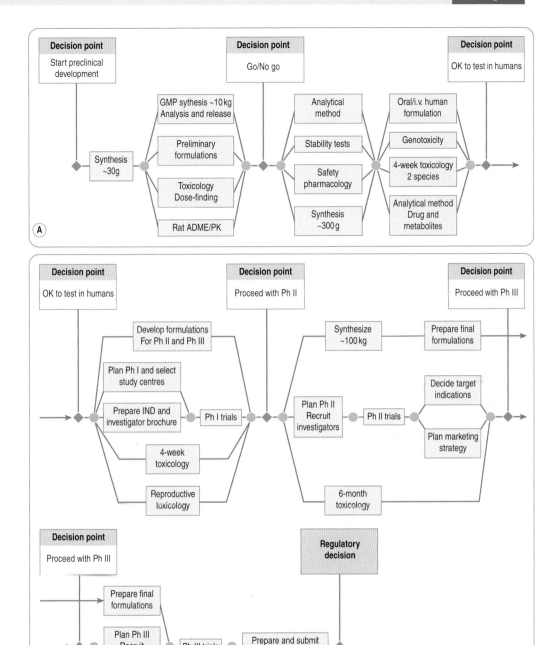

Fig. 14.4 Simplified flowchart showing the main activities involved in drug development. The nodes indicated by circles represent the start and finish points of each activity, and the diagram indicates which activities need to be completed before the next can begin. By assigning timescales to each activity, the planned overall development time can be determined and critical path activities identified. (A) Preclinical development. (B) Clinical development. *ADME*, Absorption, distribution, metabolism and excretion; *GMP*, good manufacturing practice; *IND*, investigational new drug; *i.v.*, intravenous; *Ph*, phase; *PK*, pharmacokinetics.

of unexpected delays, potentially denying patients access to useful medicines.

Fig. 14.4 is a much-simplified outline of a project plan of the development of a typical orally active drug. Each 'task', represented by an arrow, starts and ends at a circular symbol (representing an 'event'), and decision points are marked by diamond symbols. This type of graphical format, which is widely used as a project management tool and implemented in many commercially available software packages, is known as a PERT (project evaluation and review technique) chart. By assigning times—shortest possible, maximum and expected—to each task, the timing of the whole project can be assessed and the *critical path* identified. Critical path analysis is a vital component of drug development planning. Given the multifaceted nature of the process, it is important to know which deliverables will determine the overall progress. Some of these will be obvious—a clinical study cannot start if the drug product is not available, but others may be more subtle. For example, if a companion diagnostic is required, then it must be developed before pivotal (phase III) studies can start. In Fig. 14.4, the process has been reduced to a bare minimum to allow representation on a single page; in practice, each of the 'tasks' shown (e.g., develop formulations, perform phase I studies, etc.) needs to be further subdivided into a series of subtasks and timings to enable the project to be planned and monitored at the operational level. The complete diagram for a typical drug development project will be of such size and complexity as to frighten all but the most hardened project management professionals. Software tools, fortunately, are available which allow the project to be viewed in different ways, such as Gantt charts, which are bar charts set against a calendar timescale, showing the expected start and completion dates for each task, many of which will be running simultaneously on any given date.

In this section of the book, we outline the main technical and experimental parts of the work that go into drug development.

Patient safety is the first priority of anyone working in clinical research. The safety of medicines is not an absolute term but depends on two key factors: the context in which the drug is used and the benefit/risk balance for the condition for which it is used.

Vasoactive amines such as adrenaline and noradrenaline require critical care monitoring for their safe use; using them without very close monitoring of blood pressure and central venous pressure would be unsafe. On the other hand, some medicines (e.g., nonsteroidal antiinflammatory drugs [NSAIDs], H_2 antagonists) that were initially only available on prescription, can, now that enough is known about their adverse effects, be made available to consumers without prescription. In both cases, the safety profile of the drug is directly linked to the context in which it is used.

Benefit/risk is the single most important factor that regulators consider when licensing a medicine. Many of the early treatments for cancer (e.g., platinum-based chemotherapy) were associated with severe and common toxicities (e.g., bone marrow suppression, gastrointestinal tract toxicity). In the setting of a fatal condition with no alternative effective treatments, the benefit/risk was considered positive. Treatment for cancer has advanced substantially in the past 20 years, and in the context of the modern survival rates, a new treatment with a safety profile similar to early therapies would be unlikely to be considered to have a positive benefit/risk assessment now.

At the very earliest stages of drug development, benefit from treatment is an aspirational concept, and the protection of participants is of paramount importance. In Chapter 12, we have outlined the scheme for nonclinical assessment that has been developed largely to support the development of traditional (chemical) pharmaceuticals. The requirements for biological and advanced medicinal products are different and less well established. The collection and assimilation of clinical safety data are outlined in Chapter 15.

As has been outlined earlier, development of a drug requires both a package of nonclinical and clinical data relating to the actions of the drug but also development of the physical drug product. This is discussed in detail in Chapter 16.

Chapter 17 provides an overview of the clinical development process. Imaging is a particularly important tool in drug development, and its role and utility is discussed in Chapter 18.

Our current framework for discovery and development of new medicines is built on the basis of intellectual property protections (principally patents). This provides holders of patents with a period of exclusivity during which others cannot market the same product. These periods are strictly controlled and are controversial. To some, they stifle innovation by providing insufficient time to develop truly novel approaches, while to others, they are too long and allow companies to charge high prices for too long. This is a complex area and is discussed in Chapter 19.

The development and marketing of medicines is one of the most highly regulated spheres of business. Effective interactions with regulators and compliance with legal obligations are vital components of a successful development program. This is discussed in Chapter 20.

If you are successful and are granted a licence, then you may market your new medicine. This is also a highly regulated process and is discussed in Chapter 21.

Drug development has changed substantially in recent years, and in the final chapter, we look forward to the future and how it may continue to evolve.

The interface between discovery and development

For the purposes of this book, drug development is presented as an operation separate from discovery and following on from it, but the distinction is actually not clear-cut. As one moves into development, data will emerge that require a discovery-oriented evaluation in order to understand them completely. A traditional approach to discovery and development might involve the identification of an initial candidate molecule, but discovery efforts would continue to identify 'backup' molecules with enhanced potency and/or physicochemical properties. Drug development is now so expensive and time consuming that it is generally better to take additional time in the discovery process to ensure one has an optimized molecule than take forward multiple options. This is especially true for antibody development, where development of material suitable for testing in humans is especially complex and expensive. Follow-on molecules can be designed, but one needs to have a clear strategy as to what additional properties they will have or what problem with the lead they will address.

Decision points

The importance of continual reassessment of drug development projects has been emphasized earlier, but there are a number of points in the process where most companies undertake a formal detailed review, usually because these are linked to substantial investment inflection points.

The timing, nomenclature and decision-making process vary from company to company; the following is offered as a general guide:

- **Declaration of a candidate drug to progress into preclinical development studies.** In the schema outlined in Fig. 14.1, this is selection of the molecule. The discovery process is resource intensive, but throughout one has a number of options of molecules to progress. At candidate selection, one has to select a single molecule to progress and invest in. At this stage, there is an important balance between pharmacological and physicochemical properties of the molecule. In the past, pharmacological potency was prized over all other features, but many of these molecules proved not to be developable as medicines. In recent years, there has been much more focus on a balance of properties: sufficient potency but in the context of a molecule that has 'drug-like' properties, for example, soluble, low molecular weight.

The other key element reviewed at this point is the medicine vision and outline development plan. It is essential that there is agreement on the direction of travel even at this early stage, as changes can be expensive both in terms of time and resources.

- **Decision to progress into human studies.** The first human study is always a landmark for a potential new medicine. At this stage, the focus of the review is on safety. The preclinical package of pharmacology, safety pharmacology, toxicology and pharmacokinetics will be complete. It is important to ensure that the profile of the molecule remains consistent with the vision for its use in the clinic. This review will also consider the early clinical development plan to ensure that it will deliver a package of information that will be adequate to make the critical decision to commit to full development.

- **Commit to full development.** This is probably the single biggest decision in the development process. While the early development process activities may cost millions of pounds, the costs in full development are commonly measured in tens or hundreds of millions of pounds. The commit to full development review usually takes place after completion of the phase II clinical proof-of-concept study. It is essential therefore that the endpoints measured in this study provide for decision-making. Arriving at this point only to discover that the information does not support progression will introduce years of delay and substantial additional cost. This review will also scrutinize the full development plans in detail to ensure that they will deliver a package of information that will support a reimbursable medicine. This includes a detailed plan to deliver the physical drug product to the required quality.

- **Commit to file.** In an ideal world, this should be a simple decision: the phase III data show a favourable benefit/risk, and we have a robust quality drug project ready for the market. In reality, the decision is often more complex. Phase III data may show an important benefit, but with a safety signal that requires further evaluation, the drug product stability may not be what was desired, and competitors may have entered the frame with data that may displace your drug. At this stage, it is imperative to ensure that the data package really supports the medicine profile to be presented to regulators. The reputational and financial consequences of a failed marketing application are very substantial.

A couple of aphorisms are often applied to drug development, namely:

- In research, surprise = discovery; in development, surprise = disaster

- It is as valuable to stop a project as to carry one forward.

Like most aphorisms, they contain a grain of truth, but only a small one. With regard to the first, equating surprise with disaster applies, if at all, only to the technical parts of development, not to the investigational parts, which are, as discussed earlier, a continuation of research into the properties of the drug. Surprises in this arena can be good or bad for the outcome of the project. Finding, to the company's surprise, that sildenafil (Viagra) improved the sex life of trial subjects set the development project off in a completely new, and very successful, direction.

The value attached to stopping projects reflects the frustration—commonly felt in large research organizations—that projects that have little chance of ending in success tend to carry on, swallowing resources, through sheer inertia, sustained mainly by the reluctance of individuals to abandon work to which they may have devoted many years of effort. In practice, of course, the value of stopping a project depends only on the possibility of redeploying the resources to something more useful, that is, on the 'opportunity cost'. If the resources used cannot be redeployed, or if no better project can be identified, there is no value in stopping the project. What is certain is that it is only by carrying projects forward that success can be achieved. Despite the aphorism, it is no surprise that managers who regularly lead projects into oblivion achieve much less favourable recognition than those who bring them to fruition!

The need for improvement

The true cost of bringing a new medicine to market is difficult to estimate, as it a complex blend of the direct costs of that development plan and all the contemporary projects that have failed, but many estimates put this over $1 billion. This is directly reflected in the high prices of new medicines and hence limited availability. There are two principal drivers for the high cost of drug development: the low probability of success and the high cost of phase III studies. Every stage of the discovery and development process is associated with a degree of attrition (failure), but the transition from phase II to III has the lowest probability of success. Fewer than one in five medicines make it through this decision point. Drug safety remains an important reason for failure but the most common reason is a lack of or insufficient efficacy. This is an important area for research. It is vital that we ensure novel interventions are targeting processes that are important in the disease at the time we propose to intervene. The infrastructure surrounding phase III studies is not only extensive but fearsomely expensive. It is vital that we explore new ways to collect data on large numbers of patients without having to visit them individually and verify each data point manually. As healthcare records become digitized there is a real opportunity to use the routine medical record as the means to collect critical information rather than duplicate it with a complex and expensive trial data capture system.

Further reading

CDER's Regulatory Science Program Areas | FDA https://www.fda.gov/drugs/science-and-research-drugs/cders-regulatory-science-program-areas

Griffin, Posner and Barker 2013. The Textbook of Pharmaceutical Medicine, 7th Edition. London. BMJ books

Initiatives at CDER | FDA https://www.fda.gov/about-fda/center-drug-evaluation-and-research-cder/initiatives-cder#21centuryreview

Modernizing FDA's New Drugs Regulatory Program | FDA https://www.fda.gov/drugs/regulatory-science-research-and-education/modernizing-fdas-new-drugs-regulatory-program

Research and development | European Medicines Agency (europa.eu) https://www.ema.europa.eu/en/human-regulatory/research-development

Chapter | 15 |

Clinical assessment of safety

Duncan B Richards

Safety assessment in early clinical trials

All too often reports of early clinical trials conclude that the treatment was 'safe and well tolerated'. While ostensibly true, this type of statement fails to acknowledge the limitations of safety assessment in early clinical trials. These studies usually involve single-digit or low double-digit numbers of subjects given single doses or perhaps 2 weeks of dosing. It is simply not possible to draw definitive conclusions about the safety of a medicine based on this level of exposure. Nevertheless, early clinical studies are a vital step in the development of a new medicine and can provide important insights into two vital questions: (1) predictable dose-related adverse effects and (2) very common unexpected adverse effects.

A beta adrenoreceptor blocking drug would be expected to reduce heart rate in an exposure-related manner. A single-dose study in healthy subjects is an ideal opportunity to explore this in a safe manner avoiding excessive bradycardia. These studies are not, however, very informative about other risks. Not observing idiosyncratic liver toxicity in a first-in-human study is reassuring on one level, but given the small sample size, very little risk has been discharged and suitable attentiveness should be applied as the programme progresses.

The other kind of safety issue that can emerge in early studies is the very common but unexpected effect. In the worst case, this can manifest as severe adverse effects and potentially cause harm to participants. The worst disasters in early development have been associated with an incorrect or inadequate assessment of the potential for either on- or off-target effects in humans. While ostensibly unpredictable, these are in fact potentially predictable, and rigorous assessment of pharmacology as a basis for dose selection in early studies represents the most important means by which participants can be kept safe. This is further elaborated in the following section.

An approach to subject safety in early clinical studies

Keeping participants safe in early clinical studies rests on two fundamental principles: a thorough assessment of the properties of the molecule and the design of the study.

The selection of starting dose and dose range to be explored is a key decision in early clinical development. From a safety perspective, the principal considerations are laid out in Table 15.1.

Study design

The Tegenero disaster in which participants in a first-in-human study with a CD28 superagonist antibody suffered significant harm as a result of cytokine storm, highlighted the common practice of dosing participants at the same time or at short intervals. The Duff Report recommended the use of sentinel dosing in which a pair of subjects, one on active treatment and one on placebo, are dosed ahead of the rest of the cohort. This is an important means to avoid exposing large numbers of participants to an inappropriately large dose of drug, but it is also important to stagger subsequent dosing as less dramatic adverse effects may become apparent and sufficient time to assess and adapt should be built into the design. Overlapping repeat dose cohorts may confer a modest time saving, but remember that an emergent issue in one cohort has the potential to disrupt progression of all other cohorts if they overlap. Very few early development studies progress without any issue, and ensuring the design includes sufficient time to accommodate assessment of emergent issues can avoid time-consuming temporary halts.

Table 15.1 Risk assessment for first-in-human studies

	Question	Example
On-target pharmacology	Is the target itself associated with predictable risks?	Might the action of the drug result in cytokine release?
Off-target pharmacology	How selective is the drug? Has a screen for off-target effects been conducted? What are the relative concentrations at which desired pharmacology and off-target effects are seen? Is there an anticipated therapeutic index?	An antihistamine drug that blocks hERG potassium channels at therapeutic concentrations may induce ventricular arrhythmias
Safety pharmacology findings in animals	Cardiovascular, respiratory and neurological studies are standard but consider if this target or drug requires any specific studies.	Changes in heart rate are easy to measure in the clinic, but complex neurological effects may be more subtle and require specialist investigations
Toxicology findings in animals	What are the principal toxicities? Do you understand why they may occur? Are the effects reversible/avoidable, and can they be monitored in humans?	A dose-related reduction in haemoglobin is straightforward to monitor. Irreversible heart valve fibrosis is nearly impossible to monitor in the clinic, and if it were to occur, could cause lasting harm. A finding such as this may well preclude human studies.
Potential for drug–drug interactions	Consider whether the test drug could be a perpetrator or victim. How likely are the interacting drugs to be used by the target patient population?	Studies in healthy volunteers can usually avoid concomitant medication, but this simply defers the problem. If a potential interacting drug is very likely to be used in the target population (e.g., oral contraceptive pill in female patients with migraine), then an early study may be required to make patient studies practicable.
Potential for drug–disease interactions	This is less commonly considered but is of increasing importance as polypharmacy and combination therapy becomes commonplace. Is there a reason why patients may be more susceptible to the effects of a drug?	Patients with pulmonary arterial hypertension may be more susceptible to the systemic effects of a vasodilator given for their pulmonary arterial disease.

Achieving a balance between prudent and frequent safety assessments and burden on participants is a key challenge in early studies. Measuring everything all of the time is likely to generate spurious signals and likely to render the study impractical. Careful consideration of the time course of potential adverse effects is likely to be informative: direct effects on cardiac ion channels are most likely to manifest around the maximum drug concentration, while effects on the liver are likely to take at least 24–48 hours to become apparent. It is also important to distinguish between investigations that are useful in detecting adverse drug reactions (ADRs) and those that are most informative once a potential signal has been detected. For example, the ECG is a helpful screening tool for adverse cardiac effects, while cardiac MRI is most useful when deployed in those in whom a potential signal has been detected.

Phase II

Participants in clinical studies report adverse events. As development proceeds, patterns may emerge that indicate that the study drug is responsible, either because the adverse event is demonstrably more common or severe in treated subjects or because one has an increased index of suspicion based on preclinical findings. Once a causal link with the study drug is considered plausible, these events are termed ADRs. It is usually during phase II that ADRs start to be identified. Once they have been identified, it is important to take a structured approach to their evaluation and to plan how to collect more information in order to support registration.

ADR questions:

- How common is the ADR?
- Are there subpopulations that are at greater risk?
- Are there circumstances in which the event is particularly severe? Are there people who should not receive the drug? Can these people be identified prior to treatment?
- How should the ADR be treated?
- If the ADR occurs what should happen about giving the study drug? If a subject experiences this event, should they be excluded from ever receiving the drug again?

It is important to ask these questions early because, in some cases, they may require additional studies or alteration to the design of other clinical studies in order to address them adequately. In addition to the identified risks, at this stage of development, there are likely to be a number of potential risks, and a plan should be formulated to establish how these can be discharged or evaluated. For example, the potential for reproductive toxicity may not be known at this stage. When should reproductive toxicology studies be conducted? Are they needed for the phase III programme or only in time for registration? Failure to plan can mean substantial delays if oversight bodies such as regulatory authorities do not agree with your proposed risk management plans. As drug development progresses, the inclusion criteria for study participants are usually widened. This usually means that more complex patients often with substantial comorbidities will be included. Assessment of potential risks will help identify those subjects who should not be included. Phase II studies are a particular opportunity to look for adverse effects associated with abrupt withdrawal of the drug, as treatment is usually for a defined period of time.

It is important to collect as much contemporaneous information about emergent adverse events as they happen. It can be very difficult or even impossible to collect additional information after time has passed. Try to obtain as much objective information as possible, as the clinical significance of some information may only become apparent after other events have been reported. One approach is to identify certain adverse events as being of special interest. These will be flagged as soon as they are reported, facilitating contemporaneous collection of follow-up information. Structured questionnaires can be a helpful way to ensure consistent collection of detailed information. Many sponsors will also put in place special procedures for rapid assessment of specific events that are particularly associated with drugs (e.g. hypersensitivity, liver failure, seizures), whether or not these are reported as serious adverse events (SAEs).

Documentation and review

As development progresses, information relating to the drug and its target will emerge from nonclinical studies, clinical studies and the literature. This information should be summarized and reviewed in a living document that is regularly updated. This will contain information on potential and identified risks for the drug. For each of these, a plan should be made outlining how the risk can be better understood. This may involve, for example, mechanistic studies, additional nonclinical studies and literature reviews. Once a risk becomes identified, that is, there is evidence it is real, then it should be included in the development core safety information. This has a structure similar to the summary of product characteristics (SPC) and summarizes what is known about the safety of the drug in development. This information is also included in the investigator's brochure. This is important because it becomes the reference safety information used to determine whether an adverse event is expected or not. Events that are serious, suspected to be related to the drug and unexpected (suspected unexpected serious adverse reactions [SUSARs]), must be reported to regulatory authorities on an expedited basis (see later). Early in development, when information is limited, regulators may ask for serious events to be reported on the expedited basis even when they have been observed before in order to gain a better understanding of the incidence.

Serious adverse events

In drug development, the term serious adverse event (SAE) carries a specific definition. It is any untoward medical occurrence that results in death, is life-threatening, requires inpatient hospitalization or causes prolongation of existing hospitalization, results in persistent or significant disability/incapacity or may have caused a congenital anomaly/birth defect. There is a final category usually described as 'medically serious'; typically these would be events that required intervention to prevent permanent impairment or damage. The investigator is charged with making the assessment of whether an adverse event is an SAE based on these criteria. SAEs should be reported to the sponsor within 24 hours of becoming aware of the event, usually by means of an electronic or faxed paper form. The investigator is required to use their best judgement to assess causality, that is, whether they consider the event may be related to the drug or not. This is often difficult as information is limited, but an assessment is important because there are specific rules for reporting certain kinds of SAEs. A SUSAR must be reported to regulatory authorities and ethics committees within 7 days of the sponsor becoming aware of it; follow-up information should be provided within a further 8 days. These regulations have been put in place because these types of events can require the study to be stopped or amended, and it is important the information is acted upon as quickly as possible. Expectedness is another term that has a specific meaning in this setting. Only those events that are in the reference safety information (in the investigator's brochure) for a drug can be considered 'expected'.

Mechanistic investigation of adverse drug reactions

Careful description and documentation of ADRs is important to inform investigators and patients about risk, but it is increasingly important to also have a mechanistic understanding. The traditional classification of ADR identified two broad types:

- Type A—Reactions that are predictable from the drug's known pharmacology and typically result from an augmented on-target pharmacological response when given at a usual therapeutic dose.
- Type B—Reactions that are also termed idiosyncratic and are not predictable from the known pharmacological actions of the drug. These are typically rare, and safety signals are often not detected prior to marketing.

A key insight of the past 20 years has been that genetics play an important role in both types. It has been recognized for some time that polymorphisms in enzymes metabolizing drugs can alter exposure and hence pharmacology (Table 15.2). More recently, it has been observed that a high proportion of type B reactions have an immune basis, and these can be linked to particular

Table 15.2 Pharmacogenetic tests

Genetic target	Drug	Clinical relevance
HLA-B*5701	Abacavir	Severe hypersensitivity reactions to abacavir are linked to the HLA-B*5701 allele, present in up to about 10% of potential patients; avoidance of abacavir in patients with this allele markedly reduces the risk of such reactions
HLA-B*1502	Carbamazepine	Dangerous or even fatal skin reactions associated with carbamazepine are significantly more common in patients (almost exclusively with Asian ancestry) with HLA-B*1502; screen patients with ancestry from this region before starting carbamazepine, and avoid using it in those with the HLA-B*1502 allele
VKORC1/CYP2C9	Warfarin	Variants in the gene encoding vitamin K [ep]oxide reductase complex 1 (VKORC1), an enzyme complex that recycles reduced vitamin K, are associated with resistance to warfarin; patients with variants of the CYP2C9 enzyme responsible for metabolism of warfarin require much lower doses; together with age and sex, these variables explain 50% of the variation in warfarin dosage requirements
CYP2C19	Voriconazole	CYP2C19 is a polymorphically expressed enzyme, and 2.2% of the Caucasian population are poor metabolizers, who have a threefold increase in exposure to voriconazole and therefore an increased risk of adverse effects
CYP2D6	Thioridazine (withdrawn in UK)	Exposure to thioridazine is related to the number of functional CYP2D6 genes (1–3)
TPMT	Azathioprine	One in 10 of the population is heterozygous for a polymorphism that halves the activity of thiopurine methyltransferase (TPMT); 1 in 300 are homozygous and at severe risk of marrow suppression; measure TPMT activity before starting treatment; treatment with low-dose azathioprine in heterozygotes is safe and highly effective; very low doses of azathioprine (5 mg on alternate days) may be an option in homozygous deficiency
G6PD	Sulfonamides, quinolone antibiotics, most antimalarial drugs	Patients with G6PD deficiency are at increased risk of haemolytic anaemia
UGT1A1*28	Irinotecan	The (UGT1A1)*28 polymorphism reduces UGT1A1 enzyme activity (and is associated with a raised pretreatment bilirubin concentration); patients who take the usual dose are at risk of severe toxicity (neutropenia, diarrhoea); dosage reduction to account for reduced enzyme activity does not seem to adversely affect the therapeutic response
SLCO1B1	Statins	The risk of rhabdomyolysis is increased in individuals with the SLCO1B1 variant of a gene coding for an organic anion-transporting polypeptide (OATP) that regulates hepatic uptake of statins; this is too rare to be useful as a predictive test

human leucocyte antigen (HLA) genetic loci within the major histocompatibility complex region on chromosome 6. The best known of these is the association between HLA-B*57:01 and abacavir hypersensitivity. Implementation of HLA testing prior to administration of the drug has substantially reduced the incidence of severe skin reactions such as Stevens–Johnson syndrome. This is important because it allows prescribers to avoid a drug in those with elevated risk but also means that a useful drug is still available to those at low risk. An inability to identify those patients who should not receive a drug may lead to it being withdrawn and so unavailable to all. In some cases, the risk may not be linked to a single polymorphism, and there is extensive ongoing work to harness the power of genomic technology to manage the risk of ADRs.

Phase III studies

The profile of common ADRs is derived from an integrated analysis across all studies, usually comparing the incidence in those given the study drug with placebo. Because the phase III studies usually involve by far the largest number of subjects, they are the principal source of the safety profile that is presented in the initial prescribing information for a new drug. It is important to remember, however, that the information collected in the registration programme for a drug will only likely pick up the most common ADRs (Table 15.3).

By the time of seeking a licence, it is necessary to be able to speak cogently about how to use the drug safely in the different populations in which it may be used. Early in development, it may well be appropriate to exclude those about whom there is insufficient information (e.g., women of childbearing potential) or who are considered at increased risk (e.g., those with renal impairment), but as development proceeds this is no longer appropriate. Regulators will expect information to guide prescribing in all the patient groups likely to be given the drug. The

kind of information that needs to be provided needs to be carefully considered. For example, a short-term study in subjects with varying degrees of renal impairment to inform the need for dose adjustment may be adequate for a drug that is principally aimed at patients who are otherwise well with limited comorbidity. If, however, the target patient population includes 30% with renal impairment, the same study would probably not be adequate, as more information on the benefit/risk in these patients would be expected. This would probably need to be addressed by ensuring that the phase III registration studies include a sufficient proportion of patients with renal impairment to conduct an assessment.

Assessing benefit/risk

Benefit/risk should be assessed throughout the development programme as new information emerges, but it takes on critical importance at the time of registration. The simplest method is to tabulate the benefits and risks on the same page. Combined with a numerical presentation of relative risk, this can provide a helpful assessment. The most common approach is to present the benefit and safety measures with their 95% confidence intervals (forest plot). While this approach is helpful in many cases, it has its limitations, especially when the benefits and risks are very different in nature or incidence. For example, a treatment has a moderate symptomatic benefit in 50% of those treated but is associated with a severe adverse effect in 1% of those treated. In this case, there will be a particular imperative to identify markers or characteristics of the 1% who are at elevate risk and who should probably not receive the drug.

More sophisticated methods may be employed in these situations. A clinical utility index is an approach that combines a benefit and a risk outcome into a single metric by using a utility function. To derive this, the project team will consider each combination of benefit and risk (e.g., cure rate versus incidence of adverse effects) and ascribe a weight to each. This can then be used to define a minimally acceptable

Table 15.3 Number of subjects required to observe less frequent adverse drug reactions			
Incidence of adverse drug reaction	**NUMBER OF PARTICIPANTS REQUIRED[a] TO OBSERVE**		
	1 Event	**2 Events**	**3 Events**
1 in 100	300	480	650
1 in 200	600	960	1,300
1 in 1000	3,000	4,800	6,500
1 in 10,000	30,000	48,000	65,000
[a]95% chance of detecting.			

utility value that would support progression. The choice of weight involves clinical judgement and expert evaluation and requires substantial team discussion. Multiple outcomes can be combined in techniques such as multi-criteria decision analysis (MCDA). In this case, the judgement of decision makers is elicited independently, and then combined. Importantly, this kind of approach can include the views of patients which are often absent from other approaches. Bayesian methods are increasingly, applied using these types of approach to continually update the benefit–risk assessment as development proceeds and more information becomes available. This can inform decision making and identify those projects for which the proposition has drifted to a point that is no longer viable.

The summary of product characteristics

Following a successful marketing application, the most tangible output of the tens of thousands of pages of trial data, reports and so on is the SPC, a succinct document usually only two to three pages long that provides the essential information for use of the drug. A lot of the information in the SPC directly relates to the safe use of the drug (Table 15.4).

In the United States, the SPC is known as the 'drug label'.

Table 15.4 Safety information in the summary of product characteristics

SPC heading	Safety information
Therapeutic indication	Drug should only be used for their indicated populations, as these are the ones in which benefit/risk has been judged to be positive. This section should include a statement on the age range of indicated patients. There is specific legislation and procedures in places aimed at improving the quality of information generated for children, as this has often been missing.
	If a specific test is required (e.g., genotyping) it should be stated here.
Posology and method of administration	Benefit/risk can absolutely depend on dose and duration of treatment. Furthermore, some treatments require titration when initiating or discontinuing. This information should be summarized here along with any special instructions for administration, for example, time of day, with or without food, need for any premedication or any precautionary equipment that should be immediately available.
	Dose adjustments for special populations such as those with renal or hepatic impairment should be given here.
Contraindications	The contraindication section should be based on data, an absence of information would not normally lead to a contraindication. This section should be as precise as possible when defining the characteristics of patients who should not receive the drug. Some drugs and treatments should not be given together, and this should be stated here.
Special warnings and precautions for use	This is an important section but difficult to get right because it describes situations in which there is uncertainty or a lack of specific information. Phrases such as 'use with caution' are not helpful to the prescriber, as they do not describe a particular course of action. Clear instructions such as 'liver function should be monitored before initiation of treatment and monthly thereafter' are much more helpful, especially when they include specific criteria that should lead to cessation of the drug or a reduction in dose.
	This section should also include information if the drug interferes with any laboratory tests.
Interaction with other medicinal products and other forms of interaction	This section should describe clinically important interactions. This is important because some drugs change the concentration of others, but this does not have important consequences. Simply describing the change in plasma concentrations does not help the prescriber.
	Drug–drug interactions are the most common in this section, but drug–disease interactions can be clinically important and should be stated.

Table 15.4 Safety information in the summary of product characteristics—cont'd

SPC heading	Safety information
Fertility, pregnancy and lactation	In many cases, the information in this section will be largely derived from preclinical studies, as direct human data are usually sparse. Recommendations on the use of the medicinal product in women of childbearing potential should be given when appropriate, including the need for pregnancy test or contraceptive measures. Drugs are generally best avoided during pregnancy and lactation, but it is important to provide as much information to guide the prescriber when treatment may be necessary.
Effects on ability to drive and use machines	For some drugs for which a particular risk has been identified, a specific driving assessment study may be required.
Undesirable effects	This should be a summary table of adverse drug reactions associated with the drug, usually presented as a table by system organ class. The ADRs listed should be those for which there is plausible evidence of causality; a laundry list of all reported events is of little help to the prescriber or patient. This section should include an assessment of frequency. The frequency categories are somewhat broad (very common [$\geq 1/10$]; common [$\geq 1/100$ to $< 1/10$]; uncommon [$\geq 1/1000$ to $< 1/100$]; rare [$\geq 1/10,000$ to $< 1/1000$]; very rare [$<1/10,000$]), and the assessment early in a drug's life is likely to be imprecise.
	This section usually undergoes regular updates in the early postmarketing years.
	Important or serious ADRs should also be described and, whenever possible, guidance provided on how to avoid, minimize or treat the reaction.
Overdose	There is usually relatively little specific information on overdose and even less commonly a specific antidote, but if these are available, they should be stated here.
Pharmacological properties	These sections should succinctly summarize key information on the mechanism of action, pharmacokinetic and pharmacodynamics properties. This section will usually include a very brief summary of the key clinical efficacy data.
	Clinically relevant preclinical findings should be summarized here (e.g., reproductive toxicology studies).
Pharmaceutical particulars	This contains important information for safe use of the product, including a list of excipients (some patients may be allergic to some of these), shelf life, storage conditions and arrangements for safe disposal.

ADRs, Adverse drug reactions; *SPC,* summary of product characteristics.

Postmarketing surveillance

For most drugs, it is only in the postmarketing environment that the true safety profile of a drug becomes apparent. As part of the licensing process, the sponsor will be expected to propose how they propose to monitor and assess each identified risk in the postmarketing setting. The product label (SPC) is the principal means by which safety information is provided to prescribers. Patients receive a patient information leaflet and in jurisdictions such as the EU, there is a requirement to show that this has been tested for readability. In some cases, the routine information may not be considered sufficient, and the marketing authorization holder will be expected to provide additional educational materials for patients and prescribers. These must not be promotional in nature and

must be approved by regulatory authorities. For each new medicinal product, the sponsor has to submit a risk management plan at the time of licensing. This outlines how they plan to manage the major risks associated with the product and plans to address incomplete or missing information relating to the product. An important component of a risk management plan is a plan to assess the effectiveness of risk minimization or management plans. Well-intentioned but ineffective measures should be identified and modified.

Routine pharmacovigilance

During the development process, the sponsor organization is responsible for monitoring, analysing and acting upon safety signals. In this phase, the data come almost entirely from clinical trials. In the postmarketing environment, the sponsor retains these responsibilities, but in addition, regulatory authorities have responsibilities to collate and assess information that is provided to them. This is important because these authorities have access to information on drugs in the same class and therefore have the opportunity to identify safety signals that are not apparent from examination of the profile of one product.

'Routine pharmacovigilance' is the base case for monitoring products in the market, but for most new products, additional measures will be required. The marketing authorization holder is required to set up a pharmacovigilance system to enable them to receive spontaneous safety reports, as well as from ongoing clinical trials. Investigator-sponsored trials are more common once a drug comes to market and can be an important source of safety information; companies are expected to put in place proactive arrangements to receive safety information from these studies, not just ones they are sponsoring themselves. Spontaneously reported safety information can be an important source of rare adverse events, but the quality of the information supplied can be highly variable making assessment challenging.

A yearly 'periodic safety update report' (PSUR) is required in the EU (similar information is also required by the US Food and Drug Administration [FDA]) for all marketed medicines and drugs in active development. This contains important contextual information such as number of people exposed to the drug and the status of ongoing and completed trials, but in addition, it is expected to include a thoughtful and data-driven assessment of benefit/risk. This should summarize and synthesize new information (including any nonclinical data) that impacts benefit/risk. Sponsors are expected to be proactive about measures to mitigate or manage newly identified risks rather than waiting to be instructed by regulators. For example, if new data indicate that some patients are at increased risk, then there should be a plan to update the SPC with either a warning or contraindication as appropriate.

There is specific (EU) legislation relating to the systems for pharmacovigilance to ensure that companies are collecting, analysing and acting upon emergent safety date in a rigorous and auditable manner.

Managing identified risks

In some cases, simply informing the patient and prescriber is sufficient to manage and mitigate a risk. For example, being informed that a drug may cause a mild nonserious headache for the first few days of treatment may be enough to allow patients and prescribers to deal with it

appropriately. When the SPC requires a specific course of action, for example, to measure liver function tests at baseline and 6 weeks after starting treatment, then a company may be required to conduct an assessment of whether this is really happening in practice and to establish whether it prevents patients from developing hepatic impairment. This is not a typical clinical trial, but the information is important; sponsors have to consider innovative ways to collect this information. Registries have been a popular method, but these can be cumbersome and expensive, particularly when there are several products each requiring physicians to input information to a specific database. In recent years, there has been a particular focus on the use of routinely collected health data from hospitals and general practices as a means to have a more comprehensive and less onerous approach. There are complex issues relating to the use of routine health data by commercial entities, but these must be solved in the interests of patients and public health.

Missing or incomplete information

At the time of marketing, the understanding of the safety profile of most medicines is rudimentary; there is both a need for more information and in many cases specific information relating to particular risks or patient subgroups. It is usually a condition of marketing approval that an agreed list of studies/investigations will be undertaken by the sponsor. These may include measures of efficacy, for example, a drug may be authorized on the basis of an intermediate clinical endpoint but then an outcome study will be required postmarketing, but most related to studies. Postapproval safety studies (PASSs) are a formal arrangement between a company and the regulatory authority. The questions will be defined at licensing, the sponsor is then required to submit proposals as to how they will address the questions. These may be specific interventional studies (for example, a specific drug interaction study) or observational (for example, monitoring safety in those with moderate renal impairment). The progress of these studies must be tracked with the regulator, especially if changes are required, and failure to comply or make progress with these commitments can lead to withdrawal of marketing authorization. There is an increasing focus in this area that these investigations should reflect the 'real world'. The safety profile in patients in a tertiary referral specialist unit already familiar with the drug because they conducted the clinical trials may be very different from a centre where follow-up is devolved to the patient's family doctor. Again, this is an area where use of routine health record data has the potential to be transformational in terms of the scope and quality of information collected.

Further reading

Carr, D., & Pirmohamed, M. (2018). Biomarkers of adverse drug reactions. *Experimental Biology and Medicine (Maywood, NJ), 243*(3), 291–299.

EMA. *EMA guidance on good pharmacovigilance practice.* Retrieved from https://www.ema.europa. eu/en/human-regulatory/post-authorisation/pharmacovigilance/good-pharmacovigilance-practices.

EMA. *EMA guidance on pharmacovigilance.* Retrieved from https://www.ema. europa.eu/en/documents/leaflet/ pharmacovigilance_en.pdf.

Santoro, A., Genov, G., Spooner, A., Raine, J., & Arlett, P. (2017). Promoting and protecting public health: How the European Union pharmacovigilance system works. *Drug Safety, 40*(10), 855–869.

Yip, V., Alfirevic, A., & Pirmohamed, M. (2015). Genetics of immune-mediated adverse drug reactions: a comprehensive and clinical review. *Clinical Reviews in Allergy & Immunology, 48*(2–3), 165–175.

Chapter | **16** |

Pharmaceutical development

Kendall G Pitt

Introduction

Active pharmaceutical ingredients (APIs) in pharmaceutical products must be formulated into dosage forms suitable for handling, distribution and administration to patients. Common dosage forms are tablets and capsules, liquids for injection, oral inhalers, patches for transdermal administration and semisolids for dermal application. Development of dosage forms is complex, involving several stages and areas of expertise. The chemical and physicochemical properties of the drug substance are characterized in the preformulation phase. This information serves together with knowledge about the disease, intended doses and preferred route of administration, as the starting point for formulation development. Stability of the drug substance is also a key outcome of the preformulation phase. Impurities and degradation products must be identified and quantified. Hence analytical pharmaceutical chemistry methods also need to be developed and are crucial for successful formulation development. Subsequently, both mean assay and uniformity of content in unit dosage forms are vital to assure that the patient is treated with the correct dose. Similarly, release and dissolution of the APIs from the intended dosage form will need to be assessed to assure drug delivery.

This chapter describes the principal steps involved in pharmaceutical development. It is mainly illustrated with the examples of tablets and capsules, as formulation of these dosage forms contains most of the steps involved in any development. Development of solutions for injection/infusion or other sterile dosage forms are not specifically discussed in this chapter but are referred to when appropriate.

Preformulation studies

Various physical and chemical properties of the drug substance need to be investigated as a starting point to developing dosage forms. These investigations are termed *preformulation studies*. Most synthetic drugs are either weak bases (~75%) or weak acids (~20%) and will generally need to be formulated as salts for stability or solubility reasons. Salts of a range of acceptable conjugate acids or bases therefore need to be prepared and tested. Intravenous formulations of relatively insoluble compounds may need to include nonaqueous solvents or emulsifying agents. The compatibility of the APIs with commonly used excipients that are included in tablets or capsules, as well as with any parenteral additives will need to be assessed.

The main components of preformulation studies are:

- Development of a suitable spectroscopic assay method for determining concentration and purity
- Determination of solubility and dissolution rates of parent compound and salts in water and other solvents
- Chemical stability of parent compound and salts in solution and solid state
- Determination of pK_a and pH dependence of solubility and chemical stability
- Determination of lipophilicity (i.e., oil/water partition coefficient, expressed as K_d)
- Determination of particle size and shape, melting point and suitability for potential milling or other particle size reduction techniques
- Characterizations of importance for the dosage forms of choice, for example, bulk density, powder flow and compression properties.

Theoretical treatments of these molecular properties, and laboratory methods for measuring them, which are beyond the scope of this book, are described in textbooks such as Aulton (2018) or Tovey (2018). The following are some issues that commonly arise in drug development.

Solubility and dissolution rate

The question of solubility, already emphasized in Chapters 7 and 10, is particularly important in relation to the development of pharmaceutical formulations. It is measured by determining the concentration of the compound in solution after equilibration—usually after several hours of stirring—with the pure solid. In general, compounds whose aqueous solubility exceeds 10 mg/mL present no problems with formulation (Kaplan, 1972). The biopharmaceutics classification system (BCS) (Amidon et al., 1995) and the developability classification system (DCS) (Butler & Dressman, 2010) are valuable tools in classifying oral drugs for their likely absorption in humans based on their dose, solubility and intestinal permeability. Compounds with lower solubility may require conversion to salts, or the addition of nonaqueous solvents to achieve satisfactory oral absorption. The inclusion of a miscible solvent of relatively low polarity, such as 20% propylene glycol or some other biocompatible solubilizing agent, will often be required for preparing injectable formulations. This is because the extreme pH values needed to induce ionization of very weak acids or bases are likely to cause tissue damage. Complications may arise with oral formulations if the solubility is highly dependent on pH, because of the large pH difference between the stomach and the small intestine. Gastric pH can range from near neutrality in the absence of any food stimulus to acid secretion, to pH 1–2, whereas the intestinal pH is around 8. Basic substances that dissolve readily in the stomach can therefore precipitate in the intestine and so be poorly absorbed. Compounds that can exist in more than one crystal form, such as polymorphs, can also show complex behaviours. The different lattice energies of molecules in the different crystal forms mean that the intrinsic solubility of the compound is also different. Different crystal forms may correspond to different hydration states of the compound, so that a solution prepared from the unhydrated solid may gradually precipitate as hydrated crystals. An important aspect of preformulation studies is selecting the best salt to avoid these complications and to maintain chemical stability.

Compounds that have low intrinsic solubility in aqueous media can often be brought into solution by the addition of a water-miscible *solubilizing agent*, such as polysorbates, ethanol or polyethylene glycol (PEG).

Preformulation studies may therefore include the investigation of various solubilizing or stabilizing agents, such as methylcellulose or cyclodextrin.

In addition to intrinsic solubility, *dissolution rate* is important in determining the rate of absorption of an oral drug. The process of dissolution involves two steps: (a) the transfer of molecules from the solid to the immediately adjacent layer of fluid, known as the *boundary layer* and (b) escape from the boundary layer into the main reservoir of fluid, which is known as the *bulk phase* and is assumed to be well stirred so that its concentration is uniform. Step (a) is invariably much faster than step (b), so the boundary layer quickly reaches saturation. The overall rate of dissolution is limited by step (a) and depends on the intrinsic solubility of the compound, the diffusion coefficient of the solute, the surface area of the boundary layer and the geometry of the path leading from boundary layer to the bulk phase.

In practice, dissolution rates depend mainly on:

- Intrinsic solubility (since this determines the boundary layer concentration)
- Molecular weight (which determines diffusion coefficient)
- Drug particle size and dispersion of the solute (which determine the surface area of the boundary layer and the length of the diffusion path).

In pharmaceutical development, dissolution rates are often manipulated intentionally by including different polymers, such as methylcellulose into tablets or capsules, to produce 'slow-release' formulations of drugs, allowing once-daily dosage despite the drug's short plasma half-life. Wetting agents such as sodium lauryl sulfate or sodium docusate can be used with poorly soluble APIs to enhance dissolution or solubility.

Stability

A drug product for routine use is expected to have a shelf-life of at least 3 years, representing less than 5% decomposition and no significant physical change under normal storage conditions.

Accelerated stability tests are often carried out for 1–4 weeks during preformulation studies. The chemical stability of the solid is measured at temperatures ranging from 4°C to 75°C, and moisture uptake at different relative humidities is also assessed.

Measurements of stability in solution at pH values ranging from 1 to 11 at room temperature and at 37°C will be performed, including formulations with solubilizing agents where appropriate. Sensitivity to ultraviolet (UV) and visible light, and to exposure to oxygen, is also measured.

The rate of degradation in short-term studies under these accelerated harsh conditions is used to give a preliminary estimate of the likely rate of degradation under normal storage conditions. Sensitivity to low pH means that degradation is likely to occur in the stomach, requiring measures to prevent release of the compound until it reaches the intestine.

These preformulation stability tests serve mainly to warn that further development of the compound may be challenging. Definitive tests of the long-term (typically 3 years) stability of the formulated preparation will be required at a later stage of development for regulatory purposes.

Particle size and morphology

Ideally, for incorporation into a tablet or capsule, the drug substance needs to exist in small, uniformly sized particles, forming a smoothly flowing powder that can be uniformly blended with the excipient material. Rarely, the compound will emerge from the basic research chemistry laboratory with these ideal properties. More often, it will take the form of an amorphous, waxy solid, and additional work will be needed to isolate it in a salt form suitable for incorporation into a dosage form.

Preformulation studies are designed to show how far the available material falls short of this ideal and to indicate potential approaches to help overcome these challenges. Various laboratory methods are available for analysing particle size and morphology, but at the preformulation stage, simple microscopic observation will often suffice.

Particles with variable particle size or shapes are difficult to handle and mix uniformly. Hygroscopic materials and polymorphic crystal forms are a disadvantage. If liquid formulations are used in phase I, then these particle issues are unlikely to matter. However, these adverse properties will need to be addressed and controlled as development progresses to other dosage forms for later stages of clinical development.

Routes of administration and dosage forms

The administration route to be selected has to be effective and convenient for the patient. The preferred dosage form for therapeutic agents is almost always an oral tablet or capsule dosed as few times a day as possible. However, there are many dosage forms available, and Table 16.1 lists some of the main ones. An important consideration is whether it is desirable to achieve *systemic exposure* (i.e., distribution of the drug to all organs via the bloodstream) or *selective local exposure* (e.g., to the lungs, skin or rectum). In most cases, systemic exposure is required and

Table 16.1 The main routes of administration and dosage forms

Exposure required	Routes of administration	Dosage forms	
Systemic	Oral	Tablet, capsule, solution, suspension, emulsion	Liquid forms are particularly suitable for children, and for patients unable to swallow tablets. Unsuitable for foul-tasting medicines
	Parenteral		
	Injection (intravenous, subcutaneous, intramuscular), needle-free injection	Solution, emulsion, suspension, implant	Examples: cytotoxic drugs liable to damage GI tract, drugs needed for unconscious patients, drugs unstable in GI tract (e.g., peptide hormones)
	Percutaneous	Skin patches	
	Inhalation	Gas, vapour	Applicable mainly to anaesthetic agents
	Intranasal	Aerosol	Used for some hormone preparations that are not absorbed orally, e.g., vasopressin analogues, gonadotropin-releasing hormone
Topical	Skin	Ointment, cream, gel, aerosol	
	Respiratory tract	Aerosol, inhaled powder	
	Rectum, vagina	Suppository	
	Eye	Solution, ointment	

GI, Gastrointestinal.

an oral capsule or tablet will be the desired final dosage form. Even so, an intravenous formulation will normally be required for use in safety pharmacology, toxicology and pharmacokinetic studies in humans. In addition, macromolecules such as peptides, proteins and antibodies will need to be administered by injection, as they are not stable to oral ingestion and are too big to penetrate the skin.

The main routes of administration for drugs acting systemically, apart from oral and injectable formulations, are *transdermal, intranasal* and *oromucosal. Rectal, vaginal* and *pulmonary* routes are also used in some cases, though these are used mainly for drugs that act locally.

Transdermal administration of drugs formulated as small adhesive skin patches has considerable market appeal, even though such preparations are much more expensive than conventional formulations. To be administered in this way, drugs must be highly potent, lipid soluble and of low molecular weight. Examples of commercially available patch formulations include *nitroglycerin, scopolamine, fentanyl, nicotine, testosterone* and *estradiol*. The main limitation is the low permeability of the skin to most drugs and the small area covered, which mean that dosage is limited to a few milligrams per day, so only very potent drugs can be given systemically via this route of administration. Variations in skin thickness affect the rate of penetration, and the occurrence of local skin reactions is also a problem with some drugs. Various penetration enhancers, mainly surfactant compounds of the sort discussed above, are used to improve transdermal absorption. Intranasal drug administration (Illium, 2002, 2003) is another route that has been used successfully for a few drugs. The nasal epithelium is much more permeable than skin and allows the transfer of peptide drugs, as well as low-molecular-weight substances. Commercially available preparations have been developed for peptide hormones, such as *vasopressin analogues, calcitonin, buserelin* and others, as well as for conventional drugs such as *triptans, opioids* and so on. The main disadvantages are that substances are quickly cleared from the nasal epithelium by ciliary action, as well as being metabolized, and the epithelial permeability is not sufficient to allow most proteins to be given in this way. Ciliary clearance can be reduced by gel formulations, and surfactant permeability enhancers can be used to improve the penetration of larger molecules. The possibility of administering insulin, growth factors or vaccines by this route is the subject of active research efforts but has so far proved not to be commercially viable (Rohrer et al., 2018). Some studies have suggested (Illium, 2003) that substances absorbed through the nasal epithelium reach the brain more rapidly than if they are given intravenously, possibly bypassing the blood–brain barrier by reaching the central nervous system (CNS) directly via the nerves to the olfactory bulb.

Oromucosal delivery (Hearnden et al., 2012), especially utilizing the buccal and sublingual mucosa as the absorption site, is a drug delivery route that promotes rapid absorption and almost immediate pharmacological effect. The sublingual mucosa, especially, is highly vascularized, and this route bypasses the gastrointestinal tract and thus first-pass metabolism. However, few drugs can be efficiently absorbed through the oral mucosa because of physicochemical properties or enzymatic breakdown of the drug, and the amount of drug that could be absorbed is limited to a few milligrams. The drug has to be soluble, stable and able to easily permeate the mucosal barrier at the administration site, so it tends to be lower molecular weight, typically below 200. Also some formulation aspects have to be taken into consideration. A prerequisite for a rapid onset of effect using a tablet formulation is a fast disintegration and dissolution in the oral cavity, resulting in an optimal exposure of active substance to the small volume of dissolving fluids. An optimized formulation using this administration route has the potential for very fast absorption (Kroboth et al., 1995) and obtaining peak blood levels within 10 to 15 minutes. It is thereby potentially a more comfortable and convenient alternative to the intravenous route of administration.

Formulation

Formulation of an active substance into a dosage form involves careful designing, using good science and common sense. This systematic approach is usually referred to as Quality by Design (QbD) and is fully recognized by regulators and extensively described by Schlindwein and Gibson (2018). The 'ideal' drug substance intended for use as an oral preparation has the following characteristics:

- Water solubility
- Chemical stability (including stability at low pH)
- Permeability across the gastrointestinal epithelium
- Good access to site of action (e.g., blood–brain barrier penetration, if intended to work in the brain)
- Resistance to first-pass metabolism.

Tablets and capsules are the most common dosage form due to a combination of convenience for the patient and a cost-effective manufacturing process. The majority of APIs alone will have a combination of inadequate flow, poor compression properties and poor disintegration or dissolution. This usually requires additional functional materials, termed excipients, to be used in the formulation of APIs into medicines. A range of excipients is needed even for a tablet without special requirements for its drug release profile. A tablet needs to be sufficiently mechanically strong enough to withstand handling but also to have the ability to disintegrate after oral intake to release the drug.

Inert diluents or fillers, such as sugars (e.g., lactose or mannitol) or cellulosics (e.g., microcrystalline cellulose or modified starches), are added to produce tablets of a manageable size (generally, 50–500 mg). The filler should have good tabletability and flow properties, be nonhygroscopic and have acceptable taste. Binders, such as cellulose and other polymeric materials, may be needed to assist compaction into a solid tablet that will not crumble. A binder could be added either in dry form or in the granulation liquid depending on the manufacturing process. Disintegrating agents, such as starch and cellulose, ensure that the tablet disintegrates rapidly in the gastrointestinal tract. For a very fast disintegration, 'super disintegrants' could be used such as cross-linked polyvinyl pyrrolidone, sodium starch glycollate and croscarmellose that act by producing extensive swelling. Lubricants, such as magnesium stearate, may be needed to ensure that the powder runs smoothly in the tablet machine. These lubricants act by reduction of friction between particles and between particles and parts of the machine in contact. The tablet may need to be coated with a cellulosic or sugar to disguise its taste.

Capsule formulations are often used for initial clinical trials, as they are generally simpler to develop than compressed tablets but are less suitable for controlled-release formulations. A two-piece gelatin or hydroxypropyl methylcellulose (HPMC) capsule can be used to contain formulations also in semisolid or liquid form. Other advantages are that capsules are easy to swallow and provide effective taste-masking without any additional coating step. The choice of excipients and the manufacturing process is very much dependent on the characteristics of drug substance and the desired properties of the dosage form. Drug release profile is just one aspect, while the homogeneity or uniformity of content is another. If the drug substance is very potent and cohesive, then mixing a small amount of drug with a high amount of filler could lead to poor content uniformity. This problem is most severe if the drug particles are micronized to improve the dissolution rate. Different processes used in drug development and manufacturing are described in textbooks such as Aulton (2018) and Tovey (2018). A logical approach to process selection for the given API properties using the manufacturing classification system (MCS) is described by Leane et al. (2015). More extensive examples including continuous manufacturing considerations are given by Leane et al. (2018).

The shelf-life of the drug product should preferably be at least 3 years. The presence of moisture is one of the main contributors to the degradation of the drug substance. Tablets normally have a longer shelf-life than other formulations such as oral and parental liquids since they are a dry dosage form. However, it is important to choose excipients that are not hygroscopic since small amounts of moisture could decrease the stability of the drug. In addition, selection of the tablet or capsule packaging material is also an important aspect to take into consideration. For example, moisture-sensitive, freeze-dried wafers are often packed in almost impenetrable aluminium blisters.

Formulation development has to take into account the properties of the drug substance, the desired delivery system and the form of the final product. For example, in developing a new nitrate preparation for treating angina, the preferred delivery system might be a skin patch to be packaged in a foil sachet, or a nasal spray to be packaged as a push-button aerosol can. Although a simple oral tablet preparation may be feasible, the medical need and patient convenience might require the development of different dosage forms. Hence the development plan would have to be directed towards these more complex dosage forms.

Principles of drug delivery systems

Drug delivery systems in recent years have become progressively more sophisticated for three main reasons. First, biopharmaceuticals represent an increasing proportion of new drugs. They are very unlikely to conform to the 'ideal' profile summarized earlier, and so complex formulation is often needed to turn them into viable products (Haussecker, 2014; Wlodarczyk et al., 2018). Second, there is increasing emphasis on selective targeting of drugs to sites of disease via the use of specialized delivery systems. This is particularly relevant for anticancer drugs. Third, controllable delivery systems are being developed for specific indications. A further step is to incorporate sensors (e.g., for blood glucose concentration) into devices that control the delivery of insulin, in order to provide feedback control of blood glucose.

Polymers and surfactants

Combining the drug substance with different polymers and surfactants permits it to adopt states that are intermediate between the pure solid and a free aqueous solution. Polymers in colloidal, gel or solid form can be used to entrap drug molecules and have many applications in drug formulations (Kim et al., 2009; Savic et al., 2010; Torchilin, 2001):

- Polymers and surfactants in liquid form give rise to micelles or emulsions, which can greatly enhance the solubility of drug molecules, while at the same time protecting them from chemical degradation, and sometimes improving permeation through tissue barriers, such as the gastrointestinal epithelium and the blood–brain barrier.

- Polymers that form soft hydrated gels are used mainly in topical dermatological preparations.
- Solid gel formulations can be used as implantable depot preparations that can be inserted under the skin to give sustained release of the drug. Skin patches can be made from sheets of such a flexible polymer, loaded with the drug substance.
- Polymers are commonly used in tablets and capsules for several purposes, either to facilitate the manufacturing process or for a specific drug release profile, for example, binders, disintegrants and film coating agents.

There are a range of polymers available for drug formulation. Micelle formation is encouraged by combining hydrophilic and hydrophobic domains in a single polymer, for example, poloxamers. The inclusion of acidic or basic side chains enables polymers to bind oppositely charged drug molecules, thereby increasing their effective solubility.

Micelles

Micelles (Fig. 16.1) consist of aggregates of a few hundred *amphiphilic* molecules that contain distinct hydrophilic and hydrophobic regions. In an aqueous medium, the molecules cluster with the hydrophilic regions facing the surrounding water and the hydrophobic regions forming an inner core. Micelles typically have diameters of 10–80 nm, small enough not to sediment under gravity, and to pass through most filters. Micelle-forming substances have limited aqueous solubility, and when the free aqueous concentration reaches a certain point—the *critical micelle concentration*—typically in the millimolar range, micelles begin to form; further addition of the substance increases their abundance. With some compounds, as the density of micelles increases a gel is formed, consisting of a loosely packed array of micelles interspersed with water molecules. Lipophilic drug molecules often dissolve readily in the inner core allowing concentrations to be achieved that greatly exceed the aqueous solubility limit of the drug. Amphiphilic substances also tend to associate with micelles, as do high-molecular-weight substances such as peptides and proteins, which have an affinity for surfaces, on account of the large surface area that micelles present.

Micelle formation is a natural property of bile acids, which are secreted into the duodenum under physiological conditions and which play an important role in fat absorption by the intestine. Micellar drug formulations are thus an extension of a normal physiological process. Micelle formation is a general property of amphiphilic molecules, and many chemical forms have been developed for pharmaceutical use. Some examples are shown in Fig. 16.1, and additional information on the many types of polymers used in pharmaceutical formulation

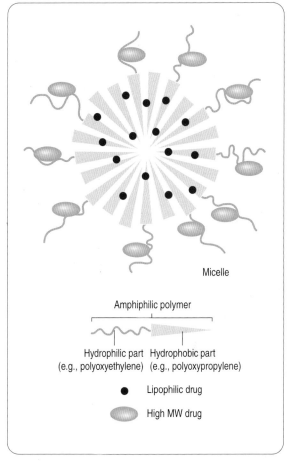

Fig. 16.1 Structures of some common pharmaceutical polymers. *MW*, Molecular weight.

is given in many textbooks (e.g., Aulton, 2018; Tovey, 2018). A particularly versatile group is that of *copolymers*, containing more than one type of polymer unit, one of which, typically, is hydrophilic (e.g., PEG), whereas the other is hydrophobic (e.g., polypropylene glycol). Alternating blocks of these two units form a copolymer (Fig. 16.1), which is commonly used in drug formulations. Copolymers of this sort at low concentrations form a liquid micellar suspension, but at higher concentrations the micelles may aggregate in an ordered array to form a water-containing gel. Such gel formulations are commonly used to prepare controlled-release preparations. The polymer components may include anionic or cationic groups, which have the effect of altering their affinity for charged drug molecules, and also of altering their pharmacokinetic behaviour.

Micelles and other drug vehicles, such as cyclodextrins and liposomes, have a considerable—and generally beneficial—effect on the pharmacokinetic properties of the drug. Often, but not invariably, absorption from gastrointestinal tract is improved, though the reasons for this are not well understood. Parenteral circulating micelles protect the drug from metabolic degradation, so the plasma half-life is generally prolonged. Micelles are too large to cross 'tight' capillary endothelium, so transfer across the blood–brain barrier is not increased. They are able to cross the fenestrated capillaries that occur in most tissues, but the rate of permeation is less than that of the uncomplexed drug. Malignant tumours and inflamed tissues generally have rather leaky capillaries with large fenestrations, so that transfer of micellar drug complexes into such tissues is more rapid than into normal tissues. This mechanism results in a degree of selectivity in the distribution of the drug to diseased tissues, a phenomenon known as *passive targeting*.

Liposomes

Liposomes were first discovered in 1965 and proposed as drug carriers soon afterwards (see Kraft et al., 2014 for a short review). They are microscopic vesicles formed when an aqueous suspension of phospholipid is exposed to ultrasonic agitation. Depending on the conditions, large, multilayered vesicles 1–5 μm in diameter, or small, single-layered vesicles 0.02–0.1 μm in diameter, may be formed. The vesicles are bounded by a phospholipid bilayer, which is impermeable to nonlipophilic compounds. They can act as drug carriers in various ways (Fig. 16.2):

- Nonlipophilic drugs are carried in solution in the aqueous core, by adding them to the aqueous medium in which the liposomes are produced. Techniques for introducing drug molecules into preformed liposomes have also been described.
- Lipophilic drugs occupy the phospholipid membrane phase
- Some peptides and proteins, as well as amphiphilic drugs, can be sequestered at the lipid–water interface.

The main purpose of using liposomes is to improve the pharmacokinetic behaviour of drugs. Liposomes are not generally suitable for oral administration, as they are destroyed by enzymes and bile acids in the small intestine. They do not cross the blood–brain barrier, so they cannot be used to improve the access of drugs to the brain. Despite an extensive literature acclaiming liposomes as the answer to almost every imaginable formulation problem, the application of liposome technology in commercial products is so far limited to a very few examples in the field of anticancer and antifungal drugs.

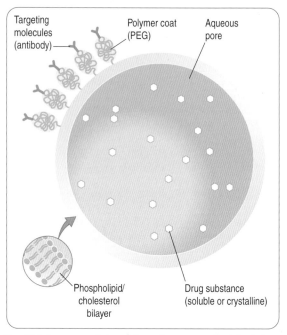

Fig. 16.2 Structure of drug delivery liposome. *PEG*, Polyethylene glycol.

Nanotechnology

Nanotechnology, using materials in the nanometre scale, is a growing scientific field. The first approved products using formulations based on nanoparticles were liposomes, polymer–protein conjugates, polymeric substances or suspensions. Medical applications of nanotechnology (nanomedicine) have also been suggested to have the potential to create new 'intelligent materials' in nanoscale to be used as diagnostic materials, in stents with and without drugs. In drug development, the technology has been suggested to have a great potential for targeted drug delivery in the treatment of cancer and organ-specific drug delivery, for example, to CNS (Singh & Lillard, 2009). Several new drug delivery technologies using a number of materials such as polymers, metals and ceramics are under development where surfaces or pores in nanoscale are loaded with pharmaceutical substances. The drug release is rate-determined or programmed using nanotechnology and conventional pharmaceutical formulation principles in combination (Flühmann et al., 2019). Besides the size, other physicochemical properties, such as surface properties, particle morphology and structure and drug release are of importance for understanding and interpreting in vivo results (Putheti et al., 2008). Table 16.2 exemplifies drug delivery applications of nanotechnology.

Table 16.2 Drug delivery applications of nanotechnology

Drug delivery system	Application
Liposomes	Targeting drug/oligonucleotide/gene delivery
Micelles	Targeting drug/oligonucleotide/gene delivery
Nanoemulsions and nanogels	CNS disorders, targeted across blood–brain barrier
Nanoparticles, e.g., metallic, mesoporous silica, solid lipids	Carrier, site-specific delivery and contrast agents in cancer therapy oligonucleotides
Nanoprobes	Biomarkers

CNS, Central nervous system.

Modified-release drug formulations

The most common challenge in drug formulation is to shorten the time to onset of action or prolong the duration of action of a drug. In either situation, the rate of absorption must be determined by the rate of release of the active substance from the dosage form. The most common method is to delay the rate of release of the drug substance from the dosage form, causing it to be absorbed gradually. Ideally, the rate of absorption should reach a steady level that is maintained for hours or days, depending on the application, until the reservoir is used up. This is known as *sustained release*. It is widely used to produce once-daily oral preparations, or long-lasting depot injections (e.g., contraceptives, hormone replacements, antipsychotic drugs), where the drug effect is required to last for weeks or months.

Other types of modified release include *delayed release*, used mainly for oral drugs that are unstable at the low pH of the stomach, and *controlled release*, produced by specialized devices that allow the rate of release to be adjusted according to need.

There are many different ways of modifying the release from oral preparations, some of which are shown in Fig. 16.3. Oral-modified release dosage forms can either be monoliths (e.g., tablets) or multiparticulates such as pellets. Monoliths can be composed of water-absorbing polymer gels that slowly become hydrated and eroded, thereby controlling drug release by a combination of diffusion and erosion (Patel et al., 2011). Alternatively, monoliths can employ osmotic technologies to expel the drug via prepared pores in an insoluble film coat (Verma & Garg, 2004). Pellets also tend to rely on coating technology to control release of the APIs (Siepmann et al., 2007).

Injectable implants operate in a similar manner of diffusion and erosion. Depot injections of drugs dissolved in oil can also be used to provide long-lasting sustained release, but these generally produce a less constant rate of administration and cannot be removed.

Controlled release represents a stage beyond sustained release and involves exploiting a sensing mechanism responding to changes in temperature or pH, for example, to the drug release mechanism. An example is the pH-sensitive system, which can be used to delay the release of acid-sensitive drugs (particularly peptides) until they have passed beyond the stomach. Drug delivery can also, in principle, be targeted to regions of low pH, such as inflamed or hypoxic tissues, by the use of pH-sensitive polymers. A particularly ingenious approach is to incorporate insulin into pH-sensitive gels loaded with glucose oxidase (commonly referred to as *GOD-gels*). If the ambient glucose concentration increases, enzymic oxidation causes a fall in pH and the release of insulin. For more details of 'responsive' polymers and their application in controlled drug delivery, see Kim et al. (2009) and Zhang et al. (2013).

Delivery and formulation of biopharmaceuticals

Biopharmaceutical drugs are large molecules and tend to be protein-based, built up of amino acid chains and structurally complex with many functional groups. Examples are human insulin in diabetes therapy, different vaccines and interferons in, for example, lung cancer, leukaemia and hepatitis therapy (see Chapters 12 and 13), as well as antibodies (see Chapter 8). The diffusional transport across epithelial barriers in the gastrointestinal tract is slow since these molecules are large, and enzymes present there result in fast degradation of the molecules. A majority of the biotech drugs are therefore delivered via the parenteral route. Despite that, the market for biotech products is growing.

Formulation of proteins and peptides is a real challenge since they are usually more unstable compared with small molecules, and the formulation strategy needs a high focus on stabilization. The structures are often both chemically and physically unstable. These molecules are often designed for specific mechanisms of action. Loss of activity can arise with, for example, increased temperature or a change in pH and therefore heating should obviously be avoided, and the right pH conditions need to be selected. Biopharmaceuticals also have fast degradation in aqueous solutions, and therefore freeze-drying is a common technique to transfer them into a dry state for longer shelf-life. However, it is important to select the right temperature and pressure to avoid damage of the molecule during the process. Further instability problems that could arise with

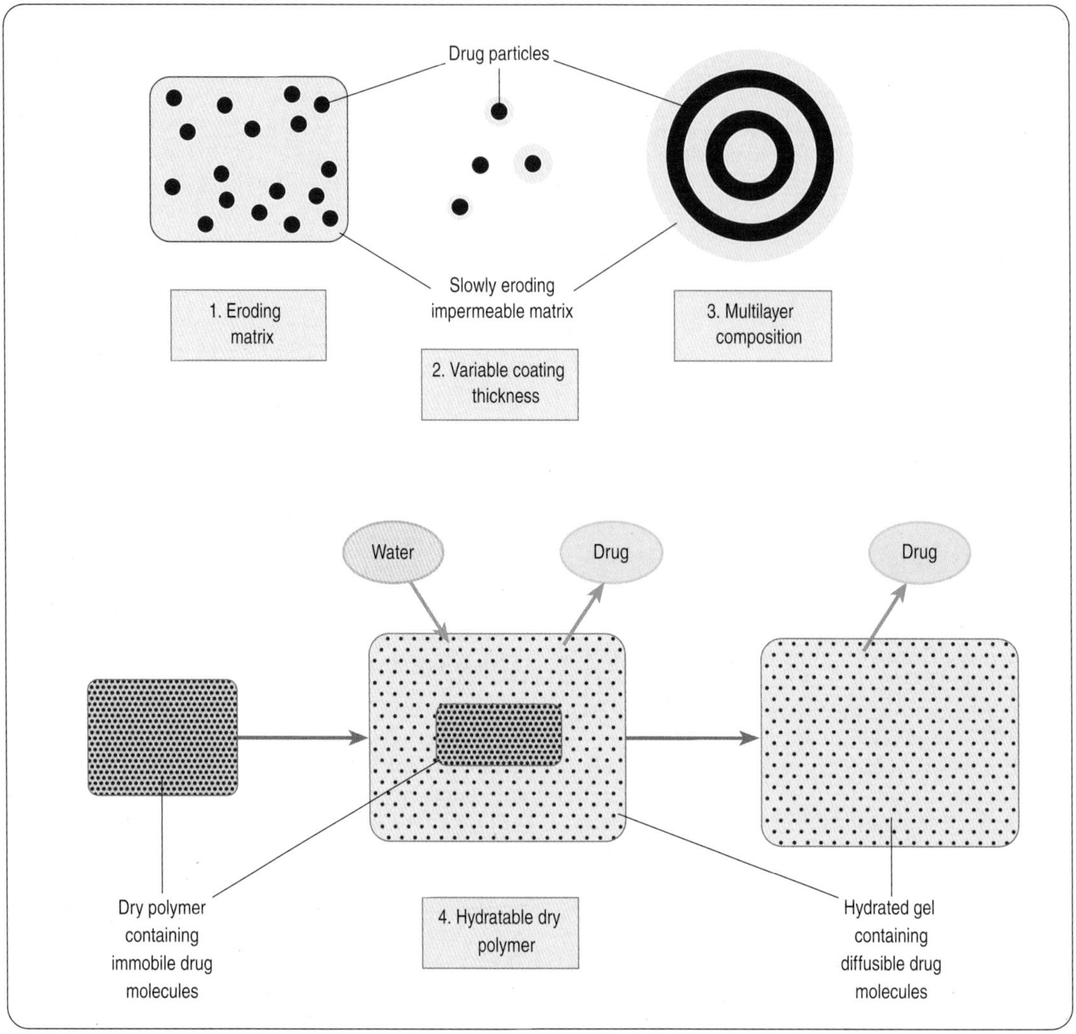

Fig. 16.3 Types of sustained-release preparation.

biopharmaceuticals are protein aggregation and oxidation. Micelles, liposomes and the addition of polymers and surfactants are used to overcome these stability problems with biopharmaceuticals. Antibody–drug conjugates can also be particularly challenging from both formulation and stability perspectives, as they have antibody, linker and payload components in the same complex (Duerr & Friess, 2019).

Drug delivery to the central nervous system

Brain capillaries, unlike those in most parts of the body, are nonfenestrated, so that drug molecules must traverse the endothelial cells, rather than passing between them, to move from circulating blood to the extracellular space of the brain (see Chapter 10). Three main routes of access are important (Scherrmann, 2002):

- Lipophilic compounds of low molecular weight cross the membrane of endothelial cells very easily and comprise the great majority of CNS-acting drugs. Peptides, proteins, nonlipophilic or ionized drugs are, for the most part, unable to cross the endothelial cell membrane.
- The endothelial cells also possess various active transport mechanisms that can allow certain non-lipophilic compounds to enter the brain. Examples include *levodopa*, used for treating Parkinson's disease,

baclofen, a Gamma-aminobutyric acid (GABA) analogue used to treat spasticity and the cytotoxic drug *melphalan*, all of which are transported across the blood–brain barrier by the amino acid transporter. Attempts have been made to couple other drugs with amino acids or sugars that are carried via this transport system. Despite being successful in animal models, however, such compounds have not been developed for clinical use. Active transport out of the brain also occurs with many compounds, including drugs such as *penicillins*, which are able to enter passively.

- Molecules can be carried as endocytotic vesicles across the endothelial cells. This type of transcytosis occurs with molecules that are bound to receptors or other proteins on the endothelial cell surface.

Approaches for improving drug delivery to the brain are described in more detail by Bicker et al. (2014), Patel et al. (2009) and Pardridge (2010).

Enabling impermeant drugs to reach the brain represents a major challenge for formulation chemists, and there are actually very few examples where it has been overcome. Most often, the drug molecule has to be redesigned to increase its lipophilicity. Formation of a lipid-soluble prodrug is one strategy but is rarely effective in this context because conversion to the active, nonlipophilic compound is likely to take place in the circulation before the drug reaches the brain.

Summary

Pharmaceutical development comprises all the activities needed to turn a therapeutic drug substance into a marketable product that will perform reliably when used in real life. Preformulation studies consist of a series of chemical and physicochemical investigations on the drug substance that indicate the kinds of formulation that are likely to be satisfactory. In some cases, problems (e.g., poor solubility or chemical instability) will emerge at this stage, requiring modification of the drug molecule before development can proceed. Therefore it is important to run preformulation activities in parallel with early drug development of new chemical entities.

The process of formulation will depend greatly not only on information from preformulation activities, but also on the medical condition and on the intended route of administration of the drug. In most cases, where the intention is to produce a tablet or capsule for oral use, an intravenous formulation will also be developed for use in clinical trials, and the oral form used in initial efficacy trials (clinical phase II) may not be the same as the intended marketed form.

Formulation studies require considerable time and resources even in cases where no problems are encountered. The end result has to be a product that can be manufactured on a large scale and meet strict quality-control standards and can be transported and stored in thousands of homes under varying conditions of temperature and humidity without significant deterioration.

Very often, pharmaceutical development is called on to improve the characteristics of the drug substance, for example, by improving its solubility using amorphous substances or new salts, disguising its taste, increasing its plasma half-life or reducing unwanted effects. Work of this kind increases the value of a substance clinically and commercially. Increasing use is being made of colloidal systems, such as micelles, polymers and liposomes as vehicles for drug molecules. Such formulations have a considerable effect on the drug's pharmacokinetic properties and can also be used to achieve a degree of targeting of the drug to the tissues on which it is required to act. Drug targeting based on antibodies is also increasingly being used, for example, as drug antibody complexes. In these cases, antibodies are raised, for example, to a particular specific cancer protein and are coupled to a chemotherapeutic molecule, thereby targeting the molecule at the cancer cell. The principles have proved applicable so far to anticancer and antifungal drugs, but many more applications are expected in the foreseeable future.

Work on more sophisticated formulations, new routes of administration and new delivery systems, for currently available drugs and biopharmaceuticals, is thought likely to contribute as much to improved therapeutics as the discovery of new drugs.

References

Amidon, G. L., Lennernas, H., Shah, V. P., & Crison, J. R. (1995). A theoretical basis for a biopharmaceutic drug classification: The correlation of in vitro drug product dissolution and in vivo bioavailability. *Pharmaceutical Research, 12*, 413–420.

Aulton, M. E. (Ed.). (2018). *Aulton's pharmaceutics. The design and manufacture of medicines* (5th ed.). Edinburgh: Churchill Livingstone.

Bicker, J., Alves, G., Fortuna, A., & Falcão, A. (2014). Blood–brain barrier models and their relevance for a successful development of CNS drug delivery systems: A review. *European Journal of Pharmaceutics and Biopharmaceutics, 87*, 409–432.

Butler, J. M., & Dressman, J. B. (2010). The developability classification system: Application of biopharmaceutics concepts to formulation development. *Journal of Pharmaceutical Sciences, 99,* 4940–4954.

Duerr, C., & Friess, W. (2019). Antibody-drug conjugates—stability and formulation. *European Journal of Pharmaceutics and Biopharmaceutics, 139,* 168–176.

Flühmann, B., Ntai, I., Borchard, G., Simoens, S., & Mühlebach, S. (2019). Nanomedicines: The magic bullets reaching their target? *European Journal of Pharmaceutical Sciences, 12,* 73–80.

Haussecker, D. (2014). Current issues of RNAi therapeutics delivery and development. *Journal of Controlled Release, 195,* 49–54.

Hearnden, V., Sankar, V., Hull, K., Juras, V., Greenberg, M., Kerr, A. R., et al. (2012). New developments and opportunities in oral mucosal drug delivery for local and systemic disease, 2012. *Advanced Drug Delivery Reviews, 64,* 16–28.

Illium, L. (2002). Nasal drug delivery: New developments and strategies. *Drug Discovery Today, 7,* 1184–1189.

Illium, L. (2003). Nasal drug delivery—possibilities, problems and solutions. *Journal of Controlled Release, 87,* 187–198.

Kaplan, S. A. (1972). Relationships between aqueous solubility of drugs and their bioavailability. *Drug Metabolism Reviews, 1,* 15–32.

Kim, S., Kim, J. H., Jeon, O., Kwon, I. C., & Park, K. (2009). Engineered polymers for advanced drug delivery. *European Journal of Pharmaceutics and Biopharmaceutics, 71,* 420–430.

Kraft, J. C., Freeling, J. P., Wang, Z., & Rodney, J. Y. H. (2014). Emerging research and clinical development trends of liposome and lipid nanoparticle drug delivery systems. *Journal of Pharmaceutical Sciences, 103,* 29–52.

Kroboth, P. D., McAuley, J. W., Kroboth, F. J., Bertz, R. J., & Smith, R. B. (1995). Triazolam pharmacokinetics after intravenous, oral, and sublingual administration. *Journal of Clinical Psychopharmacology, 15,* 259–262.

Leane, M., Pitt, K. G., & Reynolds, G. (2015). A proposal for a drug product manufacturing classification system (MCS) for oral solid dosage forms. *Pharmaceutical Development and Technology, 20,* 12–21.

Leane, M., Pitt, K. G., Reynolds, G. K., Dawson, N., Ziegler, I., Szepes, A., et al. (2018). Manufacturing Classification System in the real world: Factors influencing manufacturing process choices for filed commercial oral solid dosage formulations, case studies from industry and considerations for continuous processing. *Pharmaceutical Development and Technology, 23,* 964–977.

Pardridge, W. M. (2010). Biopharmaceutical drug targeting to the brain. *Journal of Drug Targeting, 18,* 157–167.

Patel, H., Panchal, D. R., Patel, U., Brahmbhatt, T., & Suthar, M. (2011). Matrix type drug delivery system: A review. *Journal of Pharmaceutical Sciences Research and Bioscientific Research, 1,* 143–151.

Patel, M. M., Goyal, B. R., Bhadada, S. V., Bhatt, J. S., & Amin, A. F. (2009). Getting into the brain: Approaches to enhance brain drug delivery. *CNS Drugs, 23,* 35–58.

Putheti, R. R., Okigbo, R. N., Sai advanapu, M., & Chavanpatil, S. (2008). Nanotechnology importance in the pharmaceutical industry. *African Journal of Pure and Applied Chemistry, 2,* 27–31.

Rohrer, J., Lupo, N., & Bernkop-Schnurch, A. (2018). Advanced formulations for intranasal delivery of biologics. *International Journal of Pharmaceutics, 553,* 8–20.

Savic, S., Tamburic, S., & Savic, M. M. (2010). From conventional towards new—natural surfactants in drug delivery systems design: Current status and perspectives. *Expert Opinion on Drug Delivery, 7,* 353–369.

Scherrmann, J. M. (2002). Drug delivery to brain via the blood–brain barrier. *Vascular Pharmacology, 38,* 349–354.

Schlindwein, W. S., & Gibson, M. (2018). *Pharmaceutical quality by design, a practical approach* (1st ed.). Chichester, UK: John Wiley & Sons.

Siepmann, F., Hoffmann, A., Leclercq, B., Carlin, B., & Siepmann, J. (2007). How to adjust desired drug release patterns from ethylcellulose-coated dosage forms. *Journal of Controlled Release, 119,* 182–189.

Singh, R., & Lillard J. W., Jr. (2009). Nanoparticle-based targeted drug delivery. *Experimental and Molecular Pathology, 86,* 215–223.

Torchilin, V. (2001). Structure and design of polymeric surfactant-based drug delivery. *Journal of Controlled Release, 73,* 137–172.

Tovey, G. A. (Ed.). (2018). *Pharmaceutical formulation* (1st ed.). London: Royal Society of Chemistry.

Verma, R. K., & Garg, S. (2004). Development and evaluation of osmotically controlled oral drug delivery system of glipizide. *European Journal of Pharmaceutics and Biopharmaceutics, 57,* 513–525.

Zhang, Y., Chan, H. F., & Leong, K. W. (2013). Advanced materials and processing for drug delivery: The past and the future. *Advanced Drug Delivery Reviews, 65,* 104–120.

Wlodarczyk, S. R., Custódio, D., Pessoa, A., & Monteiro, G. (2018). Influence and effect of osmolytes in biopharmaceutical formulations. *European Journal of Pharmaceutics and Biopharmaceutics, 131,* 92–98.

Chapter | **17** |

Clinical development

Duncan B Richards

Introduction

The purpose of the clinical phase of drug development is to generate sufficient understanding of the safety and efficacy of a new therapy such that a regulatory authority can consider granting marketing authorization. The word *sufficient* is important here because the development programme for new drugs will only provide a preliminary understanding of safety; rare, including potentially serious, adverse effects are unlikely to be identified by the initial development programme. While the clinical development package needs to provide robust information on the efficacy of the therapy, very few development programmes will establish the place of the therapy within the treatment pathway for the disease. These questions must be addressed by postmarketing pharmacovigilance and further clinical studies. The postmarketing package is commonly more extensive than the original development package.

The information generated by the clinical development plan is captured at authorization in the summary of product characteristics (SPCs); this is called the product label in the United States. The headings of the sections of the SPC are summarized in Fig. 17.1.

Despite the limitations of clinical development programmes, they are enormously time consuming and costly. Estimates vary, but it is now estimated that costs exceed $1 bn per new medicine. The total cost of developing a medicine is much higher (estimated to be $2.5 bn) because of considerable attrition, which means the majority of potential new medicines never reach the market.

Traditional schemes of drug development give the impression that it is a linear process divided into stages, and success at each stage will propel the project on to the next (Table 17.1). This is an oversimplification; a better way to think about development is as a series of questions leading to a body of information to support the safe use of the medicine in a defined population of patients to achieve a desired therapeutic effect. The size and nature of the programme to achieve this will vary enormously depending on the intervention and disease under study. For example, for a common disease such as type 2 diabetes, it is no longer sufficient to show an improvement in glycaemic control; evidence that the improvement in glycaemic control is not at the expense of increased cardiovascular risk is required. This may necessitate a large outcome trial involving several thousand subjects monitored for several years. By contrast, the package for a rare and rapidly fatal disease may be much more modest and may even be granted marketing authorization on the basis of a surrogate endpoint.

Although not discussed in detail here, clinical development must proceed in parallel with the development of the physical drug product, such that by the time of marketing authorization, the product is manufactured by a robust, controlled process, and that this material has been used in the registration efficacy trials. Ensuring the right material is ready at the right time is highly complex and an important contributor to the overall human and financial resources required for successful development.

Question-based drug development

Early clinical development (phase I and II in the traditional scheme) is about learning. Questions addressed during this stage of development include: what is the relationship between exposure to the drug and pharmacological effect, can a pharmacologically active dose be administered with an acceptable safety profile, is exposure to the drug predictable, and do we understand the principal determinants of this? The confirming phase of drug development (phase III) addresses questions such as: what proportion of the selected population derive a therapeutic benefit from the medicine, and what are the

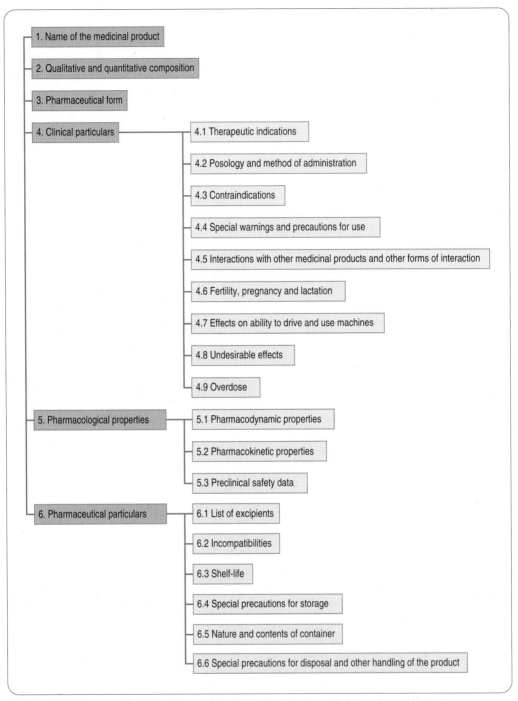

Fig. 17.1 Content of a summary of product characteristics. (From the European Medicines Agency https://www.ema.europa.eu/en/documents/scientific-guideline/revised-guideline-summary-product-characteristics-antimicrobial-products_en.pdf accessed 9 apr 2021.)

Table 17.1 Phases of clinical development

Clinical phase	General aim	Subjects/design	Data collected	Approx. number of subjects	Approx. time for clinical phase
I	Exploratory; safety, tolerability and PK to support patient studies. PD may be included (e.g., human challenge models)	Healthy subjects, in most cases, may include patient cohorts. Escalating single- and repeat-dose, placebo-controlled, randomized, double-blind	Adverse events; vital signs and ECG; laboratory safety measures. PK parameters. PD measures (sometimes)	40–60	6–12 months
IIa	Exploratory; preliminary safety and efficacy to support go/no-go decision	Patients; intended clinical dose and regimen based on phase I results. Usually placebo-controlled, randomized, double-blind, but sometimes open-label	Adverse events PK parameters. Preliminary evidence of efficacy. 'Proof of concept'	50–200	9 months–2 years
IIb	Confirmatory; dose selection to support registration	Patients in one or more indications. Selected dose levels/regimens compared with placebo and/or standard treatment, randomized double-blind	Statistically rigorous analysis of dose–response relationships. Confirmation of clinical dose and regimen for optimum efficacy, safety and tolerability	200–500	2–3 years
III	Confirmatory; efficacy and safety data to support registration; may include pharmacoeconomic evaluation	Patients in target indication(s) but including different groups (age, ethnicity, etc.). Selected dose level compared with placebo and/or standard treatment(s) randomized double-blind	Statistically rigorous measurements demonstrating safety and efficacy in comparison with placebo or existing therapies. May include pharmacoeconomic analysis	500–1000+ per study	2–5+ years
IV	Postmarketing studies to provide additional information on 1. Safety 2. Long-term outcome	Treated patients	Adverse events. Survival; long-term clinical outcomes (e.g., cardiovascular outcomes)	10,000+	2–4+ years

PD, Pharmacodynamic; *PK*, pharmacokinetic.

most common adverse effects associated with the treatment? Moving from learning to confirming assumes that what has been learned in the first phase directly informs the second. This highlights one of the most challenging aspects of modern drug development, that of translational risk. This is illustrated by the following example. Histamine type 2 (H_2) antagonists reduce stomach acid and therefore promote healing of peptic ulcers. Phase II studies

for this type of treatment identified patients with peptic ulcer by endoscopy, gave them a course of treatment, and measured the rate of ulcer healing by a second endoscopy after 6 weeks. The endpoint for phase III (registration) studies is essentially the same, but the study is larger. In this situation, the risk that a phase III study would be negative following a positive phase II study is small, so one can proceed with confidence. By contrast, the phase II endpoint for a new treatment for Alzheimer's disease might be based on an imaging endpoint such as brain volume. While this can be assessed precisely, the risk that this does not translate into a clinically meaningful effect on mental function scores or activities of daily living in phase III is high. The identification of endpoints in phase II that are predictive of clinical outcome in phase III is one of the most important areas of research in drug development today.

The limitations of the traditional development scheme are acknowledged, but it does provide a helpful framework to understand the development path and will now be discussed.

Phase I: clinical pharmacology

This first phase of drug development has the objective of developing a preliminary understanding of the clinical pharmacology of a new treatment. That said, a traditional, first in human (FIH) study conducted in healthy volunteers focuses on safety and pharmacokinetics (PK) rather than the pharmacology of the drug. This is a missed opportunity, and most phase I FIH studies will now include a measure of pharmacology.

A typical clinical development programme will include a number of other clinical pharmacology studies that are somewhat confusingly also referred to as phase I studies, although they are usually conducted much later in development. These studies will be discussed later in this chapter.

First in human studies

Before administering a new potential medicine to humans, a body of preclinical data must be assembled to evaluate the pharmacology, toxicology and drug metabolism characteristics. This must be presented to and approved by a regulatory authority and ethics committee before the study can proceed.

Study design

Most FIH studies begin with the single ascending dose (SAD) part. Although subject safety is paramount, administration of single doses will only identify the most prominent dose-related acute effects of a drug. The principal information this part of the study will generate is an understanding of exposure to the drug and whether this increases linearly with dose.

The SAD phase of the study commonly explores 6–10 dose levels with subjects organized into two or more cohorts. Subjects typically receive four dose levels with a

sufficient washout interval in between. The washout interval should take into account the PK half-life of the drug (usually five half-lives) but also the pharmacodynamic (PD) duration of action. Each cohort consists of 6–10 subjects, most will receive the study drug but usually a couple of subjects are randomized to placebo. The subject and investigator are usually blinded to the treatment allocation in order to reduce the risk of bias when assessing safety. It should, however, be noted that with these very small numbers, it is not possible to conduct any statistical assessment of the relative incidence of adverse events. Sentinel dosing is usually employed (see Chapter 15), whereby a pair of subjects (one on active and one on placebo) are dosed before the rest of the cohort. Even after sentinel dosing, it is generally prudent to split the dosing of the rest of the cohort to ensure time to evaluate any emergent safety signals prior to dosing more subjects in the cohort.

Following the SAD phase of the study, most FIH protocols will proceed to a multiple ascending dose phase. The duration of dosing should encompass PK steady state (five half-lives) but may also be informed by the duration of PD action and what will be required to enable the next (phase II) study. Subjects in FIH studies are usually resident in the phase I unit for the dosing periods in order to facilitate close safety supervision in a controlled environment.

Dose range to be explored

In principle, the administration of the very first dose of a new agent to humans should not produce observable pharmacological effects. The calculation of the starting dose should take into account the mechanism of action and the concentration−effect relationships observed in vitro and in vivo. The underlying PK/PD relationships should be derived by modelling and simulation techniques, including prediction of target occupancy versus concentration in humans in vivo. This approach to starting dose is termed the 'minimal anticipated biological effect level' (MABEL) and is recommended by most regulatory authorities as the most robust approach. It is considered more reliable than empirical thresholds that correspond to no effect (no observable effect level, NOEL), no adverse effects (no observable adverse effect level, NOAEL) or in some cases, the lowest observed adverse effect level (LOAEL) in animals. These thresholds are still used for reference but are considered unreliable as the sole means to define a dose because interspecies differences can lead to very different biological effects at similar exposures.

Dose escalation within the FIH study should be guided by all available information. A review meeting should be held at each dose level to review safety and PK data in order to select the next dose. Whenever possible, the dose decision should also be informed by PD information. Administering doses that are supramaximal for the primary pharmacology will not increase the desired effect and carry a risk of off-target effects that can be serious.

Study population

Most FIH studies continue to be conducted in healthy volunteers. Healthy volunteers provide a stable and consistent baseline from which to detect any changes that might represent a safety signal. Healthy subjects can also be easily organized into cohorts and have flexibility over their availability, both of which facilitate efficient progress of these studies. Criteria for inclusion into the study based upon medical history, physical examination, use of concomitant medications, alcohol, cigarettes and recreational drugs, as well as the results of blood testing, 12-lead ECG, blood pressure and heart rate are laid out in the study protocol. Male subjects are generally preferred because at this early stage of development, reproductive toxicology testing in animals will not usually have been completed, and the risk to the foetus of female subjects, who might be pregnant or become pregnant shortly before or after the study, has not been characterized. There has been criticism of this approach and involvement of women early in development is now encouraged, although they usually have to be of nonchildbearing potential. Once the segment 2 reproductive toxicology has been completed (see Chapter 12), female subjects of nonchildbearing potential, that is, postmenopausal, surgically sterilized, sexually abstinent or using effective methods of contraception, may be included in European studies. In the United States, female subjects may be included prior to reproductive toxicology data being available if they are of nonchildbearing potential. In some cases, it is not appropriate to use healthy young men, for example, studies of female hormone products or products for oncology, and in these cases, the subjects will be selected from the appropriate population.

Healthy subjects participating in such studies usually receive payment in recognition for time and inconvenience. The amount is agreed in advance with the reviewing ethics committee to ensure that it represents appropriate compensation, but not an inducement to participate. One vital point is that payment must only reflect time and inconvenience; it is not a payment for risk. It is the responsibility of the study team to ensure that risk to participants is minimal. Many volunteers who participate in early clinical studies do so on a regular basis. This has the advantage that they are familiar with the restrictions and requirements associated with participation, but it does carry a risk of overvolunteering and insufficient washout between studies. For this reason, many clinical units

participate in a confidential volunteer register to prevent simultaneous participation in multiple studies.

Some kinds of potential new medicine cannot be safely administered to healthy subjects. Cytotoxic anticancer therapies are obvious examples, but careful consideration should be given for any new treatment. For example, a treatment that has a significant and potentially long-lasting effect on the immune system may not be appropriate to administer to healthy subjects. Involvement of patients in early clinical trials requires careful planning. Subjects must be sufficiently well to be able to participate in study procedures, but most will not derive clinical benefit from participation, thus informed consent is particularly important. Making a clear distinction between participation in the study and receipt of clinical care is a particularly important aspect. Arrangements for ongoing treatment in the event of clinical benefit should also be clear and adequately resourced.

Safety measures

A framework for the assessment of the safety of new medicines in their first human trials is outlined in Chapter 15. In practical terms, in FIH studies, the principal means of assessment safety is close observation. Most studies are conducted in a residential setting with frequent measurement of vital signs, ECG and clinical laboratory parameters. The assessment of safety in this setting is based on analysis of trends and patterns rather than traditional medical diagnosis. For example, anaemia would be medically diagnosed based on a haemoglobin value less than 9 g/dL, whereas in a clinical study observing that four out of six participants have a drop of 2 g/dL would represent an important signal, even though all values remain in the reference range. This example—also illustrative of the key challenges in this stage of development—establishes whether a signal is real or not. All parameters are associated with variability; careful repeat measurement and seeking corroborative evidence from other related parameters is important to establish whether a signal is real or spurious. These studies usually include some subjects treated with placebo, but numbers of subjects are so small that formal statistical analysis cannot usually be performed.

The timing of assessments is important and should be determined by a careful assessment of when a safety signal may appear. For example, a drug that has the potential to interfere with potassium or sodium ion channels might be expected to reveal an effect around its peak concentration in the blood. By contrast, effects on liver function may be delayed and not apparent until after dosing has been completed. Intense monitoring at the wrong time or of the wrong kind is likely to miss important signals and give false reassurance.

Early studies also give an opportunity to assess the safety of abruptly stopping the drug. Careful measurement during the follow-up period can identify any rebound phenomena.

Pharmacokinetic measures

Measurement of exposure to the drug is often the key quantitative output from an FIH study. Exposure in the blood is the usual measure, although it is important to consider whether this is the most relevant compartment. For example, exposure in the skin for a dermatological product or in cerebrospinal fluid for a central nervous system product may be more relevant. Obtaining a good estimate of the exposure to the drug is important, and cohort size can be adjusted to ensure this is based on the measured PK variability.

The plasma or serum PK parameters usually derived are:

- C_{max}: peak drug and/or metabolite(s) concentration
- T_{max}: time to peak drug and/or metabolite(s) concentration
- $AUC_{0-\infty}$: area under the concentration–time curve of the drug and/or metabolite(s), extrapolated to infinity
- AUC_{0-T}: area under the concentration–time curve of the drug and/or metabolite(s), calculated to a specific time point T
- $t_{1/2}$: time taken for levels of drug and/or metabolite(s) to decrease by half (a measure of the rate of elimination of the drug from plasma).

Other PK parameters may also be determined, including:

- V_D: volume of distribution of drug and/or metabolite(s)
- Cl: clearance of drug and/or metabolite, i.e., the volume of plasma/serum cleared of drug and/or metabolite(s) per unit time, for example, mL/min, L/h
- MRT: mean residence time, i.e., the average time a drug molecule remains in the body after rapid intravenous (i.v.) injection.

Specialist pharmacokineticists perform the calculation of these parameters.

A comparison of the PK parameters at each dose level, for example, AUC_{∞}', C_{max}, will indicate whether they increase proportionately (linear kinetics) or disproportionately (nonlinear kinetics) with increasing dose. This information will influence the selection of dose levels, regimen and duration of dosing for the multiple, ascending repeat-dose study (MAD). The single-dose PK data can also be used to predict the drug/metabolite(s) concentrations expected on repeated dosing, based on the assumption that the kinetics do not change with time. Poorly soluble drugs may exhibit absorption saturation, whereby the amount of drug absorbed does not increase beyond a certain point at which the absorption processes are saturated. Saturation of clearance processes may result in prolonged exposure to a drug following a relatively modest increase in dose. The risk of this is increased for drugs that have a single route of elimination. In many cases, these unfavourable features would be designed out in the preclinical phase.

Phase II studies

The phase II study is usually the first opportunity to study the drug for efficacy in the target patient population. Safety information is limited at this stage, and it may not be possible to study the full range of patients with the condition. Those with the mildest disease may not experience disease progression within the study period, while those with the most severe disease may not be well enough to participate in the study. For this reason, the phase II population is necessarily a subset of what might become the final target population. This carries a risk that as development progresses, the benefit risk may not be the same in the different subpopulations.

Phase II may be split into a small-scale proof of concept study (POC), phase IIa, and formal dose ranging, phase IIb.

Proof of concept studies

The POC study is the make-or-break study for most drugs in development. For a small company, it may also make or break the whole enterprise. Although POC is a readily recognizable concept, it can vary greatly depending on the indication under study. For example, a novel antihypertensive drug would be expected to show a reduction in blood pressure in a cohort of about 50 subjects treated for a month. By contrast, a study to show disease modification in a heterogeneous disease such as rheumatoid arthritis may require a study of several hundred subjects studied for 6 months to a year. The costs of a definitive study in phase II can be very high, and in some cases, prohibitive. This can lead to underpowered studies or use of unreliable surrogate endpoints. This in turn is an important contributor to inefficiency in the drug development process, as this carries risk later into development where failure is even more costly.

The traditional approach to development is to demonstrate preliminary efficacy in phase II and to defer questions about differentiation from existing therapies to later in development. There are now relatively few areas in which there are not exiting treatments and so differentiation is becoming a more and more prominent question. Head-to-head studies in phase II remain very uncommon, but in an increasingly crowded marketplace, evidence of differential efficacy may be required to secure the investment required to proceed into full-scale development.

Phase II proof of concept study designs

The most common approach remains the double-blind placebo-controlled study, as this provides the most robust unbiased assessment of efficacy. This approach works well when the intervention can be properly blinded, and there is a robust, objective assessment that can be applied to all subjects equally. This is straightforward for measures such as blood pressure but is less so for measures such as radiographic evidence of joint erosion. These more complex measures are increasingly common and ensuring objective and consistent assessment is vital to the credibility of the study data. Many cardiovascular studies will employ a 'core lab' to analyse all the echocardiographic data from a study using a common analysis algorithm. This approach can assist with blinding, but success requires that the data are captured in the same way across all the study sites. Achieving this is a major logistical challenge.

The ideal phase II endpoint is a clinical one, as this provides the greatest confidence that the drug will confer genuine clinical benefit. It is, however, not practical for all indications. Symptomatic treatments where a short-term benefit is expected to be apparent early are less and less common; many modern therapies are aimed at altering the course of the underlying disease process, and this can take a long time to become apparent. This drives the use of surrogate markers. Some surrogates such as blood pressure for cardiovascular risk are very well established and robust; however, that a change in a circulating marker of fibrosis will correctly predict a reduced rate of progression to liver cirrhosis is much less certain.

Many modern drug targets modulate cellular processes that could have clinical value in a number of diseases. This would favour a different approach to phase II based around experimental medicine. In this approach, the focus of the study is to examine the impact of treatment on key disease processes in patients rather than on demonstrating efficacy per se. The value of this approach is that it can provide critical insight into how the drug interacts with the disease process, and use this to define the future development path. This approach can also be applied across the disease states of interest to identify which may be the most responsive. For example, immune disease may be characterized by inflammation, pain and fibrosis, and an experimental medicine study might be used to identify that the drug effect is greatest on fibrosis. This would lead to a very different development programme compared with that if the principal effect was observed on pain.

Phase IIb studies

The traditional approach for phase IIb studies has been to examine a high (probably supramaximal), medium (optimal) and low (subtherapeutic) dose. Done well, this kind of study can provide a large amount of information. The high dose establishes whether an increased dose is associated with increased efficacy and how the safety profile is altered by this higher dose. Maximizing efficacy is usually the main driver for development programmes; because safety data during development are limited, this has tended to result in the registration of high doses which turn out to have a less favourable safety profile in the long term. It is not uncommon for recommended doses to be reduced in the postmarketing arena. Identifying markers of patient responsiveness is an increasing priority in drug development. The establishment of the 'minimally' effective dose is therefore important and is the reason for the inclusion of the 'low' dose in this design. While this kind of design can be highly informative, success is predicated on the selection of doses that are sufficiently differentiated to address the principal questions. Again, the availability of a suitable clinical or PD measure is required.

The role of pharmacokinetic/pharmacodynamic modelling

Integration of PK data with PD data, usually in a mathematical model, is now a vital part of most drug development programmes. Although biological systems are complex, they can usually be adequately described by a mathematical model, providing one understands the principal determinants of response. Exploring and characterizing these through preclinical and clinical experiments can be a key enabling activity. Having to generate clinical data for every possible dose level and dosing regimen can be prohibitively time consuming and expensive for most programmes. There are now several examples of programmes where the optimal dose to be taken into registration (phase III studies) has not been formally tested in phase II but has been selected based on modelled data from the phase II study. It is an aspiration that better understanding of pathway biology coupled with machine learning techniques could allow modelling for a much more significant part of drug development with substantial efficiency benefits. See Chapter 10 for more information on this topic.

Phase III development

Phase III studies are those that principally support registration of a new medicine. As such, they are expected to provide 'substantial' evidence of safety and efficacy in order to support a robust assessment of risk/benefit during the registration assessment.

In most cases, the phase III programme will need to support registration in the major markets. In the past, this will have been the United States and Europe, but markets and development programmes are changing. In the past, many Western-based companies would only seek registration in Japan following establishment of the market in the United States and Europe and by means of a separate development programme. Increasingly, Japan is now included in initial registration programmes as development becomes more global. Regulatory review times in China have traditionally been very long, this and the requirement for a local study have delayed registration of new medicines in this country. Recent substantial changes in the regulatory environment in China to promote early registration of new products is substantially altering development strategies, with some new medicines being licensed in China first.

Traditionally, phase III studies have taken the form of replicate placebo-controlled, double-blind clinical studies. Clearly, true replicate studies would provide the most robust evidence, but, although phase III protocols may have the same design, they are usually conducted in different geographical regions. This will affect both the ethnic background of the participants and may involve substantial differences in the standard of background medical care. These have the potential to have a material effect on the results, so it is important to ensure that important subsets are of sufficient size to allow a meaningful assessment of risk benefit.

Inclusion criteria in phase III studies are vital because they usually directly translate into the indicated population for the registered product. For example, an indication for all patients with type 2 diabetes would be commercially very attractive, but this represents a very wide population, ranging from the newly diagnosed to those with severe microvascular and macrovascular complications. It is probably unrealistic for a phase III programme to be able to demonstrate robust benefit risk for such a wide range. Most programs will therefore identify a subpopulation in which the benefit risk is most favourable and study this first with a view to expanding the indication through phase IV studies. In this case, the initial indication might be for patients poorly controlled on metformin alone. The definition of poor control needs to be precise—regulators are particularly wary of vague definitions of previous treatment failure which favour the new treatment, while alternatives have not been properly explored.

The selection of a primary endpoint for a phase III study is the other critical factor. The primary endpoint will usually determine the indication statement for the medicine. In most cases, failure to meet the primary endpoint will mean the medicine will not be approved even if secondary endpoints are positive. When comparing against placebo, the study must be adequately powered to show a clinically meaningful difference. This clinically meaningful difference is vital. One needs to show a statistically robust difference, but with sufficient numbers of subjects, it is possible to show a statistically significant but clinically irrelevant difference. In most therapeutic areas, there are likely to be existing therapies, and increasingly regulators will be looking for comparison against current therapy in phase III studies. This is particularly true in Europe and many development programmes will now have a placebo-controlled study run in the United States and a sister study against an active comparator run in Europe. When comparing to an active comparator, it may be sufficient for registration to show noninferiority (i.e., not worse than) with the active comparator, but this may not be a strong platform for commercial success unless there are other clear differentiating factors.

Data integrity is vital throughout the drug development process, but in phase III, it takes on a special significance, as a marketing licence may be granted on the basis of these data. A robust, auditable chain from the source data through the case record to the final analysis is required. The types of endpoint favoured by regulatory authorities in phase III studies are those that are best aligned with this process, that is, those that are discrete variables that are readily verified and open to an absolute minimum of interpretation. When clinical events such as myocardial infarction or stroke are measured, there is now an expectation these will be independently adjudicated to ensure the veracity of the diagnosis. Vital though these types of endpoint are to the drug registration process and to give confidence of efficacy, they do not fully capture the patient experience. For example, reducing the rate of myocardial infarction is important, but for an individual patient, quality of life and functional measures may mean more to them. It is therefore vital that phase III studies also capture these other wider aspects of patient experience. To date, no new therapy has been approved based on a quality of life primary endpoint, but it is likely that this will be seen in the future.

Because of the critical importance of phase III studies, it is usual to meet with regulators before the start of the programme in order to agree that the proposed study population, design and endpoints would support registration if the studies are positive.

In an ideal world, the phase III studies should be 'confirming' the observation made in the phase II studies, but as discussed above, early studies often rely on surrogates, whereas clinical endpoints are required for registration. This is a major contributor to failure in phase III, that is, the promise suggested in phase II fails to translate into a clinically meaningful benefit.

Other studies supporting registration of a new medicine

The phase III studies provide the principal evidence of safety and efficacy for a new medicine, but there are other important pieces of information that are required for successful registration (Table 17.2).

Table 17.2 Examples of supporting clinical pharmacology studies			
Study type	**Information provided and relevance to the prescriber**	**Typical study design**	**Possible alternatives to the typical study**
Food effect	How does food affect the absorption of the drug—can it increase or decrease it? What advice should be given to patients on when to take the medicine—how long before or after food?	A single-dose crossover study in the fed and fasted state.	Food effects tend to be more marked with drugs with poor solubility. A preliminary assessment can be incorporated into FIH studies, often in the repeat-dose cohorts, by administering the drug fed and fasted on different days.
Renal impairment	Is a dose adjustment required in those with mild, moderate or severe degrees of impairment? What is the effect of dialysis?	Single-dose administration in those with mild, moderate and severe renal impairment.	If renal excretion is not an important route, then a specific study may not be required. If the patient population has varying degrees of renal impairment, then a meta-analysis of exposure in the study population may be more informative.
Hepatic impairment	Most drugs are metabolized by the liver, and liver impairment may affect drug metabolism and thus exposure. The standard classification of liver impairment is the Child–Pugh score which principally refers to degrees of cirrhosis. There are, however, many other forms of liver impairment (e.g., due to congestion in heart failure) that are not well captured by this classification.	A single-dose study in subjects with Child–Pugh class A, B and C liver impairment.	If the proposed study population includes those with liver impairment, especially when this is not related to cirrhosis, then a meta-analysis of exposure may be more informative.
Thorough QT	Inhibition of the hERG potassium channel by some drugs can induce the rare but potentially fatal arrhythmia torsade des pointes. Regulators may require a thorough QT study to discharge.	A study in healthy volunteers dosed to PK steady state with the study drug at the therapeutic dose(s) and a supratherapeutic dose. Careful regular 12-lead ECGs with manual over reading of the QT interval. The objective is to characterize whether there is a dose-related prolongation of QT and to define the magnitude of the increase to guide prescribing.	Because this is a known liability, it is now usually excluded at the molecule design stage. Modern (wireless) ECG technology can allow a detailed assessment of QT in the FIH study and in some low-risk cases may be sufficient to fulfil regulatory requirements.

Continued

Table 17.2 Examples of supporting clinical pharmacology studies—cont'd

Study type	Information provided and relevance to the prescriber	Typical study design	Possible alternatives to the typical study
Bioequivalence	The clinical efficacy of most drugs is related to its exposure profile. If the formulation used changes, then it is necessary to show that the exposure profile is the same as the original in order to avoid having to repeat efficacy studies.	A single-dose crossover study in healthy volunteers with detailed PK sampling. The regulatory definition of bioequivalence is that the 90% confidence intervals of key PK parameters (usually C_{max} and AUC) of the new formulation must be within 80%–125% of the reference.	The regulatory definition of bioequivalence is tight and, for many drugs with substantial variability, unachievable. There is therefore increased focus on avoiding formulation changes during development. Early clinical studies will often be conducted with a simple formulation (powder in bottle, hand-filled capsule), and if data are encouraging, then substantial effort will be made to develop a final formulation to take into account efficacy studies with the intent of avoiding late changes.
Drug interaction studies	Most patients take multiple medications. Drugs may interact through physical, PK and PD mechanisms. Drugs may be 'perpetrators' or 'victims' of such interactions. In some cases, combinations should be contraindicated, in others, a dose adjustment may be required.	A typical package would include a suite of studies (often 5–6) examining the potential for metabolic interactions that alter PK. These would often be single-dose studies in healthy volunteers.	Advances in modelling and simulation mean that it is often possible to predict which interactions could be clinically significant, and so refine the number and design of these studies. Other approaches with probe drugs with known routes of metabolism can also provide insight. Traditional drug interaction studies focused on PK interaction, but PD interactions (positive and negative) are of increasing importance, especially in fields such as oncology. These require a different approach commonly involving full-scale clinical trials with efficacy endpoints.

AUC, Area under the curve; *C_{max}*, peak drug and/or metabolite(s) concentration; *FIH*, first in human; *PD*, pharmacodynamic; *PK*, pharmacokinetic.

These are sometimes called phase I studies because they address clinical pharmacological questions but are better described as clinical pharmacology studies, as they are usually conducted well into development and often in parallel with phase III studies. Traditional development programmes would commonly have a large number of such studies (15–20), but many of the questions they address can also be addressed by modelling and simulation approaches. For this reason, the number of supporting clinical pharmacology studies is falling.

Phase IV

Phase IV studies are about maximizing the potential of a medicine. They fall into two broad categories: those studies required by regulatory authorities that usually focus on safety, and those initiated by the sponsor that are usually aimed at extending the indications for the medicine.

At the time of registration of a new medicine, the safety database will be limited. In most cases, regulatory authorities will ask for additional safety information to be provided in the postmarketing environment. Routine pharmacovigilance is expected for all medicines, but specific information may also be requested. If there is a specific safety concern, then a specific study may be required. For example, the registration database may be primarily made up of patients with mild renal impairment; the number with moderate or severe renal impairment may be limited. In this case, a safety study may be required to establish whether the safety profile of the medicine is similar in these patients or whether it is less favourable. In rare diseases, the number of patients in registration clinical trials may be very limited, and so there is greater uncertainly about the general safety profile. In this case, a registry or other method of following treated patients in the marketplace may be required to build a more comprehensive picture of the safety profile.

Most medicines will have a pretty restricted indication at first registration. The licence holder will want to maximize their revenue over the life cycle of the medicine. Expanding the indication for a medicine can be in several different directions. For example, a new cancer medicine may initially be licensed for second- or third-line use; studies supporting first-line use would expand its proportion of the market. In other cases, the first indication may be restricted to patients with severe disease; showing that it also is beneficial in those with less severe disease will expand the eligible population within the disease state. Another means to expand to eligible populations is to seek entirely new indications. For example, selective serotonin reuptake inhibitors (SSRIs) were initially licensed for major depression but over time additional indications including obsessive–compulsive disorder, panic disorder and posttraumatic stress disorder were added.

In some cases, the initial registration may be based on a functional or symptomatic benefit. A phase IV study may follow patients for much longer to establish whether a treatment is associated with a survival advantage. This kind of information can be important in diseases where there are several treatment options. The treatment with the most robust long-term data is most likely to be recommended by payer organizations.

The scale and duration of the phase IV studies are often much greater than the original registration package. There is good evidence that products that benefit from extensive phase IV programmes are those that maximize their commercial potential.

Paediatric drug development

Drug development programmes have traditionally focused on adults because in most cases this is the main commercial market. There has often been a dearth of information to support safe and effective prescribing in children, and major regulators have legislated to address this. The approach is different in the United States and Europe. In the United States, the approach is one of a 'carrot'—successful completion of an agreed paediatric development programme can confer an additional 6 months of data exclusivity. In Europe, the approach is more that of a 'stick'—new marketing applications will not be accepted unless an agreed paediatric investigation plan (PIP) is in place. The plan should usually start once phase I development is complete. In conditions prevalent in children (e.g., asthma), there is an expectation that the programme will be complete at initial registration, but in most cases, it needs to be ongoing at registration. One critical element of paediatric development programmes is that they need to address possible uses in children, not just whether the adult indication also occurs in children. This can mean that the disease under study in the PIP is different from that being sought in adults. Some diseases and targets do not occur in children (e.g., Alzheimer's disease), and for these, a waiver from paediatric development can be granted. In some cases, more information is needed from the adult development programme before paediatric development should start. This might be when there is a particular safety concern that requires better evaluation. Again, this needs to be agreed with the paediatric development committee.

Despite these efforts, the available information to support safe and effective prescribing in children remains patchy and incomplete. All too often, paediatric studies are suboptimally designed with limited operational effort leading to very slow recruitment. Studies may drag on for years, during which time standard of care changes, confounding the interpretation of results. This is an area where modelling and simulation can play a major role by linking drug exposure profiles in children to those in adults, and linking this to efficacy, thus providing important prescribing information with a study design that is much easier to implement and so delivers in a meaningful timeframe.

Phase 0 (microdose) studies

Many FIH studies will be supported by toxicology studies of 28-day duration because this will support up to 14 days' dosing in humans. Administration of pharmacologically active doses will also require safety pharmacology packaging. In some cases, however, there are questions about a new drug that can be answered by the administration of a single microdose. For example, it may be vital to the profile of the medicine that it has a half-life that would support once-a-day dosing. In this case, an estimate of the PK from a microdose could establish whether a candidate molecule has the right properties to be taken forward. In another example, localized administration of a very low dose could elicit a local pharmacological response that would build confidence in the mechanism of action, and so trigger investment in a full development programme. The advantage of these approaches is that under guideline ICHM3(R2), the preclinical package required is much less extensive. The key to success with these studies is to ensure that one has assays of sufficient sensitivity to be able to make a go/no-go decision.

The future and adaptive pathways

This chapter has followed the traditional scheme of drug development; while this remains the general approach for most medicines, it is very compartmentalized and may not suit the development of many therapeutic products. Specific examples include oncology, where treatment routinely extends until the patient no longer derives benefit from the start of the development process, and rare diseases, where the small patient pool and lack of alternatives make the traditional schema unattractive. Outside these more familiar situations, there is increasing social frustration with the time it takes to develop new medicines and a demand to fast-track the most promising. The challenge for regulators is to support potentially transformative products, while ensuring there is robust evidence of benefit and an adequate assessment of risk. The two main factors limiting long-term administration of most drug products is a lack of toxicology data of sufficient duration and the supply of physical drug product. It is an expectation that registration 'pivotal' studies will be conducted with the final drug product to ensure that the profile observed will reflect that to be expected in the market. Traditional manufacturing alters the method of production significantly according to scale; advanced manufacturing techniques allow for the drug product to be made on a small scale in much the same way as it is on a large scale, reducing the potential for variation in performance and so enabling a more seamless approach to drug development. Adaptive pathways are becoming formalized within regulatory authorities and are likely to become a more prominent feature of future development. A comparison of the expedited programmes available from the US Food and Drug Administration (FDA) are summarized in Table 17.3; some of these incorporate

Table 17.3 Comparison of FDA's Expedited Programs for Serious Conditions

Program	Fast track	Breakthrough therapy	Accelerated approval	Priority review
Qualifying criteria	A drug that is intended to treat a serious condition AND nonclinical or clinical data demonstrate the potential to address unmet medical need OR a drug that has been designated as a qualified infectious disease product	A drug that is intended to treat a serious condition AND preliminary clinical evidence indicates that the drug may demonstrate substantial improvement on a clinically significant endpoint(s) over available therapies	A drug that treats a serious condition AND generally provides a meaningful advantage over available therapies AND demonstrates an effect on a surrogate endpoint that is reasonably likely to predict clinical benefit or on a clinical endpoint that can be measured earlier than IMM that is reasonably likely to predict an effect on IMM or other clinical benefit (i.e., an intermediate clinical endpoint)	An application (original or efficacy supplement) for a drug that treats a serious condition AND if approved, would provide a significant improvement in safety or effectiveness OR any supplement that proposes a labelling change pursuant to a report on a paediatric study under section 505A of the Food, Drugs and Cosmetics Act. OR an application for a drug that has been designated as a qualified infectious disease product OR any application or supplement for a drug submitted with a priority review voucher

Table 17.3 Comparison of FDA's Expedited Programs for Serious Conditions—cont'd

Program	Fast track	Breakthrough therapy	Accelerated approval	Priority review
When to apply	With IND or after Ideally, no later than the pre-BLA or pre-NDA meeting	With IND or after Ideally, no later than the end-of-phase II meeting	The sponsor should ordinarily discuss the possibility of accelerated approval with the review division during development, supporting, for example, the use of the planned endpoint as a basis for approval and discussing the confirmatory trials, which should usually be already underway at the time of approval	With original BLA, NDA or efficacy supplement
Key features	Actions to expedite development and review Rolling review Designation may be rescinded if it no longer meets the qualifying criteria	Intensive guidance on efficient drug development Organizational commitment Rolling review Other actions to expedite review Designation may be rescinded if it no longer meets the qualifying criteria	Approval based on an effect on a surrogate endpoint or an intermediate clinical endpoint that is reasonably likely to predict a drug's clinical benefit	Shorter clock for review of marketing application (6 months compared with the 10-month standard review)

BLA, Biologics license applications; *IMM,* irreversible morbidity or mortality; *IND,* investigational new drug; *NDA,* new drug applications.

an adaptive element. A key element of adaptive pathways is a more regular and collaborative scheme of interaction between the regulator and developer. This is of course attractive but represents a substantial resource commitment for both parties. Large and complex organizations such as pharmaceutical companies and regulatory authorities may find it challenging to achieve the rapid internal alignment that intense iterative dialogue requires. Because of the commitment required, adaptive pathways schemes are restricted to those interventions showing the greatest early promise and/or which address substantial unmet medical need.

A central concept of adaptive development is that benefit–risk will be reassessed more frequently than in traditional development schemes and the plans adjusted accordingly. This provides for accelerated access for promising new products, but the converse also applies—medicines that fail to deliver on their early promise will be required to show additional evidence or may be removed from the market. It is worth noting that in the EU, the legal framework supporting adaptive pathways is not new legislation but the existing scientific advice, compassionate use and conditional approval rules. While this may impose some constraints, it does highlight the important point that adaptive development is precisely that—an adaption to the specific circumstances rather than an entirely alternative approach to drug development. The concept of question-based drug development was introduced at the beginning of this chapter, and it is fitting to highlight its importance at the end. Each new potential medicine is unique, and its development programme should be constructed to answer the critical efficacy and safety questions pertinent to that product rather than contorting it into some traditional prescribed schema.

Further reading

Darendorf, H., & Schmidt, S. (2019). *Rowland and Tozer's clinical pharmacokinetics and pharmacodynamics: Concepts and applications.* Philadelphia: Lippincott Williams & Wilkins.

European Medicines Agency. (2020). *Paediatric medicines: Research and development.* Retrieved from https://www.ema.europa.eu/en/human-regulatory/research-development/paediatric-medicines-research-development.

European Medicines Agency. (2020). *Adaptive pathways*. Retrieved from https://www.ema.europa.eu/en/human-regulatory/research-development/adaptive-pathways.

European Medicines Agency. (2017). *Guideline on strategies to identify and mitigate risks for first-in-human and early clinical trials with investigational medicinal products*. Retrieved from https://www.ema.europa.eu/en/documents/scientific-guideline/guideline-strategies-identify-mitigate-risks-first-human-early-clinical-trials-investigational_en.pdf.

The World Medical Association, Inc. (2008). *Declaration of Helsinki. Ethical principles for medical research involving human subjects*. 59th WMA General Assembly Seoul, October 2008. Retrieved from https://www.wma.net/what-we-do/medical-ethics/declaration-of-helsinki/doh-oct2008/.

Chapter | **18** |

Clinical imaging in drug development

Philip Stephen Murphy, Paul M Matthews

Introduction

Clinical imaging continues to make significant contributions across all drug development stages. Established imaging methods are routinely applied to neuroscience and oncology drug development. Innovative methods are increasingly being incorporated. In other therapeutic areas (e.g., immuno-inflammation), the importance of imaging techniques already is recognized for a wide range of disease applications.

Clinical phase failure has been a dominant factor limiting pharmaceutical industry productivity, but new drug development paradigms are emerging to deliver more informed approaches to early drug development (Cook et al., 2014; Morgan et al., 2012, 2018; Owens et al., 2015). To further reduce attrition, more direct translation of an understanding of biology across levels of complexity and physical scales, from cells to animal models, and then to humans, is needed. Imaging technologies hold particular promise as tools. They can enable the translation of molecular measurements at the cell level to in vivo preclinical imaging approaches that can often be extended directly to humans.

One approach to instantiating this has been through the introduction of 'experimental medicine' to drug development. As a complement to traditional phase II studies' designs, experimental medicine relies on using multiple small, shorter, information-rich clinical studies to validate targets in human disease and characterize new molecule pharmacokinetics (PK) and pharmacodynamics (PD). Imaging methods are providing an ever-growing array of clinical measurements for experimental medicine that complement biomarker- and tissue-based evaluations.

However, translating technology solutions for drug development poses challenges with each application. First is the conceptual challenge: how can imaging contribute to solving the problem? A useful broad framework for considering potential roles for imaging tools in clinical drug development is in terms of how they could address any of the major questions in any new drug development effort:

1. **Target validation:** does the chosen therapeutic target potentially play a central role in determining the disease or symptom of interest?
2. **Biodistribution:** does the molecule reach the tissue of interest in potentially pharmacologically active concentrations?
3. **Target interactions:** does the molecule interact with the target of interest? What is the relationship between administered dose and interaction with the target?
4. **Pharmacodynamics:** what are the effects of the drug, and how long do they last?
5. **Patient stratification and precision medicine (PM):** how can the most responsive patient population be identified for more efficient clinical trials? How can a medicine be given in the clinic targeted to those patients who will experience the greatest benefit?

The 'three pillar' concept has highlighted how linked evidence regarding new molecule delivery, target interactions and PD alone can translate into a substantial reduction in late programme failure (Morgan et al., 2012). This chapter will provide a brief overview of clinical imaging applications in drug development, outlining the bases of major clinical imaging technologies, current and potential applications and challenges integrating these techniques into a modern drug development plan.

Imaging methods

Positron emission tomography

Positron emission tomography (PET) imaging relies on either radiolabelled ligands that can bind selectively to a target of interest or metabolic substrates relevant to disease biology. PET ligands are most typically labelled with

259

Table 18.1 Some examples of PET radioisotopes useful in drug development applications

Radioisotope	Half-life
^{15}O	2 minutes
^{11}C	20 minutes
^{68}Ga	68 minutes
^{18}F	109 minutes
^{89}Zr	3.3 days

PET, Positron emission tomography.

positron-emitting radioisotopes that decay with a relatively short half-life, although some applications demand long-lived isotopes (Table 18.1). A short half-life allows a sufficient dose to be administered for a strong imaging signal, while minimizing long-term risks associated with the ionizing radiation.

PET imaging is based on the principle that emitted positrons collide with local electrons to produce pairs of photons that travel at 180 degrees to each other and can be detected as coincident events by γ detectors surrounding the subject. The relative positions of detected coincident events and their precise timing enable localization of the original annihilation events for reconstruction of the spatial distribution of the radiolabelled ligand. By following the time course of the emissions (and appropriate instrument corrections) across different tissues, the rates of delivery of the radiotracer and the amount retained can be modelled.

Only microdoses of radioligands or other radiolabelled molecules need to be used; PET is so exquisitely sensitive that even nanomoles of labelled material (e.g., with ^{11}C-labelling) can be detected. However, spatial resolution is limited intrinsically by the distance over which the annihilation event occurs (and, in practice, is typically ~4 mm).

A majority of PET scans are performed on a PET-CT (computed tomography [CT]) scanner that enables both PET and CT acquisitions during a single session. The CT component provides both co-registered structural images and corrections to the PET data to reduce artefacts. Co-registration of PET with magnetic resonance imaging (MRI) is typically achieved through software. The more recent advent of PET-MRI scanners enables these data to be integrated from a single scanning session. In principle, integrated PET-MRI scanners offer a range of new opportunities, such as MRI-based motion correction of the PET images (Hope et al., 2019) or for functional studies (e.g., arterial spin labelling [ASL] cerebral perfusion by MRI) to better inform the modelling of PET radiotracer binding (Scott et al., 2019).

Magnetic resonance imaging

MRI conventionally relies on the interaction of the weak magnetic dipole of the hydrogen nucleus with a strong applied magnetic field varying in a well-defined way across the body. Energy in the radiofrequency range modulates this with a specific frequency that depends on the precise magnetic field at each point in the body. As most hydrogen atoms in the body are in water (or fat), the frequencies of the mix of signals detected can be used to reconstruct tissue morphology as an image. Additional information comes from the intensity and duration of the signal detected. These are determined by the concentration of hydrogen atoms (e.g., how much water or fat) and their local environment, respectively.

The effect of the environment of the hydrogen atoms is expressed as two parameters: the T_1 and T_2 relaxation times. Changes in the way in which the radiofrequency is applied and the signal is received by the scanner mix the relative contributions of T_1 and T_2 parameters to the signal in different ways. This allows image contrast (grey scale variation) between different tissues (e.g., grey matter and white matter in the brain) or regions of a heterogeneous tissue to be generated. Images thus allow tissue size and shape to be measured and are sensitive to the state of tissue (e.g., changing with evolution of the pathology of stroke in the brain).

The unique attribute of MRI is the almost limitless potential to modulate tissue contrast through both endogenous contrast mechanisms and the delivery of contrast agents to further change the signal. This provides a wide range of methods to image structure, function and tissue composition within a single scanning session. This information-rich toolset is particularly attractive for drug development. A review of all relevant techniques is beyond the scope of this chapter, but three of the major techniques being applied in drug development include structural, contrast-enhanced and functional MRI (fMRI).

Structural MRI

The variety of tissue contrasts that can be generated during the MRI acquisition enables a wide range of structural evaluations. For example, abnormal structures (e.g., tumour) can be readily measured in three dimensions and reproducibly monitored over time. Subtly changing structural features such as joint cartilage thickness can be reliably monitored over a period of months or years. The structural measurement can be extended further to inform on tissue composition. For example, by studying the relative signal of fat to water, the progression of certain disease processes can be monitored (e.g., nonalcoholic steatohepatitis) (Caussy et al., 2018) and Duchenne muscular dystrophy (Mankodi et al., 2016).

Contrast-enhanced MRI

The signal of blood relative to tissue can be enhanced on a T_1-weighted image by intravenous injection of a paramagnetic chelate that alters local relaxation properties of water in blood. This can simply increase contrast of normal to abnormal tissue (e.g., defining a brain tumour due to a disrupted blood–brain barrier) or can be extended to measure tissue microvascular parameters. Quantitatively measuring signal change following injection of a contrast agent provides one way by which MRI can measure blood volume, flow and vascular permeability. These techniques have been extensively applied to drug development where altered vasculature can be pharmacologically modified (e.g., rheumatoid arthritis and cancer).

Functional MRI

fMRI is based on indirect measures of neuronal response by being sensitive to changes in relative blood oxygenation (Jezzard et al., 2001). Increased neuronal activity is associated with a local haemodynamic response involving both increased cerebral blood flow and blood volume. This neurovascular coupling appears to be a consequence predominantly of presynaptic neurotransmitter release and thus reflects local signalling.

The most commonly used fMRI imaging method applies blood oxygenation level-dependent (BOLD) contrast. MRI is sensitive to changes in blood oxygenation because deoxyhaemoglobin is paramagnetic and therefore locally distorts the static magnetic field used for MR imaging. In the MRI magnet, the magnetic field is made highly homogeneous, but the presence of deoxyhaemoglobin leads to small magnetic field inhomogeneities around blood vessels, the magnitude of which increases with the amount of paramagnetic deoxyhaemoglobin. A relationship between neuronal activation and blood oxygenation is observed because blood flow increases with higher neuronal activity, and this increase in blood flow is larger than is needed simply for increased oxygen delivery with greater tissue demands: the local oxygen extraction fraction decreases with synaptic activity. The BOLD signal therefore is not a direct measure of blood flow. Note also that these signal changes are small (typically, 0.5%–5% at 3 T).

fMRI can be used to assess PD (pharmacologic magnetic resonance imaging [pHMRI]). A typical experiment would involve acquisition of a series of brain images during infusion of a drug or over the course of a changing cognitive state (e.g., performing a visually presented working memory task versus attending to a simple matched visual stimulus). Regions of significant signal change with drug infusion or between cognitive states then are defined by statistical analysis of the time series of signal change.

Quantitative measurement of this change allows measures relevant to drug action on the brain to be defined.

Clinical MRI typically enables measurement volumes between 1 and 5 mm^3. Morphological measures can be conducted with high precision because of the high soft-tissue contrast. Acquisition methods for these can be combined with those for functional and molecular data. Moreover, the method is nonionizing and without known health risks. However, emerging concern regarding the risk of paramagnetic contrast agents (for contrast-enhanced MRI) in certain settings should be noted (Fraum et al., 2017). This should be considered in the context of MRI contrast agent use in clinical trials where multiple, repeat injections may be necessary.

Computed tomography

X-rays are differentially absorbed by different tissue densities, allowing the most basic imaging technique, the 'X-ray', to provide rapid, low-cost scans to study bone, for example. Such simple methods have been used in clinical trials of rheumatoid arthritis to measure changes in joint morphology associated with disease progression. CT is the cross-sectional extension of the X-ray that enables multiple image slices to be derived. A beam of X-rays is rapidly rotated around the moving patient, building up multiple image slices through the anatomy being studied. With the high-speed, low-cost and high-quality structural imaging delivered by CT, it is considered the radiology workhorse. In drug development, CT is one of the most widely used methods through the structural evaluation of solid tumours. In such applications, it is used from phase I to phase III to measure response and progression of disease. In addition, CT of the lung can provide structural trial endpoints in studies of chronic obstructive pulmonary disease (COPD) and lung fibrosis in addition to cardiac applications. Further technology developments—for example, high-resolution peripheral CT, are providing important microstructural interrogations of bone lesion repair in rheumatoid arthritis (Finzel et al., 2019).

Other techniques

Beyond PET, MRI and CT, other methods continue to be used in specific settings and will likely deliver further applications in the future. For example, ultrasound has a relatively limited breadth of applications to drug development to date. It is used to monitor cardiac function (echocardiography) in trials where there may be potential cardiac toxicities. Beyond that, despite the wide availability and diagnostic use, it remains limited for drug development. High variability of measurement is often quoted as a limiting factor. Optical imaging using light to measure normal tissue contrasts (e.g., as in optical coherence tomography for examinations of the retina) or exploiting molecularly targeted exogenously administered contrast agents have shown potential value in specific applications for drug development (Linssen et al., 2019). The main advantages of optical imaging include high sensitivity and microscopic resolution. However, due to the limitations of light scattering through tissue, applications of these techniques are limited to those involving superficial tissues, such as for assessing ocular pathology associated with neuroinflammatory disease, monitoring the progression of diseases manifesting in the skin (e.g., systemic scleroderma). Evaluating lesions in remote tissue compartments (e.g., lung or gut) has been made possible using functionalized endoscopes with advanced optical imaging capabilities (Seth et al., 2016; van der Sommen et al., 2018).

The drug development community will continue both to monitor available technologies and support the development of new applications for some of those in the course of their validation as PD measures. Drug development in the future is likely to benefit further from two distinct technology trajectories: (1) complex, information-rich molecular and functional methods applicable to small studies at single centres and (2) democratization of technologies such as ultrasound to allow regular, low-cost monitoring of large cohorts of subjects.

Human target validation

Confidence in progression of drug development simply on the basis of target validation in preclinical models (e.g., by demonstration of a phenotype plausibly related to the human disease with knockout of the gene of interest) is limited in the absence of prior human genetic or other secure evidence regarding aetiology. Progression of a promising target on the basis of animal model data alone arguably is particularly problematic for chronic diseases, for complex diseases that are determined by the interaction of multiple biological factors and the environment and particularly for those with uniquely human phenotypes (which include many neurological and perhaps all psychiatric disorders). This has brought an increasing interest in validation of new therapeutic targets based on experimental medicine in human disease 'models'. Clinical imaging methods can provide strong support for this by enabling noninvasive assessments of molecular interactions and tissue biochemistry and physiology in humans.

Human models also may usefully support target validation and development concepts for drugs intended for symptom management. For example, sleep deprivation has been used as a model for mild cognitive impairment. In this case, fMRI has been applied to characterize physiological changes specific to sleep deprivation-associated cognitive impairment and to test for their modulation by test agents interacting with new therapeutic targets of interest (Chuah & Chee, 2008). In this instance, the nature of the impairments with the sleep deprivation challenge, coupled to the ability of fMRI to report quantitatively on physiological modulation in specific functional anatomical regions relevant both to cognitive impairment and the model (e.g., the hippocampus), lends considerable specificity to associated behavioural measures. Modulation of impaired hippocampal activation during memory tasks after sleep deprivation by a new molecule provides compelling evidence supporting validation of the molecule target(s) for symptomatic treatment of disorders of memory.

An alternative concept for target validation in humans involves testing for modulation of disease-related brain systems by allelic variation at candidate target loci. This approach employs structural MRI or fMRI outcomes as endophenotypes (heritable quantitative traits) (Elliott et al., 2018). For example, indirect evidence has suggested that glycogen synthase kinase-3 beta (GSK3β) and canonical Wnt pathway function contribute to the molecular pathology of major depressive disorder (MDD). Brain structural changes also have been associated with MDD. To test the hypothesis that GSK3β is relevant to the disease, variations in brain grey volume were associated with GSK3β polymorphisms in a mixed population of healthy controls, and MDD patients were provided as evidence of the influence of genetic variation in GSK3β and MDD (Inkster et al., 2010). Supporting evidence for functional associations also can come from similar analyses linking brain structural variation to genetic polymorphisms related to genes encoding multiple proteins contributing to the same signalling pathway (Inkster et al., 2010). With the recent availability of large imaging datasets linked to genotyping of subjects, opportunities for this kind of work have expanded greatly (Elliott et al., 2018; Mollink et al., 2019).

Functional imaging methods can be used in similar ways. Patients with a history of affective disorders carrying the S allele of the common 5-HTTLPR polymorphism in the serotonin transporter gene (SLC6A4) have an exaggerated fMRI response (in the amygdala) to environmental threat relative to L allele homozygotes (Hariri et al., 2002). Other work has supported hypotheses regarding genetic variation associated with other disorders. For example, polymorphisms linked to the genes DISC1, GRM3 and COMT all have been related to imaging endophenotypes for schizophrenia and associated with altered hippocampal structure and function (Callicott et al., 2005), glutamatergic fronto-hippocampal function and prefrontal dopamine responsiveness (Egan et al., 2004), respectively.

Application of fMRI approaches that define neurobiological bases for general cognitive processes (such as in the context of psychiatric disease, motivation or reward) facilitates understanding of the general importance of targets relevant to more than one disease. For example, fMRI approaches have contributed to the current appreciation for neural mechanisms common to addictive behaviours across a wide range of substance abuse states. Studies of cue-elicited craving have defined similar activities of the mesolimbic reward circuit in a range of addictions (e.g., nicotine [David et al., 2005]). Combination of fMRI with PET receptor mapping on the same subjects has the potential to relate systems-level dysfunction directly with the molecular targets of drug therapies to further speed target validation in appropriate circumstances (Deco et al., 2018).

With the potential to define the relationship between in vivo molecular pathology and disease expression, the relevance of a target can be inferred more confidently in some instances than is possible based on postmortem studies only. For example, central to current therapeutic hypotheses for schizophrenia is targeting of dopamine receptor signalling. PET imaging with a receptor-specific radiotracer allows the receptor densities and distributions to be mapped in vivo in patient and healthy control populations. Using this approach, D_2/D_3 binding potential (BP) values have been shown to be abnormal in people with schizophrenia in both striatal and extrastriatal regions and to vary with age (Kegeles et al., 2010).

A limitation of the PET measure, however, is that it does not distinguish between effects of abnormal receptor availability or dopamine release (and neurotransmitter occupancy of the receptor that reduces the free receptor available for binding to the radiotracer). To more specifically test the therapeutic hypothesis that dopamine receptor antagonism is relevant to schizophrenia, dynamic changes in receptor BP can be studied before and after an intervention modulating dopamine release. For example, dopamine depletion leads to a larger increase in PET D_2 receptor availability in patients with schizophrenia than in healthy controls, suggesting a higher synaptic dopamine concentration in the patients (Kegeles et al., 2010). Similar approaches have been developed for studying other neurotransmitter systems, for example, for studying endogenous opioid or serotonin release (Colasanti et al., 2012; Tyacke & Nutt, 2015).

The relevance of a target to symptoms or behaviours can be validated in a similar fashion. For example, because dopamine is known to be an important mediator of the reinforcing effects of cocaine, it was hypothesized that alterations in dopamine function are involved in cocaine dependence. To validate dopamine receptor modulation as a therapeutic target for the treatment of drug dependence, pre- and postsynaptic dopamine functions were characterized by assessing the receptor-specific binding of a PET radiotracer in recently detoxified cocaine-dependent subjects and related directly to drug-seeking behaviour in the same group of subjects (Martinez et al., 2007).

Biodistribution

Microdialysis can provide accurate measurements of the free concentration of a drug in the brain or other organs or direct assays of tissue uptake can be performed on biopsies or performed postmortem. However, because of its relative inaccessibility, whether a drug intended for a central nervous system (CNS) target crosses the blood–brain barrier in sufficient amounts to be pharmacologically active can be very difficult to answer early in new drug development using conventional approaches to phase I and IIa studies (see also Chapter 10). Confidence in extrapolation of measures directly from rodents to humans is limited (Fig. 18.1). Recognized species differences in blood–brain barrier penetration are related to species-specific patterns of expression of transport enzymes, for example. Beyond the CNS, evaluation of whole-body distribution of drug can also be important. In cancer, for example, differences in the microenvironment (including interstitial fluid pressure and the nature of the tumour stroma) may impact drug levels (Fuso Nerini et al., 2014). Methods able to systemically survey multiple lesion sites to study differential response of lesions are required.

PET imaging using a radiolabelled drug provides the most general method for assessing drug distribution non-invasively (for a short, clear review of methods, see Gunn & Rabiner, 2017).

Imaging biodistribution can answer the question: does a molecule reach the tissue of interest in concentrations high enough to be potentially pharmacologically active? In addition, confirming absence of uptake in a given tissue (e.g., CNS) can de-risk future toxicity, minimizing undesired impacts in some therapeutic applications.

The principles for a PET biodistribution study are straightforward. The time course of data from the blood and tissue allows the clearance from plasma to tissue (a function of the blood flow and the tissue extraction of the molecule from the blood) to be estimated. If the tissue uptake is low, then separate estimates of the blood volume and allowance in the kinetics for the amount of the labelled molecule in the blood at any point are needed. An important caution, however, is that it is only the distribution of the positron-emitting isotope 'label' that is being measured with PET. Information also is needed regarding the concentration and the nature of any metabolites carrying the isotope that are generated during the imaging period and appropriate corrections made to the uptake model.

Molecules in the tissue will distribute to varying extents into tissue 'free' and 'bound' compartments. Binding can be either specific (e.g., binding to a receptor) or nonspecific, reflecting, for example, lipophilic interactions or the action of nonspecific uptake mechanisms. In the general case, a nonlinear relationship between the relative tissue distribution of a molecule and the amount that is specifically bound is

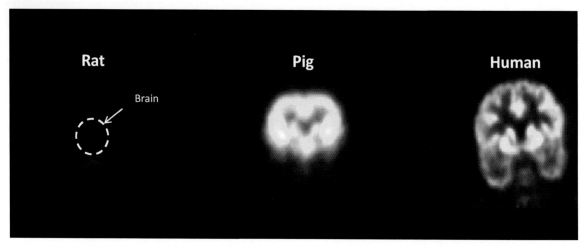

Fig. 18.1 Species differences in blood–brain barrier penetration. A novel central nervous system (CNS) active molecule was labelled with ^{11}C for PET biodistribution studies in a rodent, pig and human. The studies illustrate how poorly predictive rodent studies can be regarding distribution into the human brain. The small rodent brain lies at the *arrowhead*. A detected signal scale (standardized uptake value or SUV) is shown to the *right*.

expected. To define this, a kinetic analysis of the tissue compartment signal change over time is needed, ideally with respect to another compartment in which there is similar nonspecific, but no specific, binding (a 'reference' region).

Moreover, if the plasma free concentration of the labelled molecule is measured, and it is assumed that the molecule distributes passively, measures over the time course to a steady-state distribution allow an estimation of the tissue free concentration (Slifstein & Laruelle, 2001). Defining the volume of distribution of a molecule along with measurement of the plasma free concentration allows the occupancy of a receptor (OR) to be estimated if the assumption that the in vitro and in vivo K_D are equivalent, where:

$$OR = C_{\text{free plasma}}/(C_{\text{free plasma}} + K_D)$$

The passive distribution assumption can be tested with separate, invasive preclinical experiments (ideally, in a nonhuman primate for brain studies), exploring the relationship between plasma concentration of the molecule and the concentration in the tissue of interest as demonstrated by microdialysis.

The passive distribution model does not hold in situations in which there is high expression of active transporters for the molecule of interest, such as P-glycoprotein, at the blood–brain barrier. Evidence for transporters can be derived from demonstration of exclusion of tracer doses of the radiolabelled molecule but increasing tissue uptake with increasing plasma concentrations of the unlabelled molecule or after a transporter inhibitor is administered (Loscher & Potschka, 2005).

Reaching the tissue of interest in amounts sufficient to have a pharmacological effect is such a fundamental

requirement for drug action that, if there is uncertainty, biodistribution data should be acquired at the earliest stages of new drug development. Relative biodistribution can be a factor contributing to selection of the lead molecule for development at candidate selection. Preclinical studies can be performed efficiently prior to filing for registration of a labelled drug molecule as an investigational medicinal product (IMP). However, as the labelled drug molecule is used in microdoses only, toxicity testing for IMP filing can be limited to studies in a single species, allowing even human volunteer studies to progress early in a drug development programme.

While the greatest application of biodistribution studies thus far has been in the development of CNS drugs, biodistribution studies should also play an important role in optimizing anticancer drugs. Although the molecular mechanisms of anticancer drug resistance have been studied, the uptake of drug into the tumour is of fundamental importance in exerting a therapeutic effect (Minchinton & Tannock, 2006). Upregulation of pumps and tumour microenvironmental parameters can modulate tumour drug uptake.

Although a small proportion of anticancer agents in drug development pursue a PET biodistribution study, there now exists an extensive list of agents that have been studied (de Vries et al., 2019). Although the radiochemistry can be complex, small, definitive studies can be delivered. For example, ^{11}C-labelled lapatinib, a dual epidermal growth factor, was studied in six subjects with metastatic breast cancer (Saleem et al., 2015). It was concluded that at therapeutic serum concentrations of ^{11}C-lapatinib, there was no significant uptake of the drug through the intact blood–brain barrier, only in metastases. See Fig. 18.2

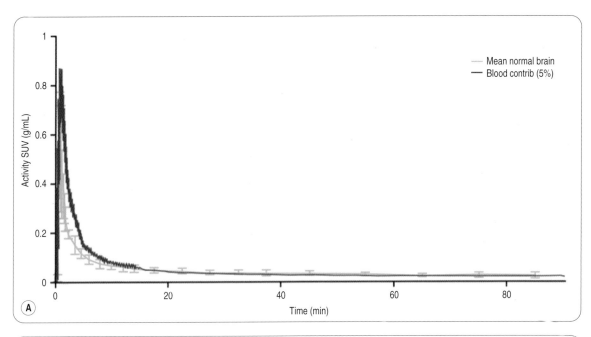

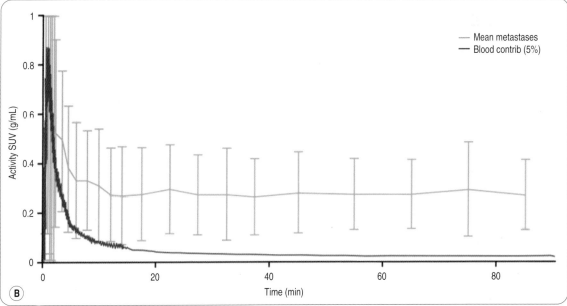

Fig. 18.2 Summary of blood volume contribution to total activity. Mean radioactivity time curves for (A) normal brain and (B) brain metastases. This demonstrates the signal in normal brain does not significantly deviate from the blood contribution, whereas the disrupted blood–brain in metastases facilitates uptake. *SUV*, Standardized uptake value (Reproduced with permission from EJNMMI Research. Saleem, A., Searle, G. E., Kenny, L. M., Huiban, M., Kozlowski, K., Waldman, A. D., et al. (2015). Lapatinib access into normal brain and brain metastases in patients with Her-2 overexpressing breast cancer. *EJNMMI Research*, 5, 30.).

summarizing the mean activity time curves derived from (A) normal brain and (B) metastases. With a disrupted blood–brain barrier present in metastases, the activity can be seen elevated relative to the blood contribution.

There is potential for integration of PET with conventional drug metabolism and pharmacokinetic (DMPK) radiotracer studies of new molecules, although it is not an approach that has been used widely. Subjects can be administered both [11]C- and ^{14}C-labelled molecules simultaneously. The radiation burden added by the ^{14}C-labelled molecule at radiotracer doses is small. The long half-life of [14]C (5700 years) means that there is no time pressure on sample handling for the additional analyses! This potentially allows the ^{14}C to be used to provide more detailed information on PK behaviour, which can improve modelling in the PET experiment. An alternative would be to use ^{13}C label with gas chromatography-mass spectrometry (GC-MS), allowing additional information on molecule absorption, distribution, metabolism and excretion (ADME) to be obtained. The value of the information can be enhanced by performing the study after administering varying pharmacological doses of the unlabelled 'cold' drug. However, the cost of this combined approach is high, limiting its use to specialized applications.

A creative extension of the traditional biodistribution experiment was demonstrated in use of the differential distribution of alternatively labelled molecules to provide information on drug metabolism directly from the PET experiment. The approach demands extensive radiochemistry to deliver two radiolabelled molecules but provides an elegant reminder that what is measured by PET is the distribution of the label, not the molecule specifically. Temozolomide undergoes decarboxylation and ring opening in the 3–4 position to produce the highly reactive methyldiazonium ion that alkylates DNA. To evaluate this directly in humans, a dual radiolabelling strategy was employed in which [11C]temozolomide was radiolabelled separately both in the 3-N-methyl and 4-carbonyl positions. [11]C in the C-4 position of [4-^{11}C-carbonyl]temozolomide will be converted to [11C]CO_2 and an inactive metabolite. Paired studies were performed with both forms of [11C]temozolomide in six patients with gliomas. A third PET scan was performed with ^{11}C-radiolabelled bicarbonate to provide data allowing quantitative modelling of the labelled CO_2 release from the independently performed temozolomide experiment. Data were obtained on activities of [11C]temozolomide and [11C]metabolites in plasma collected during scanning, and [11C]CO_2 was measured in the expired air. Greater amounts of [11C]CO_2 in the plasma and exhaled air and lower tumour [11C]temozolomide signal with the [4-^{11}C-carbonyl]temozolomide relative to that labelled in the 3-N-methyl position confirmed ring opening as a

mechanism for metabolic activation of temozolomide (Saleem et al., 2003).

Monoclonal antibodies (mAbs) and other biopharmaceuticals now represent an established therapeutic modality across a range of diseases. Characterizing biodistribution is equally important in biopharmaceutical development. A range of methods for labelling large molecules with positron-emitting isotopes have been established with the term ImmunoPET commonly applied (Van Dongen et al., 2015). Due to the much longer tissue distribution times for these large molecules, long-lived position emitters such as zirconium-89 are considered more compatible to enable mAbs to be followed over days rather than hours. Protocols for robust chelating approaches using desferrioxamine (DFO) are now considered reliable and typically result in one chelate per antibody, ensuring the properties of the mAb are maintained (Vosjan et al., 2010). Routine and standardized methods have been established to good manufacturing practice (GMP) including quality control steps to ensure labelled mAbs maintain functionality.

Developments continue in the labelling approaches (Bhatt et al., 2018), quantification aspects and experimental design to maximize the information gained from these studies. Radiation dosimetry should be carefully considered. Due to the long half-life of zirconium-89, radiation dosimetry should be carefully managed to balance image quality with radiation exposure. Experience of method and protocol optimization now extends from cancer patients into other therapeutic settings and even healthy volunteers (Thorneloe et al., 2019). Through the growth in marketed therapeutic mAbs and other large-molecule modalities in development pipelines, these clinical methodologies are becoming an established tool for biopharmaceutical characterization.

These are important methodologies providing biodistribution information not available by other means. This can be achieved in small cohorts studied in a single centre. The techniques have been extensively applied to neuroscience and in the last decade extended into other application areas such as cancer. However, they remain underused in drug development. In part, this is because they are arguably the most complex imaging studies to conduct and relatively few PET imaging centres have the resources needed to deliver them. Although radiochemistry options are broadening, the chemistry can be challenging, and studies are time-consuming and costly to set up (Murphy et al., 2017; Saleem et al., 2014). Identifying radiolabelling needs must be considered early in the drug development lifecycle to ensure methods are ready to add value to development milestones. To ensure this occurs, strong links are required between the drug development community and expert academic centres able to translate these complex techniques into high-quality clinical studies.

Target interaction

Does a potential drug interact with the intended target to an extent that could be pharmacologically active? What is the relationship between plasma concentrations (and thus administered dose) and the target interaction?

Direct demonstration of interaction of a molecule with the tissue target confirms distribution into the tissue. Target interaction studies also allow estimation of relevant tissue binding of a molecule without making assumptions regarding correspondences between in vivo and in vitro measures or between human and preclinical in vivo receptor affinities.

Target interaction studies are more informative if there is a strong hypothesis concerning the degree of target interaction needed for a pharmacological effect. In such cases, data relating plasma concentration to target occupancy can guide dose selection directly. For example, for inhibitors of G-protein coupled receptors, preclinical (and clinical) studies suggest that free concentrations sufficient to provide at least 70% receptor occupancy are needed. By demonstrating the relationship between plasma concentration and target interaction, doses sufficient to achieve this degree of interaction can be defined. If this information is available before dose-ranging studies, the range of doses that need to be explored is reduced, allowing the number of volunteers exposed to the experimental molecule (and cost) to be minimized at this early stage.

Target interaction studies demand availability of a radioligand that has good affinity and relative specificity for the target (Cunningham et al., 2005). The selected radioligand with relative target selectivity then can be used for imaging the extent of target available before and after a pharmacological dose of the molecule of interest. The ratio of the specifically bound radioligand to its free concentration (estimated from the plasma free concentration) in the tissue is termed the BP. The estimated BP at equilibrium is the ratio of the target availability (B_{avail}) relative to the radioligand dissociation constant from the receptor (B_{avail}/K_D). With prior administration of the unlabelled (drug) molecule that binds to the same target, the measured BP varies with the local concentration and the affinity of the unlabelled molecule. Over a range of doses of the unlabelled molecule, the variation in radioligand BP thus allows binding affinity of the unlabelled molecule to be estimated. As a rule of thumb, the radiotracer BP before any drug administration should be greater than about 0.5 for sufficient signal to detect binding changes.

Estimates of in vivo BP for alternative candidate molecules for a target can provide particularly important information if there are dose-limiting toxicities (Fig. 18.3). In such cases, the BP measures and simultaneous measures of plasma concentration allow estimation of the pharmacologically active dose range, the upper limit of which can be measured. The percentage changes in binding ($\Delta BP(ND)$) following challenges with antipsychotic drugs were measured. A regression model, based on published values of regional D_2 and D_3 fractions of $[^{11}C]$ PHNO BP(ND) in six brain regions, then was used to infer the specific occupancy separately on the D_2 and D_3 receptors (Girgis et al., 2011).

Target interaction studies typically have been conducted with single-dose studies for experimental convenience. A follow-up study, informed by the prior data, then is possible after repeat dosing to confirm dose–occupancy relationships with more chronic drug administration. However, if it is known (or can reasonably be assumed) that repeat dosing does not induce changes in receptor expression or availability, a consistent relationship between plasma concentration and target occupancy can be assumed and repeat-dose brain target occupancy can be estimated based on the basis of the combined occupancy data obtained after administration of a single dose and PK data. The principles behind this kind of analysis were illustrated with a study of single- and repeat-dose target interactions for the antidepressant duloxetine. Integrated plasma concentration-time-target occupancy models were fitted to the single dose data to characterize the model parameters, and then applied to an estimated repeat-dose duloxetine plasma time course to predict the 5-HTT (5-hydroxytryptamine transporter) occupancy after repeat dosing (Abanades et al., 2011).

Pharmacodynamics

Imaging methods can provide information on in vivo tissue structure, physiology and biochemistry. Based on questions derived from the pharmacological hypotheses for the study, these approaches thus can be used to provide PD information for proof of principle or molecule differentiation. The full range of imaging methods has been—or could be—applied with the common objective of answering the question: does a molecule exert a pharmacological effect on the biological system of therapeutic interest? A range of potential applications is illustrated by some general principles and specific examples (Box 18.1).

Early phase development

The advent of experimental medicine as a drug development paradigm is increasing the demands on first-in-patient studies to generate evidence of pharmacology. Information-rich studies in small cohorts with a short

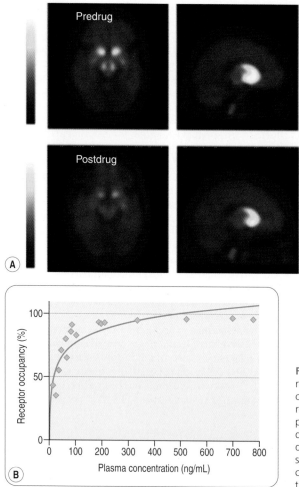

Fig. 18.3 (A) Images illustrating the specific binding of a receptor-specific radioligand before and after administration of pharmacological doses of a drug targeting the same receptor binding site. The reduced specific signal on the positron emission tomography (PET) scans after dosing reflects decreased receptor site availability in the presence of the drug. (B) Quantitative modelling of the PET signal to measure specific binding of the radioligand as a function of plasma concentration for the drug allows the in vivo receptor affinity of the drug to be estimated.

treatment duration have the potential to address multiple knowledge gaps. Imaging has an established role in some indications and treatment settings, providing endpoints proximal and distal to the drug action. For example, structural responses in a small number of subjects in a phase I oncology trial provide direct evidence for antitumour activity and confidence to proceed to further studies. Although such structural responses are downstream from the pharmacological action, it demonstrates disease modification.

Pharmacological studies of neurological disease have been a particularly important area for the development of new imaging PD markers, in part, simply because brain tissue can only be accessed under exceptional circumstances, and development of circulating biomarkers has been challenging because of the relative compartmentalization of the brain. However, MRI fundamentally changed how clinical trials in multiple sclerosis (MS) were performed (Tur et al., 2018). An initial therapeutic development goal was the limitation of acute relapses, which are associated with new CNS inflammatory lesions, and gadolinium enhancement of T_1-weighted images and persistent hyperintensity on T_2-weighted images in the acute and chronic stages. The observation that the frequency of new gadolinium enhancement is as much as 10-fold the rate of disease relapse (Arnold & Matthews, 2002) and validation of the correlation between changes in these imaging markers and changes in relapse rate with treatments (Sormani et al., 2009) have given confidence that early phase trials with MRI endpoints for antiinflammatory therapies can be reliably informative, demand smaller numbers of patients for meaningful endpoints and can be completed more quickly than trials with clinical outcome measures. More recent studies of the progression of disability have

Box 18.1 **Selected applications of imaging in drug development**

Safety and toxicity

- Imaging biomarkers as noninvasive, in vivo surrogates for direct, ex vivo studies of tissues and their translation from preclinical to clinical studies
- Confirmation molecule does not accumulate in nontarget sites of potential toxicity
- Surveillance of potential safety signals in large-scale trials

Early phase clinical development

- Biodistribution studies confirming molecule reaches the target tissue
- Target pharmacokinetic (PK) (dose–target occupancy) measurements guiding dose selection
- Pharmacodynamic (PD) biomarkers for proof of pharmacology, stronger 'reasons to believe' or contributing key rationale for proof of concept
- Translational preclinical imaging to identify or validate new imaging biomarkers or provide early differentiation between candidates based on target PK or PD responses

Late phase clinical development

- Surrogate markers of response more sensitive than clinical measures for accelerated approval
- Stratification of patients based on potential for treatment efficacy
- Pharmacological differentiation of asset from marketed drugs or new competitor compounds

Marketed drugs

- Differentiation between available treatments
- Indication expansion
- Earlier detection of disease or associated pathology:
  - Improved disease classification/diagnosis
  - Diagnosis of presymptomatic or minimally symptomatic disease
  - Improved identification of chronic disease exacerbation/recurrence
  - Patient stratification based on disease subphenotype or early treatment response

associated it with chronic inflammation, also amenable to monitoring by MRI or PET (Matthews, 2019) and quantitative MRI measures of brain volume loss (atrophy) or tissue rarefaction (Filippi et al., 2019). In such cases, the costs and complexity of serial MRI scans for the evaluation of the frequency of new enhancing lesions or the volume of T_2 hyperintense lesions is well offset by the gains in trial efficiency and informativeness. Additional endpoints are now in various stages of validation, allowing other

specific neuropathological changes to be monitored to report on PD for therapeutics targeting remyelination or neuronal preservation, for example. In 'real world' drug use, the risks of the most highly effective medicines can be mitigated by use of MRI to monitor people with greater immunosuppression for development of (ideally, preclinical) progressive multifocal leukoencephalopathy (PML).

Alzheimer's disease (AD) has been a major recent area of imaging marker research aiming to discover and validate neuropathological measures applicable in shorter term drug trials, because of the slow rate of clinical progression of the disease. The most striking neuropathological feature of AD is the progressive brain atrophy related to neuronal dystrophy (retraction of the extensive ramification of neurites extending from the neuronal cell body) and death. This is reflected in shrinking of the cortex (and other grey matter), which leads to generalized brain atrophy. Measurement of the rate of brain atrophy provides a PD index related to neurodegeneration (Chandra et al., 2019). Robust, automated brain MRI measures of volume and volume change (Smith et al., 2009) provide reproducible indices for which the relationship with neurodegeneration and the progression of disease have strong face validity. Much interest has focussed on development of similarly robust approaches for the measurement of regional brain volumes defining atrophy, for example, specifically of the hippocampus, which promise higher sensitivity. Disease-associated changes in measures reflecting microstructural differences in grey or white matter also have promise as measures of progression (Mak et al., 2017). Molecular imaging of the abnormal protein aggregates that are the target for new therapeutics using PET radiotracers also has been applied in proofs of principle for PD measures in trials targeting brain amyloid, for example, Rinne et al. (2010). Unfortunately, reductions in PET measures of amyloid aggregates appear not to be strong predictors of clinical benefit, at least after clinical expression of the disease. More recent work focussed on developing direct measures of synaptic density using PET as an approach for finding biomarkers more directly relating neurodegenerative pathology and symptoms (Chen et al., 2018).

PD biomarkers ideally should be tailored specifically to the drug development question. For example, a number of preclinical and pilot clinical studies had suggested that peroxisome proliferator activated receptor-gamma (PPAR-γ) agonism could reverse bioenergetic defects related to abnormal insulin signalling and reduced glucose uptake in AD that might be contributing to neurodegeneration. The brain has a high metabolic rate and glucose is the preferred substrate. A reduced rate of glucose utilization, particularly in the hippocampus and temporal-parietal cortex, is an early discriminant of people at risk of developing AD. This prior and related knowledge allowed a precise PD hypothesis to generate a proof-of-principle study of the efficacy of the PPAR-γ agonist rosiglitazone in AD: efficacious treatment enhances uptake of the glucose analogue [^{18}F]-fluorodeoxyglucose (FDG) and enhanced FDG uptake may predict slowing of the clinical disease. A novel multicentre FDG-PET trial with 80 subjects found only a trend for an improvement in FDG uptake over the first month of treatment and provided no evidence for slowing of the progression of metabolic dysfunction or neurodegeneration (Tzimopoulou et al., 2010; Fig. 18.4). These data were consistent with the negative results from two large phase III trials (involving many hundreds of patients) that had been conducted in parallel. The experience suggests that well-selected imaging PD markers, rigorously measured in a well-powered study, may predict clinical outcomes related to treatment. With greater confidence in them and their earlier staging, there could have been major cost and trial efficiency gains.

The combination of PD molecular imaging with clinical studies also provides lessons regarding the pathophysiology of the disease of interest. This now has been well illustrated by a recent study of antiamyloid antibody treatment effects on amyloid aggregates in the brains of people with AD (Liu et al., 2015). Brain amyloid deposits can be assessed by PET measures of brain binding of the radiotracer [^{11}C]-Pittsburgh compound B (PIB) and related radiotracers that bind to the beta sheet structure of the deposits. In phase IIa studies with both antibodies, time- and dose-dependent reductions in radiotracer binding in the brain were reported (Rinne et al., 2010). However, subsequent follow-up of a larger population in phase III trials did not suggest an effect on clinical outcome. This argues that the relevant toxic species may not be the amyloid aggregate itself and thus is not correlated with deposition of the amyloid aggregate. For example, these PET radiotracers do not report on amyloid oligomers or tau deposition, both of which may be more directly mediating neurodegeneration (Zott et al., 2019). While amyloid PET provided PD evidence consistent with the mechanistic hypothesis underlying the antibody development programme, with hindsight, it seems clear that amyloid tracer uptake does not provide a useful measure of clinical progression in the established disease, whereas tau deposition appears to provide a stronger correlation (Hanseeuw et al., 2019).

For specific applications, fMRI may provide imaging PD markers for drugs that have actions—direct or indirect—on brain activity, for example, for measurement of brain activity correlated with a symptom of interest such as pain (Sanders et al., 2015). The method is of particular interest

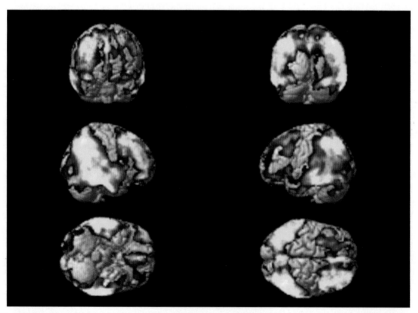

Fig. 18.4 FDG-PET as an imaging biomarker for the neuropathology in Alzheimer's disease. Rendering of the location of the voxels with significant decreases in glucose metabolism (*red*) over a 12-month period is overlaid on the surface of a reference brain (*grey*). Changes in the rate of decrease of brain glucose metabolism can be used as a pharmacodynamic marker for therapies intended to slow neurodegeneration (Tzimopoulou et al., 2010). *FDG-PET*, Fluorodeoxyglucose-positron emission tomography.

as a way of providing an objective, neurophysiological measure of brain events related to subjective experiences. This could be of special value in patients who are unwilling or—as for those with AD—unable to report accurately. An advantage of fMRI is that similar imaging approaches can be adapted to address a broad range of PD questions simply by applying them in the context of different behavioural task challenges.

An emerging alternative to fMRI conducted while performing a task is the use of resting state fMRI, which probes the continuing functional interactions—or connectivity—between brain regions (Zhang & Raichle, 2010). There is a continued background activity in the brain, the modulation of which is measured with task-related fMRI-assessed differences in brain activity between different task-related states, and resting state fMRI measures the intrinsic background activity of fMRI signal fluctuations that occur at low frequencies (0.01–0.05 Hz) without stimulation. Coherent changes in these are found even between widely separated brain regions. These consistent spatiotemporal coherence patterns define common activity networks that correspond functional anatomically with those engaged by task-constrained activations (Smith et al., 2009). Changes in the coherence measures before and after administration of a drug can define those brain regions directly or indirectly modulated by the drug (Cole et al., 2010). Nonetheless, fMRI still is immature as a trial endpoint measure, in part because of the lack of standardization of methods for data acquisition and analysis across trials (Sadraee et al., 2019).

Oncology

Structural monitoring of disease is considered a fundamental component in the study of new treatments for solid tumours. This is usually based on CT scanning to measure disease at baseline and throughout treatment. Radiological evaluation of the scans is typically performed using well-established response criteria, frameworks that specify how lesions are selected, measured and combined to evaluate response (Eisenhauer et al., 2009). Although these approaches are coarse from an imaging science perspective, the simplicity ensures measurements can be readily achieved across centres in complex disease with lesions in multiple anatomical sites. More refined structural imaging (e.g., high-resolution volumetric lesion scanning) has been successfully applied in specific disease settings in phase II studies. In such settings, imaging can be optimized to reliably study small volumetric changes, for example, high-resolution lung CT in non–small cell carcinoma (Altorki et al., 2010) and MRI for studying brain metastases (Lin et al., 2009). In many disease settings, volumetrically measuring small metastases reliably in multiple anatomical locations is problematic.

Beyond structure, a growing 'toolkit' of imaging markers for activity of biological processes commonly altered by many therapies is becoming available. For example, quantitative FDG-PET provides a marker for the elevated glucose metabolism in tumours as a consequence of the upregulation of glycolysis (the 'Warburg' effect). Changes in FDG uptake can reflect specific effects on insulin signalling and glucose uptake (e.g., of use with Akt or PI3 kinase-specific inhibitors), as well as nonspecific effects on glycolytic enzyme expression or cell viability. Due to the broad diagnostic role of FDG-PET, the technique is available at the majority of cancer centres participating in clinical trials. For this reason, it is also a technique that can be applied in a range of cancer applications, from small, well-controlled quantitative studies through to use in large phase II or phase III studies used as an adjunct to structural imaging.

Beyond FDG, multiple tracers with potential to measure pharmacology have been studied, for example, tracers targeting apoptosis (Wang et al., 2017), proliferation (Bollineni et al., 2016), hypoxia (Fleming et al., 2015) and integrins (Haubner et al., 2014). However, despite clinical testing and some promise, none of these methods have emerged as having generic importance in early phase oncology trials.

Functional and microstructural imaging with MRI has demonstrated success with techniques like dynamic contrast-enhanced (DCE)–MRI and diffusion MRI. DCE-MRI uses the time course of signal change in a tumour after injection of a bolus of a gadolinium contrast agent into the circulation to model tissue blood volume, perfusion and the microvascular permeability, which is increased with tumour neoangiogenesis. PD effects of angiogenesis inhibitors have been demonstrated across tens of trials (O'Connor et al., 2012). An example is shown in Fig. 18.5, in which an antiangiogenic effect is shown in a patient with hepatocellular carcinoma after only 3 weeks of treatment within a dose-finding study of pazopanib (Yau et al., 2011). PD effects measured with DCE-MRI have been consistently shown across many developmental agents in different tumour types, and responses can be seen within days of commencing treatment.

PD measures can be integrated with those for biodistribution to define PK-PD relationships directly. This innovative strategy was applied to the characterization of a novel antisense oligonucleotide strategy for tumour treatment. The antisense oligonucleotide was labelled with ^{11}C and a PET biodistribution study performed to demonstrate its accumulation within the tumour tissue, while biochemical studies performed on samples obtained from biopsies of the same tumours were used to relate these measures to direct tests of the PD hypothesis (Talbot et al., 2010).

Through innovation in imaging science, the range of methods available to study disease response in early

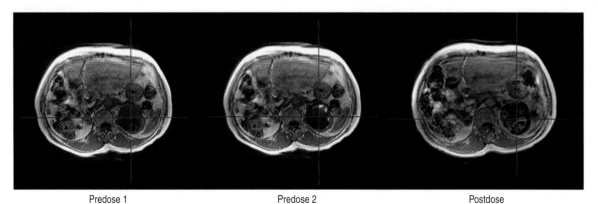

| Predose 1 | Predose 2 | Postdose |

Fig. 18.5 An example of DCE–MRI-defined pharmacological response in a patient with hepatocellular carcinoma. Two predose scans (predose 1 and predose 2) were performed to evaluate reproducibility. The structural scans are overlaid with coloured functional maps describing vascular permeability. The postdose scan was performed 3 weeks after treatment with pazopanib. *DCE-MRI,* Dynamic contrast enhanced magnetic resonance imaging. (Yau, T., Chen, P. J., Chang, P., Curtis, C. M., Murphy, P. S., Suttle, A. B., et al. (2011). Phase I dose-finding study of pazopanib in hepatocellular carcinoma: Evaluation of early efficacy, pharmacokinetics, and pharmacodynamics. *Clinical Cancer Research, 17,* 6914–6923.)

clinical trials will broaden. For example, the advent of cancer immunotherapies has seen a parallel emergence of molecular methods with potential sensitivity to detect relevant tissue cell populations. It is important to note that still few PD markers are confidently applied relative to the potential breadth of technologies available. New technologies will only become established PD methodologies through robust clinical testing. Early phase clinical trials with well-phenotyped patients, biopsies and biomarkers provide an ideal framework to incorporate exploratory endpoints to qualify for the benefit of future studies. In addition, drug developers must clearly communicate drug development challenges to imaging scientists to develop timely solutions.

Patient stratification and precision medicine

A critical issue in early drug development is to establish an appropriate level of confidence in the potential of a new molecule to become a therapy. One way in which this can be facilitated is by better controlling for intrinsic variations in therapeutic responses between individuals. As well demonstrated in oncology, stratification of patients based on specific disease characteristics can allow for more powerful trial designs. Consider, hypothetically, the difference in outcomes of trials first for a population in which a new molecule has a 50% treatment effect in 20% of patients (leading to a 10% net treatment effect), and then in a stratified population enriched so that 70% are responders (net 35% treatment effect). If it is able to

predict potential responders, imaging could suggest ways of best selecting optimal patient groups for applications of new molecules. Of course, developing such a strategy is predicated on having an understanding of pharmacology sufficient to make useful guesses regarding the selection of stratification criteria.

Imaging-based stratification is already applied in clinical practice to better ensure efficacy and limit adverse outcomes, for example, to limit surgical treatments to patients with localized neoplastic disease, or tissue plasminogen activator (tPA) therapy to patients presenting within a few hours after ischaemic stroke. Enrichment of clinical trials based on imaging indices also is well established in specific areas, for example, enrichment of MS trial populations for active inflammatory disease by screening for gadolinium-enhancing lesions at trial entry.

There are obvious cautions to the use of enrichment or stratification methods. First, they can increase trial cost or complexity to an undesirable extent. Individual scans and the additional demands for image data management, quality control and expert support in analysis add complexity and cost. The demands of research imaging in busy clinical settings can limit times for scheduling subjects in a trial, introducing constraints that make trial execution more difficult. Information sheets for volunteers and consent forms inevitably become more difficult to understand as imaging procedures and their safety concerns are explained, potentially reducing recruitment. Specialized types of imaging (e.g., PET scanning with advanced radiotracers) are typically only available at a very limited number of sites. A consequence can be less efficient trial design and execution. These consequences need to be factored into decisions to use imaging for stratification.

Optimally efficient statistical methods able to evaluate likelihoods of causality to derive maximum utility from the data and an understanding of the clinical relevance of strategies add value. In situations where image-derived metrics derived from routine clinical imaging can be used for stratification, immediate gains may be expected.

However, the gains may be lower than might initially be expected. There are a number of reasons for this. One is that use of quantitative imaging methods demands explicit consideration of ways of controlling for inter-session or inter-site variance in measurements with a care that generally is not used even for good quality diagnostic imaging. One report also has highlighted the possibility that a stratified population may behave differently from the general population, so that gains from the investment in stratification are reduced, for example, modelling showed that an increase in outcome variance in a subgroup of patients with mild cognitive impairment selected according to proposed criteria significantly offset the gains expected from the population as a whole (Schneider et al., 2010).

Imaging methods have been used successfully to predict treatment with existing therapies, often in small studies at single centres. Seldom have methodologies been translated into use in drug development, and therefore they remain underused. This may be due to the practical reasons outlined, but also the imaging methods must be compelling to add clear value to stratification criteria.

Towards precision medicine

PM is an extension of the concept of stratification of patients in trials to their stratification in medical care delivery. It is about tailoring of medical treatment to the individual characteristics of each patient. The intent is for treatments to be concentrated on those who will benefit, sparing expense and side effects for those who will not.

The concepts underlying PM are not novel. Healthcare delivery has long relied on physiological or pathological indices, as well as their clinical assessments to optimize (personalize) the diagnosis and treatment of patients. Current efforts in PM are evaluating the use of new biomarkers (including imaging-based measures), together with an understanding of both pharmacology and disease to make more rational treatment choices for individual patients. Potential applications of this approach in an imaging context would include:

- Selection of patients for a treatment based on imaging
- Dose adjustment based on imaging measures
- Identification of risks or early markers of adverse events with use of the drug based on imaging
- Using imaging to monitor treatment responses
- Selection of presymptomatic people with developing pathology for treatment based on imaging criteria.

To date, a number of drugs have been filed using companion biomarkers to select patients most likely to achieve a successful outcome. Broader use of these concepts will undoubtedly have a positive impact on healthcare systems. PM approaches ultimately will demand a common vision from all stakeholders including the pharmaceutical industry and regulatory agencies. These approaches are likely to be successful if integrated early into new drug development. Stakeholders continue to engage on steps required to make personalized medicine successful with a significant focus on biomarker qualification (Arnold, 2018).

Imaging represents some unique challenges to enable PM strategies. Methods most likely to deliver the right information to support treatment based on target-specific information (e.g., imaging human epidermal growth factor receptor 2 (HER2)-positive breast cancer with PET) represent some of the most complex techniques to scale to widespread use. For example, tracer cost and availability are likely to be limited. Also, scanning acquisition and analysis protocols would need to be carefully controlled to ensure consistent utility of derived metrics. Efforts will need to focus on image method scalability and standardization to ensure imaging can be deployed to accompany drug treatment decisions.

Imaging as a surrogate marker

Enthusiasts of imaging in drug development often explain the benefits of any imaging approach through its potential to become a surrogate marker for clinical treatment responses in pivotal trials. However, the instances in which this will be possible are likely to be rather limited.

The Food, Drug and Cosmetic Act is interpreted by the US Food & Drug Administration (FDA) as demanding evidence that the drug confers a clinical benefit. This establishes a clear need to acquire data for efficacy, as the usual, most meaningful clinical measures that, in general, are not expressed simply as imaging outcomes. Although still uncommon, there are circumstances in which registration studies are based on some imaging component. For example, radiological assessments of tumour size can contribute to progression-free survival endpoints in some cancer studies (Clinical Trial Endpoints for the Approval of Cancer Drugs and Biologics Guidance for Industry, 2018 https://www.fda.gov/media/71195/download).

There could be special situations in which imaging may provide a primary outcome measure and may be considered within the provisions of subpart H, 21 CFR 314.50 of the Accelerated Approval provision, which allows approval on the basis of a surrogate marker likely to predict clinical benefit. However, a central tenet of this regulation is that it is applied in a situation in which there is an 'inability' to assess a clinical outcome with a feasible trial. Applications to the evaluation of treatments for rare diseases with known pathophysiological mechanisms, for which there are well-established imaging markers, may be the most obvious areas for immediate application, for example, in rare storage disorders such as adrenomyeloneuropathy.

Even in such situations, for the first agent in a new therapeutic class, the use of imaging markers is unlikely to meet generally acceptable criteria as a measure of efficacy. The most obvious example of how such an approach would be developed would be to follow imaging observational studies of the disease and validation of the biomarker against usual measures of progression or even against a 'gold standard' intervention. However, a simple correlation between the natural history of progression and a measure will not establish predictive likelihood in the context of a new treatment. Even validation against a 'gold standard' treatment does not establish the general relationship because of the potential for multiple mechanisms or therapeutic effects other than those originally postulated.

Use of imaging as a stratification measure to define a population in which a drug may have higher efficacy is more likely to be possible, as long as the imaging stratifier is clinically meaningful and feasible in the real world. Of course, if used for registration of a drug, this could limit the population to those able to be imaged and with imaging findings consistent with the specific stratified class. Imaging also could be used for an approved drug to provide PD evidence of potential benefits that may add perceived value for its use in a case for its reimbursement.

Imaging in the real world— challenges to implementation

As with any aspect of trial conduct, conceptually elegant, robust implementation of clinical imaging in the context of a new drug trial brings substantial challenges. While imaging markers can have a high statistical power in some pharmacological applications, the measures are quantitative, continuous and often dependent on multiple factors. Controlling for variance in data between sites or even between examinations at a single site can be demanding. Reasonable prior estimates of the expected treatment effect size and the reproducibility of measures is needed to estimate the potential study power. Progression of overpowered studies incorporating complex and expensive outcomes will be not be sustainable.

In general, studies with designs based on reproducibility of measures within a single site can substantially underestimate true variance. For example, structural measures based on MRI are dependent on the homogeneity

and linearity of the MR gradients, which can vary between instruments and installations of even the same instruments. Fortunately, considerable effort has been expended in standardizing measurements (Shukla-Dave et al., 2019). In analogous ways, the performance of PET scanners varies (Boellaard et al., 2015). In both cases, calibrations with standard phantoms used across sites can be used to minimize variances. Even so, instrument or site bias in measurements can be introduced in many ways, for example, differences in radiofrequency coil coupling for MRI, detection mode for PET scanners or injection timing for radiopharmaceuticals or contrast agents. Analysis of results allowing for confounding of site-to-site variation helps to ensure that site bias can be recognized and optimally accounted for.

In single centres, acquisition and analysis can be carefully standardized through quality assurance, training and analysis workflows including quality control. Translating methods even to more than three centres can be problematic without careful attention, oversight and clear communication with site imaging experts. Significant resource is required to coordinate these activities, without which expensive imaging examinations costing hundreds of thousands of pounds will contribute nothing to trial decision-making. Scaling to tens and hundreds of centres creates even more challenges, and there is generally an acceptance that imaging variability can be high at such scale. Prescribing even basic imaging parameters, such as minimum CT slice thickness, can be unsuccessful and add considerable variability to studies.

Fig. 18.6 summarizes scanning variability in a large phase III study incorporating FDG-PET into multiple centres (PSM, personal contribution). One of the basic parameters to standardize in FDG-PET is the time of scan start following injection of the tracer. Poor control of this will add significant variability of the measured signal, limiting ability to compare subjects and study response within a subject. In this case, 60 min +/− 10 min was prescribed in the protocol. Reviewing the timing, it is apparent that many scanning sessions fell outside of this window (or in some cases, perhaps the value was recorded incorrectly). Continued activity is required through professional bodies (e.g., Society of Nuclear Medicine, European Association of Nuclear Medicine) to promote high quality, consistent scanning to benefit diagnostic applications and clinical trial applications. Failing to address this will limit the value imaging can bring to clinical trials.

More fundamentally, introduction of more sophisticated imaging endpoints will limit the availability of sites. Training on specialized techniques may not be accessible widely, for example, cardiac MRI demands cardiologist and radiographer training and ongoing experience to maintain skills if it is to be performed well. Some methods may be implemented only at institutions with

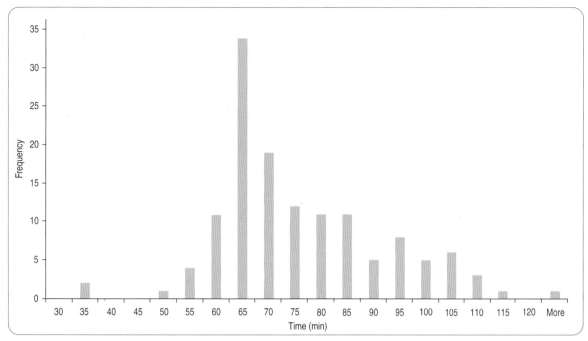

Fig. 18.6 Lack of fluorodeoxyglucose-positron emission tomography (FDG-PET) standardization from a phase III clinical trial. The parameter represented here is the time from injection to scan start that was recommended to be 60 minutes. Significant and in some cases very high deviations were recorded.

relevant research interests. PET methods relying on molecular probes, other than the few that are obtainable commercially, are only available at a limited number of sites, and shorter-lived isotopes (e.g., for [^{11}C] PET radiotracers) can only be used where there are radiopharmaceutical manufacturing facilities and a cyclotron is accessible on site.

The outcomes from many methods depend on precisely how they are implemented. Consensus criteria have been developed to minimize site variation in DCE-MRI measures, for example, Leach et al. (2012). Analytical techniques can be designed that are relatively robust to many aspects of patient or site variability. The issues have been discussed before in different contexts, for example, for precision in the assessment of brain atrophy rates or dynamic changes in FDG measures of brain glucose utilization in AD (Smith et al., 2009; Tzimopoulou et al., 2010).

Imaging approaches are variably complex (or can confer additional health risks) for patients or volunteers. These factors limit volunteer interest and complicate recruitment. MRI studies can be as short as 7–10 minutes (e.g., a whole body scan for fat–water assessment) or less, but multisequence studies demand cooperation for periods of 30–60 minutes in what to the volunteers may be the alien environment of the high field magnet bore and

with the sometimes distressing noise from the MR gradients. Prior familiarization of subjects with both the magnet and the noise, and attentive support from staff, can reduce complaints of claustrophobia and increase tolerance of more extended procedures. Contrast or radiopharmaceutical injections demand placement of intravenous catheters, so are not strictly noninvasive. While intravenous catheters are generally well tolerated, the intraarterial (typically placed in the radial artery) cannulation needed for serial blood sampling to allow accurate estimation of the input function for fully quantitative PET can be uncomfortable. Finally, all of the imaging methods using ionizing radiation carry some estimated additional health risks for subjects. It is important therefore to minimize demands on volunteers to those strictly needed to answer the question(s) of interest and to ensure that the procedures and risks are explained well, that procedures are optimized to give subjects the best experience possible and that they are conducted by highly trained staff to minimize risk or discomfort.

Some clinical studies for drug development already are incorporating imaging routinely to provide data for development decisions because of the demands of usual clinical care delivery or the need for imaging-based safety readouts. For these, the extra care in site setup and data analysis needed for quantitative imaging endpoints may add minimally to either trial cost or complexity. However, in other instances, imaging endpoints typically add substantially to cost and trial complexity and can make recruitment more difficult. Feasibility of the design of any imaging-supported clinical trial needs to be carefully explored with potential trial sites. Sometimes, relatively small issues—such as the extra time needed in the clinical centre for a full imaging examination—add so much to the burden of the trial for patients communicating into a research centre, that recruitment within desired time frames is not possible. It is important therefore that the value of the imaging outcome is high, commensurate with these direct and indirect costs. In the planning stage, designs and development plans that do not rely on imaging need to be considered to balance the information available with respect to both ease of implementation by the sites and participation by volunteers.

Imaging-supported clinical drug development is still an immature field and experience is limited. Validation of methods in the context of novel targets or classes of therapeutic molecules is even more limited. Potential applications need to be anticipated sufficiently and investments made well in advance of need if imaging is to be applied most powerfully in these contexts. This is most easily illustrated by considering molecular imaging markers. PET biodistribution studies demand the site-specific labelling and quantitative modelling of the distribution of signal in the tissues of interest. Implementation demands evaluation of labelling feasibility under the constraints of automated or semiautomated radiochemical methods, tailored for the appropriate half-life and the development and validation of the specific radiopharmaceutical and metabolite quantitative analysis methods for the radiotracer of interest. While timelines are highly variable and depend on both the molecule and on particular capabilities of the imaging centre, typical estimates from our experience with recent molecules suggest that even an optimal progression timeline demands at least 3–4 months for feasibility to be established, and 3 months for validation of a novel-labelled molecule. Thus the decision to incorporate a PET biodistribution study needs to be made well in advance of the need for information. Fortunately, as a microdosing experiment, this planning can be done and implementation completed as one of the earliest experiments in the sequence of clinical development studies.

Target occupancy studies are more demanding, especially if a radioligand suitable for use as a reporter for the target needs to be developed. Radioligand development is as challenging as the first stages of any drug development programme, as affinity and specificity need to be balanced for the molecule. Candidate radioligands show high attrition along the course of development and validation. Limiting nonspecific binding is a particular challenge. In general, useful radioligands should be lipophilic enough to diffuse well between tissue compartments without being so lipophilic that they accumulate in fatty tissues to a substantial extent. However, advances in design-based biomathematical modelling approaches (Guo et al., 2009) and the great potential for radioligand development to benefit from medicinal chemistry experience in the syntheses of related drug candidates suggest that there are substantial opportunities for more efficient development in the future.

Pharmacological fMRI offers the advantages of a potentially general marker for brain PD studies and has been used for a broad range of applications in healthy volunteers and patients. However, major challenges to the meaningful quantitative interpretations of pHMRI measures remain. First, the relationship of blood flow changes with altered presynaptic activity depends on the physiological (and, potentially, pharmacological) context. Even the direction of changes in relative activation in pathological states may be difficult to interpret precisely. For example, reduced activation in the ageing brain may reflect either brain functional impairment or improved efficiency. Experimental designs need to accommodate this, for example, by studying dose–response relations and behavioural correlates in individual studies. Additionally, BOLD signal changes arising from any direct (or indirect, e.g., with changes in ventilation rate [Wise et al., 2004]) need to be controlled. While experience has shown that fMRI provides pharmacologically discriminative measures (Matthews, 2009) and that studies can be implemented across multiple sites and the resulting data meaningfully integrated (Bosnell et al., 2008), there still is a lack of standardization of methods and availability of robust metrics.

However, there is real potential for realizing this. For example, direct measures of brain–blood flow can be made using noninvasive ASL-MRI methods that have greater stability over time for better assessment of slow (of the order of a minute or more) changes in brain responses and now can be implemented robustly (Xie et al., 2010). These measures are also expressed in absolute terms using scales that can be harmonized across sites. With care for safety issues and correction of the artefacts induced by the shifting magnetic field gradients used for MRI, high-quality electro-encephalography (EEG) now can be obtained simultaneously during an fMRI examination (Lemieux, 2004), allowing simultaneous pHMRI and pharmaco-EEG studies. Variance in measures can be reduced by correcting for variations in P_{CO_2} across the ventilatory cycle (Wise et al., 2004). Advances in positron detection methods also have led to combined human PET/MRI scanners (Mannheim et al., 2018) that allow integrated experiments examining target occupancy in addition to detailed characterizations of PD (Kelly-Morland et al., 2017).

Summary

Clinical imaging has an important role in drug development. The utility already has been well demonstrated in several applications reviewed here. It can facilitate more seamless transitions from preclinical to clinical development. Imaging also will facilitate answering critical questions earlier in development and directly with human studies, adding to confidence in decision-making. While implementation of imaging-supported protocols can add to trial complexity and cost per patient, where imaging has greater sensitivity, the gains can translate into smaller numbers of subjects in trials. This would have a particularly large impact on the potential to pursue studies for rare diseases for which it may be possible to recruit only small numbers of subjects or for highly stratified populations among even prevalent diseases for which personalized medicine is sought.

There now is an opportunity to substantially extend the range of situations in which, and the extent to which, imaging is used in clinical drug development. However, optimal use will demand the development of preclinical and clinical imaging strategies to support molecule development from the earliest stages of programme planning to ensure that methods are validated and ready to be implemented as critical decision points in projects are being approached. Wider use in development should catalyse new applications for imaging-based PM to better ensure that the right medicine is used by the right patient.

Imaging innovation for drug development is likely to follow multiple paths. In one direction, methods will increase in complexity, for example, with novel detection methods, multimodal evaluations, reference to large imaging biobanks, multiplexed molecular imaging and novel probes. In the opposite direction, simplification of imaging methods (e.g., low-cost ultrasound, optical measurements) will offer 'democratized' technologies with the potential to provide frequent measures and to be applied in patient populations in which imaging was not feasible previously. The integration of imaging and nonimaging endpoints particularly through better workflows and advanced analytics will be vital. So too will the use of imaging across measurement scales, for example, using advanced tissue techniques to validate our in vivo measurements.

An active dialogue is needed between drug developers and innovators of imaging in order that a flow of technologies can confidently deliver information-rich trial endpoints for a more successful drug development.

References

Abanades, S., Van Der Aart, J., Barletta, J. A., Marzano, C., Searle, G. E., Salinas, C. A., et al. (2011). Prediction of repeat-dose occupancy from single-dose data: Characterisation of the relationship between plasma pharmacokinetics and brain target occupancy. *Journal of Cerebral Blood Flow and Metabolism, 31,* 944–952.

Altorki, N., Lane, M. E., Bauer, T., Lee, P. C., Guarino, M. J., Pass, H., et al. (2010). Phase II proof-of-concept study of pazopanib monotherapy in treatment-naive patients with stage I/II resectable non-small-cell lung cancer. *Journal of Clinical Oncology, 28,* 3131–3137.

Arnold, D. L., & Matthews, P. M. (2002). MRI in the diagnosis and management of multiple sclerosis. *Neurology, 58,* S23–S31.

Arnold, M. E. (2018). An industry perspective on the US FDA biomarker qualification effort. *Bioanalysis, 10,* 913–916.

Bhatt, N. B., Pandya, D. N., & Wadas, T. J. (2018). Recent advances in zirconium-89 chelator development. *Molecules, 23,* 638.

Boellaard, R., Delgado-Bolton, R., Oyen, W. J., Giammarile, F., Tatsch, K., Eschner, W., et al. (2015). FDG PET/CT: EANM procedure guidelines for tumour imaging: version 2.0. *European Journal of Nuclear Medicine and Molecular Imaging, 42,* 328–354.

Bollineni, V. R., Kramer, G. M., Jansma, E. P., Liu, Y., & Oyen, W. J. (2016). A systematic review on [(18)F]FLT-PET uptake as a measure of treatment response in cancer patients. *European Journal of Cancer, 55,* 81–97.

Bosnell, R., Wegner, C., Kincses, Z. T., Korteweg, T., Agosta, F., Ciccarelli, O., et al. (2008). Reproducibility of fMRI in the clinical setting: Implications for trial designs. *NeuroImage, 42,* 603–610.

Callicott, J. H., Straub, R. E., Pezawas, L., Egan, M. F., Mattay, V. S., Hariri, A. R., et al. (2005). Variation in DISC1 affects hippocampal structure and function and increases risk for schizophrenia. *Proceedings of the National Academy of Sciences of the United States of America, 102,* 8627–8632.

Caussy, C., Reeder, S. B., Sirlin, C. B., & Loomba, R. (2018). Noninvasive, quantitative assessment of liver fat by MRI-PDFF as an endpoint in NASH trials. *Hepatology, 68,* 763–772.

Chandra, A., Dervenoulas, G., & Politis, M. (2019). Alzheimer's disease neuroimaging initiative, magnetic resonance imaging in Alzheimer's disease and mild cognitive impairment. *Journal of Neurology, 266,* 1293–1302.

Chen, M. K., Mecca, A. P., Naganawa, M., Finnema, S. J., Toyonaga, T., Lin, S. F., et al. (2018). Assessing synaptic density in Alzheimer disease with synaptic vesicle glycoprotein 2A positron emission tomographic imaging. *JAMA Neurology, 75,* 1215–1224.

Chuah, L. Y., & Chee, M. W. (2008). Cholinergic augmentation modulates visual task performance in sleep-deprived young adults. *Journal of Neuroscience, 28,* 11369–11377.

Colasanti, A., Searle, G. E., Long, C. J., Hill, S. P., Reiley, R. R., Quelch, D., et al. (2012). Endogenous opioid release in the human brain reward system induced by acute amphetamine administration. *Biological Psychiatry, 72*, 371–377.

Cole, D. M., Beckmann, C. F., Long, C. J., Matthews, P. M., Durcan, M. J., & Beaver, J. D. (2010). Nicotine replacement in abstinent smokers improves cognitive withdrawal symptoms with modulation of resting brain network dynamics. *NeuroImage, 52*, 590–599.

Cook, D., Brown, D., Alexander, R., March, R., Morgan, P., Satterthwaite, G., et al. (2014). Lessons learned from the fate of AstraZeneca's drug pipeline: A five-dimensional framework. *Nature Reviews. Drug Discovery, 13*, 419–431.

Cunningham, V. J., Parker, C. A., Rabiner, E. A., Gee, A. D., & Gunn, R. N. (2005). PET studies in drug development: Methodological considerations. *Drug Discovery Today. Technologies, 2*, 311–315.

David, S. P., Munafo, M. R., Johansen-Berg, H., Smith, S. M., Rogers, R. D., Matthews, P. M. et al. (2005). Ventral striatum/nucleus accumbens activation to smoking-related pictorial cues in smokers and nonsmokers: A functional magnetic resonance imaging study. *Biological Psychiatry, 58*, 488–494.

de Vries, E. G. E., Kist De Ruijter, L., Lub-De Hooge, M. N., Dierckx, R. A., Elias, S. G., & Oosting, S. F. (2019). Integrating molecular nuclear imaging in clinical research to improve anticancer therapy. *Nature Reviews. Clinical Oncology, 16*, 241–255.

Deco, G., Cruzat, J., Cabral, J., Knudsen, G. M., Carhart-Harris, R. L., Whybrow, P. C., Logothetis, N. K., et al. (2018). Whole-brain multimodal neuroimaging model using serotonin receptor maps explains non-linear functional effects of LSD. *Current Biology, 28*, 3065–3074.e6.

Egan, M. F., Straub, R. E., Goldberg, T. E., Yakub, I., Callicott, J. H., Hariri, A. R., et al. (2004). Variation in GRM3 affects cognition, prefrontal glutamate, and risk for schizophrenia. *Proceedings of the National Academy of Sciences of the United States of America, 101*, 12604–12609.

Eisenhauer, E. A., Therasse, P., Bogaerts, J., Schwartz, L. H., Sargent, D., Ford, R., et al. (2009). New response evaluation criteria in solid tumours: Revised RECIST guideline (version 1.1). *European Journal of Cancer, 45*, 228–247.

Elliott, L. T., Sharp, K., Alfaro-Almagro, F., Shi, S., Miller, K. L., Douaud, G., et al. (2018). Genome-wide association studies of brain imaging phenotypes in UK Biobank. *Nature, 562*, 210–216.

Filippi, M., Bruck, W., Chard, D., Fazekas, F., Geurts, J. J. G., Enzinger, C., et al., (2019). Association between pathological and MRI findings in multiple sclerosis. *Lancet. Neurology, 18*, 198–210.

Finzel, S., Kraus, S., Figueiredo, C. P., Regensburger, A., Kocijan, R., Rech, J., et al. (2019). Comparison of the effects of tocilizumab monotherapy and adalimumab in combination with methotrexate on bone erosion repair in rheumatoid arthritis. *Annals of the Rheumatic Diseases, 78*, 1186–1191.

Fleming, I. N., Manavaki, R., Blower, P. J., West, C., Williams, K. J., Harris, A. L., et al. (2015). Imaging tumour hypoxia with positron emission tomography. *British Journal of Cancer, 112*, 238–250.

Fraum, T. J., Ludwig, D. R., Bashir, M. R., & Fowler, K. J. (2017). Gadolinium-based contrast agents: a comprehensive risk assessment. *Journal of Magnetic Resonance Imaging, 46*, 338–353.

Fuso Nerini, I., Morosi, L., Zucchetti, M., Ballerini, A., Giavazzi, R., & D'incalci, M. (2014). Intratumor heterogeneity and its impact on drug distribution and sensitivity. *Clinical Pharmacology & Therapeutics, 96*, 224–238.

Girgis, R. R., Xu, X., Miyake, N., Easwaramoorthy, B., Gunn, R. N., Rabiner, E. A., et al. (2011). In vivo binding of antipsychotics to D3 and D2 receptors: A PET study in baboons with [^{11}C]-(+)-PHNO. *Neuropsychopharmacology, 36*, 887–895.

Gunn, R. N., & Rabiner, E. A. (2017). Imaging in central nervous system drug discovery. *Seminars in Nuclear Medicine, 47*, 89–98.

Guo, Q., Brady, M., & Gunn, R. N. (2009). A biomathematical modeling approach to central nervous system radioligand discovery and development. *Journal of Nuclear Medicine, 50*, 1715–1723.

Hanseeuw, B. J., Betensky, R. A., Jacobs, H. I. L., Schultz, A. P., Sepulcre, J., Becker, J. A., et al. (2019). Association of amyloid and tau with cognition in preclinical Alzheimer disease: A longitudinal study. *JAMA Neurology, 76*, 915–924.

Hariri, A. R., Mattay, V. S., Tessitore, A., Kolachana, B., Fera, F., Goldman, D., et al. (2002). Serotonin transporter genetic variation and the response of the human amygdala. *Science, 297*, 400–403.

Haubner, R., Maschauer, S., & Prante, O. (2014). PET radiopharmaceuticals for imaging integrin expression: Tracers in clinical studies and recent developments. *BioMed Research International, 2014*, 871609.

Hope, T. A., Fayad, Z. A., Fowler, K. J., Holley, D., Iagaru, A. H., Mcmillan, A., et al. (2019). State of the art PET/MRI: Applications and limitations—summary of the first ISMRM/SNMMI co-provided workshop on PET/MRI. *Journal of Nuclear Medicine, 60*, 1340–1346.

Inkster, B., Nichols, T. E., Saemann, P. G., Auer, D. P., Holsboer, F., Muglia, P., et al. (2010). Pathway-based approaches to imaging genetics association studies: Wnt signaling, GSK3beta substrates and major depression. *NeuroImage, 53*, 908–917.

Jezzard, P., Matthews, P. M., & Smith, S. (2001). *Functional magnetic resonance imaging: Methods for neuroscience.* Oxford: Oxford University Press.

Kegeles, L. S., Abi-Dargham, A., Frankle, W. G., Gil, R., Cooper, T. B., Slifstein, M., et al. (2010). Increased synaptic dopamine function in associative regions of the striatum in schizophrenia. *Archives of General Psychiatry, 67*, 231–239.

Kelly-Morland, C., Rudman, S., Nathan, P., Mallett, S., Montana, G., Cook, G., et al. (2017). Evaluation of treatment response and resistance in metastatic renal cell cancer (mRCC) using integrated (18)F-Fluorodeoxyglucose ((18)F-FDG) positron emission tomography/magnetic resonance imaging (PET/MRI); The REMAP study. *BMC Cancer, 17*, 392.

Leach, M. O., Morgan, B., Tofts, P. S., Buckley, D. L., Huang, W., Horsfield, M. A., et al. (2012). Imaging vascular function for early stage clinical trials using dynamic contrast-enhanced magnetic resonance imaging. *European Radiology, 22*, 1451–1464.

Lemieux, L. (2004). Electroencephalography-correlated functional MR imaging studies of epileptic activity. *Neuroimaging Clinics of North America, 14*, 487–506.

Lin, N. U., Dieras, V., Paul, D., Lossignol, D., Christodoulou, C., Stemmler, H. J. et al. (2009). Multicenter phase II study of lapatinib in patients with brain metastases from HER2-positive breast cancer. *Clinical Cancer Research, 15*, 1452–1459.

Linssen, M. D., Ter Weele, E. J., Allersma, D. P., Lub-De Hooge, M. N., Van Dam, G. M., Jorritsma-Smit, A., et al. (2019). Roadmap for the development and clinical translation of optical tracers cetuximab-800CW and trastuzumab-800CW. *Journal of Nuclear Medicine, 60,* 418–423.

Liu, E., Schmidt, M. E., Margolin, R., Sperling, R., Koeppe, R., Mason, N. S., et al. (2015). Amyloid-beta 11C-PiB-PET imaging results from 2 randomized bapineuzumab phase 3 AD trials. *Neurology, 85,* 692–700.

Loscher, W., & Potschka, H. (2005). Role of drug efflux transporters in the brain for drug disposition and treatment of brain diseases. *Progress in Neurobiology, 76,* 22–76.

Mak, E., Gabel, S., Mirette, H., Su, L., Williams, G. B., Waldman, A., et al. (2017). Structural neuroimaging in preclinical dementia: From microstructural deficits and grey matter atrophy to macroscale connectomic changes. *Ageing Research Reviews, 35,* 250–264.

Mankodi, A., Bishop, C. A., Auh, S., Newbould, R. D., Fischbeck, K. H., & Janiczek, R. L. (2016). Quantifying disease activity in fatty-infiltrated skeletal muscle by IDEAL-CPMG in Duchenne muscular dystrophy. *Neuromuscular Disorders, 26,* 650–658.

Mannheim, J. G., Schmid, A. M., Schwenck, J., Katiyar, P., Herfert, K., Pichler, B. J., et al. (2018). PET/MRI hybrid systems. *Seminars in Nuclear Medicine, 48,* 332–347.

Martinez, D., Narendran, R., Foltin, R. W., Slifstein, M., Hwang, D. R., Broft, A., et al. (2007). Amphetamine-induced dopamine release: Markedly blunted in cocaine dependence and predictive of the choice to self-administer cocaine. *The American Journal of Psychiatry, 164,* 622–629.

Matthews, P. M. (2019). Chronic inflammation in multiple sclerosis—seeing what was always there. *Nature Reviews. Neurology, 15,* 582–593.

Matthews, P. M. (2009). Pharmacological applications of fMRI. In M. Filippi (Ed.), *fMRI techniques and protocols.* Heidelberg and New York: Springer-Verlag.

Minchinton, A. I., & Tannock, I. F. (2006). Drug penetration in solid tumours. *Nature Reviews. Cancer, 6,* 583–592.

Mollink, J., Smith, S. M., Elliott, L. T., Kleinnijenhuis, M., Hiemstra, M., Alfaro-Almagro, F., et al. (2019). The spatial correspondence and genetic influence of interhemispheric connectivity with white matter microstructure. *Nature Neuroscience, 22,* 809–819.

Morgan, P., Brown, D. G., Lennard, S., Anderton, M. J., Barrett, J. C., Eriksson, U., et al. (2018). Impact of a five-dimensional framework on R&D productivity at AstraZeneca. *Nature Reviews. Drug Discovery, 17,* 167–181.

Morgan, P., Van Der Graaf, P. H., Arrowsmith, J., Feltner, D. E., Drummond, K. S., Wegner, C. D., et al. (2012). Can the flow of medicines be improved? Fundamental pharmacokinetic and pharmacological principles toward improving Phase II survival. *Drug Discovery Today, 17,* 419–424.

Murphy, P. S., Patel, N., & Mccarthy, T. J. (2017). Has molecular imaging delivered to drug development? *Philosophical Transactions. Series A, Mathematical, Physical, and Engineering Sciences, 375,* 20170112.

O'connor, J. P., Jackson, A., Parker, G. J., Roberts, C., & Jayson, G. C. (2012). Dynamic contrast-enhanced MRI in clinical trials of antivascular therapies. *Nature Reviews. Clinical Oncology, 9,* 167–177.

Owens, P. K., Raddad, E., Miller, J. W., Stille, J. R., Olovich, K. G., Smith, N. V., et al. (2015). A decade of innovation in pharmaceutical R&D: The Chorus model. *Nature Reviews. Drug Discovery, 14,* 17–28.

Rinne, J. O., Brooks, D. J., Rossor, M. N., Fox, N. C., Bullock, R., Klunk, W. E., et al. (2010). 11C-PiB PET assessment of change in fibrillar amyloid-beta load in patients with Alzheimer's disease treated with bapineuzumab: A phase 2, double-blind, placebo-controlled, ascending-dose study. *The Lancet. Neurology, 9,* 363–372.

Sadraee, A., Paulus, M., & Ekhtiari, H. (2019). fMRI as an outcome measure in clinical trials: A systematic review in clinicaltrials.gov *medRxiv.*

Sadraee, A, Paulus, M., & Ekhtiari, H. (2021). fMRI as an outcome measure in clinical trials: A systematic review in clinicaltrials.gov Brain and Behaviour, e02089.

Saleem, A., Brown, G. D., Brady, F., Aboagye, E. O., Osman, S., Luthra, S. K., et al. (2003). Metabolic activation of temozolomide measured in vivo using positron emission tomography. *Cancer Research, 63,* 2409–2415.

Saleem, A., Murphy, P., Plisson, C., & Lahn, M. (2014). Why are we failing to implement imaging studies with radiolabelled new molecular entities in early oncology drug development? *The Scientific World Journal, 2014,* 269605.

Saleem, A., Searle, G. E., Kenny, L. M., Huiban, M., Kozlowski, K., Waldman, A. D., et al. (2015). Lapatinib access into normal brain and brain metastases in patients with Her-2 overexpressing breast cancer. *EJNMMI Research, 5,* 30.

Sanders, D., Krause, K., O'muircheartaigh, J., Thacker, M. A., Huggins, J. P., Vennart, W., et al. (2015). Pharmacologic modulation of hand pain in osteoarthritis: A double-blind placebo-controlled functional magnetic resonance imaging study using naproxen. *Arthritis & Rheumatology, 67,* 741–751.

Schneider, L. S., Kennedy, R. E., & Cutter, G. R. (2010). Alzheimer's disease neuroimaging initiative. Requiring an amyloid-beta1-42 biomarker for prodromal Alzheimer disease or mild cognitive impairment does not lead to more efficient clinical trials. *Alzheimer's & Dementia, 6,* 367–377.

Scott, C. J., Jiao, J., Melbourne, A., Burgos, N., Cash, D. M., De Vita, E., et al. (2019). Reduced acquisition time PET pharmacokinetic modelling using simultaneous ASL-MRI: Proof of concept. *Journal of Cerebral Blood Flow and Metabolism, 39,* 2419–2432.

Seth, S., Akram, A. R., Mccool, P., Westerfeld, J., Wilson, D., Mclaughlin, S., et al. (2016). Assessing the utility of autofluorescence-based pulmonary optical endomicroscopy to predict the malignant potential of solitary pulmonary nodules in humans. *Scientific Reports, 6,* 31372.

Shukla-Dave, A., Obuchowski, N. A., Chenevert, T. L., Jambawalikar, S., Schwartz, L. H., Malyarenko, D., et al. (2019). Quantitative imaging biomarkers alliance (QIBA) recommendations for improved precision of DWI and DCE-MRI derived biomarkers in multicenter oncology trials. *Journal of Magnetic Resonance Imaging, 49,* e101–e121.

Slifstein, M., & Laruelle, M. (2001). Models and methods for derivation of in vivo neuroreceptor parameters with PET and SPECT reversible radiotracers. *Nuclear Medicine and Biology, 28,* 595–608.

Smith, S. M., Fox, P. T., Miller, K. L., Glahn, D. C., Fox, P. M., Mackay, C. E., et al. (2009). Correspondence of the brain's functional architecture during activation and rest. *Proceedings of the National Academy of Sciences of the United States of America, 106,* 13040–13045.

Sormani, M. P., Bonzano, L., Roccatagliata, L., Cutter, G. R., Mancardi, G. L., & Bruzzi, P. (2009). Magnetic resonance imaging as a potential surrogate for relapses in multiple sclerosis: A meta-analytic approach. *Annals of Neurology*, 65, 268–275.

Talbot, D. C., Ranson, M., Davies, J., Lahn, M., Callies, S., Andre, V., et al. (2010). Tumor survivin is downregulated by the antisense oligonucleotide LY2181308: a proof-of-concept, first-in-human dose study. *Clinical Cancer Research*, 16, 6150–6158.

Thorneloe, K. S., Sepp, A., Zhang, S., Galinanes-Garcia, L., Galette, P., Al-Azzam, W., et al. (2019). The biodistribution and clearance of AlbudAb, a novel biopharmaceutical medicine platform, assessed via PET imaging in humans. *EJNMMI Research*, 9, 45.

Tur, C., Moccia, M., Barkhof, F., Chataway, J., Sastre-Garriga, J., Thompson, A. J., et al. (2018). Assessing treatment outcomes in multiple sclerosis trials and in the clinical setting. *Nature Reviews Neurology*, 14, 75–93.

Tyacke, R. J., & Nutt, D. J. (2015). Optimising PET approaches to measuring 5-HT release in human brain. *Synapse*, 69, 505–511.

Tzimopoulou, S., Cunningham, V. J., Nichols, T. E., Searle, G., Bird, N. P., Mistry, P., et al. (2010). A multi-center randomized proof-of-concept clinical trial applying [(1)(8)F]FDG-PET for evaluation of metabolic therapy with rosiglitazone XR in mild to moderate Alzheimer's disease. *Journal of Alzheimer's Disease*, 22, 1241–1256.

van der Sommen, F., Curvers, W. L., & Nagengast, W. B. (2018). Novel developments in endoscopic mucosal imaging. *Gastroenterology*, 154, 1876–1886.

Van Dongen, G. A., Huisman, M. C., Boellaard, R., Harry Hendrikse, N., Windhorst, A. D., Visser, G. W., et al. (2015). 89Zr-immuno-PET for imaging of long circulating drugs and disease targets: why, how and when to be applied? *Quarterly Journal of Nuclear Medicine and Molecular Imaging*, 59, 18–38.

Vosjan, M. J., Perk, L. R., Visser, G. W., Budde, M., Jurek, P., Kiefer, G. E., et al. (2010). Conjugation and radiolabeling of monoclonal antibodies with zirconium-89 for PET imaging using the bifunctional chelate p-isothiocyanatobenzyl-desferrioxamine. *Nature Protocols*, 5, 739–743.

Wang, X., Feng, H., Zhao, S., Xu, J., Wu, X., Cui, J., et al. (2017). SPECT and PET radiopharmaceuticals for molecular imaging of apoptosis: From bench to clinic. *Oncotarget*, 8, 20476–20495.

Wise, R. G., Ide, K., Poulin, M. J., & Tracey, I. (2004). Resting fluctuations in arterial carbon dioxide induce significant low frequency variations in BOLD signal. *NeuroImage*, 21, 1652–1664.

Xie, J., Clare, S., Gallichan, D., Gunn, R. N., & Jezzard, P. (2010). Real-time adaptive sequential design for optimal acquisition of arterial spin labeling MRI data. *Magnetic Resonance in Medicine*, 64, 203–210.

Yau, T., Chen, P. J., Chan, P., Curtis, C. M., Murphy, P. S., Suttle, A. B., et al. (2011). Phase I dose-finding study of pazopanib in hepatocellular carcinoma: Evaluation of early efficacy, pharmacokinetics, and pharmacodynamics. *Clinical Cancer Research*, 17, 6914–6923.

Zhang, D., & Raichle, M. E. (2010). Disease and the brain's dark energy. *Nature Reviews. Neurology*, 6, 15–28.

Zott, B., Simon, M. M., Hong, W., Unger, F., Chen-Engerer, H. J., Frosch, M. P., et al. (2019). A vicious cycle of beta amyloid-dependent neuronal hyperactivation. *Science*, 365, 559–565.

Chapter 19

Intellectual property in drug discovery and development

Brian Cordery, Claire Phipps-Jones

As is clear from the rest of this book, it costs a great deal of effort and money to discover and develop a new drug. No one would make such an investment if the results could simply be copied by an imitator who had invested nothing. The best way to protect the investment is by obtaining patent protection that can cover, among other things the drug, its formulation, mode of administration, purpose and/or dosing regimen. In this chapter, we will look at what patents are, what kinds of inventions can be patented and how a patent may be obtained and enforced.

Patents are not the only form of intellectual property (IP), but they are by far the most important for the pharmaceutical industry and can be used alongside regulatory data protection and data exclusivity to protect an invention. Many patents that are filed and granted prove to be worth nothing, but a patent protecting a blockbuster drug against generic competition may be worth millions of dollars for each day that it is in force. An unexpected loss of patent protection may have a large effect upon the market value of the company holding the patent.

What is a patent?

A patent is the grant by a nation state or supranational body of the exclusive right to commercialize an invention in that state for a limited time. During that time (the 'term' of the patent, usually 20 years from the filing date, although this may be extended by up to 5 years in cases where an marketing authorisation (MA) is not granted for some time after patent grant, and by a further 6 months in the case of meeting certain paediatric criteria), the patent owner can go to the courts and enforce its rights by suing an infringer. An owner who wins the infringement suit can generally obtain a court order (an injunction) to stop any further infringement, damages or other compensation, costs, an order for destruction of infringing goods, declarations relating to the validity of the patent and publication of the result. Note that although the state grants the patent right, the state does not check whether the right is being infringed—the patent owner must do that.

It is important to realize that the rights given by a patent do not include the right to practice the invention, but only to exclude others from doing so. This right can be exercised so as to achieve a monopoly market, or alternatively, may be used to obtain a revenue stream by way of licence/royalty fees. Many inventors and business managers think that having a patent gives them freedom to operate, but this is not so. The patentee's freedom to use the invention may be limited by laws or regulations having nothing to do with patents, or by the existence of other patents. For example, owning a US patent for a new drug does not give the right to market that drug in the United States without permission from the US Food & Drug Administration (FDA) (see Chapter 20). Similarly, an EP patent does not give the right to market that drug in Europe without approval from the European Medicines Agency (EMA) or similar national authority.

What is less obvious is that having a patent does not give the right to infringe an earlier existing patent. To take a simple example, if A has a patent for a process using an acid catalyst, and B later finds that nitric acid (not disclosed in A's patent) gives surprisingly good results, B may be able to get a patent for the process using nitric acid as catalyst. However, because this falls under the broad description of acid catalysis covered in A's patent, B is not free to use its invention without the permission of A. On the other hand, A cannot use nitric acid without a licence from B, and in this situation, cross-licensing may allow both parties to use the improved invention.

Patents are important to industry because they give the innovator a period of exclusivity during which the investment in R&D can be recovered. They are of particular importance to the pharmaceutical industry because once the chemical structure of a drug is published, it is usually rather easy to copy the product, and because the manufacturing cost of a pharmaceutical is only a small part of the selling price, an imitator who has no R&D costs to recover can sell the product cheaply and still make a profit. The situation is not quite so stark in respect of biological medicines, which over time are becoming increasingly important to many life sciences companies.

The patent specification

A patent (which strictly speaking is just a one-page certificate of grant) is in most countries published with a printed *patent specification*, which typically will be 10–100 pages long, or even more. The patent specification consists of three parts: the bibliographic details and abstract, the description and the claims. Each part has a different purpose.

Bibliographic details

The title page usually sets out the bibliographic details, giving information, such as the names of the inventors, the owner or assignee of the patent, the title, the dates of priority, filing, publication and grant and the name of the attorney, if any, who acted for the patentee. It may also give the international search classification, and a list of prior published documents considered by the Patent Office when examining the application. Generally, it will also have an abstract summarizing the invention; this is meant as a tool for searching purposes and is not used in determining the scope of protection given by the patent.

Description

The longest part of the specification is the description, the purpose of which is to give enough information about the invention to enable a skilled person who is technically qualified in the relevant field to reproduce it. This ensures that when the patent is no longer in force, the invention will be fully in the public domain and able to be used by anyone having the necessary skills. The description will usually start with a brief account of the background to the invention, followed by a summary of the invention, then present full details, with actual examples where appropriate. There may also be figures (drawings, structural formulae, graphs, photographs, etc.), and if DNA or amino acid sequences are disclosed, there will be sequence identifiers in standard form.

Claims

At the end of the specification come one or more claims, which have the legal purpose of setting out exactly what is covered by the scope of the exclusionary right. The claims must not be interpreted in light of the other parts of the specification, and so it is unsafe to rely only on the wording of the claims absent the wider context. Readers who see that what they wish to do clearly falls within the claims of someone else's patent are put upon notice that if they go ahead, they may be sued for infringement, and will have to stop their activities unless they can prove that the patent is invalid. Unfortunately, the reverse situation is not so clear. In many countries, particularly the United States, even an activity that does not fall within the literal wording of a patent claim may nevertheless be held to infringe by 'equivalence'. The consequence is that before doing anything in the United States that is even close to the claims of a granted US patent, you must make sure that you get a written opinion from a US patent attorney that you are not infringing any valid claims. If you do not, and infringement is found, you may find yourself having to pay triple damages for 'wilful infringement'. Various European countries have similar concepts of equivalence, although the damages position is less clearly defined.

What can be patented?

There are basically only two categories of subject matter that can be patented—*products* and *processes*. Products are broadly anything having physical reality, including machines, manufactured articles, chemical compounds, compositions comprising a mixture of substances and even living organisms. A process may be a process for manufacturing an article or synthesizing a compound, or may be a method of using or testing a product. However, a patent for a process for making something, for example, a chemical compound, also covers the direct product of that process. A patent claiming simply 'the compound of formula X' covers X however it is made, but a process claim to 'a method of production of X by reacting Y and Z' covers X only when made by that process, and not in any other way. A claim to the compound itself covers the compound not only however it is made but also however it is used. Thus a claim to a compound invented as a dyestuff will also cover the compound when used as a pharmaceutical.

There are also some types of subject matter for which the grant of patents is specifically excluded, and these exclusions vary from country to country. For example, some countries do not grant patents on any plants or animals, whereas in Europe, only specific plant and animal varieties are excluded, and in the United States, there is no such restriction. Similarly, the United States allows patents for methods of surgical or medical treatment or diagnosis, whereas most other countries do not. Nevertheless, the invention that a known drug may be used for a new indication may usually be protected in these countries by patents having a different form of claim. Generally, patents will not be granted in any country for aesthetic creations, mathematical and scientific theories and discoveries without any practical application.

Pharmaceutical inventions

Within the pharmaceutical field, patentable inventions may include not only new chemical compounds of known structure, but also, for example, biopolymers and mixtures the structure of which has not been fully elucidated. Isolated DNA sequences and genes are also patentable as chemical compounds, although in some countries the scope of protection given by the patent is limited to the disclosed use. Even if a chemical compound is already known, it may be possible to patent variants, such as new optical isomers and crystal forms of the compound, as well as new galenic formulations, mixtures with other active ingredients, manufacturing and purification processes, assay processes and so on.

If a known compound, not previously known to have any pharmaceutical use, is found to be useful as a drug, this invention may be protected by claiming a pharmaceutical composition containing the compound, or, in Europe, the specific pharmaceutical use of the compound. If the invention is that a known drug has a new and unexpected indication, such an invention may be protected in the United States by a 'method of medical treatment' claim ('method of treating a human suffering from disease Y by administering an effective amount of a compound X'), or in Europe, by a use claim ('use of compound X for the treatment of disease Y').

Requirements for patentability

For an invention in any of the above categories to be patentable, it must meet three basic criteria and not be specifically excluded from patentability by statute:
- It must be *novel*
- It must involve an *inventive step* (must not be obvious)
- It must be *industrially applicable* (must have utility).

Novelty

The first and clearest requirement is that nothing can be patentable which is not new. If a patent were to be granted for something already known, then the grant of a patent in respect of this information would violate the fundamental principle that a patent cannot deprive the public of rights that it already has. There are, however, different definitions of 'novelty'. An invention is new if it is not part of the 'state of the art', the state of the art being defined as everything that was available to the public by written or oral publication, use or any other way, in any country in the world, before the priority date of the invention. For example, if it could be proved that the invention had been described before that date in a public lecture (or even a nonconfidential conversation) given in the Mongolian language in Ulan Bator, a European patent application for the invention would lack novelty even if no European had heard or understood the lecture.

Although historically the United States took a different position, all countries now operate a 'first-to-file' system, whereby if two persons make the same invention, the first one to file a patent application gets the patent. For this reason, it is important for inventors to file a patent application before publishing any results.

Inventive step (nonobviousness)

Whereas the concept of novelty is (or should be) an objective matter, the question of whether or not something involves an inventive step is intrinsically much more difficult, as subjective judgement is involved. The basic principle to remember is that the reason for requiring the presence of an inventive step is that ordinary workers in that field should remain free to apply their normal skills to making minor variations of old products.

Thus the person to whom the invention must be nonobvious in order to be patentable is the 'person skilled in the art', that is, a worker who is competent but lacks imagination or inventive capability. In pharmaceutical chemistry and biotechnology, the 'person skilled in the art' may be considered to be a team of highly qualified scientists.

It is a legal fiction to suppose that such a team could be competent but noninventive, considering that its members would, if employed in industry, be expected by their company to make inventions, and academic scientists would be expected by their university to produce original scientific work, which amounts to much the same thing. The point is that obviousness should be judged by a person with qualifications and imagination that are average for those in the field. It may be obvious to a genius, but the real question is whether it is obvious to the normal worker in the field.

It is often very easy to reconstruct an invention with the benefit of hindsight, as a series of logical steps from the prior art, but it does not necessarily follow that the invention was obvious, especially if there is evidence that the invention was commercially successful, or satisfied a need. The question 'If the invention was so obvious, why did no one do it before?' may, in some circumstances, be a relevant one to ask. It may also be relevant to ask what choices the skilled person or team had at the priority date of the patent and whether there was an expectation of success in respect of any of them.

Industrial applicability (utility)

In Europe, it is a requirement that the invention should be capable of industrial application, which is broadly defined and includes making or using the invention in any kind of industry, including agriculture.

Patent issues in drug discovery

The strategies that should be used to obtain patent protection for a compound in development are described later in this chapter. However, some patent issues need to be considered at an earlier stage. Here, we consider issues that concern the selection of a compound as a development candidate.

The two questions that need to be answered before significant sums are invested in development activities are:

- What sort of protection can we get for this compound?
- What patent rights of others could prevent us from marketing this compound?

These are two completely different issues. As explained earlier, it is perfectly possible to have strong patent protection for one's own invention, yet still to be blocked by earlier dominating patent rights owned by someone else. The 'patent situation' for a compound should attempt to give the answers to both questions.

The state of the art

The answers to the two basic questions depend upon the *state of the art*—patent jargon for all material relating to the technical field that has been published at the relevant date. The state of the art (sometimes called the *prior art*) includes not only published scientific papers, but also, for example, what is in textbooks, manufacturers' brochures, newspaper articles, web pages on the Internet and oral presentations at conferences. It also includes patent documents, which may be either granted patents or published patent applications that have not been examined as of the date of publication.

The requirements that a patentable invention must be *novel* and must have an *inventive step* mean that nothing can be patented that is already part of the state of the art,

and that anything that is very close to the state of the art may be very difficult to patent.

Patent documents as state of the art

A granted patent is not only a description, which, like any kind of prior publication, is part of the state of the art. It also contains *claims* defining the scope of protection. Published patent applications also contain claims, but these are often much broader than the claims (if any) that will finally be granted.

Patent documents in the state of the art are therefore important in answering the second basic question, which concerns *freedom to operate*. Granted patents may be invalidated by a court, but as a rule, they have a presumption of validity that is hard to challenge. Patent applications do not give exclusionary rights but may act as a warning flag for rights that may be granted in the future.

Evaluation by the patent professional

A professional evaluation of the patent situation of a new chemical entity (NCE) needs to be made at about the same time that the filing of a patent application is being considered. The timing of this will depend upon the patent policy of the company or organization owning the invention, but will usually be at the time the compound is ready to enter the development process, that is, at the time of transition of the compound to 'drug candidate' status.

The patent situation must be established on the basis of a search of the scientific and patent literature. Ideally, the search should be carried out by a professional patent searcher and evaluated by a patent solicitor (UK)/attorney (US) or patent attorney (UK)/agent (US). However, it is becoming more and more easy for a patent professional or a scientist to carry out searches online, and while these are unlikely to be as complete as those done by a professional searcher, such a 'quick and dirty' search may be all that is required at this early stage if it identifies relevant patent or scientific literature. If not, it is advisable to conduct further, detailed searches. At some stage after a patent application has been filed, searches will be carried out in the major patent offices, and these can be used to supplement the search made at the time of filing.

More complete 'freedom to operate' searches must be made at later stages, for example, to ensure that the proposed manufacturing process and the chosen pharmaceutical formulation are also free from third-party patent rights.

Sources of information

For patent literature, there are now a number of databases available online that allow full-text searching by keywords. One, available on the website of the US Patent and Trademark Office (http://www.uspto.gov), contains fully searchable texts of all US patents since 1976, as well as image files of all US patents back to 1790. A similar database (Espacenet) available through the home page of the European Patent Office (http://www.epo.org) allows searching of European patent applications, patent cooperation treaty (PCT) applications and various other jurisdictions, such as the UK and Japan. For Japan, the Japan Platform for Patent Information database, available through the website of the Japanese Patent Office (http://www.jpo.go.jp), gives English-language abstracts of all Japanese early published applications from 1976 onwards. Use of these databases is free.

Other databases, maintained by commercial firms that charge user access fees, add value by high-quality abstracts and additional indexing possibilities, and downloading and printing information from these may be quicker and easier than it is from public domain Internet databases.

Chemical Abstracts (CAs), a product of the American Chemical Society and available through the SciFinder and STN databases, abstracts both patents and scientific literature in the chemical field. The information retrieval system is based on a CA registry number allocated to every published chemical compound; once this has been identified, abstracts of all patents or literature articles mentioning the compound can be listed, and printed out if required.

Clarivate Analytics provides a wide range of abstracting and information retrieval systems for both scientific and patent literature. The latter includes the WPI (World Patent Index) database, covering all patents in the major countries issued since 1974. Searches can be made on the basis of keywords, or of partial structures of chemical compounds.

Results of the evaluation—new chemical entities

If the search shows that the compound lacks novelty, that is, it has already been published, then the best course is to pick a different one for development. Even though it may be possible to obtain some form of secondary patent protection, for example, the use of the compound as a medicament if it was previously known for a nonpharmaceutical use, most companies will prefer to invest in the development of a compound where it is possible to patent the compound itself.

If the NCE appears to be novel, but the search shows that very similar compounds are known, the compound may lack an inventive step. If the compound has unexpected, superior properties compared to the known product, these may be used to establish the inventive step. However, it would be necessary to show that the difference between the two compounds was not obvious to the person skilled in the art.

If the NCE, despite being apparently novel and inventive, appears to be covered by a third-party patent, the advice would be to go ahead only if the third-party patent appears to be invalid or will have expired before your product can reach the market, or if you are sure that you will be able to obtain a licence on acceptable terms.

Obtaining patent protection for a development compound

Filing a patent application

When to file

For pharmaceutical inventions, the decision when to make a first filing will depend on a number of factors, including the intensity of competition in the relevant field. Given that in most countries, including the United States, the first to file an application gets the patent, it would seem to make sense to file as early as possible as soon as an invention is made. It is not quite as simple as this, however. For one thing, the earlier a patent is filed the earlier it will expire, and particularly in the pharmaceutical field, the last year or two of patent life for a major product can be worth hundreds of millions of dollars. For another, a patent application filed at a very early stage may lack sufficient enabling disclosure to support claims of the desired scope. In order to be valid, a patent must be plausible—that is, the skilled person reading the patent must have reason to suspect that the invention may work. Too much delay, however, and another party may have filed an earlier application or published a paper that destroys the novelty of the invention. Finding the sweet spot in which to file the patent application is a delicate issue and will vary depending on the molecule and the disease to be treated.

Where to file

Normally, a single filing in one country will be made, which, under the Paris Convention for the Protection of Industrial Property, can form the basis for a claim to priority in other countries. Some national laws, such as those of the United States and France, require that, for reasons of national security, an application for any invention made in that country must first be filed in that country (unless special permission is obtained). Therefore it is best to check the law in the country in which the invention is made. The UK now limits this requirement to certain categories of inventions, but it may be safer to file all UK-originating inventions in the UK first.

The Paris Convention, now adhered to by the great majority of countries, provides that a later application filed for the same invention in another Convention country within 12 months of the first filing in a Convention country may claim the priority of the original application. This means that the first filing date (the *priority date*) is treated for prior art purposes as if it were the filing date of the later application, so that a publication of the invention before the later application but after the priority date does not invalidate claims for the same invention in the later application. If it were not for the Paris Convention, it would be necessary to make simultaneous filings in all the countries of interest at a very early stage, which would be extremely wasteful of time and money. Instead, a single priority filing may be made and a decision taken before the end of the priority year on what to do with the application.

During the priority year, work on the invention will normally continue, and, for example, further compounds will be made and tested, new formulations compounded or new process conditions tried. All this material can be used in preparing the patent applications to be filed abroad, and, where possible, a subsequent application in respect of the country of first filing. It is also possible to file new patent applications for further developments made during the priority year, and then at the foreign filing stage to combine these into a single application. However, it will only be possible to claim priority (i.e., to assess the novelty/inventiveness of the invention at the priority date) for these aspects of the invention disclosed in the original application.

The foreign filing decision

There are four options to be considered:
- Abandon
- Abandon and refile
- Obtain a patent in the country of first filing only
- File corresponding applications in one or more foreign countries.

Abandonment. If there is no commercial interest in the invention at all, or if a search has shown that it lacks novelty, one can simply do nothing. Sooner or later a fee must be paid or some action taken to keep the application in being, and when this is not done, the application will lapse. It is best not to withdraw the application explicitly, as such a positive abandonment is usually irrevocable, and applicants have been known to change their minds.

If applicants want to ensure that they retain freedom to operate, and that no one else can patent the invention, they should have it published, either by continuing an application in their home country long enough for it to issue as a published application (see later) or by sending it to a journal such as *Research Disclosure*, in which any disclosure may be rapidly published for a reasonable fee.

Refiling. It frequently happens that by the time the foreign filing decision must be taken, it is not yet possible to decide whether or not to invest time and money in foreign patenting. Commercial interest may be low but could increase later, more testing may have to be done or the inventors may not have done any more work on the invention since the first application was filed. In such cases, the best solution is to start from the beginning again. The existing application is abandoned, a new application is filed and the 12-month countdown starts all over again. In this case, it is essential to meet the requirements of the Paris Convention that the first application be explicitly abandoned before the second application is filed.

Of course, refiling always entails a loss of priority, usually of 8–10 months, and if someone else has published the invention or filed a patent application for it during this time, the refiled application cannot lead to a valid patent. Consequently, in a field where competitors are known to be active, refiling may involve an unacceptable risk, and, naturally, if there has been any known publication of the invention since the priority date, abandonment and refiling is ruled out. Such publication most frequently arises from the inventor himself. Most inventors know that they should not publish inventions before a patent application is filed; it is not so generally realized that publication within the priority year can also be very damaging.

Home-country patenting. If the applicant is an individual or a small company having no commercial interests or prospects of licensing outside the home country (which will usually be the country in which the first filing is made), the expense of foreign filing would be wasted, and the applicant will wish only to obtain a patent in the home country. Even where the applicant is a larger company that would normally file any commercially interesting case in several countries, individual applications may be of such low interest that protection in the home country is all that is needed. This option is, of course, more attractive if the home country is a large market such as the United States, rather than a small country such as Switzerland.

Foreign filing. Finally, if an invention appears likely to be commercially important, the decision may be to file corresponding applications in a number of other countries.

For the pharmaceutical industry, one can assume that the costs of patent protection would be small compared with the value of protection for any compound that actually reaches the market, but at the time when a foreign filing decision must be taken, it is usually impossible to estimate the chance that the product in question will progress that far. Accordingly, one must rely upon some rule of thumb such that if the product is being developed further, foreign filing should be carried out as a matter of course. High patenting costs are a necessary part of the high research overheads of the pharmaceutical industry.

Procedures on foreign filing

National filings. It is possible to file patent applications (in the local language) in the national patent offices of each selected country individually. This involves a large outlay of money at a relatively early stage, and also means that all necessary translations must be prepared in good time before the end of the priority year. It is also very labour intensive, as the application must be prosecuted separately before each national patent office. Fortunately, there are ways to simplify the procedure.

Regional patent offices. One is that there are certain regional patent offices by which patents in a number of countries can be granted based on a single application filed and prosecuted in one patent office. By far the most important of these is the European Patent Office, which as of April 2019, grants patents for a total of 38 countries. These are all the 28 current EU states plus Albania, Iceland, Liechtenstein, Northern Macedonia, Monaco, Norway, San Marino, Serbia, Switzerland and Turkey. The European application can be filed in English, French or German, and translations into other languages may be required at the time of grant under the provisions of The London Agreement. Once the European patent is granted, opposition to the patent may be filed by any other party within 9 months of the date of grant. If the opposition is wholly or partly successful, the patent is invalidated or limited in scope for all of the designated countries.

Although the European Patent Convention provides for a central filing, grant and opposition procedure, once the European patent is granted, it is treated as if it were a bundle of national patents in the designated contracting states, so that, for example, the European patent may be invalidated by the courts in one country without directly affecting its validity in other countries. Significant progress has been made towards establishing the Unitary Patent (UP), a unitary right covering all participating EU countries. However, whether, and if so when, UPs will be available remains unclear as at the start of 2019.

Other regional patent offices are the Eurasian Patent Office (Russia and certain former Soviet countries), and ones for English-speaking and French-speaking African countries.

Patent cooperation treaty. The PCT allows rights to be established in a large number of countries (152 as of 1 April 2019) by a single international application. Search and optional preliminary examination are carried out before the application goes to the national or regional patent offices. This system gives the maximum flexibility and allows the costs associated with translations and so on to be significantly postponed. There are now very few economically significant countries that are not members of the PCT, of which the most important is Taiwan. An initial international phase, in which a search and possibly also a preliminary examination is carried out, is followed after 18 months by a national phase, in which selected national or regional patent offices conclude the examination process and grant (or refuse) the patent. The PCT procedure is described in more detail in Box 19.1.

Selection of countries. In deciding the list of countries in which patent protection should be obtained, the main criteria are the strength of patent protection in the country and the size of the market. Now that most countries have joined the World Trade Organization and are obliged by the TRIPs (Trade-Related Aspects of Intellectual Property Rights) agreement to introduce strong patent protection; the most important criterion has become market size. There is no point in filing patents in a country if the size of the market does not justify the costs, no matter how strong its patent laws may be. Nevertheless, for an NCE that may become a market product, filing in 40–60 countries is normal practice. To avoid long discussions each time a decision must be taken, the use of standard filing lists to cover most situations makes a lot of sense.

Maintenance of patents. In nearly all countries, periodic (usually annual) renewal fees must be paid to keep a patent in force. These generally increase steeply towards the end of the patent term, thus encouraging patent owners who are not making commercial use of their patents to make the invention available to the public earlier than would otherwise be the case. To save costs, pharmaceutical patents should be abandoned as soon as they no longer provide protection for a compound that is on the market or is being developed. Maintaining a collection of patents that are not being used is an expensive luxury.

Extension of patent term. The standard patent term provided in the TRIPs agreement is at least 20 years from the filing date. However, because it takes a long time to bring a drug to market, the effective term (the term during which a drug is sold with patent protection) is much less than this. To compensate for these regulatory delays, a

---

Box 19.1 PCT procedure

International phase

Filing

An international application can be filed by any national or resident of a PCT country, at a national or regional patent office competent to act for that applicant, or at the International Bureau (World Intellectual Property Office, or WIPO) in Geneva. A single filing fee can give rights in all Contracting States.

International publication and search report

The PCT application is published 18 months from the first priority date, and the search report drawn up by the International Searching Authority (selected from one of a number of patent offices including the US Patent and Trademark Office [USPTO] and the European Patent Office [EPO]) is published at the same time or as soon as possible afterwards. At the same time, a Written Opinion on Patentability is drawn up, indicating on the basis of the search report whether or not the invention appears to be new and nonobvious. If no further steps are taken, this will be issued as the International Preliminary Report on Patentability (IPRP).

International preliminary examination

If applicants wish to contest the findings of the Written Opinion, they may, within 22 months from the priority date, file a *Demand for International Preliminary Examination*, pay a fee and respond to the Written Opinion, possibly also making amendments. This will then be taken into account in the final form of the IPRP.

National phase

After 30 months from the priority date, the application may be sent to any of the national or regional patent offices, translated into the local language as necessary. The individual patent offices may rely on the international search and examination reports to any extent they choose in deciding whether or not to grant a patent. This varies from offices that usually ignore the IPRP altogether (e.g., the USPTO), to those that will grant a patent without further examination only if the IPRP is positive (e.g., Turkey), to Singapore, which will automatically grant a patent on any PCT application with an IPRP, whether it is positive or negative. Singapore very sensibly puts the burden on the applicants, who, if they wish to enforce the patent, would have to prove to the court that the negative IPRP was incorrect.

---

number of countries, including EU states, the United States, Switzerland and Japan, allow for patent term extensions of up to 5 years for pharmaceutical (and sometimes agricultural) products. In the United States, patent term extension is one part of the Hatch–Waxman Act, in which the interests of the innovative companies are balanced against those of the generic companies. The former get a longer patent term, the latter are allowed to carry out testing for FDA approval during the patent term, so that they can come on the market as soon as patent protection expires. In Europe, extension is provided by means of a separate form of IP right known as a Supplementary Protection Certificate (SPC). An SPC can be further extended by 6 months (known informally as a paediatric extension), where the marketing approval application contains results and information in compliance with an agreed plan following completion of a Pediatirc Investigation Plan (PIP). As at 2019, China is seriously contemplating the introduction of a patent term extension regime.

Enforcement of patent rights. Governments grant patents but do not enforce them. The patent owner must take action against infringement by suing an infringer in the civil courts. If successful, the patentee can often obtain an injunction to restrain further infringement, as well as other remedies such as damages and costs. Usually the alleged infringer will counterclaim that the patent is invalid, and if the patentee loses the case, the patent may be revoked. This risk, as well as the high cost of litigation, must be weighed against the benefit gained if the infringer is forced out of the market. As an alternative to litigation, the patentee may choose to exploit the patent by granting exclusive or nonexclusive licences for royalties or other forms of compensation, or in exchange for a cross-licence.

Although the procedure for obtaining a patent has been harmonized to a large extent by the PCT and other means, the procedure for enforcement, as well as the cost and the chance of success, varies enormously from one country to another. In the United States, patent infringement cases are heard at first instance in the Federal District Courts, in which the judges are not specialized in IP law and in which many cases are decided by jury verdicts. At the appeal stage, however, the Court of Appeals for the Federal Circuit is a specialized and technically competent court. In England, on the other hand, patent cases are heard either in the Intellectual Property Enterprise Court (for lower value disputes) or, more usually, in the Patents Court, which is part of the High Court. Both of these are specialized courts with technically literate judges. Appeals are heard by panels of three judges in the Court of Appeal, one of whom will usually have a technical background.

In both the United States and the English systems issues of patent validity are dealt with by the same court that deals with the issue of infringement, and this is also the case in the majority of European and Asian countries. In Germany, Japan, China and Korea, however, these issues are kept separate, and a patent may be invalidated only by a special court or by a branch of the patent office.

It is a problem in many parts of the world that even if the country has a good patent law on paper, enforcement of patent rights may be very difficult for a number of reasons, ranging from lack of experienced judges to inefficiency and even corruption.

Other forms of intellectual property. A *trademark* is a word, design, shape or colour used to distinguish the goods of the trademark owner from those of another manufacturer. Unlike patents, registered trademarks may be renewed at the end of their term and may be kept alive indefinitely, although they may be liable to cancellation if they are not used. Thus, once a patent for a drug has expired, a competitor will be able to sell a generic version but must sell it under the International Non-proprietary Name (INN) or its own trademark, not that of the originator. Special rules exist regarding brand names used for pharmaceutical products.

Additional forms of IP include *copyright* (e.g., for the text of advertisements and package inserts), design rights and *Internet domain names*, which may, for example, incorporate the name of a product and may be a useful marketing tool.

Further protection can be obtained by exploiting regulatory data protection and data exclusivity.

Further reading

Useful websites

Patent offices

EPO: https://www.epo.org
UK: https://www.gov.uk/topic/intellectual-property/patents
USA: https://www.uspto.gov

Japan: https://www.jpo.go.jp
WIPO: https://www.wipo.int

Professional organizations

Chartered Institute of Patent Attorneys: http://www.cipa.org.uk

European Patents Institute: https://www.patentepi.com
American Intellectual Property Law Association: https://www.aipla.org

Lists of links

https://www.bl.uk/collection-guides/patents

Chapter | **20** |

Regulatory affairs

Chris Parkinson

Introduction

This chapter introduces the role of the regulatory affairs (RA) department of a pharmaceutical company, outlining the process of developing and getting a drug approved. It emphasizes the importance of interactions of RA professionals with the external regulatory authorities, and with other functions within the company.

To keep this chapter reasonably succinct, the examples given illustrate the first registration of a new chemical compound. The same reasoning also applies, however, to any subsequent change to the approval of products. Depending on the magnitude of the change, the new documentation that needs to be compiled, submitted and approved by health authorities is variable, ranging from a few pages of pharmaceutical data (e.g., for an update to product stability information) to a complete new application for a new clinical use in a new patient group with a new pharmaceutical form. We have also included a section on the specific considerations for biopharmaceuticals and advanced therapy medicinal products (ATMPs).

Please note that, as every drug substance and every project is unique, the views expressed represent the opinion of the authors and are not necessarily shared by others active in the field.

Brief history of pharmaceutical regulation

Control of pharmaceutical products has been the task of authorized institutions for thousands of years, and this was even the case with the apothecaries of ancient Greece and Egypt.

From the Middle Ages, control of drug quality, composition purity and quantification was achieved by reference to authoritative lists of drugs, their preparation and their uses. These developed into official pharmacopoeias, of which, the earliest was possibly the New Compound Dispensatory of 1498 issued by the Florentine guild of physicians and pharmacists.

The pharmacopoeias were local rules, applicable in a particular city or district. During the 19th century, national pharmacopoeias replaced local ones, and since the early 1960s, regional pharmacopoeias have successively replaced national ones. Now work is ongoing to harmonize—or at least mutually recognize—interchangeable use of the US Pharmacopeia, the European Pharmacopoeia and the Japanese Pharmacopoeia.

As described in Chapter 1, the advances in experimental pharmacology and chemistry during the second half of the 19th century revealed that the effect of the main botanical drugs being used was due to chemical substances in the plants. The next advance, synthetic chemistry, made it possible to manufacture active chemical compounds. More recently, the development of biotechnology has allowed the production of proteins, antibodies and cell-based therapeutics that present specific challenges for regulatory processes.

Lack of adequate drug control systems or methods to investigate the safety of new chemical compounds became a much greater risk as prefabricated drug products became broadly and freely distributed. In the United States, as long ago as 1906, the struggle to control the adulteration of food, drink and drugs led to the passing of the US Pure Food and Drug Act. The Act required improved declaration of contents, prohibited false or misleading statements and required content and purity to comply with labelled information. Two decades later, the US Food and Drug Administration (FDA) was established to control US pharmaceutical products. Safety regulations in the United States were, however, not enough in 1937 to prevent the sale of a paediatric *sulfanilamide* elixir containing the toxic solvent diethylene glycol. One hundred and seven people, both adults and children, died as a result of ingesting the elixir, and in 1938, the Food Drug and Cosmetic Act was passed, requiring for the first time the approval by the FDA before marketing of a new drug product.

The *thalidomide* disaster highlighted gaps in the evaluation of medicines before they were made widely available to the public. Thalidomide (Neurosedyn, Contergan) was launched during the last years of the 1950s as a nontoxic treatment for a variety of conditions, such as colds, anxiety, depression, infections and so on, both alone and in combination with a number of other compounds, such as analgesics and sedatives. Once on the market, it was also noted to be effective against morning sickness in pregnant mothers, a use that became widely recommended.

The compound was initially regarded as harmless due to the lack of acute toxicity after high single doses. After repeated long-term administration, however, signs of neuropathy developed, with symptoms of numbness, paraesthesia and ataxia. But the horrifying effects of thalidomide were the gross malformations in infants born to mothers who had taken thalidomide during pregnancy: their limbs were partially or totally missing, a hitherto extremely rare malformation called *phocomelia* (seal limb). Altogether, approximately 12,000 infants were born with the defect in those few years before thalidomide was withdrawn from the market in 1961/1962.

This catastrophe became a strong driver to develop animal test methods to assess drug safety before administering compounds to humans. Moreover, it was the trigger for a rigorous revision by national authorities to introduce comprehensive legal requirements for control procedures before marketing of pharmaceutical products (Cartwright & Matthews, 1991).

Dr Frances Kelsey, a reviewer at the FDA, has been accredited with keeping thalidomide off the US market, thereby protecting the US population from the tragedy. This led to strong public support in the United States for more effective drug regulation. The US Kefauver-Harris Drug Amendments of 1962 introduced the requirement for evidence of efficacy as well as safety as a condition for registration. In addition, formal approval was required by the FDA for patients to be included in clinical trials of new drugs. In Europe, the UK Medicines Act 1968 made safety assessment of new drug products compulsory. The Swedish Drug Ordinance of 1962 defined the medicinal product and required a clear benefit–risk ratio to be documented before approval for marketing. All European countries established similar controls during the 1960s. In Japan, the Pharmaceutical Affairs Law enacted in 1943 was revised in 1961 (and again in 1979 and 2005) to establish the current drug regulatory system, with the Ministry of Health, Labour and Welfare assessing drugs for quality, safety and efficacy.

The 1960s and 1970s saw a rapid increase in laws, regulations and guidelines for reporting and evaluating the risk versus benefit of new medicinal products. At a time when the pharmaceutical industry was becoming more international and seeking new global markets, the registration of medicines remained a national and increasingly complex undertaking. Although different regulatory systems were based on the same key principles, the detailed technical requirements diverged over time, often for traditional rather than scientific reasons, to such an extent that the industry found it necessary to duplicate tests in different countries to obtain global regulatory approval for new products. This was a waste of time, money and animals' lives, and it became clear that harmonization of regulatory requirements was needed.

European efforts to harmonize requirements for drug approval across the European Economic Community (EEC) began in 1965 with Council Directive 65/65/EEC, establishing and maintaining a common European approach alongside the expansion of the European Union (EU). The EU harmonization principles have also been adopted by Norway, Iceland and Liechtenstein. This successful European harmonization process gave impetus to discussions about harmonization on a broader international scale (Cartwright & Matthews, 1994).

International harmonization

The international harmonization process started in 1990, when representatives of the regulatory authorities and industry associations of Europe, Japan and the United States (representing the majority of the global pharmaceutical industry) met to plan an International Conference on Harmonization (ICH). The meeting actually achieved more, suggesting *terms of reference* for ICH, and setting up an ICH Steering Committee representing the three regions.

The task of ICH was agreed as, '...increased international harmonization, aimed at ensuring that good quality, safe and effective medicines are developed and registered in the most efficient and cost-effective manner. These activities are pursued in the interest of the consumer and public health, to prevent unnecessary duplication of clinical trials in humans and to minimize the use of animal testing without compromising the regulatory obligations of safety and effectiveness' (Tokyo, October 1990).

ICH has remained a very active organization, with substantial representation at both authority and industry level from the founding members, the EU, the United States and Japan. In 2015, ICH began an evolution towards a more global initiative. It is now constituted by 16 members and 28 observer countries.

ICH conferences, held every 2 years, have become a forum for open discussion and follow-up of the topics that are at the heart of drug development. The important

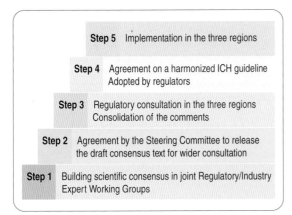

Step 5   Implementation in the three regions

Step 4   Agreement on a harmonized ICH guideline
Adopted by regulators

Step 3   Regulatory consultation in the three regions
Consolidation of the comments

Step 2   Agreement by the Steering Committee to release
the draft consensus text for wider consultation

Step 1   Building scientific consensus in joint Regulatory/Industry
Expert Working Groups

Fig. 20.1 Five steps in the International Conference on Harmonization (ICH) process for harmonization of technical issues.

achievements so far are the scientific guidelines agreed and implemented in the national/regional drug legislation, not only in the ICH territories but also in other countries around the world. Guidance for new technologies, such as continuous drug manufacturing processes, and addressing consistent interpretation of guidelines across the expanding membership are just some of the topics being tackled today. For a complete list of ICH guidelines and their status, see the ICH website (website reference 1). The five-step process for harmonization of guidelines under ICH is summarized in Fig. 20.1. That regulators and the pharmaceutical industry collaborate from the start of discussions on ICH topics increases the efficiency of the process and ensures mutual understanding across regions and functions; this is a major factor in the success of ICH. However, regulatory consensus does not always bring regulatory innovation. An example of this is the requirement for long-term toxicity studies having a duration of 9 months in nonrodent species that was a compromise between 12 months required for the United States and 6 months for Europe and Japan prior to the ICH guideline. Regulatory innovation is rather in the domain of academia or organizations, such as the Centre for Innovation in Regulatory Science (http://www.cirsci.org/).

Roles and responsibilities of health authority, regulatory authority and company

The basic division of responsibilities for drug products is that the health authority promotes public health by making new drug products available to patients within their jurisdiction. The regulatory agency is a body appointed by the health authority to ensure the efficacy, safety and quality of drug products. The regulatory authority grants an authorization for a pharmaceutical product that permits marketing and is a binding agreement between the regulatory authority and the pharmaceutical company. The pharmaceutical company is responsible for all aspects of manufacture and testing of the drug product, including the conduct of clinical trials in human subjects. This evidence generated throughout the development of the approved medicine is set out in a dossier that is submitted to the health authority in an application for marketing authorization. When the application is authorized, the key aspects of the dossier are condensed in the prescribing information (the 'label'). Any change to the prescribing information that is planned must be submitted to the regulatory authority for approval before being implemented.

To protect the public health, regulatory authorities also develop regulations and guidelines for companies to follow in order to ensure a favourable balance between the possible risks of treatment and the therapeutic benefit the treatment offers to patients.

The authorities' work is partly financed by fees paid by pharmaceutical companies. Fees may be reduced, under certain conditions, to stimulate research. This may be driven, for example, by company size or prevalence of the disease intended for treatment.

In summary, the regulatory authority:
- approves applications to conduct clinical trials
- gives procedural and scientific advice to companies during drug development
- grants marketing authorizations for drugs that have been scientifically evaluated to provide evidence of a satisfactory benefit/risk ratio
- monitors the safety of the marketed product, based on: (1) reports of adverse reactions from healthcare providers and (2) from compiled and evaluated safety information from the company that owns the product
- can withdraw the licence for marketing when the benefit–risk assessment is no longer considered positive. It may also withdraw a licence if a company fails to supply and act upon emergent information.

The company:
- owns the data that form the basis for assessment, documents the data and is responsible for its accuracy and correctness, for keeping it up to date and for ensuring that it complies with standards set by current scientific development and the regulatory authorities
- collects, compiles and evaluates safety data, and submits reports to the regulatory authorities at regular intervals—and takes rapid action in serious cases. The requirement to analyse is important; regulatory authorities have the ability to compare data across related products, but the primary responsibility to continuously assess and propose actions to address

emergent issues lies with the manufacturer. Actions might involve the withdrawal of the entire product or of a product batch (e.g., tablets containing defects in the product or the product packaging), or a request to the regulatory authority for a change in prescribing information

- has a right to appeal and to remediate cases of non-compliance.

The role of the regulatory affairs department

The ultimate goal for the RA department of a pharmaceutical company is to be responsible for obtaining authorization for new pharmaceutical products and ensuring that the authorization is maintained for as long as the company wants to keep the product on the market.

RA serves as the interface between the regulatory authorities and the project team and is the channel of communication with the regulatory authorities as the project proceeds in drug development. It is critical that RA ensures that the project plan correctly anticipates what the regulatory authorities will require to support each stage in development of the product from entry into human clinical trials to submission of the marketing authorization application. During the development process, sound working relations with authorities, particularly within the framework of seeking scientific advice, are essential. Topics for discussion with authorities may include issues such as divergence from guidelines, the design of the clinical development programme and pharmaceutical formulation development.

It is the responsibility of RA to keep abreast of current legislation, guidelines and other regulatory intelligence Such rules and guidelines often allow some flexibility, and the regulatory authorities expect companies to take responsibility for deciding how they should be interpreted. The RA department plays an important role in giving advice to the project team on how best to interpret the rules.

Most companies assess and prioritize new projects based on an intended target product profile (TPP). The RA professional plays a key role in advising on what will be realistic prescribing information (the 'label') for the intended product. The RA department reviews all documentation from a regulator's perspective, ensuring that it is clear, consistent and complete, and that its conclusions are explicit and founded on robust data. RA also drafts the core prescribing information that is the basis for global approval and will later provide the platform for marketing. The documentation takes multiple forms, including clinical trials applications, paediatric investigation plans, regulatory agency briefing documents, as well as the submissions for marketing authorization of new products and for changes to approved products. The latter—licence maintenance—is a major commitment and accounts for about half of the work of the RA department.

An important proactive task of RA is to provide input when legislative changes are being discussed and proposed, for example, the extensive European Commission and European Medicines Agency (EMA) consultations leading to the European Clinical Trial Regulation (CTR) 536/2014 (see Clinical trials later). In the ICH environment, there is a greater opportunity to exert influence at an earlier stage of guideline development.

The drug development process

An overview of the process of drug development is given in Chapters 14–18 and summarized in Fig. 20.2. As already emphasized, the sequential approach, designed to minimize risk by allowing each study to start only when earlier studies have been successfully completed, is now giving way to a partly parallel approach in order to save development time.

All studies in the nonclinical area—chemistry, pharmacology, pharmacokinetics, pharmaceutical development and toxicology—aim to establish indicators of safety and potential efficacy sufficient to allow investigations in humans. According to ICH nomenclature, documentation of chemical and pharmaceutical development relates to *quality* assessment, animal studies relate to *safety* assessment and studies in humans relate to *efficacy*.

Quality assessment (chemistry and pharmaceutical development)

The *quality module* of a submission documents purity and assay for the drug substance, and purity data for all the inactive ingredients. The formulation must fulfil requirements for consistent quality and allow storage at predetermined environmental conditions, and the container must be shown to be fit for purpose. The aspects of quality of a pharmaceutical product have to be kept under control throughout the development process, not least because toxicology and pharmacology results only support human exposures to substances of comparable or higher purity. Large-scale production, improved synthetic route, different raw material supplies and so on may produce a substance somewhat different from the first laboratory-scale batches. All substantial changes must be known and documented. Although this applies to all medicinal products, it can be a particular challenge for biopharmaceuticals in that changes to the scale and process of manufacturing can, for example, alter the glycosylation profile of an immunoglobulin molecule, and in so doing, alter its properties.

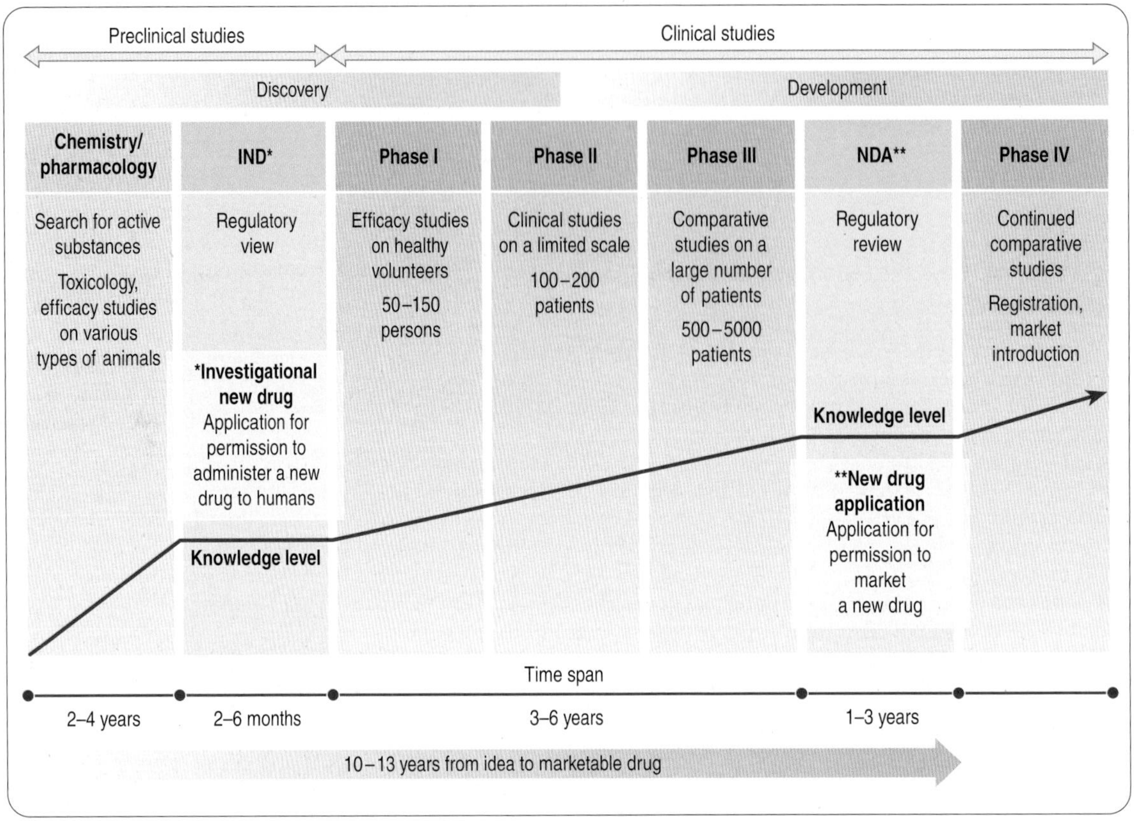

Fig. 20.2 The drug development process. *IND*, Investigational new drug; *NDA*, new drug application.

The evolution of the physical drug product from prototype formulations used in early studies through to the final product to be used in the market is complex and has to be managed in parallel with the emerging clinical profile. For initial human studies, simple formulations, such as intravenous (i.v.) and oral solutions are commonly used to assess safety and pharmacology. These are rarely suitable for longer-term studies to assess safety and efficacy in patients (often across multiple sites in several countries), and considerable work is often required to produce a formulation suitable for phase II studies. Ideally, this would be the final formulation, but often this is not possible. There is an expectation that the formulation used in phase III registration studies is the final formulation to ensure that key safety and efficacy data were generated with the formulation that will be used in the market. At each stage of this evolution, regulatory authorities will closely examine the impact of any changes to assess the extent to which the previous safety and efficacy data can be considered relevant to the next study. In the past, this often involved the use of bridging studies to show the pharmacokinetic equivalence of the new formulation with previous ones. This approach assumes that previous studies used the optimal dose. More sophisticated use of modelling and simulation to link drug exposure with effect has shifted the emphasis to defining the desired pharmacokinetic profile for future studies and linking that to the profile of the proposed formulation rather than showing direct equivalence per se. This interdependency highlights the need for close collaboration between the clinical and drug product teams; failure to link these two elements can lead to studies having to be repeated, delaying delivery of new treatments to patients and substantially increasing development costs. It is also important to consider early enough in development if there will be a need for market- or region-specific formulations that are driven by prescribing patient preferences or cultural preferences.

The analytical methods used and their validation must be described. Manufacturing processes and their validation are also required to demonstrate interbatch uniformity. However, full-scale validation may be submitted when production of commercial product has started.

Studies on the stability of both drug substance and product under real-life conditions are required, covering the full time of intended storage. Early in development, preliminary stability data are sufficient for the start of clinical studies. The allowable storage time will be increased as supportive data are gathered and submitted. Extrapolation of stability data generated under accelerated conditions of higher temperature and humidity is a widely accepted approach for assigning longer shelf-life than supported by real-time stability results. Even marketing authorizations can be approved on less than real-time storage information, but there is a requirement to submit final data when available.

Inactive ingredients, as well as active substances need to be documented, unless they are well known and already documented. Even then, a risk assessment should be carried out specific to its use in a new drug product. It may subsequently be necessary to perform additional animal studies to support novel uses of commonly used additives.

The details of requirements and the many changes needed during development and maintenance of a product make the quality dossier the most resource intensive from a regulatory perspective. Also, legislation differs across countries most in this area, so it will often be necessary to adapt the documentation for the intended regional submission. It is the role of RA professionals to justify to regulatory authorities in submissions or in agency meetings that any deviation from a strict following of the local regulations carries no additional risk to patients.

As stated earlier, all changes to the originally submitted dossier must be made known to the approving regulatory authority. Many of these changes are made in the quality section. To avoid the high volume of submissions for minor quality changes, legislation now allows the submission of annual reports documenting those changes that have no impact on quality.

Safety assessment (nonclinical pharmacology and toxicology)

Next, we consider how to design and integrate pharmacological and toxicological studies in order to produce adequate documentation to support the first studies in humans. ICH guidelines define the information needed from animal studies in terms of doses and time of exposure, to allow clinical studies, usually first in healthy subjects and later in patients. The principles and methodology of animal studies are described in Chapter 12. The questions discussed here are *when* and *why* these animal studies are required for regulatory purposes.

Primary pharmacology

The primary pharmacology studies conducted in laboratory animals or human-derived cells provide the first evidence that the compound has the pharmacological effects that might give rise to a therapeutic benefit. It is a clear regulatory aim to use validated animal models to establish a theory for the mechanism of action. Ideally, an animal model that mirrors the biological mechanism of the human disease will meet that expectation. This will not always be possible in every case and, without those nonclinical supporting data, a very strong case must be made to justify taking the drug into clinical trials.

General pharmacology

General pharmacology[1] studies investigate effects other than the primary intended therapeutic effects. Safety pharmacology studies (see Chapter 12), which must conform to good laboratory practice (GLP) standards, are focussed on identifying the effects on physiological functions that in a clinical setting are unwanted or harmful. Particularly important are studies designed to detect effects on the cardiovascular, central nervous and respiratory systems.

Although the study design will depend on the properties and intended use of the compound, general pharmacology studies are normally of short duration (i.e., acute, rather than chronic, effects are investigated), and the dosage is increased until either a clear adverse effect occurs or there are signs of general toxicity. The studies may also include comparisons with known compounds whose pharmacological properties or clinical uses are similar.

When justified, for example, when pharmacodynamic effects occur only after prolonged treatment, or when effects seen with repeated administration give rise to safety concerns, the duration of a safety pharmacology study needs to be prolonged. Indeed, this used to be a routine requirement for the nonclinical safety pharmacology package for Japan before their requirements came into line with ICH guidelines. The route of administration should, whenever possible, be the route intended for clinical use. An appropriate exception to this would be when insufficient exposure to the drug is observed in animals (usually by the inhaled or oral route) such that i.v. dosing in the animals is warranted.

There are cases when a secondary pharmacological effect has, eventually, been developed into a new indication. *Lidocaine*, for example, was developed as a local anaesthetic agent, and its cardiac effects after overdose were considered a hazard. Later, that cardiac effect was exploited as a treatment for ventricular arrhythmia.

All relevant safety pharmacology studies must be completed before studies can be undertaken in humans. Complementary studies may still be needed to clarify unexpected findings in later development stages as clinical data emerge.

---

[1]There are a number of widely used terms with similar meanings, for example, secondary pharmacology, safety pharmacology, high-dose pharmacology, regulatory pharmacology and pharmacodynamic safety.

Pharmacokinetics: absorption, distribution, metabolism and excretion

Preliminary pharmacokinetic tests to assess the absorption, plasma levels and half-life (i.e., exposure information) are performed in rodents in parallel with the preliminary pharmacology and toxicology studies (see Chapter 10).

Initial studies in humans normally start with supporting data from limited short-term animal studies, and only if the results from human studies are acceptable, detailed animal and human absorption, distribution, metabolism and excretion (ADME) studies are performed.

Plasma concentrations observed in animals are used to predict the concentrations that may be efficacious/tolerated in humans, under the assumption that similar biological effects should be produced at similar concentrations of drug interacting with the target across species. This is a reasonable assumption provided the in vitro target affinity is similar across species; quantitative pharmacology models are important in establishing this link.

Investigations during the toxicology programme give the bulk of the pharmacokinetic information because of the long duration of drug exposure and the wide range of doses tested in several relevant species. They also provide information about tissue distribution and possible accumulation in the body, including placental transfer and exposure of the fetus, as well as excretion in milk.

Metabolic pathways differ considerably between species, often quantitatively but sometimes also qualitatively. Active metabolites can influence the effect of a drug, especially after repeated use. A toxic metabolite with a long half-life may accumulate in the body and thereby pose a considerable risk. The characterization and evaluation of metabolites are long processes and may be the last studies to be completed in a development programme.

Toxicology

The principles and methodology of toxicological assessment of new compounds are described in Chapter 12. Here, we consider the regulatory aspects.

In contrast to the pharmacological studies, toxicological studies generally follow standard protocols. Active comparators are not used, but the effects of the drug substance are compared at various dose levels to a vehicle control, given by the intended route of administration. The choice of species must be justified but commonly used species are preferred (e.g., rat, dog), as there are most comparative data available to provide context for these species.

Single and repeated-dose studies. The acute toxicity of a new compound must be evaluated prior to the first human exposure.

This information is obtained from dose-escalation studies or dose-ranging studies of short duration. Lethality is no longer an ethically accepted endpoint. The toxicology requirements to support the first exploratory studies in humans are described in the ICH guideline M3 (see website reference 1). Table 20.1 shows the duration of repeated-dose studies recommended by ICH, to support clinical trials and therapeutic use for different periods.

Table 20.1 Duration of repeated-dose toxicity studies
Recommended Minimum Duration of Repeated-Dose Toxicity Studies

Maximum duration of clinical trials	TO SUPPORT CLINICAL TRIALS		TO SUPPORT MARKETING	
	Rodents	Nonrodents	Rodents	Nonrodents
Up to 2 weeks	2 weeks[a]	2 weeks	1 month	1 month
>2 weeks to 1 month	Same as the clinical trial[b]	Same as the clinical trial[b]	3 months	3 months
>1 month to 3 months			6 months	3 months
>3 months to 6 months			6 months[c]	9 months[c,d]
>6 months	6 months[b,c]	9 months[b,c,d]		

[a]In the United States, as an alternative to 2-week studies, single-dose toxicity studies with extended examination can support single-dose human trials.
[b]Data from 3-month studies in rodents and nonrodents may be sufficient to start clinical trials longer than 3 months provided longer-term data are made available before extension of the clinical trial.
[c]If paediatric patients are the target population, long-term toxicity studies in juvenile animals may be required.
[d]Studies of 6 months duration are acceptable in nonrodents in certain cases, for example, intermittent treatment of migraine, chronic treatment to prevent recurrence of cancer, indications for which life expectancy is short, animals cannot tolerate the treatment.

Genotoxicity. Preliminary genotoxicity evaluation of gene mutation and chromosomal damage (see Chapter 12) is needed before the drug is given to humans. If results from those studies are ambiguous or positive, further testing is required. The entire standard battery of tests needs to be completed before phase II (see Chapter 12).

Carcinogenicity. The objective of carcinogenicity studies is to identify any tumorigenic potential in animals, and they are required only when the expected duration of therapy, whether continuous or intermittent, is 6 months or more. Examples include treatments for conditions such as allergic rhinitis, anxiety or depression.

Carcinogenicity studies are also required when there is particular reason for concern, such as chemical similarities to known carcinogens, pathophysiological findings in animal toxicity studies or positive genotoxicity results. Compounds found to be genotoxic by in vitro as well as in vivo tests are presumed to be transspecies carcinogens with hazards to humans. Such properties in a new medicine would almost certainly prevent its use in anything but severe and life-threatening diseases.

Carcinogenicity studies normally run for the lifespan of the test animals. They are performed quite late in the development programme and, with the agreement of regulatory authorities, may not necessarily be completed when the application for marketing authorization is submitted. Indeed, for products for which there is a great medical need in the treatment of certain serious diseases, the regulatory authority may agree that submission of carcinogenicity data can be delayed until after marketing approval is granted.

Reproductive and developmental toxicity. These studies (see Chapter 12) are intended to reveal effects on male or female fertility, embryonic and fetal development and peri- and postnatal development.

An evaluation of effects on the male reproductive system is performed in the repeated-dose toxicity studies, and this histopathological assessment is considered more sensitive in detecting toxic effects than are fertility studies. Men can therefore be included in phase I–II trials before the male fertility studies are performed in animals.

Women may enter early studies before reproductive toxicity testing is completed, provided they are of nonchildbearing potential, and provided repeated-dose toxicity tests of adequate duration have been performed, including the evaluation of female reproductive organs.

For women of childbearing potential, there is a high regulatory and ethical concern regarding unintentional fetal exposure, and there are regional differences (Box 20.1) in the regulations about including women of childbearing potential in clinical trials. Generally speaking, women of childbearing potential may be included in short-to-moderate

---

Box 20.1 Requirement for reproduction toxicity related to clinical studies in fertile women

EU	Embryo/fetal development studies are required before phase I, and female fertility should be completed before phase III
United States	Careful monitoring and pregnancy testing may allow fertile women to take part before reproduction toxicity is available. Female fertility and embryo/fetal assessment to be completed before phase III
Japan	Embryo/fetal development studies are required before phase I, and female fertility should be completed before III

---

duration clinical trials if they use two forms of highly effective contraception.

Local tolerance and other toxicity studies. The purpose of local tolerance studies is to ascertain whether medicinal products (both active substances and excipients) are tolerated at sites in the body that may come into contact with the product in clinical use. This could mean, for example, ocular, dermal or parenteral administration. Other studies may also be needed, for example, studies on immunotoxicity, antigenicity studies on metabolites or impurities. The drug substance and the intended use will determine the relevance of other studies.

Efficacy assessment (studies in humans)

When the preclinical testing is sufficient to start studies in humans, the RA department compiles a clinical trial submission, which is sent to the regulatory authority and the ethics committee (see Regulatory procedures, later).

The clinical studies, described in detail in Chapter 17, are classified according to Table 20.2.

Human pharmacology

Human pharmacology studies refer to the earliest human exposure in volunteers, as well as any pharmacological studies in patients and volunteers throughout the development of the drug.

The first study of a new drug substance in humans has essentially three objectives:

- To investigate *tolerability* over a range of doses with extensive safety monitoring to detect common severe adverse effects
- To obtain information on *pharmacokinetics*, and to measure bioavailability and plasma concentration–effect relationships

Table 20.2 ICH classification of clinical studies

Type of study	Study objectives	Traditional terminology
Human pharmacology	Assess tolerance; describe or define pharmacokinetics/pharmacodynamics; explore drug metabolism and drug interactions; estimate activity	Phase I
Therapeutic exploratory	Explore use for the targeted indication; estimate dosage for subsequent studies; provide basis for confirmatory study design, endpoints, methodologies	Phase II
Therapeutic confirmatory	Demonstrate or confirm efficacy; establish safety profile; provide an adequate basis for assessing benefit–risk relationship to support licensing (drug approval); establish dose–response relationship	Phase III (a and b)
Therapeutic use	Refine understanding of benefit–risk relationship in general or special populations and/or environments; identify less common adverse reactions; refine dosing recommendations	Phase IV

- To examine the *pharmacodynamic activity* over a range of doses and obtain a dose–response relationship, provided a relevant effect can be measured in healthy volunteers or patients.

Further human pharmacology studies are performed to document pharmacodynamic and pharmacokinetic effects. The clinical data needed to support progressing to trials in patients include the complete pharmacokinetic evaluation and the performance of bioavailability/bioequivalence studies during the development of new formulations or drug-delivery systems. Information is also obtained on the possible influence of food on absorption, and that of other concomitant medications, that is, drug interaction. Exploration of metabolism is also performed early in the clinical development process.

Special patient populations need particular attention because they may be particularly sensitive or resistant to treatment regimens acceptable to a less-at-risk adult population. One obvious category is patients with renal or hepatic impairment, who may be unable to metabolize or excrete the drug effectively. The metabolic pattern and elimination route are important predictors for such patients, and these subjects are not typically included in clinical trials until late in development.

Sex differences may also occur and should be investigated by the inclusion of women at the dose-finding stage of clinical trials.

A drug interaction is an alteration in the pharmacodynamic or the pharmacokinetic properties of a drug caused by factors such as concomitant drug treatment, diet, social habits (e.g., tobacco or alcohol), age, sex, ethnic origin and time of administration.

Interaction studies should be performed, where possible, in healthy volunteers in order to minimize the risk to the trial participants. These studies look at possible metabolism changes when co-administering compounds that share the same enzymatic metabolic pathway. Also, changes in pharmacokinetic behaviour can be investigated in combinations of drugs that are expected to be used together. Such studies are performed when clinical findings require clarification or if the company wishes to avoid standard warning texts on the product label that would otherwise apply. Drug–disease interactions (e.g., the impact of tumour lysis in cancer or a pulmonary vasodilator on systemic blood pressure) are complex and do not lend themselves to studies in healthy subjects; nonetheless, they should be considered and studies designed to evaluate their impact. Failure to address these issues may lead to regulatory contraindications or warnings that preclude practical use of the drug in clinical practice.

Therapeutic exploratory studies

After relevant information in healthy volunteers has been obtained, safety conclusions from combined animal and human exposure will be assessed internally. If favourable, initial patient studies can begin. There is an inherent tension here, to obtain the most consistent results, and the patient population should be as homogeneous as possible; however, the final target population may be much more diverse. Initial clinical studies are used primarily to establish efficacy measured against no treatment, so the design should be placebo controlled when ethically justified. Also for ethical reasons, only a limited number of closely monitored patients take part in these studies and, since lasting benefit is not expected, should be of the shortest duration needed to identify a therapeutic effect.

Studies in special populations: elderly, children, ethnic differences

Clinically significant differences in pharmacokinetics between the elderly and the young are due to several factors related to ageing, such as impaired renal function, which can increase the variability in drug response, as well as increasing the likelihood of unwanted effects and drug interactions. Bearing in mind that the elderly are the largest group of consumers of medicines, this category should be studied as early as possible in clinical trials.

Clinical trials in children. Studies in children are supported through experience from adult human studies, provision of information on the pharmacokinetic profile of the substance and clinical evidence of benefit of the drug. Placebo-controlled studies in children are generally regarded as unethical. Because of the difficulties of conducting these studies, and the often small commercial return, companies in the past seldom considered it worthwhile to test drugs in children, and then to seek regulatory approval for marketing drugs for use in children. Nevertheless, drugs were, and still are, often prescribed 'off-label' for children, on the basis of clinical experience suggesting that they are safe and effective. Such off-label prescribing is undesirable, first as clinical experience is less robust than formal clinical trials data as a guide to efficacy and safety, and second because it leaves the clinician, rather than the pharmaceutical company, liable for any harm that may result. More recently, regulations to include a paediatric population in clinical development plans have forced the development of new guidance as to how to include children in clinical development. Market exclusivity prolongation has been successfully tried for some years in the United States, and in July 2003, the Federal Food, Drug and Cosmetic Act was amended to request paediatric studies in a new submission unless omission is justified. In September of 2007, the Paediatric Research Equity Act replaced the 2003 Act, and an assessment was made to evaluate the quality of the studies submitted. The results have been positive: between September 2007 and June 2010, more than 250 clinical trials had been conducted, and since 2012, over 350 further studies have been undertaken (see website reference 2).

In Europe, the European Commission adopted the Paediatric Regulation in February 2007 (see website reference 3). This stipulates that no marketing approval will be granted unless there is an agreed paediatric investigation plan in place or, alternatively, there is a waiver from the requirement because of the low risk that the product will be considered for use in children. The paediatric studies may, with the agreement of the regulatory authority, be performed after approval for other populations. For new compounds or for products with a Supplementary Protection Certificate or SPC (see section on Patent protection), paediatric applications will be given a longer market exclusivity period, and off-patent products can be given a special paediatric use marketing authorization (PUMA); funds will be available for paediatric research in these products.

To further encourage paediatric research, Authority scientific advice is free. Paediatric clinical data from the EU and elsewhere are collected in a common European database to avoid repetition of trials with unnecessary exposure in children. The US FDA and the EMA in Europe exchange information on paediatric clinical research.

Ethnic differences. In order for clinical data to be accepted globally, the risk of ethnic differences in safety, efficacy and pharmacokinetics of a drug must be assessed. ICH efficacy guideline E5 defines a bridging data package that would allow extrapolation of foreign clinical data to the population in the new region. A limited programme may suffice to confirm comparable effects in different ethnic groups.

Ethnic differences may be genetic in origin, as in the example described in Chapter 17, or related to differences in environment, culture or medical practice.

Therapeutic confirmatory studies

The therapeutic confirmatory phase of drug development is intended to confirm efficacy results from controlled exploratory efficacy studies, but now, in a more realistic clinical environment and with a broader population. These are very large, very expensive studies and should only be embarked upon following regulatory authority advice from all the regions intended for marketing.

In order to document convincingly that the product is efficacious, there are some 'golden rules' to be aware of in terms of the need for statistical power, replication of the results and so on. Further, for a product intended for long-term use, its performance must be investigated during long-term exposure.

Evidence is considered to be more robust if treatment effects across the trials in the application, as well as in relevant subgroups within one trial, are consistent.

All these aspects will, however, be influenced by what alternative treatments there are, the intended target patient population, the rarity and severity of the disease, as well as other factors and must be evaluated case by case.

Clinical safety profile

An equally important function of this largest and longest section of the clinical documentation is to capture all adverse events and other safety information to enable evaluation of the relative benefit–risk ratio of the new

299

compound. Meta-analysis across studies may help to identify rarer adverse drug reactions, but in most cases rare adverse effects will not be apparent from the initial development package. To document clinical safety, the ICH E1 guideline on products intended for chronic use stipulates that a minimum of 100 patients be treated for at least 1 year, and 300–600 treated for at least 6 months. In reality, however, several thousand patients usually form the database for safety evaluation for marketing approval.

Not until several similar studies can be analysed together can a real estimate be made of the clinical safety of the product. For common diseases, this is an expected requirement of the initial registration package, but for rare diseases, such meta-analysis may only be practical in the postmarketing setting.

Typically, the collected clinical database should be analysed across a sensible selection of variables, such as sex, age, race, exposure (dose and duration), as well as concomitant diseases and concomitant pharmacotherapy. This type of integrated data analysis is a rational and scientific way to obtain necessary information about the benefits and risks of new compounds.

To further emphasize the accountability for the product by the pharmaceutical company, a more proactive legislation for risk evaluation has been introduced in the United States, the EU and Japan. The term risk evaluation and mitigation strategy (REMS) in the United States is matched by the risk management system in the EU and Japan.

The key difference here is that rather than reporting and reacting to adverse reactions that have occurred, possible or potential risks should be foreseen or identified early, and mitigation/minimization activities be planned in advance. The risk management plan is generally part of the regulatory approval and follows the product's entire lifecycle. The true risk profile will develop along with the increased knowledge base. The goal is that it should be possible to demonstrate how and why the treatment benefits outweigh the risks at any time rather than relying on intermittent review (see website references 4 and 5).

Regulatory aspects of novel types of therapy

As emphasized in earlier chapters, the therapeutic landscape is moving ever more towards biological and biopharmaceutical treatments, as well as various innovative, so-called advanced therapies. There are also broadening definitions of what constitutes medical devices. The regulatory framework established to ensure the quality, safety and efficacy of conventional synthetic drugs is not entirely appropriate for many biopharmaceutical products, and even less so for the many gene- and cell-based products currently in development. Recombinant proteins have been in use since 1982, and the regulatory process for such biopharmaceuticals is now well established, hence this chapter will mainly focus on these. The EU also has, for example, new legislation in force since December 2008 specifically on ATMPs, meaning somatic cell therapy, gene therapy and tissue engineering. This involves requirements for the applicant, as part of a marketing authorization, to establish a risk management system. In addition to the standard requirements in terms of safety follow-up for an approved product, this system should also include an evaluation of the product's effectiveness (see website reference 6). In the United States, there are a number of FDA guidelines relating to cellular and gene therapies. The regulatory framework for even newer therapeutic modalities relating, for example, to nanotechnologies is not yet clearly defined, and the regulatory authorities face a difficult task in keeping up with the accelerating pace of technological change.

Biopharmaceuticals

Compared with synthetic chemical compounds, biopharmaceuticals can show great structural diversity, and their production methods are also diverse, including complex fermentation and recombinant techniques, as well as techniques involving the use of transgenic animals and plants. All of these elements pose new challenges for the robust demonstration of quality control. This has necessarily led to a fairly pragmatic regulatory framework. Quality, safety and efficacy requirements have to be no less stringent, but procedures and standards are flexible and generally established on a case-by-case basis. This adds a level of uncertainty for the sponsoring pharmaceutical company; flexible approaches may deliver an early approval, but differences of opinion about data can introduce lengthy and difficult-to-resolve delays.

Published guidelines on the development of conventional drugs need to be considered to determine what parts are relevant for a particular biopharmaceutical product. In addition, there are, to date, seven ICH guidelines that deal exclusively with biopharmaceuticals—Q5A–E, Q6B and S6—as well as numerous FDA and Committee for Medicinal Products for Human Use (CHMP) guidance documents. These deal with quality aspects and, in one case, preclinical safety aspects. The definition of what is included in the term 'biopharmaceutical' varies somewhat between documents and therefore needs to be checked. The active substances include proteins and peptides, their derivatives and products of which they are components. Examples include (but are not limited to) cytokines, recombinant plasma factors, growth factors, fusion proteins, enzymes, hormones and monoclonal antibodies (see also Chapters 8 and 9).

Advanced therapy medicinal products. The advent of ATMPs in the late 1990s heralded a new kind of medicine that could not follow the usual regulatory pathway to licensing, yet still had to follow the key principles of establishing quality, safety and efficacy for licensing. This manipulation of genes or introduction of altered cells or tissues into the body in order to change the course of disease was a scientific, ethical and legislative challenge to regulators.

In the United States, about 70% of investigational new drug (IND) applications for gene therapy submitted to the FDA are for rare diseases. Most of these conditions are diagnosed in childhood and are life-threatening. However, conducting a clinical trial with the traditional design using large numbers of subjects with inclusion of a control arm is practically impossible. In addition, control of the manufacture of ATMPs has raised new problems regarding quality, including how the products might be affected by changes in the manufacturing process. Much of the initial research on ATMPs has been conducted by academia and small start-up companies that lack the experience of producing high-quality therapies that can be scaled up to produce commercial volumes.

Faced with these rapid advances in biology and therapeutic delivery technologies, the EMA and the FDA were the first agencies to establish new guidelines for development and licensing. These guidelines adapt the good manufacturing practice (GMP), GLP and good clinical practice (GCP) requirements to the specific characteristics of ATMPs and address the novel and complex manufacturing scenarios utilized for these products. They foster a risk-based approach to the manufacture and testing of such products—FDA has some 29 cellular and gene therapy guidances dating from 1998 to the present.

The EMA has also set up an Innovation Task Force to provide a forum for informal dialogue between EMA and developers of ATMPs in the early stages of the medicine development process. Registered small- and medium-sized enterprises (SMEs) are encouraged to approach the SME office to request meeting to discuss their planned regulatory strategy. In addition, the EMA has established the EU Innovation Network, to support drug developers seeking national and EMA advice. In addition, regulatory agencies are seeking to provide more guidance on emerging therapies such as gene editing; the EMA and the FDA are working together on this to avoid digressions in the advice proffered by the two.

One milestone in May 2016 was the EMA's approval of Strimvelis, developed by GlaxoSmithKline, and the first ex vivo stem cell gene therapy to treat patients with the very rare disease ADA-SCID (severe combined immunodeficiency due to adenosine deaminase deficiency). ADA-SCID is estimated to occur in approximately 15 patients per year in Europe. Later, in December 2017, the first FDA approval was granted for an in vivo gene therapy product, Luxturna, filed by Spark Therapeutics. Luxturna treats a rare, inherited eye condition caused by mutations to a gene called *RPE65* that can cause blindness.

EU legislation also provides for scientific and financial incentives to encourage research and development in the area of advanced therapies. Developers of ATMPs can obtain reductions in the fees payable to EMA of: 65% fee reduction for a request for scientific advice for ATMPs (90% for SMEs) and a 90% fee reduction for the certification procedure.

Quality considerations. Viruses are commonly used as vectors in the manufacture of biopharmaceuticals. A unique and critically important feature for biopharmaceuticals is the need to ensure and document viral safety aspects, as adventitious virus contamination of manufacturing environments is of high concern. Furthermore, there must be preparedness for potentially new hazards, such as infective prions. Therefore strict control of the origin of starting materials and expression systems is essential. The current battery of ICH quality guidance documents in this area reflects these points of particular attention.

At the time when biopharmaceuticals first appeared, the ability to analyse and exactly characterize the end product was not possible. Therefore their efficacy and safety depended critically on the manufacturing process itself, and emphasis was placed on 'process control' rather than 'product control'.

Since then, much experience and confidence has been gained. Bioanalytical technologies for characterizing large molecules have improved dramatically. Bioassays to demonstrate the pharmacological potency of the final product are a specific feature of biopharmaceuticals and are an important difference from chemical entities, where characterization relies on physical structure. Advances in technological assessment of biopharmaceuticals mean that the quality packages are less different from chemical entities than they used to be, but the inherent complexity of biopharmaceuticals usually means the package has to be more extensive.

Today the concept of 'comparability' has been established, and approaches for demonstrating product comparability after process changes have been outlined by regulatory authorities. This is an important step, as it has allowed licensing of biosimilar versions of biopharmaceuticals akin to a 'generic' version of a chemical pharmaceutical product. A legal framework was established first in the EU, in 2004, and the first such approvals (somatropin products) were seen in 2006. Japan followed in 2009 with its first biosimilar (again somatropin). Approvals were behind in the United States since there was not a regulatory pathway for biosimilars until such provisions were signed into law in March 2010 (see website reference 7). The FDA approved the first US biosimilar filgrastim in March 2015, after years of debate and regulatory hurdles. The first monoclonal antibody biosimilar followed in April 2016, with infliximab being approved for all eligible indications of the reference product, Janssen's REMICADE.

Safety considerations. The expectations in terms of performing and documenting a nonclinical safety evaluation for biotechnology-derived pharmaceuticals are well outlined in the ICH guidance document S6. This guideline was revised in 2011, and a further addendum added in 2016, all driven by scientific advances and experience gained since publication of the original guidance. It indicates a flexible, case-by-case and science-based approach but also points out that a product needs to be sufficiently characterized to allow the appropriate design of a preclinical safety evaluation.

Generally, all toxicity studies must be performed according to GLP. However, for biopharmaceuticals, it is recognized that some specialized tests may not be able to comply fully with GLP. The guidance further comments that the standard toxicity testing designs in the commonly used species (e.g., rats and dogs) are often not relevant because these species are pharmacologically unresponsive to humanized proteins.

To make it relevant, a safety evaluation should include a species, often a nonhuman primate, in which the test material is pharmacologically active. Further, in certain justified cases, one relevant species may suffice, at least for the long-term studies. If no relevant species at all can be identified, the use of transgenic animals expressing the human receptor or the use of homologous proteins may be considered.

Other factors of particular relevance with biopharmaceuticals are potential immunogenicity and immunotoxicity. Long-term studies may be difficult to perform, depending on the possible formation of neutralizing antibodies in the selected species. For products intended for chronic use, the duration of long-term toxicity studies must, however, always be scientifically justified. While the formation of (neutralizing) antibodies may be a feature of the cross-species immune response, antidrug antibodies may also form in humans. The package for biopharmaceuticals should include preclinical studies assessing the potential for antibody formation and clinical assessment during human studies. Regulatory guidance also states that standard carcinogenicity studies are generally inappropriate, but that product-specific assessments of potential risks may still be needed, and that a variety of approaches may be necessary to accomplish this.

In 2006, disastrous clinical trial events took place with an antibody (TGN 1412), where healthy volunteers suffered life-threatening adverse effects. These effects had not been anticipated by the company or the authority reviewing the clinical trial application (CTA). The events triggered intense discussions on risk identification and mitigation for so-called first-in-human clinical trials, and in particular, for any medicinal product that might be considered 'high risk'. Since then, specific guidelines for such CTAs have been issued by the regulatory authorities. These guidelines have been further updated to include guidance on the inclusion of assessments of pharmacodynamic response following deaths and harm to subjects participating in a study in Rennes, France who were given doses that were very much higher than needed to maximize the desired pharmacological effect.

Efficacy considerations. The need to establish efficacy is in principle the same for biopharmaceuticals as for conventional drugs, but there are significant differences in practice. The establishment of a dose–response relationship can be difficult, as there may be an 'all-or-none-effect' at extremely low levels. Establishing a maximum tolerated dose (MTD) in humans is considered less useful these days, as the emphasis is on measuring pharmacology, but it is particularly unhelpful for biopharmaceuticals, as many will not evoke any dose-limiting side effects. Measuring pharmacokinetic properties may be difficult, particularly if the substance is an endogenous mediator. Biopharmaceuticals may also have very long half-lives compared with small molecules, often in the range of weeks rather than hours, especially if they form a complex with their target which then persists. Establishing the pharmacokinetics in terms of free and bound product can be important to understand the therapeutics response but is often technically challenging.

For any biopharmaceutical intended for chronic or repeated use, there will be extra emphasis on demonstrating long-term efficacy. This is because the medical use of proteins is associated with potential immunogenicity and the possible development of neutralizing antibodies, such that the intended benefit may be reduced or even disappear with time. Repeated assessment of immunogenicity may be needed, particularly after any process changes.

To date, biopharmaceuticals have typically been developed for serious diseases or where there is an unmet need for new medicines. Certain types of treatments, such as cytotoxic agents or immunomodulators, cannot be given to healthy volunteers. In such cases, the initial dose-escalation studies will have to be carried out in a patient population rather than in healthy volunteers.

Regulatory procedural considerations. In the EU, only the centralized procedure can be used for marketing authorization of biopharmaceuticals, including biosimilars (see Regulatory procedures, later). This process involves a single submission to the EMA, and if granted, the licence applies in all EU member states. In the United States, biopharmaceuticals are in most cases approved by review of Biologics License Applications (BLAs), rather than New Drug Applications (NDAs).

Personalized therapies

It is recognized that an individual's genetic makeup influences the effect of drugs. As long ago as the 1950s, the inherited differences in response to drugs such as isoniazid and succinylcholine were recognized. Terminology used in this area can be confusing; pharmacogenetics typically refers to the way that genetic differences alter the pharmacokinetic properties of a drug, while pharmacogenomics refers to how genetic differences alter the response to drugs.

Pharmacogenetic research has focussed on the observation that some patients were more susceptible to adverse effects of drugs, and this had a genetic basis. One of the best described examples is the association of severe hypersensitivity reactions to the antiretroviral drug abacavir and their association with the human Leukocyte antigen (HLA) B*5701 allele. Patients are now tested for this before starting this drug. There are several other examples now adopted into clinical practice.

Incorporating pharmacogenomic concepts into therapeutic practice is still at a relatively early stage, but it is advancing rapidly. In 2018, the FDA licensed a drug for the treatment of paediatric cancer on the basis of the underlying genetic mutation rather than the physical location of the tumour (Vitrakvi [larotrectinib]). Delivering this kind of approach requires a suitably validated assay to be available to test prospective patients for the biomarker or genetic mutation. Development of a 'companion' diagnostic adds a considerable level of complexity to the development process, as it must be developed, validated and made commercially available in parallel with the development of the drug product. In many cases, the company developing the assay will be different from the company developing the drug. This approach remains in its infancy but is relatively common in cancer therapy and is now branching out into other therapeutic areas. Specific patient selection information is increasingly used in the indication statement. The Tykerb indication, for example, includes the statement '. . . for the treatment of patients with advanced or metastatic breast cancer whose tumours overexpress HER2'.

In the EU, there are two guidelines, one adopted in April 2010 on the use of pharmacogenetic methodologies in the pharmacokinetic evaluation of medicinal products, and the second adopted in 2016 on good pharmacogenomic practice.

Orphan drugs

Orphan medicines are those intended to diagnose, prevent or treat rare diseases; in the EU, being further specified as life-threatening or chronically debilitating conditions. The concept also includes therapies that are unlikely to be developed under normal market conditions, where the company can show that a return on research investment will not be possible. To qualify for orphan drug status, there should be no satisfactory treatment available or, alternatively, the intended new treatment should offer a 'significant benefit' (see website references 8 and 9). In order to justify the assumption of significant benefit, the sponsor should be able to provide some supportive clinical evidence in their orphan drug request.

To qualify as an orphan indication, the prevalence of the condition must be fewer than 5 in 10,000 individuals in the EU, fewer than 50,000 affected in Japan or fewer than 200,000 affected in the United States. Financial and scientific assistance is made available for products intended for use in a given indication that obtain orphan status. Companies developing orphan drug benefit from financial benefits including a reduction in or exemption from fees; in some cases, regulatory authorities and other government agencies may provide some direct funding towards the development costs as well. Specialist groups within the regulatory authorities provide scientific help and advice on the execution of studies. The normal requirements to demonstrate safety and efficacy still apply, but agencies have some discretion to apply pragmatic approaches that reflect the rarity of the condition. For example, only one phase III study may be required for licensing, and the standard expectations for numbers of subjects treated at each stage of development may be reduced.

The most important benefit stimulating orphan drug development is market exclusivity for 7–10 years for the product, for the designated medical use. In the EU, the centralized procedure (see Regulatory procedures, later) is compulsory for orphan drugs.

The orphan drug incentives are fairly recent. In the United States, the legislation dates from 1983, in Japan from 1995 and in the EU from 2000. The US experience has shown that this has certainly stimulated drug research for rare diseases; a review of the first 25 years of the Orphan Drug Act showed 326 marketing approvals, the majority of which are intended to treat rare cancers or metabolic/endocrinological disorders.

Environmental considerations

Environmental risk evaluation of the finished pharmaceutical products originated as a requirement for veterinary medicines, and then later became a requirement for human pharmaceuticals in the United States and the EU. The main concern relates to the risk of contamination of the environment by the compound or its metabolites. The environmental impact of the manufacturing process is a separate issue that is regulated by legislation relating to manufacturing rather than medicines per se.

The US requirement for environmental assessment (EA) applies in all cases where action is needed to minimize environmental effects. An Environmental Assessment Report is then required, and the FDA will develop an Environmental Impact Statement to direct necessary action. Drug products for human or animal use can, however, be excluded from this requirement under certain conditions (see website reference 10), for example, if the estimated concentration in the aquatic environment of the active substance is below 1 part per billion, or if the substance occurs naturally. In Europe, a corresponding general guideline was implemented in December 2006 for human medicinal products (see website reference 11).

Regulatory procedures

Clinical trials

In 1747, James Lind conducted an experiment on 12 sailors suffering from scurvy. There were six treatment groups, each of the two sailors given various potions to consume. The two sailors who were given oranges and lemons were the only ones to improve. This early step in the advancement of systematic clinical research was nevertheless completely unregulated. The evolution of CTRs, like other drug regulations, has tended to be in response to events resulting in harm to patients. It is evident that clinical trials can pose risks to humans, but scientific advances in the field of medicine will always bring with them the possibility of new, unthought of risks: the earlier in the development process, the greater the risk.

The ethical basis for all clinical research is the Declaration of Helsinki (see website reference 12), which was an international response to the crimes of human experimentation that took place during World War II. It states that the primary obligation for the treating physician is to care for the patient. It also says that clinical research may be performed provided the goal is to improve treatment. Furthermore, the subject must be informed about the potential benefits and risks and must consent to participate. The guardians of patients who for any reason cannot give informed consent (e.g., small children) can agree to participation.

During the development process, regulatory authorities are primarily concerned with the safety of subjects/patients involved and the scientific basis of the intended study protocol. Regulatory authorities require all results of clinical trials approved by them to be reported back, whether or not the results will be part of a future marketing application. Ethics committees also review clinical trials of potential treatments (see later).

All clinical research in humans should be performed according to the internationally agreed Code of Good Clinical Practice, as described in the ICH guideline E6 (see website reference 1).

Europe

Until relatively recently, the regulatory requirements to start and conduct clinical studies in Europe have varied widely between countries, ranging from little or no regulation to a requirement for complete assessment by the health authority of the intended study protocol and all supporting documentation.

The efforts to harmonize EU procedures led to the development of a Clinical Trial Directive implemented in May 2004 (see website reference 13). The main benefits are that both regulatory authorities and ethics committees must respond within 60 days of receiving clinical trial applications, and the requirements for information to be submitted are defined and published in a set of guidelines. Much of the information submitted to the regulatory authority and ethics committee is the same; however, the emphasis of the review by these two bodies is somewhat different. The ethics committees are primarily focussed on the impact of the research on the rights and the wellbeing of the subject, the information they receive and their consent. The regulatory agency's main concern is the management of risk to the subjects such that there is a favourable balance of benefit versus risk for the subjects.

In spite of the Clinical Trial Directive, however, some national differences in format and information requirements have remained, and upon submission of identical clinical trial protocols in several countries, the national reviews may reach different conclusions. This led to the EU Heads of Agencies setting up the clinical trials facilitation group (CTFG; see http://www.hma.eu/ctfg.html), a body composed of experts from the national regulatory agencies in the EU with the remit to foster a more harmonized regulatory framework for clinical trials in Europe. The CTFG set up the voluntary harmonization procedure (VHP) for clinical trials involving at least three EU member states. This comprises two steps, where in the first round, one coordinating regulatory authority manages national comments on the application and provides the applicant with a consolidated list of comments or questions. In the second step, the usual national applications for the clinical trial are submitted, but national approval must then be gained very rapidly without any further requests for change. Substantial amendments to the CTA should also be submitted through the VHP to maintain a harmonized authorization. Additional EU countries may also be added via a second-round VHP should there be the need to expand the countries participating in the clinical trial.

Notwithstanding the efforts of the EU member states to harmonize clinical trials in Europe, dissatisfaction on the lack of harmonization within the clinical trial sponsor community and the European Commission led to the adoption of a new CTR 536/2014. As a regulation rather than a directive, the CTR applies uniformly in all member states except for the aspects of ethical approval, national laws on ethical matters having precedence over EU regulation. The CTR includes an EU portal for electronic submission of a single dossier to all concerned member states. The development of this EU portal has proven to be a difficult information technology project run by the EMA and, at the time of going to press, is still under construction and is not expected to be available until sometime in 2021.

The United States

An IND application must be submitted to one of the review divisions of the FDA before a new drug is given to humans. The application is relatively simple (see website reference 14), and to encourage early human studies, it is not necessary to submit complete, final preclinical study reports. The toxicology safety evaluation can be based on draft and unaudited reports, provided the data are sufficient for the FDA to make a reliable assessment. However, complete study reports must be made available to the FDA within 60 days of the initial submission.

Unless the FDA has questions, or even places the product on 'clinical hold', the IND is considered opened 30 days after it was submitted, and from then on new study protocols are added to it for every new study planned. New scientific information must be submitted whenever changes are to be made, for example, updates to chemistry, manufacturing and controls (CMC) or preclinical information, new patient categories or new indications that fall within the scope of the same review division. For a new protocol in an indication that is the remit of a different review division, a new IND needs to be submitted to that review division. The IND process requires an annual update report describing project progress and additional data obtained during the year. The annual Development Safety Update Report (DSUR) fulfils this requirement globally.

As well as the 'safe to proceed' from the FDA, approval from the Institutional Review Board (IRB) is needed for every institution where a clinical study is to be performed.

Japan

Historically, because of differences in medical culture, treatment traditions and the possibility of significant racial differences, clinical trials in Japan had not been useful for drug applications in the Western world. Also, for a product to be approved for the Japanese market, repetition of clinical studies in Japan was necessary, often delaying the availability of products in Japan.

With the introduction of international standards under the auspices of ICH, data from Japanese patients are increasingly becoming acceptable in other countries. The guideline on bridging studies to compensate for ethnic differences (ICH E5; see website reference 1) may allow Japanese studies to become part of global development.

The requirements for beginning a clinical study in Japan are similar to those in the United States or Europe. Scientific summary information is generally acceptable, and ethics committee approval is necessary.

Application for marketing authorization

The application for marketing authorization (MAA in Europe, NDA in the United States and JNDA in Japan) is compiled and submitted as soon as the drug development programme has been completed and judged satisfactory by the company. Different authorities have differing requirements as to the level of detail and the format of submissions, and it is the task of the RA department to collate all the data as efficiently as possible to satisfy these varying requirements with a minimum of rework. Presubmission meetings with the reviewing agencies in the EU, United States and Japan are essential.

The US FDA in general requires raw data to be included, allowing them to make their own analysis, and thus they request the most complete data of all authorities. European authorities require a condensed dossier containing critical evaluations of the data, allowing a rapid review based on conclusions drawn by named scientific experts. These may be internal or external and are selected by the applicant.

Japanese authorities have traditionally focussed predominantly on data generated in Japan, studies performed elsewhere being supportive only. However, it has become increasingly common for Japanese patients to take part in global phase III programmes rather than in bespoke Japan-only studies.

The procedures adopted in these three regions are described later in more detail.

Europe

Several procedures are available for marketing authorization in the EU (Fig. 20.3, see website reference 13):
- *National procedure*, in which the application is evaluated by one regulatory authority. This procedure is allowed for products intended for that country

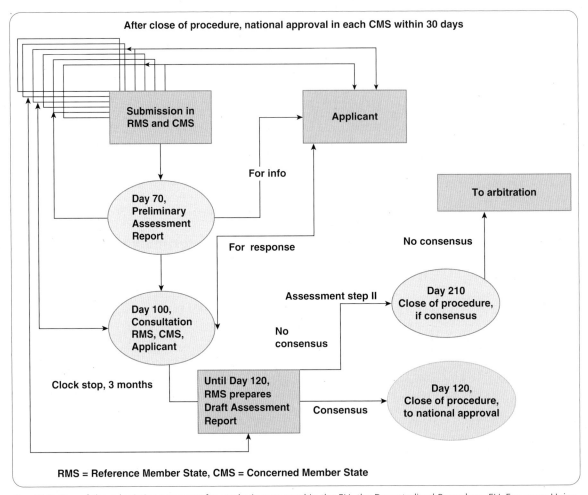

Fig. 20.3 One of the submission processes for marketing approval in the EU, the Decentralized Procedure. *EU*, European Union.

only. Also, it is the first step in a mutual recognition procedure.

- *Mutual recognition*, in which a marketing approval application is assessed by one national authority, the Reference Member State (RMS), which subsequently defends the approval and evaluation in order to gain mutual recognition of the assessment from other European authorities. The pharmaceutical company may select countries of interest. These, the Concerned Member States, have 90 days to recognize the initial assessment. The mutual recognition procedure is used for harmonization and conversion of nationally approved products. After mutual recognition, the final marketing authorizations are given as national decisions, but the scientific assessment is quicker and requires fewer resources from all national authorities. In the case of nonagreement, referral to EMA for

arbitration is done as a last resort. But before arbitration is considered, the Coordination Group for Mutual Recognition and Decentralized Procedures (CMDh/CMDv) will try to resolve outstanding issues. This is a group composed of expert members from European regulatory authorities. The worst outcome of an arbitration would be that the marketing authorizations obtained are withdrawn in all EU countries, including the RMS.

- *Decentralized procedure* is similar to the mutual recognition procedure. It is a modernization, the aim of which is to share the work among authorities earlier in the process, with the possibility of a decision being reached before 120 days have passed from receipt of a valid submission. It is the procedure of choice for a new chemical entity when not following the centralized procedure.

- *Centralized procedure* is a 'federal' procedure carried out by the EMA, with scientists selected from CHMP to perform the review, the approval body being the European Commission. This procedure is mandatory for biotechnological products, biosimilars, orphan drugs, as well as products intended to treat diabetes, AIDS, cancer, neurodegenerative disorders, autoimmune diseases and viral diseases.
- The centralized procedure starts with the nomination of one CHMP member to act as *rapporteur*, who selects and leads the assessment team. A selected *co-rapporteur* and team make a parallel review. The European Commission approves the application based on a CHMP recommendation, which in turn is based on the assessment reports by the two rapporteur teams. Products approved in this way can be marketed in all EU countries with the same prescribing information, packs and labels.

CHMP is prepared to give scientific advice to companies in situations where published guidance on the European position is not available, or when the company needs to discuss a possible deviation from guidelines. Such advice, as well as advice from national regulatory authorities, may be very valuable at any stage of the development programme and may later be incorporated in new guidelines. Providing advice requires considerable effort from CHMP specialists, and fees have to be paid by the pharmaceutical company.

The United States

The FDA is more willing than other large authorities to take an active part in planning the drug development process. Some meetings between the FDA and the sponsoring company are more or less compulsory. One such example is the so-called end-of-phase II meeting. This is in most cases a critically important meeting for the company in which clinical data up until that point are presented to the FDA together with a proposed remaining phase III programme and the company's target label. The purpose is to gain FDA feedback on the appropriateness of the intended NDA package and whether the anticipated clinical data to be gained from phase III are likely to enable approval of a desirable product label. At the same time, these discussions may make it possible in special cases to deviate from guidelines by prior agreement with the FDA. Furthermore, these discussion meetings ensure that the authority is already familiar with the project when the dossier is submitted.

The review time for the FDA has decreased substantially in the last few years (see Chapter 22). Standard reviews should be completed within 10 months, and priority reviews of those products with a strong medical need within 6 months.

The assessment result is usually communicated either as an approval or as a complete response letter. The latter is a request for additional information or data before approval.

Japan

In Japan, the regulatory authority is today available for consultation, allowing scientific discussion and feedback during the development phase. These meetings tend to follow a similar pattern to those in the United States and the EU and have made it much easier to address potential problems well before submission for marketing approval is made.

These changes have meant shorter review times and a more transparent process. The scientific review in Japan is performed by the Pharmaceuticals and Medical Devices Agency (PMDA), and the ultimate decision is made by the Ministry of Health, Labour and Welfare (MHLW) based on the Evaluation Centre's report.

It is worth mentioning that health authorities, in particular in the ICH regions, have well-established communication channels and often assist and consult each other.

The common technical document

Following the good progress made by ICH in creating scientific guidelines applicable in the three large regions, discussions on standardizing document formats began in 1997. The aim was to define a standard format, called the Common Technical Document (CTD), for the application for a new drug product. It was realized from the outset that harmonization of *content* could not be achieved, owing to the fundamental differences in data requirements and work processes between different regulatory authorities. Adopting a common *format* has, nonetheless, been a worthwhile step forward.

The guideline was adopted by the three ICH regions in November 2000 and subsequently implemented, and it has generally been accepted in most other countries. This saves much time and effort in reformatting documents for submission to different regulatory authorities. The structure of the CTD (see website reference 1) is summarized in Fig. 20.4.

Module 1 (not part of the CTD) contains regional information such as the application form, the suggested prescribing information, the application fee and also other information that is not considered relevant in all territories, such as EA (required in the United States and Europe but not in Japan). Certificates of different regional needs are also to be found in Module 1, as well as patent information not yet requested in the EU.

Module 2 comprises a very brief general introduction, followed by summary information relating to quality,

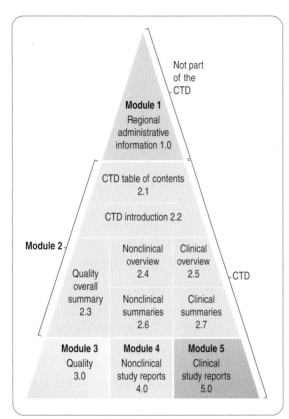

Fig. 20.4 Diagrammatic representation of the organization of the Common Technical Document (CTD).

safety (i.e., nonclinical studies) and efficacy (i.e., clinical studies). Quality issues (purity, manufacturing process, stability, etc.) are summarized in a single document of a maximum 40 pages. The nonclinical and clinical summaries each consist of a separate *overview* (maximum 30 pages) and *summaries of individual studies*. The overviews in each area are similar to the previous EU Expert Reports, in that they present critical evaluations of the programme performed. Detailed guidelines (see website references 1, 13 and 14), based on existing US, European and Japanese requirements, are available to indicate what tabulated information needs to be included in these summaries, and how the written summaries should be drafted. The nonclinical section has been fairly noncontroversial. The guidance is very similar to the previous US summary, with clear instructions on how to sort the studies regarding animals, doses, durations of treatment and routes of administration.

The clinical summary is similar to what was required by the FDA, incorporating many features taken from the Integrated Summaries of Efficacy (ISE) and Safety (ISS). ISE will generally fit in the clinical summary document.

The ISS document has proved very useful in drawing conclusions from the clinical studies by sensible pooling and integration but is too large (often more than 400 pages in itself) to be accepted in the EU and Japan. This problem can be resolved by including the ISS as a separate report in Module 5.

Modules 3, 4 and 5 comprise the individual study reports. Most reports are eligible for use in all three regions, possibly with the exception at present of Module 3, Quality, which may need regional content.

There has been a transformation to fully electronic submissions—known as e-CTD—in place of the large quantities of paper that composed an application for marketing approval. Experimental data are lodged in databases, allowing the information to be transferred from pharmaceutical companies to regulatory authorities much more easily. The electronic structure also greatly facilitates navigation within the dossier. Guidelines on the structure and interface between databases in the industry setting and those at the authorities are available.

Administrative rules

Patent protection and data exclusivity

Patent protection

A patent is a form of protection issued by a government authority to an inventor to exclude others from making, using, offering for sale or selling the same invention for a limited period of time, in exchange for public disclosure of the invention when the patent is granted. Early in the life of a medicine, the inventor will apply for a patent. Generally, the term of a new patent is 20 years from the date on which the application for the patent was filed. During the 1980s, the time taken to develop and obtain marketing approval for a new drug increased so much that the period of market exclusivity established by the original patent could be too short to allow the company to recoup its R&D costs. To overcome this problem (see Chapter 19), the EU Council, in 1992, introduced rules allowing companies to apply for an SPC, matching similar legislation in the United States and Japan. An SPC extends the duration of a patent. It enters into force after expiry of a patent upon which it is based and in Europe it has a maximum 5-year term.

The application for an SPC has to be submitted within 6 months of first approval anywhere in Europe, within or outside the EU, and from then on the clock starts. It is thus strategically important to obtain first approval in a financially important market for best revenue.

Nonpatent regulatory exclusivity

Nonpatent regulatory exclusivity, also called data exclusivity, should not be confused with patent protection. Pharmaceutical companies are granted exclusive marketing rights by a government authority upon approval of a drug that can run concurrently with a patent or not. The protection of the originators' data means that generic products cannot be approved by referring to the originator product documentation until the exclusivity period has ended. The length of nonpatent regulatory exclusivity varies depending on the country and the type of exclusivity. Types of data exclusivity include new chemical entity, paediatric, orphan and biologic.

Pricing of pharmaceutical products—'the fourth hurdle'

The 'fourth hurdle' or 'market access' are expressions for the ever-growing demand for cost-effectiveness in pharmaceutical prescribing. Payers, whether health insurance companies or publicly funded national institutions, require stringent justification for the normally high price of a new pharmaceutical product. This means that, if not in the original application, studies have to demonstrate that the clinical benefit of a new compound is commensurate with the suggested price, compared with the previous therapy of choice in the country of application.

To address this concern, studies in a clinical trial programme from phase II onwards normally include health economic measures (see Chapter 17). In the United States, certainly, it is advantageous to have a statement of health economic benefit approved in the package insert, to justify reimbursement. A favourable benefit–risk evaluation is no longer sufficient: value for money must also be demonstrated in order to have a commercially successful product (see also Chapter 21). However, because of the different national reference pricing systems in place around the world, there is the need for local postapproval studies to provide the necessary evidence to support the reimbursement claims.

List of abbreviations

CHMP	Committee for Medicinal Products for Human Use, the new name to replace CPMP early 2004
CTD	Common Technical Document
CMDh/ CMDv	Coordination Group for Human/Veterinary Medicinal Products for Mutual Recognition and Decentralized Procedure (EU)
EC	Ethics committee (EU), known as institutional review board (IRB) in USA
eCTD	Electronic Common Technical Document
EMA	European Medicines Agency
ERA	Environmental Risk Assessment (EU)
EU	European Union
FDA	Food and Drug Administration; the US regulatory authority
GCP	Good clinical practice
GLP	Good laboratory practice
GMP	Good manufacturing practice
ICH	International Conference on Harmonization
IND	Investigational New Drug application (US)
IRB	Institutional Review Board (US), equivalent to Ethics Committee in Europe
ISS	Integrated Summary of Safety (US)
JNDA	Japanese New Drug application
MAA	Marketing authorization application (EU), equivalent to NDA in USA
MHLW	Ministry of Health, Labour and Welfare (Jpn)
MTD	Maximum tolerated dose
NDA	New Drug application (USA)
SPC	Supplementary Protection Certificate
WHO	World Health Organization

References

Cartwright, A. C., & Matthews, B. R. (1991). *Pharmaceutical product licensing requirements for Europe*. London: Ellis Horwood.

Cartwright, A. C., & Matthews, B. R. (Eds.). (1994). *International pharmaceutical product registration*. London: Taylor and Francis.

Website references
1. http://www.ich.org/
2. http://www.fda.gov/Drugs/DevelopmentApprovalProcess/DevelopmentResources/ucm049867.htm
3. http://ec.europa.eu/health/files/eudralex/vol-1/reg_2006_1902/reg_2006_1902_en.pdf
4. http://www.fda.gov/downloads/Drugs/GuidanceComplianceRegulatoryInformation/Guidances/UCM184128.pdf
5. https://www.ema.europa.eu/en/documents/regulatory-procedural-guideline/guidance-format-risk-management-plan-rmp-eu-integrated-format-rev-201_en.pdf

6. http://www.ema.europa.eu/docs/
en_GB/document_library/Regulatory_
and_procedural_guideline/2009/10/
WC500006326.pdf

7. https://www.fda.gov/vaccines-blood-
biologics/general-biologics-guidances/
biosimilars-guidances

8. https://www.ema.europa.eu/en/
documents/regulatory-procedural-
guideline/recommendations-elements-
required-support-medical-plausibility-
assumption-significant-benefit-orphan_
en.pdf

9. http://www.fda.gov/ForIndustry/
DevelopingProductsforRareDiseases
Conditions/default.htm

10. https://www.fda.gov/regulatory-
information/search-fda-guidance-
documents/environmental-assessment-
human-drug-and-biologics-applications

11. http://www.ema.europa.eu/docs/
en_GB/document_library/Scientific_
guideline/2009/10/WC500003978.pdf

12. https://www.wma.net/policies-post/
wma-declaration-of-helsinki-ethical-
principles-for-medical-research-
involving-human-subjects/

13. http://ec.europa.eu/health/documents//
eudralex/index_en.htm

14. https://www.fda.gov/

Chapter | 21 |

The role of pharmaceutical marketing

Vincent M Lawton

Introduction

This chapter puts pharmaceutical marketing into the context of the complete life cycle of a medicine and the continually evolving process of market access (MA). It describes the old role of marketing and contrasts with its continually evolving function in a rapidly changing environment and its involvement in the drug development process. It examines the move from the product-centric focus of the 20th century to the customer-centric focus of the 21st century and the critical challenge for all stakeholders to successfully achieve MA for much needed medicines for the benefit of patients.

Pharmaceutical marketing increased strongly in the 10–15 years following World War II, during which time thousands of new molecules entered the market, 'overwhelming' physicians with new scientific facts to learn in order to safely and appropriately prescribe these breakthroughs to their patients. There was a great dependence on the pharmaceutical companies' marketing departments and their professional sales representatives to give the full information necessary to support the prescribing decision.

The basis of drug discovery is research and verifiable data obtained from it. Logically, pharmaceutical marketing needs evidence drawn from data to be credible, effective and ethical. Evidence-based marketing is the basis of pharmaceutical marketing. That is based on data and research, with rigorous examination of all plans and follow-up to verify the success of programmes. Management guru Peter F. Drucker claimed that marketing 'is so basic it cannot be considered a separate function. … It is the whole business seen from the point of view of its final result, that is, from the customer's point of view'.

Pharmaceutical marketing is the way important and accurate information on the safety, efficacy and cost-effectiveness of new and established medicines is conveyed to the physician, the payer and healthcare providers in order that the right patient receives the right and most effective treatment. A key point of controversy for the health authorities that pay for the medicines is the 'high' cost that seems to be rising year on year as new and more expensive treatments come to the market. From the point of view of the pharmaceutical industry, the drive is towards discovery and development of medicines for the benefit of the patients. In order to attain that goal, there is a considerable investment over a decade or more of around $1.5 billion to bring a drug to market. Only 3 out of 10 medicines recover that investment. The industry is adapting to the new reality of the 'barriers to market access' that have been constructed to lower the cost of providing treatment advances for patients.

Pharmaceutical marketing—background

Medical innovation accelerated in the 1950s and early 1960s with more than 4500 new medicines arriving on the market during the decade beginning in 1951. By 1961, around 70% of expenditure on drugs in the United States was on these newly arrived compounds. Pharmaceutical companies marketed the products vigorously and competitively. The tools of marketing used included advertising, mailings and visits to physicians by increasing numbers of (largely) well-trained and knowledgeable professional sales representatives.

Back in 1954, Bill Frohlich, an advertising executive, and David Dubow, a visionary, set out to create a new kind of information company that could enable organizations to make informed, strategic decisions about the marketplace. They called their venture Intercontinental Marketing Services (IMS), and they introduced it at an opportune time, when pharmaceutical executives had few data to consult when in the throes of strategic or tactical planning. By 1957, IMS had published its first European syndicated research study, an audit of pharmaceutical sales within the West German market. Its utility and popularity prompted IMS to expand into new geographies—Great Britain, France, Italy, Spain and Japan among them. Subsequent acquisitions in South Africa, Australia and New Zealand strengthened the IMS position, and by 1969, IMS, with an annual revenue of $5 million, had established the gold standard in pharmaceutical market research in Europe and Asia. IMS (now IQVIA) remains the largest supplier of data on drug use to the pharmaceutical industry, providers, such as health maintenance organizations (HMOs) and health authorities, and payers, such as governments.

Medical associations were unable to keep the doctors adequately informed about the vast array of new drugs. It fell, by default, upon the pharmaceutical industry to fill the knowledge gap. This rush of innovative medicines and promotion activity was named the 'therapeutic jungle' by Goodman and Gilman in their famous textbook (Goodman & Gilman, 1960). Studies in the 1950s revealed that physicians consistently rated pharmaceutical sales representatives as the most important source in learning about new drugs. The much valued 'detail men' enjoyed lengthy, in-depth discussions with physicians. They were perceived as a valuable resource to the prescriber, often as 'part of the team'. This continued throughout the following decades.

A large increase in the number of drugs available necessitated appropriate education of physicians. Again, the industry gladly assumed this responsibility. In the United States, objections about the nature and quality of medical information that was being communicated using marketing tools (Podolsky & Greene, 2008) caused controversy in medical journals and Congress. The Kefauver–Harris Drug Control Act of 1962 imposed controls on the pharmaceutical industry that required that drug companies disclose to doctors the side effects of their products, allowed their products to be sold as generic drugs after having held the patent on them for a certain period of time, and obliged them to prove on demand that their products were, in fact, effective and safe. Senator Kefauver also focussed attention on the form and content of general pharmaceutical marketing and the postgraduate pharmaceutical education of the nation's physicians. A call from the American Medical Association (AMA) and the likes of Kefauver led to the establishment of formal Continuing Medical Education (CME) programmes, to ensure physicians were kept objectively apprised of new development in medicines. Although the thrust of the change was to provide medical education to physicians from the medical community, the newly respectable CME process also attracted the interest and funding of the pharmaceutical industry. Over time, the majority of CME around the world has been provided by the industry (Ferrer, 1975).

The marketing of medicines continued to grow strongly throughout the 1970s and 1980s. Some marketing techniques, perceived as 'excessive' and 'extravagant', came to the attention of the committee chaired by Senator Edward Kennedy in the early 1990s. This resulted in increased regulation of the industry's marketing practices, much of it self-regulation (Todd & Johnson, 1992).

The size of pharmaceutical sales forces increased dramatically during the 1990s, as major pharmaceutical companies, following the dictum that 'more is better', bombarded doctors' surgeries with its representatives. Seen as a competitive necessity, sales forces were increased to match or top the therapeutic competitor, increasing frequency of visits to physicians and widening coverage to all potential customers. This was also a period of great success in the discovery of many new 'blockbuster' products that addressed unmet clinical needs. In some countries, representatives were given targets to call on 8 to 10 doctors per day, detailing three to four products in the same visit. In an average call on the doctor of less than 10 minutes, much of the information was delivered by rote with little time for interaction and assessment of the point of view of the customer. By the 2000s, there was one representative for every six doctors. The time available for representatives to see an individual doctor plummeted, and many practices refused to see representatives at all. With shorter time to spend with doctors, the calls were perceived as less valuable to the physician. Information gathered in a 2004 survey by Harris Interactive and IMS Health (Nickum & Kelly, 2005) indicated that fewer than 40% of responding physicians felt the pharmaceutical industry was 'trustworthy'. Often, they were inclined to mistrust promotion in general. They granted pharmaceutical sales representatives less time, and many closed their doors completely, turning to alternative forms of promotion, such as e-detailing, peer-to-peer interaction and the Internet.

Something had to give. Fewer 'blockbusters' were hitting the market, regulation was tightening its grip and the downturn in the global economy was putting pressure on public expenditure to cut costs. The size of the drug industry's US sales forces had declined by 10% to about 92,000 in 2009, from a peak of 102,000 in 2005 (Fierce Pharma, 2009). This picture was mirrored around the world's pharmaceutical markets. ZS Associates, a sales strategy consulting firm, predicted another drop in the United States—this time of 20%—to as low as 70,000 by 2015. It is of interest, therefore, that the US pharmaceutical giant Merck ran a pilot programme in 2008, under which regions cut sales staff by up to one-quarter and continued to deliver results similar to those in other, uncut, regions. A critical cornerstone of the marketing of pharmaceuticals, the professional representative, is now under threat, at least in its former guise.

Product life cycle

It is important to see the marketing process in the context of the complete product life cycle, from basic research to generalization at the end of the product patent. A typical product life cycle can be illustrated from discovery to decline as follows (William & McCarthy, 1997) (Fig. 21.1).

The product's life cycle period usually consists of five major steps or phases:

- Product development
- Introduction
- Growth
- Maturity
- Decline.

Product development phase

The product development phase begins when a company finds and develops a new product idea. This involves translating various pieces of information and incorporating them into a new product. A product undergoes several changes and developments during this stage. With pharmaceutical products, this depends on efficacy and safety. Pricing strategy must be developed at this stage in time for launch. In a number of markets for pharmaceuticals, price approval must be achieved from payers (usually government agencies). **Marketing plans**, based on market research and product strengths, for the launch and development of the product, are established and approved within the organization. Research on expectations of customers from new products should form a significant part of the marketing strategy. Knowledge, gained through market research, will also help to segment customers according to their potential for early adoption of a product. Production capacity is geared up to meet anticipated market demands.

Introduction phase

The introduction phase of a product includes the product launch phase, where the goal is to achieve maximum impact in the shortest possible time, to establish the product in the market. Marketing promotional spend is highest at this phase of the life cycle. Manufacturing and supply chains (distribution) must be firmly established during this period. It is vital that the new product is available in all outlets (e.g., pharmacies) to meet the early demand.

Growth phase

The growth phase is the time when the market accepts the new entry and when its market share grows. The maturity of the market determines the speed and potential for a new entry. A well-established market hosts competitors who will seek to undermine the new product and protect its own market share. If the new product is highly innovative relative to the market, or the market itself is relatively new, its growth will be more rapid.

Marketing becomes more targeted and reduces in volume when the product is well into its growth. Other aspects of the promotion and product offering will be released in stages during this period. A focus on the efficiency and profitability of the product comes in the latter stage of the growth period.

Maturity phase

The maturity phase comes when the market no longer grows, as the customers are satisfied with the choices available to them. At this point the market will stabilize, with little or no expansion. The exception is when new therapeutic indications and academic research can expand usage of these products. New product entries or product developments can result in displacement of market share towards the newcomer, at the expense of an incumbent product. This corresponds to the most profitable stage for a product if, with little more than maintenance marketing, it can achieve a profitable return. A product's branding and positioning, synonymous with the quality and reliability demanded by the customer, will enable it to enjoy a longer maturity phase. The achievement of the image of 'gold standard' for a product is the goal. In some pharmaceutical markets around the world, the length of the maturity phase is longer than in others, depending on the propensity of physicians to switch to new medicines. For

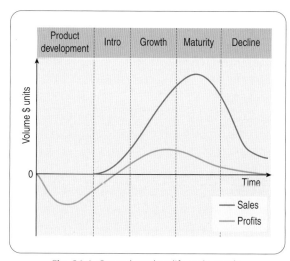

Fig. 21.1 General product life cycle graph.

example, French doctors are generally early adopters of new medicines, where British doctors are slow.

Decline phase

The decline phase usually comes with increased competition, reduced market share and loss of sales and profitability. Companies, realizing the cost involved in defending against a new product entry, will tend to reduce marketing to occasional reminders, rather than the full-out promotion required to match the challenge. With pharmaceutical products, this stage is generally realized at the end of the patent life of a medicine. Those companies with a strong R&D function will focus resources on the discovery and development of new products.

Pharmaceutical product life cycle (Fig. 21.2)

As soon as a promising molecule is found, the company applies for patents. A patent gives the company intellectual property rights over the invention for around 20 years. This means that the company owns the idea and can legally stop other companies from profiting by copying it. Sales and profits will enable the manufacturer to reinvest in R&D:

- For a pharmaceutical product, the majority of patent time could be over before the medicine even enters the market.
- Once it is produced, it takes some time for the medicine to build up sales and so achieve market share; in its early years, the company needs to persuade doctors to prescribe and use the medicine.
- Once the medicine has become established, then it enters a period of maturity; this is the period when most profits are made.
- Finally, as the medicine loses patent protection, copies (generic products) enter the market at a lower cost, therefore sales of the original medicine decline rapidly.

The duration and trend of product life cycles vary among different products and therapeutic classes. In an area of unmet clinical need, the entry of a new efficacious product can result in rapid uptake. Others, entering into a relatively mature market, will experience a slower uptake and more gradual growth later in the life cycle, especially if experience and further research results in newer indications for use (Grabowski et al., 2002).

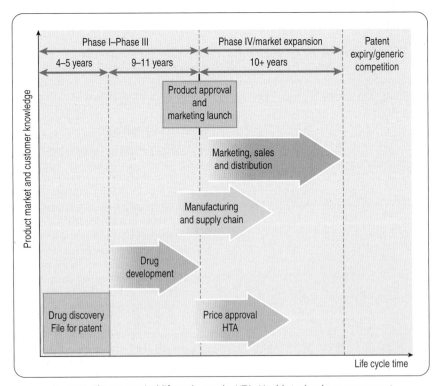

Fig. 21.2 Pharmaceutical life cycle graph. *HTA*, Health technology assessment.

Traditional pharmaceutical marketing

Clinical studies

Pharmaceutical marketing depends on the results from clinical studies. These premarketing clinical trials are conducted in three phases before the product can be submitted to the medicines' regulator for approval of its licence to be used to treat appropriate patients. The marketing planner or product manager will follow the development and results from these studies, interact with the R&D function and specialists in the treatment area. Marketing plans are developed accordingly. The three phases (described in detail in Chapter 17) are as follows.

Phase I trials are the first stage of testing in human subjects.

Phase II trials are performed on larger groups (20–300) and are designed to assess how well the drug works, as well as to continue phase I safety assessments in a larger group of volunteers and patients.

Phase III studies are randomized controlled multicentre trials on large patient groups (300–3000 or more depending upon the disease/medical condition studied) and are aimed at being the definitive assessment of how effective the drug is, in comparison with current 'gold standard' treatment.

Marketing will be closely involved in the identification of the gold standard, through its own research. It is common practice that certain phase III trials will continue while the regulatory submission is pending at the appropriate regulatory agency. This allows patients to continue to receive possibly life-saving drugs until the drug can be obtained by purchase. Other reasons for performing trials at this stage include attempts by the sponsor at 'label expansion' (to show the drug works for additional types of patients/diseases beyond the original use for which the drug would have been approved for marketing), to obtain additional safety data or to support marketing claims for the drug.

Phase IV studies are done in a wider population after launch to determine if a drug or treatment is safe over time or to see if a treatment or medication can be used in other circumstances. Phase IV clinical trials are done after a drug has gone through phases I, II and III, has been approved by the regulator and is on the market.

Phase IV is one of the fastest-growing areas of clinical research today, at an annual growth rate of 23%. A changing regulatory environment, growing concerns about the safety of new medicines and various uses for large-scale, real-world data on marketed drugs' safety and efficacy are primary drivers of the growth seen in the phase IV research environment. Postmarketing research is an important element of commercialization that enables companies to expand existing markets, enter new markets, develop and deliver messaging that directly compares their products with the competition. Additionally, payer groups and regulators are both demanding more postmarketing data from drug companies. There is a particular interest in postmarketing surveillance studies, with the focus on safety.

Advantages of phase IV research include the development of data in particular patient populations, enhanced relationship with customers and development of advocacy among healthcare providers and patients. These studies help to open new communication channels with healthcare providers and to create awareness among patients. Phase IV data can also be valuable in the preparation of a health economics and health technology assessment (HTA) dossier, to demonstrate cost-effectiveness.

Identifying the market

At the stage when it appears that the drug is likely to be approved for marketing, the product manager performs market research to identify the characteristics of the market. The therapeutic areas into which the new product will enter are fully assessed, using data from standard sources to which the company subscribes. These data are generally historic and do not indicate what could happen nor do they contain much interpretation. The product manager must begin to construct a story to describe the market, its dynamics, key elements and potential. This is the time to generate extensive hypotheses regarding the market and its potential. Although these hypotheses can be tested, they are not extensively validated. Therefore the level of confidence in the data generated at this stage would not normally enable the marketer to generate a reliable plan for entry to the market but will start to indicate what needs to be done to generate more qualitative and quantitative data.

When the product label is further developed and tested, further **market research**, using **focus groups** (*a form of qualitative research in which a group of people are asked about their perceptions, opinions, beliefs and attitudes towards a new concept and the reasons for current behaviour*) is instituted. This might be to ask a group of physicians to examine their current prescribing practice and rationale for this behaviour. These data are extensively validated with more qualitative research. The identification of the target audiences for the new medicines is critical by this stage.

Traditionally, the pharmaceutical industry has viewed each physician customer in terms of his/her current prescribing patterns (market share for a given product) and potential market value. Each company uses basically the same data inputs and metrics, so tactical implementation across the industry is similar from company to company.

The product

Features, attributes, benefits, limitations

A product manager is assigned a product before its launch and is expected to develop a marketing plan for the product that will include the development of information about the existing market and a full understanding of the product's characteristics. This begins with **Features**, such as the specific mechanism of action, the molecular form, the tablet shape or colour. Closely aligned to this are the product **Attributes**, usually concrete things that reside in the product including how it functions. These are characteristics by which a product can be identified and differentiated. For example, these can include the speed of onset of action, absence of common side effects, such as drowsiness, or a once-per-day therapy rather than multiple doses. Then come the **Benefits** of the new product. Benefits are intrinsic to the customer and are usually abstract. A product attribute expressed in terms of what the doctor or patient gets from the product rather than its physical characteristics or features. A once-per-day therapy can lessen the intrusion of medicine-taking on patient's lives. Lack of drowsiness means the patient complies with the need to take the medicine for the duration of the illness and is able to function effectively during their working day. The benefits may also accrue to the physician as patient compliance indicates that the patient is feeling well, thanks to the actions of the doctor. It is critically important for the pharmaceutical marketer to maintain balance in promotional material. The **Limitations** of the product, where they could lead to the medicine being given to a patient for whose condition the medicine is not specifically indicated, must be clearly indicated in all materials and discussions with the doctor. The potential risk of adverse reactions of a medicine must also be clearly addressed in marketing interactions with medical professionals. Some markets encourage feedback from the treating physician on adverse reactions, such as the UK Yellow Card system.

The analysis of the product in this way enables the marketer to produce a benefit ladder, beginning with the product features and attributes, and moving to the various benefits from the point of view of the customer. Emotional benefits for the customer in terms of how they will feel by introducing the right patient to the right treatment are at the top of the ladder. It is also important for the product manager to construct a benefit ladder for competitive products in order to differentiate.

Armed with these data and the limited quantitative data, the product manager defines the market, identifies the target audience and their behaviour patterns in prescribing. Assessments are made of what must be done to effect a change of behaviour and the prescription of the new medicine once launched. A key classification of a target physician is his or her position in the **Adoption** Pattern of innovative new products. There are three broad classifications generally used:

- **Early adopters/innovators**: those who normally are quick to use a new product when it is available.
- **Majority**: most fall into this category. There are the **early majority** and the **late majority**, defined by their relative speed of adoption. Some are already satisfied and have no need for a new product. Some wait for others to try first, preferring to wait until unforeseen problems arise and are resolved. Improved products (innovative therapies) may move this group to prescribe earlier.
- **Laggards/conservatives**: this group is the slowest adopter, invariably waiting for others to gain the early experience. They wait for something compelling to occur, such as additional evidence to support the new product, or a new indication for which they do not currently have a suitable treatment.

Assessing the competition

It is critical for a product marketer to understand the competition and learn how to outmanoeuvre them. Market research is the starting point. A complete analysis of the competitive market through product sales, investment levels and resource allocation helps the marketer to develop the marketing plan for their own product. But it is important to understand the reason for these behaviours and critically evaluate their importance and success.

A comprehensive review of competitor's activities and rationale for them is also necessary. Tools are available to facilitate this in the United States, for example, PhRMA (the industry association) publishes a *New Medicines Database* that tracks potential new medicines in various stages of development. The database includes medicines currently in clinical trials or at the US Food & Drug Administration (FDA) for evaluation (PhRMA). However, it is not just a desk-bound exercise for a group of bright young marketers. Hypotheses, thus formed, must be tested against the customer perception of them.

The appearance of promotional aids, such as 'detail aids', printed glossies containing key messages, desktop branded reminder items (e.g., calendars) or 'door openers' (pens, stick-it pads, etc.) to get past the 'dragon on the door' (receptionist), is common, but do they work? In the pharmaceutical industry, for many years, marketing has been a little like the arms war. Rep numbers are doubled or tripled because that is what the competition is doing. Identical looking detail pieces, clinical study papers wrapped in a shiny folder with the key promotional messages and product label printed on it appear from all competitors. Regulations known as 'medical-legal control' are in place, internally and at a national level, to ensure that promotional messages are accurately stated, balanced and backed by well-referenced evidence, such as clinical trial data and the approved product label.

Are promotional activities being focussed on key leverage points and appropriate behavioural objectives? Before embracing what seems to be a good idea from the competition, the marketer needs to understand how this is perceived by the customer. New qualitative research needs to be conducted to gain this insight. One of the principal aims of successful marketing is to differentiate one product from another. It would therefore seem to be counterintuitive for an assessment of competitor behaviour to conclude that copying the idea of a competitor is somehow going to automatically enable you to outcompete them. Much of traditional pharmaceutical marketing implementation has been outsourced to agencies. These organizations are briefed about the product, the market into which it will enter and the key therapeutic messages the company wishes to convey. The companies retain the preparation and maintenance of the marketing plan and, in general, leave the creative, behavioural side of the preparation to the agency. It is not therefore surprising that a formulaic approach to marketing delivery has been the norm.

A classic example of this effect came in the 1990s, with direct to consumer (DTC) advertising. This form of direct marketing, in the printed media, television and radio, is legally permitted in only a few countries, such as the United States and New Zealand. Its original conception, for the first time, was to talk directly to patients about the sorts of medication that they should request from their physician. Anyone watching breakfast television in the United States will be bombarded with attractive messages about what you could feel like if you take a particular medicine. These messages always contain a balance about contraindications and possible adverse reactions. Patients are encouraged to consult their physician. This concept was original and seems to have been effective in a number of cases (Kaiser Family Foundation, 2001), with increased sales volumes. Then, practically every major company jumped on the bandwagon and competed for prime time slots and the most attractive actors to play the role of patient. The appearance of these messages is practically identical and one washes over another. Probably the only people to pay them much attention, because of the volume and sameness, are the pharmaceutical marketers and the advertising agencies that are competing for the business. As for the physicians, little attention was paid to their reaction to this visual-media–informed patient.

In assessing how successful DTC has been, early data from the United States (Kaiser Family Foundation, 2001) observed, on average, that a 10% increase in DTC advertising of drugs within a therapeutic drug class resulted in a 1% increase in sales of the drugs in that class. Applying this result to the 25 largest drug classes in 2000, the study found that every $1 the pharmaceutical industry spent on DTC advertising in that year yielded an additional $4.20 in drug sales. DTC advertising was responsible for 12% of the increase in prescription drugs sales, or an additional $2.6 billion, in 2000. DTC advertising did not appear to affect the relative market share of individual drugs within their drug class. In the decade to 2005 in the United States, spending on DTC practically tripled to around $4.2 billion (Donohue et al., 2007). This level of expenditure and impact on prescriptions has caused a great deal of controversy driven by traditional industry critics. However, some benefits have accrued, including the increased interaction between physicians and patients. In surveys, more than half of physicians agree that DTC educates patients about diseases and treatments. Many physicians, however, believe that DTC encourages patients to make unwarranted requests for medication.

From a marketing point of view, new concepts like DTC can prove helpful. Sales increase and patients become a new and legitimate customer. The cost of entry, particularly in financially difficult times, can be prohibitive for all but a few key players. For those who are in this group, it becomes imperative that they stay there, as it is still a viable though costly segment. The naysayers are successfully containing DTC to the United States and New Zealand. The clarion calls for a moratorium and greater FDA regulation have still been avoided by those who market in this way. Will the investment in this type of marketing continue to pass the test of cost-effectiveness and revenue opportunity? Competitive marketing demands a continuous critical assessment of all expenditure according to rigorous ROI (return on investment) criteria.

DTC advertising expenditure decreased by more than 20% from 2007 to 2009. Economic pressures and the global financial meltdown resulted in a tighter budgetary situation for the pharmaceutical industry. These pressures have been strongly affected by rapidly disappearing blockbuster drugs, generic competition and decreasing R&D productivity.

e-Marketing

e-Marketing is a process, using the Internet and other electronic media, of marketing a brand or concept by directly connecting to the businesses of customers.

In pharmaceuticals, electronic marketing has been experimented with since the late 1990s. As a branch of DTC, it has been limited to only a couple of markets, the United States and New Zealand. Some companies have created websites for physician-only access with some success, in terms of usage, but it is difficult to assess in terms of product uptake. Electronic detailing of physicians, using digital technology—the Internet and video conferencing— has been used in some markets for a number of years.

There are two types of e-detailing: interactive (virtual) and video. Some physicians find this type of interaction convenient, but the uptake has not been rapid or widespread, nor has its impact been accurately measured in terms of utility.

While e-Marketing has promise and theoretically great reach, the pharmaceutical industry in general has done little more than dabble in it. It is estimated to occupy around 1%–3% of DTC budgets.

CME

CME is a long-established means for medical professionals to maintain and update competence and learn about new and developing areas of their field, such as therapeutic advances. These activities may take place as live events, written publications, online programmes, audio, video or other electronic media (Accreditation Council for Continuing Medical Education). Content for these programmes is developed, reviewed and delivered by a faculty who are experts in their individual clinical areas.

Funding of these programmes has been largely provided by the pharmaceutical industry, often through Medical Education and Communications Companies or MECCs. A number of large pharmaceutical companies have withdrawn from using these sorts of third-party agencies in the United States, due to the controversy concerning their objectivity. The Swedish health system puts a cap of 50% on the level of contribution to costs of the pharmaceutical industry.

This type of activity is beneficial to the medical community and provides, if only through networking, an opportunity to interact with the physicians. The regulation of content of these programmes is tight and generally well controlled, but a strong voice of discontent about the involvement of the industry continues to be sounded. The fact is that a key stakeholder in the medical decision-making process wants and benefits from these programmes, as long as they are balanced, approved and helpful. If the pharmaceutical industry wants to continue with the funding and involvement, then it should be seen as a legitimate part of the marketing template.

Key opinion leaders

Key opinion leaders (KOLs), or 'thought leaders', are respected individuals in a particular therapeutic area, such as prominent medical school faculty, who influence physicians through their professional status. Pharmaceutical companies generally engage KOLs early in the drug development process to provide advocacy and key marketing feedback. These individuals are identified by a number of means, reputation, citations, peer review and even social network analysis.

Pharmaceutical companies will work with KOLs from the early stage of drug development. The goal is to gain early input from these experts into the likely success and acceptability of these new compounds in the future market. Marketing personnel and the company's medical function work closely on identifying the best KOLs for each stage of drug development. The KOL has a network that, it is hoped, will also get to know about a new product and its advantages early in the launch phase. The KOL can perform a number of roles, in scientific development, as a member of the product advisory board and an advisor on specific aspects of the product positioning.

The marketing manager is charged with maintaining and coordinating the company's relationship with the KOL. Special care is taken by the company of the level of payment given to a KOL, and all payments must be declared to the medical association that regulates the individual, whatever the country of origin. KOLs can be divided into different categories. *Global*, *national* and *local* categorizations are applied, depending on their level of influence. Relationships between the company and a particular opinion leader can continue throughout the life cycle of a medicine, or product franchise.

Market access

Once a pharmaceutical product has demonstrated efficacy and safety within clinical trials, the manufacturer has the task of bringing their product to a regulator that will assess the validity of data generated from these trials, such as efficacy, safety and pharmaceutical quality. If the pharmaceutical product is of an acceptable standard, then the manufacturer will receive market authorization (MAu) from the regulator. Where MAu issued by a regulator was usually enough to ensure access to patients in the past, today the hurdles to reach the patient with a new treatment are much higher.

MA is the process of ensuring that a pharmaceutical product that has achieved MAu is available to patients who would benefit in as many markets as is feasible, in an expeditious and sustained manner. MA as an integrated discipline has evolved as a result of rising healthcare costs, the management of risk and uncertainty and the need to protect and incentivize innovation. Today, MA activities fall into three converging disciplines:
- HTA
- Pricing and reimbursement
- Formulary inclusion.

These areas are of importance not only to pharmaceutical manufacturers but to payers (private health insurers, statutory health insurers, governmental health systems), providers (hospitals, healthcare trusts, accountable care organizations, integrated delivery networks, etc.), buyers (healthcare professionals) and consumers (patients).

Payers' perspective

The payers are the entities that reimburse/finance the cost of healthcare. When payers fund medicine, they fund the production of health. Their means of procuring the production of health is through the purchase of health services and medicines. The health service's or medicine's value depends on the individual perspective of the payer regarding the unmet medical needs of the market it serves and how these proposed solutions address that need. Their perspective on value will reflect the pain points and processes of the healthcare continuum of that market. Moreover, the evidence generated from clinical trials, the epidemiology and assessment of cost-effectiveness is highly important.

Payers in different markets will have different requirements for evidence of a product. This will be centred around clinical and economic value, as a payer's focus will be on assessing the value for money of a product for human health.

The steady rise of pharmaceutical expenditure and its consequence on budgets of public payers has been a growing concern for policy makers and is therefore the target of a number of cost containment measures assisted by the creation of HTA bodies. (International Pricing and Reimbursement Schemes 2015).

Pricing

Balancing the payers' objective to minimize their budget exposure while trying to extract as much as possible from the perceived value of a product is the key challenge when pricing a new pharmaceutical product. There are a number of pricing methods such as cost-based pricing (not used for a pharmaceutical product but frequently used for medical devices), value-based pricing (VBP), competition-based pricing (often used in conjunction with VBP), skimming pricing and external reference pricing (ERP). VBP and ERP are of growing relevance in today's pharmaceutical MA process.

Value and value-based pricing

The idea behind VBP is that the price of goods should reflect the value to the buyer rather than reflect the cost needed to make the product. Although this seems simple, there is no widely accepted definition with respect to pharmaceuticals. Decision-makers will generally define the health effect as the most important benefit and, therefore, factor of any assessment of value with regards to a medicine.

Towse and Barnsley described other factors that can be recognized by decision-makers when determining value (Towse & Barnsley, 2013):

- The 'value' of the health gain to society may be higher or lower depending on the patient receiving it. For example, in the UK National Institute for Health and Care Excellence (NICE) attributes a specific value weight when appraising end-of-life treatments. Additionally, orphan diseases (rare diseases) are also treated differently across health systems in that there is a willingness to pay for higher prices with lower evidence standards of therapeutic added value.
- There may be elements of benefit to the patient that are not linked to an improvement in health but perhaps to quality of life.
- Beyond the value delivered to patients and a healthcare system, there may be other costs and benefits that translate to societal impact. This could include unrelated medical costs, productivity effects and benefits experienced by the patient's family.
- Innovative attributes of a medicine may be considered to have value independent of the health gain generated.

There are of course many other factors that are taken into account when considering the value of a medicine. As each stakeholder will have their own objectives to achieve, the ability of the medicine in question to deliver on these objectives will provide the stakeholder with their own perspective of value (Fig. 21.3).

The **pharmaceutical** value proposition (Towse and Barnsley, 2013) 'starts with the raising of capital to fund R&D, concluding with the marketing and resulting sale of the products. In essence, it is about making innovative medicines that command a premium price'.

The **payer's** value system begins with raising revenue, through taxation or patient contribution. The value created for patients and other stakeholders is by managing administration and provision of healthcare. For the payer, the goal is to have a cost-effective health system and to enhance its reputation with its customers, or voters in the case of governments. It aims to minimize its costs and keep people well.

The **provider**, in this case the physician, wants to provide high quality of care, economically and for as long as necessary. This stakeholder values an assessment of the health of a given population and to know what measures can be taken to manage and prevent illness.

The convergence of these three stakeholders' value systems, as conveyed in a PwC Report, is as follows (PricewaterhouseCoopers, 2009). 'The value healthcare **payers** generate depends on the policies and practices of the providers used', whereas **providers** generate value based on the revenues from payers and drugs that pharmaceutical companies provide. As for the pharmaceutical company,

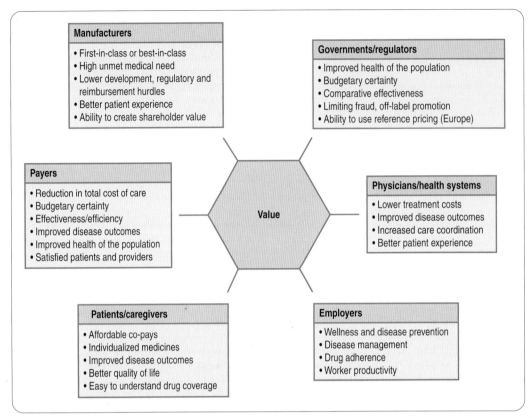

Fig. 21.3 Stakeholder values. (From Licking, E., & Garfield, S. (2016). A road map to strategic drug pricing. *In Vivo*, *34*, 3.)

the value it provides is dependent on access to the patients who depend on the payers and physicians. In this scenario, each of the partners is by definition dependent on the others. An antagonistic relationship between these parties is therefore counterproductive and can result in each of the stakeholders failing to achieve their goals. Applying VBP to a manufacturer's new medicine requires well-designed market research with payers, physicians and patients. By engaging with these stakeholders, a manufacturer can link the proposed price and/or approval of a pharmaceutical to the perceived value of its product and understand the hurdles that may have to be overcome.

Pharmacoeconomic analysis helps question cost-effectiveness and the savings that would be applied to the current management of a particular disease. By attaining this information, a manufacturer will be able to set an acceptable premium price, but this is a difficult task due to the varying practices of healthcare across the world. The cost of care can vary from payer and healthcare provider, making a unified pricing approach difficult.

The UK uses quality adjusted life years (QALYs) as the model of assessing the value of a medicine. From a

manufacturer's point of view, the main drawback will be the fact that a QALY will vary based on each payer due to differences in epidemiology, medical practice, cost of services and ways of accounting for these costs (Delagneau, 2018).

Another conundrum for the pharmaceutical industry is the acceptance from the stakeholders of their definition of innovation. Where a patient, previously uncontrolled on one statin, for example, may be well controlled by a later entry from the same class, the payer may not accept this as innovative. They are unwilling to accept the fact that some patients may prefer the newer medicine if it means paying a premium to obtain it. With the aid of HTA, the payer may use statistical data to 'disprove' the cost-effectiveness of the new statin and block its reimbursement. The pharmaceutical company will find it difficult to recoup the cost of R&D associated with bringing the drug to the market. The PwC Report (Pricewaterhouse Coopers, 2009) addresses this problem by suggesting that the industry should start to talk to the key stakeholders, payers, providers and patients during phase II of the development process. It is at this stage, they suggest, that pricing plans should start to be tested with stakeholders, rather than waiting until well into phase III/launch. It is possible to do this, but the real test of whether a medicine is a real advance comes in the larger patient pool after launch. Postmarketing follow-up of patients and phase IV research can help to give all stakeholders reassurance about the value added by a new medicine. It was in the 1990s, after the launch of simvastatin, that the 6-year-long 4S study (Scandinavian Simvastatin Survival Study Group, 1994) showed that treatment with this statin significantly reduced the risk of morbidity and mortality in at-risk groups, thus fundamentally changing an important aspect of medical practice. At phase II, it would have been difficult to predict this. With today's HTA intervention, it is difficult to see if the product would have been recommended at all for use in treatment.

External reference pricing

In the European Union (EU), each country is free to implement its own national pricing and reimbursement policies, which has resulted in a wide variety of pharmaceutical pricing regulations.

The financial crisis in 2008 resulted in a number of budget cuts, and of those cuts healthcare spending became a major target. Price reductions, changes in co-payments, in the VAT (value added tax) rates on medicines and in the distribution margins were among the most common measures (Vogler et al., 2011). Many EU member states reacted by using ERP as a cost containment tool for purchasing purposes. ERP is used regularly by several countries including Australia, Brazil, Canada, Japan, Jordan, South Africa and Turkey, which regularly refer to drug prices set by EU member states in order to derive their own.

In Europe, the UK and Sweden do not apply ERP and have instead decided to adopt VBP instead. Countries across the world use ERP for different purposes and refer to different countries (Table 21.1).

Despite its success in providing cost containment, there are a number of limitations to ERP as a pricing methodology. The first is that a referenced price was initially set to suit the characteristics of the healthcare system of that market, as well as the health needs, income and healthcare costs. Additionally, the implementation of ERP is limited, as there is a lack of transparency of drug prices set in individual markets, therefore providing a reliance on back calculations to infer a reference ex-factory price (Remuzat et al., 2015). ERP has therefore become a concern for manufacturers in their implementation of launch sequence strategies. The use of ERP in pricing negotiations has occasionally resulted in acrimonious relations between the two sides, one choosing to go with the lowest common denominator price, and the Pharma company delaying entry into the market in question as the price proposed by the buyer is unacceptable. The resultant delay in access for the patient of an advanced treatment can have adverse consequences.

Health technology assessors' perspective

HTA is a multidisciplinary field that assesses the impact of a health technology (medicines and medical devices) in a healthcare setting. Following MAu, the HTA body determines the cost-effectiveness of the medicine in question, this being the payer's primary requirement for reimbursement. The impact of a new medicine is not restricted to clinical and economic ramifications but also has organizational, social, legal and ethical consequences, all of which are assessed by an HTA body. HTA mainly aims to inform policy and clinical decision-making and can be defined as 'a systematic evaluation of the properties and effects of a medicine, addressing the direct and intended effects

Table 21.1 Use of external reference pricing in an example set of countries (Remuzat et al., 2015; Toumi, 2017)

Country	Use
Germany & Poland	Used as additional information during pricing negotiation of reimbursed medicines
Italy	To obtain additional information during price negotiation. Previously used as the primary method for assessment of new drugs
Spain	To determine the price for which there is no alternative available on the Spanish market
Belgium	To provide supporting detail for a pricing decision but also as a criterion for price cuts
Finland	Used as one criterion when approving reasonable wholesale price
Japan	To adjust price when the local price diverges significantly from the concurrent price levels in France, Germany, the UK and the United States
Australia	Used as one of several pricing methods to determine the selling price for pharmaceuticals listed under the Pharmaceutical Benefits Scheme, referencing the UK and New Zealand

of this technology as well as its indirect and unintended effects' (Oortwijn et al., 2017).

Health authorities across the world, including Western markets, are facing increasing concerns in allocating budget to the reimbursement of new premium-priced medicines (Malmström et al., 2013). Changing demographics, the rise of chronic diseases, population segmentation owing to the growing field of pharmacogenomics, the launch of high-priced medicines and increased patient expectations all act as compounding pressures for a health authority (Godman et al., 2015; WHO, 2015).

HTA's role in MA has thus become a crucial hurdle in the decision-making process of the introduction of a new medicine into the existing continuum of care.

Europe has seen an increase in reliance upon HTAs. The array of methodologies used by HTAs is adapted to the needs and standard practices of a particular health system. Each country has its own decision-making process and priorities, therefore HTA processes vary between markets. There are efforts, however, to streamline the process through cooperation like EUnetHTA (European network for Health Technology Assessment) and the adaptive pathways scheme of the European Medicines Agency (EMA).

HTA processes in differing markets

United Kingdom. Founded as a special health authority in 1999, NICE provides national guidance on the promotion of good health and the prevention and treatment of ill health (ISPOR Global Health Care Systems Road Map, 2008). Through its HTA processes, it provides national guidance on health technologies, as well as providing standards for clinical practice through its clinical guideline development processes (Cylus et al., 2015). It has been responsible for single and multiple technology appraisals making the National Health Service (NHS) aware of new medicines, as well as providing them with recommendations on the allocation of its budget.

Wales and Scotland each have their own advisory organizations that inform about cost-effectiveness. These include the AWMSG (All Wales Medicines Strategy Group) that has agreed to review all new medicines not assessed by NICE since 2009 and the SMC (Scottish Medicines Consortium) that takes precedence over NICE recommendations for NHS boards in Scotland.

The pharmacoeconomic value is assessed by NICE using incremental cost-effectiveness ratios (ICERs), expressed as a cost per QALY, where recommendations are based upon crossing thresholds of £20,000 and £30,000 per QALY. If the medicine has an ICER of less than £20,000/QALY, then the technology is deemed to be cost-effective. An ICER of between £20,000 and £30,000 per QALY would indicate that the medicine would be recommended for reimbursement

conditional upon additional factors. A stronger case will be needed for a therapy that exceeds £30,000/QALY, such as an end-of-life treatment.

France. The main HTA organization in France is the HAS (Haute Autorite de Santé). It was established by the French government in 2004 and was officially based on the legislations of the government and the SHI (Statutory Health Insurance) (Chevreul et al., 2015). Within the HAS, the Transparency Commission (*Commission de la Transparence*) is responsible for evaluating drugs.

Each of these departments assesses the product's medical benefit or absolute therapeutic value into a medical value score, which is called the SMR (Service medical Rendu). The SMR is categorized on a five-level scale: *major, important, moderate, low* or *insufficient*. Each level acts as a justification of a reimbursement rate from 0% to 100%. *Major* or *important* SMRs can lead to a 65% SHI coverage or 100% for irreplaceable medicines for serious and disabling conditions (Toumi, 2017). *Moderate* or *weak* allows for 30% coverage, and *insufficient* forbids coverage.

The product's relative medical benefit is then compared to similar options, resulting in a medical added value called the ASMR (*Amelioration du Service Medical Rendu*). It is a five-level scale ranging from ASMR I for *major improvement* or *life-saving drug* to ASMR V for *no improvement*.

Another HAS commission called the CEESP (*Commission d'Evaluation Economique et de Santé Publique*) evaluates the cost-effectiveness of the intervention and determines the nature of implementation in the healthcare system such as coverage conditions of patients or medical practices (Chevreul et al., 2015). The results of this evaluation and the uncertainty that surrounds them are presented as a recommendation to UNCAM (*Union Nationale des Caisses d'Assurance Maladie*), which provides the Ministry of Health with a final recommendation about inclusion.

Germany. In Germany, the organizations that are involved in the assessment of a medicine are the IQWiG (Institute for quality and efficiency in Health Care) and the G-BA (Federal Joint Committee) for assessment and appraisal, respectively (Busse & Blümel, 2014).

The G-BA is a multidisciplinary committee that is responsible for ensuring efficiency in the healthcare system by controlling coverage and providing limitations in prescribing. They assess new medicines and evaluate new treatment methods in order to classify them into reference pricing groups that are then presented to the Federal Ministry of Health for approval. The G-BA makes the final decision publicly available. HTAs are typically conducted by IQWiG (Kahveci et al., 2018).

Founded in 2004, IQWiG's responsibility is to assess medical efficiency, quality and effectiveness. HTA reports are prepared by IQWiG at the request of the G-BA assessing cost–benefit ratios of medicines in Germany. The criteria used in their assessment are related to patient outcomes such as quality of life, mortality and morbidity. IQWiG also has an informal collaboration with NICE and HAS, providing bilateral sharing of basic information and scientific evidence (Kahveci et al., 2018).

United States. The United States is one of the few countries in the world that does not have price controls on prescription drugs. It is the largest pharmaceutical market in the world, accounting for over 30% of worldwide consumption of pharmaceutical products (Wee, 2017). Gaining access to patients in the United States is a vastly complicated task that requires a refined strategy on the manufacturer's side. Unlike the UK, there is no universal coverage or heavy reliance on formal HTA. The financing of healthcare in the United States is fragmented and distributed across a variety of competing private entities. Coverage is distributed either through private insurance or through the government-sponsored programmes, Medicare and Medicaid. Medicare covers patients who are over 65 years of age, and Medicaid covers the poor and disabled, though the extent of coverage varies from state to state.

In 2014, 283.2 million people in the United States, 89.6% of the US population, had some type of health insurance, with 66% of workers covered by a private health insurance plan. Among the insured, 36.5% of the population received coverage through the US government through Medicare (50.5 million), Medicaid (61.65 million) and/or Veterans Administration or other military care (14.14 million) (people may be covered by more than one government plan). In 2014, nearly 32.9 million people in the United States had no health insurance (Wee, 2017).

Following the introduction of the Affordable Care Act in 2010, value-based healthcare has grown in importance. Among the wide variety of healthcare providers in the United States are Accountable Care Organizations that have grown in prominence, taking on risk that will either result in penalties should certain metrics not be achieved or shared savings made by streamlining the delivery of healthcare. Many reforms have been suggested as a means to tackle drug pricing in the United States. One of these reforms is to introduce ERP, known in the United States as International Price Indexing (IPI). Although the implementation of IPI looks less likely due to overwhelming criticism, there is still growing pressure for price controls and price transparency.

Due to the fragmented nature of healthcare coverage in the United States, HTA has been decentralized where adoption, coverage and reimbursement of health technologies are left to local payers. The government research organization, AHRQ (Agency for Healthcare Research and Quality), performs technology assessments for the Centers for Medicare and Medicaid Services (CMS) using comparative effectiveness research. These assessments, usually done in association with a university, are used by CMS to inform its national coverage decisions for the Medicare programme, as well as provide information to Medicare carriers.

Formulary decisions are influenced by a variety of stakeholders including pharmacy benefit managers (PBMs), CMS and individual health plans, where all use their own tools to regulate patient access to medicines. US payers have reported that they have minimal ability to negotiate prices for high-impact drugs and as a result express an interest in utilizing VBP methodologies (Informa, 2019).

The Institute for Clinical and Economic Review is an independent nonprofit US-based organization that assesses the cost-effectiveness of health technologies. The growing demand for VBP has caused it to rise to prominence as it continues to provide publicly available reports on new treatments. Using similar techniques to NICE, the institute has published assessments on several treatments, but payer incorporation of such reports into the decision-making process has its drawbacks. These include the fact that the institute is not regulated, and that the publication of these reports take time; however, its advent has influenced some manufacturers to form a collaboration in developing cost-effective pricing strategies for novel treatments (Informa, 2019).

Value in US healthcare is of concern to decision-makers, but its use is not explicit. The move towards value-based care means that manufacturers must demonstrate the value of their health technologies to payers. This is now increasingly occurring by differentiating their product using real-world evidence to back up claims of not only efficacy but also effectiveness.

Industry perspective

As with all stakeholders involved with the launch of new health technologies, it is in the interest of the manufacturer to gain access to patients quickly and in a sustained manner. Getting a pharmaceutical product to the point of MAu will have included many hurdles along the way, with preclinical and clinical costs that are substantial. Development of a medicinal product is a high-risk business marked by substantial financial risks, with expenditures incurred for many development projects that fall along the development pathway.

There have been a number of studies estimating the cost of bringing a drug to market, describing clinical success rates ranging from 21% in the early 2000s to approximately 12% in 2012 (DiMasi et al., 2003, 2016). Where the average cost incurred by a pharmaceutical manufacturer was estimated by DiMasi et al. to be $802 million in the early 2000s. A new study by the same group has suggested that the cost may now be $2.5 billion (DiMasi et al., 2016). Although this number has been regarded as controversial, even a cost of $1 to $2 billion is a substantial investment. It takes on average 10 years to develop a new medicine from initial discovery to launch. The incentive of the pharmaceutical manufacturers to gain an ROI is thus of paramount importance.

Securing revenues to recover the cost of development is not the only aim. A healthy revenue stream will allow a company to reinvest profits into R&D, thereby safeguarding the cost of innovation, allowing them to take the risky journey all over again.

Simply speaking, the revenue comes from looking at the addressable patient population that can be treated by this new agent, multiplied by the price per unit of that agent. There are therefore two main points for the pharmaceutical industry when launching a new product. These include:

- Maximizing patient access internationally
- Setting a price that will be reimbursed by each market.

These two objectives have their own hurdles of which regulators, HTA and formulary inclusion are members, but at the end of the day, it is whether a payer is convinced that this product is worth paying for. The marketing team, health economic analysts, financial function and global considerations are all part of the pricing plan. Cost-effectiveness analyses and calculations of benefit to the market are all factored into the equation. When a global strategy is proposed, market research is conducted along with pricing sensitivity analyses. At a time of budget constraints and cost containment strategies, it is important that a payer gets value for money. Thus it is in the manufacturer's best interests to limit the risk and uncertainty that these payers must bear.

Risk and uncertainty

Regulators assess a manufacturer's claims for their product that has undergone rigorous testing over several years, is efficacious, safe for human use and of high pharmaceutical quality.

In contrast, payers are entities that finance or reimburse the cost of health products and services. Where a regulator will be more concerned with benefit/risk ratios, payers will be more concerned with benefit/cost. Payers will need to assess the validity of clinical trial data for a new technology and determine whether the findings are in line with the real-life treatment pathways occurring in the market

in which they operate and whether it will be cost-effective for that particular healthcare system. HTA bodies enable the payer to determine the added value of the new medicine and the impact of its introduction to the system on budget.

The clinical trial data that are provided by a manufacturer to a regulator demonstrate efficacy and safety under controlled conditions in a limited population that are subject to exclusion criteria in order to achieve statistical significance. Where this type of data is a good indicator of the drug's initial value, its effects may not necessarily translate into a real-world setting. Patients in the real-world may be concurrently treated for a number of conditions, have a different pharmacogenomic profile to those assessed in the clinical trial and be treated under a different continuum of care. The payer works in a real-world setting and is therefore more interested in efficacy under normal conditions otherwise known as *effectiveness*.

In the absence of data that would prove a medicine's effectiveness in the real world, payers are forced to bear uncertainty around a new product's performance. Uncertainty in this context is the ignorance of consequences, extent of magnitude of circumstances, conditions or events that this new product may create when introduced into the healthcare system (Toumi, 2017). *Risk*, however, is the set of known outcomes of use of the new product and the probability that those outcomes will occur. Risk then can be accounted for unlike *uncertainty*, which is a strong source of fear, potentially leading to the rejection of product coverage or approval. The identification and quantification of risks, however, can be addressed in risk mitigation plans.

Healthcare is fraught with risk and uncertainty, and payers have generally accepted them. Where risk is manageable, uncertainty provides the greater level of discomfort, as it does not only relate to the product's potential effect on the patient, but its potential ineffectiveness among different cohorts of patients. At a time when payers are executing cost containment measures, they need the assurance that what they are paying for provides value for money. Effectiveness assesses whether an intervention does more good than harm when provided under usual circumstances of healthcare practice. Efficiency measures the effect of an intervention in relation to the resources it consumes ('Is it worth it?') (Cochrane, 1972). How efficacy in clinical trials translates into effectiveness, and furthermore into efficiency, and budget impact are the issues that payers must deal with (Toumi, 2017).

The populations assessed in clinical trials may not reflect the characteristics of the population that a payer is responsible for. Moreover, the clinical measures may not reflect the standards of care within a given market, providing the payer with another level of uncertainty.

Some of the clinical trial-related uncertainties are as follows:

- Population based
  - Geographic area
  - Inclusion/exclusion criteria
  - Compliance
- Outcome measures
  - Use of surrogate outcomes
  - Use of poorly or nonvalidated measures
  - Use of outcome measures not relevant to the disease being tested
- Study design
  - Small number of patients
  - Open label versus blind design
  - Blinding maintenance
  - Inappropriate study duration

- Choice of comparator drug
  - Difference between guidelines and clinical practice
  - Off-label usage
  - Differences in clinical practice between countries

Today, manufacturers are encouraged to engage with payers and HTAs earlier in the development cycle in order to determine the design of a phase III clinical trial that would satisfy both stakeholders, addressing any potential uncertainties at an earlier stage. The manufacturer must know the differences in treatment guidelines and population segmentation for each market it intends for product launch. Table 21.2 lists a number of examples relating to different types of uncertainty.

There are many aspects to consider when designing a clinical trial and HTA bodies will have different requirements for what they consider to be cost effective. It is the

Table 21.2 List of example uncertainties related to clinical trials submitted by a manufacturer to an HTA body

Drug and indication	HTA body & date	Comments
Population-related uncertainties		
Ivacaftor: cystic fibrosis	G-BA: 7 February 2013	Study submitted does not include severe patients
Pivmecillinam: urinary tract infection (UTI)	HAS: 3 April 2013	Study results performed in Nordic countries cannot be transposed to clinical practice in France, due to current resistance of *Escherichia coli* to pivmecillinam in France, which is the main germ encountered in community-acquired UTI
Vinfluinine: transitional cell carcinoma of the urothelial tract	NICE: January 2013	Uncertainty regarding the effectiveness for the licensed population in the UK due to differences in the characteristics and treatment pathways in the trial vs UK clinical practice: The study population was younger and fitter and had better renal function than the general UK patients with advanced or metastatic transitional cell carcinoma of the urothelial tract. The study excluded patients who had had adjuvant or neoadjuvant chemotherapy, even though in UK practice, many patients in the UK who are eligible to receive the second-line palliative chemotherapy will already have received two lines of treatment
Comparator-related uncertainties		
Axitinib: renal cell carcinoma	HAS: 9 January 2013	No comparative data vs alternative treatments having MAu after failure to sunitinib
Pivmecillinam: axial spondyloarthritis	HAS: 3 April 2013	No study compared pivmecillinam to antibiotics currently used in France to treat community-acquired UTIs (the company submitted one study vs active comparator [sulfamethazol] and one study vs placebo)
Linagliptin: type 2 diabetes mellitus	G-BA: 21 February 2013	Dual therapy: one potentially relevant direct comparative study, BUT issue in the study design as two different treatment strategies were compared: one strategy without a specific target level for blood glucose for linagliptin vs another strategy with a specific target for blood glucose for glimepiride (glimepiride dose up-titrated in the first phase of the study)

Continued

Table 21.2 List of example uncertainties related to clinical trials submitted by a manufacturer to an HTA body—cont'd

Drug and indication	HTA body & date	Comments
Study design-related uncertainties		
Ruxolitinib: myelofibrosis	HAS: 9 January 2013	One open-label trial and doubt on the blind maintenance in the double-blind trial due to adverse events (thrombocytopenia)
Axitinib: RCC	HAS: 9 January 2013	Weaknesses in the methodology of the phase III study submitted for the dossier: Open-labelled study whereas double-blinded study would have been possible
Aclidinium bromide: COPD	G-BA: 21 March 2013	Inadequate duration of comparative trials for a long-term therapy (<6 months)
Outcome-related uncertainties		
Ruxolitinib: myelofibrosis	HAS: 9 January 2013	Lack of validation of the instrument EORTC QLQ-C30 in this disease
Aclidinium bromide: COPD	HAS: 17 April 2013	The efficacy of aclidinium bromide on exacerbations and hospitalizations was not evaluated as an endpoint (main or secondary) even though they are considered the important criteria to assess the clinical benefit in the patient
Ruxolitinib: myelofibrosis	G-BA: 7 February 2013	The instrument used to assess the symptoms of myelofibrosis was not enough validated (symptoms were assessed using a symptom diary, MSAF v2.0 defining a total symptom score)

COPD, Chronic obstructive pulmonary disease; *EORTC*, European Organisation for Research and Treatment of Cancer; *HTA*, health technology assessment; *MAu*, market authorization; *RCC*, renal cell carcinoma.
Modified from Toumi, M. (2017). *Introduction to Market Access for Pharmaceuticals.* Boca Raton: CRC Press pp204. See this publication for more details.

responsibility of the manufacturer to minimize the uncertainty and identify the risks of a given product in order to increase the likelihood of its use by a payer.

Should an HTA make a positive recommendation to a payer, the payer will still be faced with questions regarding budget impact: How many doses per patient? How many patients? Cost per dose. In some cases, the total cost may not be feasible for the payer despite the impact it may have on patients' quality of life. In other cases, there may be a marked improvement in health outcomes with the new medicine, but the uncertainty is too large to bear.

This is where managed entry agreements (MEAs) have come into place in the assistance of managing risk and uncertainty.

Managed entry agreements

An MEA is an arrangement between a manufacturer and payer/provider that enables access to (coverage/reimbursement of) a medicine subject to specified conditions. These arrangements can use a variety of mechanisms to address uncertainty about the performance of technologies or to manage the adoption of technologies in order to

maximize their effective use or limit their budget impact (Klemp et al., 2011).

There are two categories of MEAs. Financial-based and health outcomes-/performance-based (Fig. 21.4). There are multiple advantages of MEAs, including the fact that they can help address postlicensing uncertainty and enable early access to innovative treatments (Kanavos et al., 2017). Another advantage is that they provide manufacturers with certainty regarding initial price and potential for future financial rewards thus encouraging innovation (Kanavos et al., 2017).

MEAs offer benefits for manufacturers, payers and patients with increasing potential value in oncology, rare diseases and regenerative medicine. Examples of MEAs are presented in Box 21.1.

Although the pharmaceutical industry is perhaps more in line with an outcomes-based approach, there is low appetite among European payers and HTA bodies for using agreements that involve the collection of outcomes data due to the difficulty in acquiring those data (Bouvy et al., 2018). Technological infrastructure is seen to be the main barrier for adoption of this type of agreement.

MA is constantly evolving due to the changing environment in which the pharmaceutical industry operates. For manufacturers, this ever-changing landscape has had

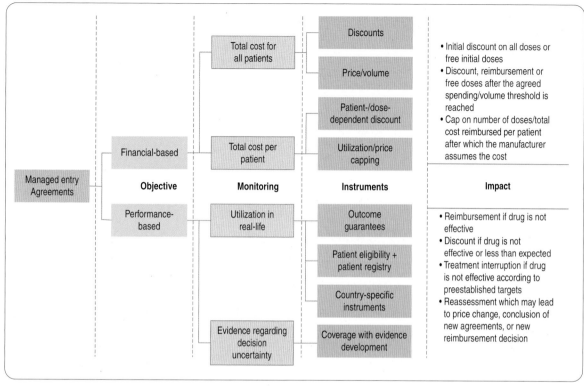

Fig. 21.4 Taxonomy of managed entry agreements. (From Ferrario, A., & Kanavos, P. (2013). *Managed entry agreements for pharmaceuticals: The European experience.* EMiNet, Brussels.)

Box 21.1 **Managed entry agreement examples**

Financial-based agreements

Price volume agreements

- In France, as part of a range of budget controls concerning high cost hepatitis C drugs, Gilead entered into an agreement to cut the list price of Sovaldi by €5k per treatment (27% discount from original price) based on a fixed volume (undisclosed)

Budget capping

- In Australia, any spending over AUS$100m on Enbrel (etanercept) will be rebated by Amgen
- In Italy, pharmaceutical companies are allocated an annual budget by Agenzia Italiana del Farmaco (AIFA), and rebate a proportion of the overspend on their products compared to the budget

Dose capping

- Roche entered into an agreement with several German insurance companies, setting a dose cap for Avastin. If the dose cap is exceeded within a set period, Roche will reimburse the patient's treatment either partially or fully
- For Novartis' treatment Lucentis, up to 14 doses per treated eye would be reimbursed by the UK National Health System NHS. For any further doses required by the patient, Novartis agreed to reimburse the treatment, as long as it was administered at the recommended frequency and in the recommended conditions

Outcomes-based agreements

Coverage with evidence development

- In the Netherlands, drugs with a lack of evidence on effectiveness (e.g., some orphan drugs) have a reevaluation of reimbursement after 4 years. In this time, data are gathered for cost-effectiveness assessment. However, reevaluation decisions are not always implemented due to public/political pressure

Continued

Box 21.1 **Managed entry agreement examples—cont'd**

Patient registry

- When Bosentan (Actelion) was reimbursed in Australia, a registry was set up to monitor patient mortality. If the observed mortality rate was shown to be higher than originally claimed, the reimbursement level of Bosentan would be lowered accordingly, managing the payer's risk of drug failure

Outcome guarantees

- An agreement between Novartis and two sickness funds in Germany entails that Novartis will recredit the money spent on Aclasta, an osteoporosis drug, if the patient breaks any bones within 12 months

Source: Bouvy et al, 2018; Ferrario and Kanavos 2013.

---

ramifications in their core business structure and in the way they operate.

Changing environment—changing marketing

Traditional pharmaceutical marketing has served the pharmaceutical industry well over the past 60 years, but less so as we move on. The development of the market over time has the majority of the industry doing the same things and effectively cancelling each other out. The importance of differentiation from the competition is still high, whether the product or market is weak or strong. How can it be achieved? (See Box 21.2.)

The philosophy of the 1990s and early 2000s was that 'more is better'. More reps, more physician visits, more samples, more congresses and so on. All the while the old customer, the physician, was closing doors on sales reps and losing trust in the industry's motives and integrity. Additionally, the physician as **provider** is losing power as the principal source of therapeutic decision-making. Within the traditional pharmaceutical marketplace, over 70% of marketing spend is focussed on physicians. Does this allocation any longer make sense? Companies are

structured and resourced in order to serve this stakeholder, not the other customers who are increasingly vital to the success or otherwise of new medicines.

The key stakeholder

Even more important, a new customer base is appearing, one of whose goals is to contain costs and reduce the rapid uptake of new medicines without any 'perceived' innovative benefit. At the time of introduction, this **payer** may be told of the 'benefit' claimed by the manufacturer. If the communicator of this message is an official of a health department, it is unlikely that they will be able, or motivated, to convince the payer of the claimed benefit. As the **payers** are rapidly taking over as the key stakeholder, it is imperative that the marketer talks directly to them. The pharmaceutical industry has viewed this stakeholder as something of a hindrance in the relationship between them and their 'real' customer, the doctor. It is likely that the feeling may be mutual. Industry has generally failed to understand the perspective and values of the payer, willing to accept an adversarial relationship during pricing and reimbursement discussions.

R&D present and future

It has been said that the primary care managed 'blockbuster' has had its day. Undoubtedly R&D productivity is going through a slow period. Fewer breakthrough treatments are appearing (IMS Intelligence, 2008).

A more optimistic perspective can be drawn from the Innovative Medicines Initiative:

> *The Innovative Medicines Initiative (IMI) works to improve health and wellbeing by speeding up the development of, and patients' access to, next-generation vaccines, medicines and therapies, especially for areas of unmet need. Funded to the tune of roughly €5bn (2008–2020), the programme represents an unprecedented collaboration between the EU (via the European Commission) and the European pharmaceutical industry (via the European Federation*

Box 21.2 **Competitive differentiation**

PRODUCT STATUS/OPPORTUNITIES	
Weak or disappearing	**Strong or emerging**
• Promotional spending and sales force size	• Market access plan/execution
• Product innovation and differentiation	• Ethical promotion and regulatory conformity
• Managed care and contracting relationships	• Utilization of medical technology
• Direct to consumer	• Internet
	• Marketing sophistication

of Pharmaceutical Industries and Associations) and is to date the world's largest public private partnership in life science.

The unique platform of the Innovative Medicines Initiative, now in its second phase, provides an invaluable opportunity for all those involved in healthcare research—from universities and Pharma companies to patient groups and medicines regulators—to exchange knowledge and work together to enhance clinical trials, improve regulation, and develop new commercial possibilities. (Meulien, 2018)

Products of the future

Generic versions of previous 'blockbuster' molecules, supported by strong clinical evidence, are appearing all the time, giving payers and providers choice without jeopardizing patient care. This is clearly the future of the majority of primary care treatment. But if a sensible dialogue and partnership is the goal for all stakeholders in the process, generics should not only provide care, but should also allow headroom for innovation.

It would seem reasonable that a shift in emphasis from primary to secondary care research will happen. It would also seem reasonable that the pharmaceutical industry will need to think beyond just drugs and start to consider complete care packages surrounding their medical discoveries, such as diagnostic tests and delivery and monitoring devices.

Marketers will need to learn new specialties and prepare for more complex interactions with different providers. Traditional sales forces will not be the model for this type of marketing. Specialist medicines are around 30% more expensive to bring to market. They treat smaller populations and will therefore demand higher prices to recoup the development cost. The debate with payers, already somewhat stressed, will become much more important. The skills of a marketer and seller will of necessity stretch far beyond those needed for primary care medicines. The structure and scope of the marketing and sales functions will have to be tailored to the special characteristics of these therapies.

The future of marketing

Global medicines expenditure is forecast to reach US $1.4 trillion by 2020, an increase of approximately 30% from 2015 (IMS Health, 2015). The development of pharmaceutical products continues to rise in cost as regulatory and HTA standards increase. Price controls are more rigorous in

Europe than in the United States, but the growing demand for affordable healthcare is influencing the rise of value-based approaches to tackle the spending on health technologies. The process of developing a new medicine and ensuring that the patient has access to it is time-consuming, costly and overcome with hurdles.

Effective strategies and well-implemented marketing plans to obtain MA is the key to getting the best possible treatment to the patient on time. It cannot be managed bit by bit, an add-on to an already outdated way of working. It should be a fully integrated process embedded in a company with a wide range of skill and multifunctional expertise, to be able to work closely with all key stakeholders.

MA is a complex and multifaceted process with many stakeholders. The discussions between the different parties have been complicated by their different goals. Pharmaceutical marketing can play a critical role in bringing different perspectives together with the focus on the well-being of the patient. It requires an integrated approach to the stakeholders, based on high-level knowledge, skill and demonstrable outcomes at a fair and affordable cost.

In the area of emerging technologies, digital health tools are now increasing in their adoption, especially regarding remote patient monitoring and management. Using the technology in a smartphone and wearable device, an application can use algorithms to capture a growing list of objective health-related outcomes such as gait, tremor, heart rate, speech disturbance and sleep disturbance. As this area grows, digital health leaders are aiming to create a multitude of clinically validated 'digital biomarkers' as a cheap alternative for healthcare purposes acting as another mechanism for gathering health-related outcomes. As this can be monitored in the outpatient setting, this could provide stakeholders with a rich real-world dataset in an inexpensive manner that might provide solutions to not only outcome-based MEAs but for streamlining the inefficiencies that occur within healthcare.

If the industry and the key stakeholders are to work more effectively together, an appreciation of each other's value systems and goals is imperative. The industry needs to win back the respect of its customers for its pivotal role in the global healthcare of the future.

The excess of overenthusiastic marketing and sales personnel in the 'more is better' days of pharmaceutical promotion has been well documented and continues to grab the headlines. Regulation and sanctions have improved the situation significantly, but there is still lingering suspicion between the industry and its customers.

The most effective way to change this is greater transparency and earlier dialogue throughout the drug discovery and development process. Marketing personnel are a vital interface with the customer groups, and it is important that they are developed further in the new technologies and value systems upon which the customer relies.

Pharmaceutical marketing must advance beyond simplistic messages and valueless giveaways to have the aim of adding value in all interactions with customers. Mass marketing will give way to more focussed interactions to communicate clearly the value of the medicines in specific patient groups.

The new way of marketing

Marketing must focus on the benefits of new medicines from the point of view of each of the customers. The past has been largely dominated by a focus on product attributes and an insistence on their intrinsic value. At one point, a breakthrough medicine almost sold itself. All that was necessary was a well-documented list of attributes and features. That is no longer the case.

It seems as if the provider physician is not going to be the most important decision maker in the process anymore. Specialist groups of key account managers should be developed to discuss the benefits and advantages of the new medicine with health authorities and other government representatives.

Payers and other stakeholders should be involved much earlier in the research and development process, possibly even before research begins, to get the customer view of what medicines are needed from their point of view. Price and value added must be topics of conversation in an open and transparent manner, to ensure full understanding.

The future of marketing is in flux. As Peter Drucker said, 'Marketing is the whole business seen from the customer's point of view. Marketing and innovation produce results; all the rest are costs. Marketing is the distinguishing, unique function of the business' (Trout, 2006). This is a great responsibility and an exciting opportunity for the pharmaceutical industry. It is in the interests of all stakeholders that it succeeds. The wellbeing of a patient is an interdependent responsibility of all stakeholders, not an insurmountable burden.

References

Bouvy, J. C., Sapede, C., & Garner, S. (2018). Managed entry agreements for pharmaceuticals in the context of adaptive pathways in Europe. *Frontiers in Pharmacology, 9*, 280.

Busse, R., & Blümel, M. (2014). Germany: Health system review. *Health Systems in Transition, 16*, 1–296.

Chevreul, K., Berg Brigham, K., Durand-Zaleski, I., Hernandez-Quevedo, C. (2015). France: Health system review. *Health Systems in Transition, 17*, 1–218.

Cochrane, A. L. (1972). *Effectiveness and efficiency: Random reflection on health services*. London: Nuffield Provincial Hospitals Trust.

Cylus, J., Richardson, E., Findley, L., Longley, M., O'Neill, C., & Steel, D. (2015). United Kingdom: Health system review. *Health Systems in Transition, 17*, 1–126.

Delagneau, B. (2018). *Is the price right? An overview of US pricing strategies*. Retrieved from http://www.pharmexec.com/price-right-overview-us-pricing-strategies.

DiMasi, J. A., Grabowski, H. G., & Hansen, R. W. (2016). Innovation in the pharmaceutical industry: New estimates of R&D costs. *Journal of Health Economics, 47*, 20–33.

DiMasi, J. A., Hansen, R. W., & Grabowski, H. G. (2003). The price of innovation: New estimates of drug development costs. *Journal of Health Economics, 22*, 151–185.

Donohue, J. M., Cevasco, M., & Rosenthal, M. B. (2007). A decade of direct-to-consumer advertising of prescription drugs. *New England Journal of Medicine, 357*, 673–681.

Ferrario, A., & Kanavos, P. (2013). *Managed entry agreements for pharmaceuticals: The European experience*. EMiNet, Brussels.

Ferrer, J. M. (1975). How are the costs of continuing medical education to be defrayed? *Bulletin of the New York Academy of Medicine, 51*, 785–788.

Fierce Pharma. (2009). *Sales force cuts have only just begun—FiercePharma*. Retrieved from http://www.fiercepharma.com/story/sales-force-cuts-have-only-just-begun/2009-01-20#ixzz15Rcr0Vn0.

Godman, B., Malmstrom, R. E., Diogene, E., Gray, A., Jayathissa, S., Timoney, A., et al. (2015). Are new models needed to optimize the utilization of new medicines to sustain healthcare systems? *Expert Review of Clinical Pharmacology, 8*, 77–94.

Godman, B., Oortwijn, W., De Waure, C., Mosca, I., Puggina, A., Specchiam, M. L., et al. (2016). *Links between Pharmaceutical R&D models and access to affordable medicines*. Retrieved from https://www.

europarl.europa.eu/thinktank/en/document.html?reference=IPOL_STU(2016)587321.

Goodman, L. S., & Gilman, A. (1960). *The Pharmacological Basis of Therapeutics: A Textbook of Pharmacology, Toxicology, and Therapeutics for Physicians and Medical Students* (2nd ed.). New York: Macmillan.

Grabowski, H., Vernon, J., & DiMasi, J. (2002). *Returns on research and development for 1990s new drug introductions, Pharmacoeconomics, 2002*. Adapted by IBM Consulting Services. Retrieved from https://dukespace.lib.duke.edu/dspace/bitstream/handle/10161/6718/Number16.pdf?sequence=1&isAllowed=y

IMS Health. (2015). *Global medicines use in 2020: Outlook and implications*. London: IMS Health.

IMS Intelligence. (2008). *360: Global pharmaceutical perspectives 2007*. Connecticut: IMS Health, Norwalk.

Informa. (2019). *Market access trends in the US, Europe, and emerging markets*. Pharma Intelligence.

International Pricing and Reimbursement Schemes. (2015). Prepared by Strategy & (Part of PWC) for the Wellcome Trust. Retrieved from https://engage.dhsc.gov.uk/acceleratedaccess/wp-content/uploads/sites/9/2015/10/Strategy-Case-Studies-Report-1.pdf.

Kahveci, R., Oortwijn, W., Godman, B., Meltem Ko√ß, E., & Tibet, B. (2018). Role of health technology assessment in pharmaceutical market access in developed countries. In A. I. Wertheimer (Ed.), *Pharmaceutical Market Access in Developed Markets* (pp. 225–256). Guvenc Kockaya, Italy.

Kaiser Family Foundation. (2001). *Understanding the effects of direct-to-consumer prescription drug advertising.* Retrieved from www.kff.org/content/2001/3197/DTC%20Ad%20Survey.pdf.

Kanavos, P., Ferraio, A., Tafuri, G., & Siviero, P. (2017). Managing risk and uncertainty in health technology introduction: The role of managed entry agreements. *Global Policy, 8,* 84–92.

Klemp, M., Frønsdal, K. B., Facey, K., & HTAi Policy Forum. (2011). What principles should govern the use of managed entry agreements? *International Journal of Technology Assessment in Health Care, 27,* 77–83.

Licking, E., & Garfield, S. (2016). A road map to strategic drug pricing. *In Vivo, 34,* 3.

Malmström, R. E., Godman, B. B., Diogene, E., Baumgärtel, C., Bennie, M., Bishop, I., et al. (2013). Dabigatran—a case history demonstrating the need for comprehensive approaches to optimize the use of new drugs. *Frontiers in Pharmacology, 4,* 394.

Meulienm, P. (2018). *Celebrating Ten Years of the Innovative Medicines Initiative.* HealthEuropa.eu. Retrieved from https://www.healtheuropa.eu/ten-years-innovative-medicines-initiative/85489/.

Nickum, C., & Kelly, T. (September 1, 2005). *Missing the mark(et).* PharmExecutive.com.

Oortwijn, W., Determann, D., Schiffers, K., Tan, S. S., & van der Tuin, J. (2017). Towards integrated health technology assessment for improving decision making in selected countries. *Value in Health, 20*(8), 1121–1130.

Podolsky, S. H., & Greene, J. A. (2008). A historical perspective of pharmaceutical promotion and physician education, *Journal of the American Medical Association, 300,* 831–833. doi:10.1001/jama.300.7.831.

PricewaterhouseCoopers. (2009). *Pharma 2020, which path will you take?* Retrieved from http://www.pwc.com/gx/en/pharma-life-sciences/pharma-2020/pharma-2020-vision-path.jhtml.

Remuzat, C., Urbinati, D., Mzoughi, O., El Hammi, Belgaied, W., & Toumi, M. (2015). Overview of external reference pricing systems in Europe. *Journal of Market Access & Health Policy.* doi:10.3402/jmahp.v3.27675.

Scandinavian Simvastatin Survival Study Group. (1994). Randomized trial of cholesterol lowering in 4444 patients with coronary heart disease: The Scandinavian Simvastatin Survival Study (4S). *Lancet, 344,* 1383–1389.

Todd, J. S., & Johnson, K. H. (1992). American Medical Association Council on Ethical and Judicial Affairs. Annotated guidelines on gifts to physicians from industry. *The Journal of the Oklahoma State Medical Association, 85*(5), 227–231.

Toumi, M. (2017). *Introduction to Market Access for Pharmaceuticals.* Boca Raton: CRC Press.

Towse, J., & Barnsley, P. (2013). Approaches to identifying, measuring, and aggregating elements of value. *International Journal of Technology Assessment in Health Care, 29,* 360–364.

Trout, J. (2006). *Tales from the marketing wars: Peter Drucker on marketing.* Retrieved from https://www.forbes.com/2006/06/30/jack-trout-on-marketing-cx_jt_0703drucker.html?sh=c0b7759555cb

Vogler, S., Zimmerman, N., Leopold, C., & de Joncheere, K. (2011). Pharmaceutical policies in European countries in response to the global financial crisis. *Southern Med Review, 4,* 69–79.

Wee, R. (2017). *Biggest pharmaceutical markets in the world by country.* WorldAtlas. Retrieved from http://www.worldatlas.com/articles/countries-with-the-biggest-global-pharmaceutical-markets-in-the-world.html.

WHO. (2015). *Access to new medicines in Europe: Technical review of policy initiatives and opportunities for collaboration and research.* Retrieved from http://www.euro.who.int/__data/assets/pdf_file/0008/306179/Access-new-medicines-TR-PIO-collaboration-research.pdf?ua=1.

William, D., & McCarthy, J. E. (1997). *Product life cycle: 'essentials of marketing'.* Richard D Irwin Company.

Chapter | 22 |

Drug discovery and development: the future?

Raymond G Hill, Duncan B Richards

In this chapter, we attempt to summarize those advances that have been made since the publication of the second edition and try to point to the key events that may be in play in the immediate future. A number of factors have come together to produce a real increase in the number of new drugs being introduced to medical practice so that worries about falling productivity in the pharmaceutical industry have receded. However, the amount of true novelty may not have increased, and one of the changes we have seen is that improvements in technology mean that multiple approaches to targets are possible. These have been exploited so that in some cases you may find antibody, oligonucleotide, cell or gene therapy and small-molecule approaches all being evaluated against the same target, but fewer new targets per se have emerged. Each of these approaches is likely to have a very different profile, making assessment of the competitive landscape more complex. To put matters in context, we discuss the costs, timelines and success rates of the drug discovery and development operations of major pharmaceutical companies. The information comes from published sources, including the websites of the Association for the British Pharmaceutical Industry (http://www.abpi.org.uk), the European Federation of Pharmaceutical Industries and Associations (http://www.efpia.eu) and the Pharmaceutical Research and Manufacturers of America (http://www.phrma.org). Details of the development process are quite well documented, because the regulatory authorities must be notified of projects in clinical development. The discovery phase is much harder to codify and quantify. Development projects focus on a specific compound, and it is fairly straightforward to define the different components, and to measure the cost of carrying out the various studies and support activities that are needed so that the compound can be registered and launched. In the discovery phase, it is often impossible to link particular activities and costs to specific compounds; instead, the focus is often on a therapeutic target, such as diabetes, Parkinson's disease or lung cancer, or on a molecular target, such as a particular receptor or enzyme, where the therapeutic indication may not yet be determined. The point at which a formal drug discovery project is recognized and 'managed' in the sense of having a specific goal defined and resources assigned to it varies greatly between companies. A further complication is that, as described in Section 2 of this book, the scientific strategies applied to drug discovery are changing rapidly, so that historic data may not properly represent the current situation. For these reasons, it is very difficult to obtain useful data on the effectiveness of drug discovery research. There are, for example, few published figures to show what proportion of drug discovery projects succeed in identifying a compound fit to enter development, whether this probability differs between different therapeutic areas, and how it relates to the resources allocated, although we do include reference to those that we have been able to find. It is clear that the situation may be changing as emerging therapies (Chapter 9) allow direct design of treatments from an understanding of the genetics of disease. We attempt to predict some trends and new approaches at the end of this chapter.

As will be seen from the analysis that follows, even with the recent increases in productivity, the most striking aspects of drug discovery and development are that: (1) failure is much more common than success, (2) it costs a lot and (3) it takes a long time (Fig. 22.1).

Recent advances in technology

A number of technology barriers have been crossed, and although efforts to use oligonucleotides as drugs have been going on for 20 years or more, the problem of making

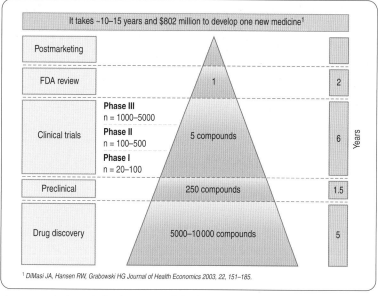

It takes ~10–15 years and $802 million to develop one new medicine[1]

Postmarketing		
FDA review	1	2
Clinical trials — **Phase III** n = 1000–5000, **Phase II** n = 100–500, **Phase I** n = 20–100	5 compounds	6
Preclinical	250 compounds	1.5
Drug discovery	5000–10 000 compounds	5

Years

[1] DiMasi JA, Hansen RW, Grabowski HG Journal of Health Economics 2003, 22, 151–185.

Fig. 22.1 The attrition of compounds through the discovery and development pipeline (PhRMA). *FDA*, US Food & Drug Administration. (From DiMasi, J. A., Hansen, R. W., & Grabowski, H. G. (2003). The price of innovation: new estimates of drug development costs. *Journal of Health Economics, 22,* 151–185.)

nontoxic and specific agents that have therapeutic activity has only recently been solved (see Chapter 9). Examples will be discussed later in this chapter, but some diseases that up to now have not been accessible with drugs are amenable to treatment using this approach. Another advance is in the use of cells as therapy, especially in cells that have been modified using the chimeric antigen receptor (CAR)-T approach (see Chapter 9). Again, this appears to be a way of treating diseases for which no previous effective treatment existed, but raises new problems of how such therapy is delivered to the patients who need it, and how it can be delivered in a cost-effective way. A feature of some of the new technologies is that they offer the opportunity for effective treatment in previously intractable conditions (e.g., neurodegeneration), and in a small number of cases, a cure. Exciting though the prospect of a cure is, it represents a challenge for an industry and reimbursement model that has been largely based on chronic treatment to mitigate disease.

We have also seen the emergence of new approaches to treatment using existing technology such as the use of immunotherapy for treating neoplastic disease using antibodies directed at targets such as programmed cell death protein 1 (PD-1) (see later). The combined use of drugs and software apps is another emerging area, and this overlaps with the increasing use of implanted biosensors in conditions such as diabetes. There is also increased use of nondrug therapies such as biostimulation for treatment of a range of conditions. These latter areas get us into topics that are at present outside the scope of this book.

Spending

Global pharmaceutical companies spent $35 billion on R&D in 1996, rising to $95.2 billion in 2009, and although spending was flat and for some companies (especially those struggling with integration postmergers or takeovers) spending actually fell for a number of years, the trend is again upwards. In 2013, spending had reached $144 billion, and in 2017, $165 billion. Fig. 22.2 shows total global R&D expenditure over the period 2010–24 using actual figures up to May 2018 and estimated trends thereafter. The R&D expenditure of the 10 largest pharmaceutical companies in 2009 averaged nearly $5 billion per company over the range of Roche at $8.7 billion to Lilly at $4.13 billion (Rang & Hill, 2013). In 2019, the top 10 pharmaceutical companies collectively spent $82 billion, with Roche being the top spender at $12.06 billion down to GSK at number 10 spending $5.62 billion (FierceBiotech, 2020). The annual increase in R&D spending in the industry over the last 20 years in most cases has exceeded sales growth, reflecting the need to increase productivity (Kola & Landis, 2004). Typically, more than 20% of sales revenues are reinvested in R&D, a higher percentage than in any other industry, except communications equipment, in the United States (Fig. 22.3). The most recent figures available show that in 2019, an increased investment in R&D is being made by the top 10 companies, with AstraZeneca topping the list at 24.8% of revenues (FierceBiotech, 2020). In

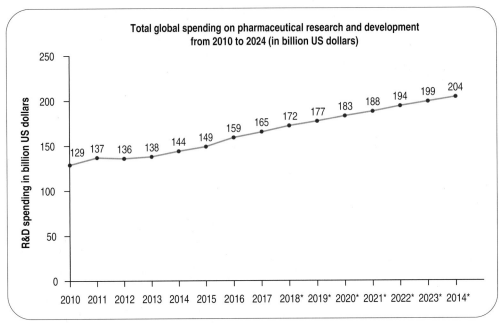

Fig. 22.2 Total global pharmaceutical R&D spending 2010–24 (*actual figures to 2018 and estimates thereafter). (From EvaluatePharma—World Preview 2019, Outlook to 2024, page 22.)

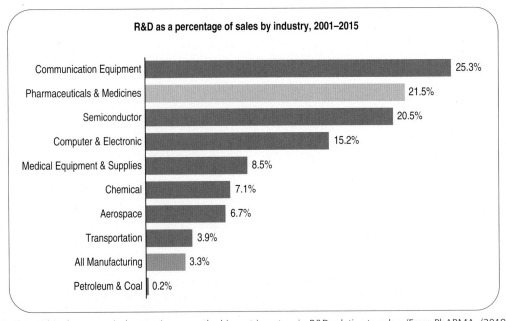

Fig. 22.3 The US biopharmaceutical sector is among the biggest investors in R&D relative to sales. (From PhARMA. (2019). *Biopharmaceuticals in perspective—slide set Summer*. Retrieved from www.phrma.com.)

2010, as mentioned earlier, the overall global R&D spending for the industry fell to $68 billion (a 3% reduction from 2009) (Hirschler, 2011). This fall reflected a growing disillusion with the poor returns on money invested in pharmaceutical R&D. In Fig. 22.4, the continued reduction in return on investment in drug discovery from 2010 to 2016 is illustrated (Mullard, 2017), although the reaction to this appears to be increased rather than decreased spending on R&D. The overall cost of R&D covers discovery research, as well as the various development functions, described in Section 3 of this book. As will be discussed later, the substantial drop-out rate

of compounds proceeding through development means that the overall costs cover many failures, as well as the few successes. The overall cost of developing a compound to launch, and how much this has increased up to 2019, is shown in Fig. 22.5 and dealt with in more detail in the next section. Although the numbers are very large, there is little consensus on the 'right' amount to spend on R&D, and indeed in terms of return on investment this spending has offered a poor return in recent years. Several commentators have suggested that large companies should focus on the development stage of the process, noting that a high proportion of medicines

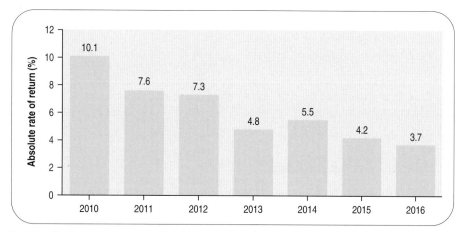

Fig. 22.4 Continuing reduction in the return on investment in drug discovery. (From Mullard, A. (2017). R&D returns continue to fall. *Nature Reviews. Drug Discovery, 16*, 9.)

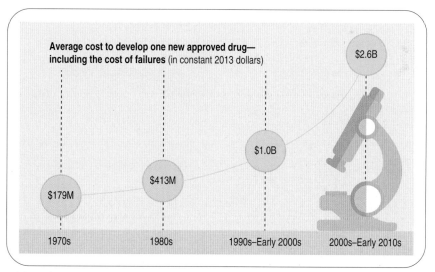

Fig. 22.5 The costs of drug development have more than doubled over the past decade. (From PhARMA. (2019). *Biopharmaceuticals in perspective—slide set Summer*. Retrieved from www.phrma.com.)

registered by the large companies have come from in-licensing activity.

Numbers of compounds in clinical development according to therapeutic classes are shown in Fig. 22.6 based on figures provided by the American research-based pharmaceutical industry and is dominated by three therapeutic areas, namely:

- Cancer, endocrine and metabolic diseases (including osteoporosis, diabetes and obesity)
- Central nervous system disorders (including Alzheimer's disease, schizophrenia, depression, epilepsy and Parkinson's disease)
- Cardiovascular diseases (including atherosclerosis, coronary disease and heart failure).

The trend in the last decade has been away from cardiovascular disease towards other priority areas, particularly cancer and metabolic disorders, and also a marked increase in research on biopharmaceuticals, whose products are used in all therapeutic areas and in emerging modalities (see Chapter 9). There is also a marked increase in the number of drugs being introduced for the treatment of rare or orphan diseases driven by enabling legislation in the United States and EU (see Chapter 20).

How much does it cost to develop a drug?

Estimating the cost of developing a drug is not as straightforward as it might seem, as it depends very much on what is taken into account in the calculation. Factors such as 'opportunity costs' (the loss of income that theoretically results from spending money on drug development rather than investing it somewhere else) and tax credits (contributions from the public purse to encourage drug development in certain areas) make a large difference and are the source of much controversy. The Tufts Centre for Drug Development Studies estimated the average cost of developing a drug in 2000 to be $802 million, increasing to $897 million in 2003 (DiMasi et al., 2003; Fig. 22.1), compared with $31.8 million (inflation-adjusted) in 1987, and concluded that the R&D cost of a new drug was increasing at an annual rate of 7.4% above inflation. The latest figures from the Tuft's group (see also Fig. 22.5) estimate that in 2016, the total cost from discovery to launch was $2.870 billion (DiMasi et al., 2016). This is admittedly a controversial area and as mentioned earlier is often difficult to get precise figures to work from. Wouters et al. (2020) recently analysed data for 63 therapeutic agents developed by 47 companies between 2009 and 2018 and arrived at the conclusion that the real cost to bring a new drug to market was $985 (median) to $1336 (mean) million. They included an adjustment based on clinical trial success rates to account for the cost of failures.

The fact that more than 70% of R&D costs represents discovery and 'failure' costs, and less than 30% represents direct costs (which, being determined largely by requirements imposed by regulatory authorities, are difficult to reduce), has caused research-based pharmaceutical companies to focus on improving (1) the efficiency of the discovery process and (2) the success rate of the

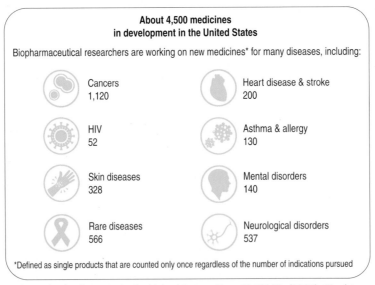

**About 4,500 medicines
in development in the United States**

Biopharmaceutical researchers are working on new medicines* for many diseases, including:

Cancers
1,120

Heart disease & stroke
200

HIV
52

Asthma & allergy
130

Skin diseases
328

Mental disorders
140

Rare diseases
566

Neurological disorders
537

*Defined as single products that are counted only once regardless of the number of indications pursued

Fig. 22.6 About 4500 medicines in development in the United States. (From PhARMA. (2019). *Biopharmaceuticals in perspective—slide set Summer*. Retrieved from www.phrma.com.)

compounds entering development (Kola & Landis, 2004). A good example of the expensive failure of a compound in late-stage clinical development after many years of study is illustrated by the experience of Pfizer, with their cholesterol ester transfer protein (CETP) inhibitor, torcetrapib, and that of other companies also developing agents with this mechanism (Mullard, 2011). This approach to treating cardiovascular disease by raising levels of the 'good' high-density lipoprotein (HDL) cholesterol had looked very promising in the laboratory and in early clinical testing, but in late 2006, development was halted when a large phase III clinical trial revealed that patients treated with torcetrapib had an increased risk of death and heart problems. At the point of termination of their studies, Pfizer had already spent $800 million on the project. The impact extended beyond Pfizer, as both Roche (dalcetrapib) and Merck (anacetrapib) also had compounds acting on this mechanism in clinical development. It was necessary to decide if this was a class effect of the mechanism or whether it was just a compound-specific off-target effect limited to torcetrapib. Intensive comparisons of these agents in collaboration with academic groups and a published full analysis of the torcetrapib clinical trial data allowed the conclusion that this was most likely to be an effect limited to torcetrapib, possibly mediated by aldosterone, and it was not seen with the other two CETP blockers (Mullard, 2011). Roche and Merck were able to restart their clinical trials, but using very large numbers of patients and focussing on clinical outcomes to establish efficacy and safety. The Pfizer experience probably added 4 years to the time needed to complete development of the Merck compound anacetrapib and made this process more expensive (e.g., the pivotal study that started in 2011 recruited 30,000 patients), with no guarantee of commercial success. In addition, the patent term available to recover development costs and to make any profit was now 4 years shorter (see Chapter 19). In 2018, it was shown that (after three compounds with the same mechanism had already failed in phase III clinical trials), in the 30,000 patient REVEAL trial, anacetrapib decreased coronary heart disease when added to statin therapy (Tall & Rader, 2018), and it was suggested that CETP inhibition could provide another treatment option for those patients needing further reduction in low-density lipoprotein (LDL). The latest twist in the CETP story is that anacetrapib has been shown to accumulate in adipose tissue, and regulatory approval is not being sought, so bringing to an end a long and expensive development process for the pharmaceutical industry with the conclusion that CETP inhibition does not provide sufficient cardiovascular benefit for routine use (Armitage et al., 2019). This case is illustrative of a key feature of modern drug development: the eye-watering cost of large multinational late-stage clinical trials. It is not unusual for a single study to

cost several hundred million dollars. This is an important driver of the price we all pay for new medicines, and several groups are examining how novel approaches can be applied to dramatically decrease the costs. The increased use of electronic patient records offers one way to collect information on a patient's clinical course without the traditional case record form and its associated infrastructure. These approaches raise important questions about privacy and data security, but the rewards for a more streamlined approach to late-stage development are enormous.

The saga of new cholesterol-lowering treatments continues, and the hot target at present is proprotein convertase subtilisin kexin 9 (PSK9), and as with CETP, it arose from observations in patients with aberrant gene expression and those with a loss of function mutation appear to have a lower lifetime risk of atherosclerotic disease (Rosenson et al., 2019). Unlike CETP where all the drugs tested in human subjects were small organic molecules, the drugs targeting PSK9 that first entered clinical evaluation were monoclonal antibodies (mAbs), and these have been followed by vaccines (to generate endogenous antibodies and thus have a longer treatment interval than monoclonals), small molecules (which will have the advantage of oral administration) and a small interfering RNA (siRNA) (Dorey, 2015). This is thus an extremely competitive area with mAbs clearly demonstrating clinical efficacy and being marketed widely; the siRNA inclisiran is in the last stages of phase III clinical trial and expected to be filed for regulatory approval before the end of 2020 (Nishikido & Ray, 2019). This underlines the complexity of modern drug discovery, with multiple technical approaches rapidly leading to innovative but costly new treatments. Clinicians are faced with the decision of whether to treat patients with generic statins at minimal cost, achieve better control of cholesterol with a PSK9 monoclonal with the inconvenience of up to 26 injections a year and very much higher cost or to wait for inclisiran, which will require only two injections per year but potentially at an even higher cost than the monoclonals (see Chapter 21).

Sales revenues

Over the past 25 years, the overall sales of pharmaceuticals have risen steadily. In the period 1999–2004, the top 14 companies showed an average sales growth of 10% per year, whereas in 2004–09, growth was still impressive but at a lower rate of 6.7% per year. Loss of exclusivity as patents expire is the most important reason for reduced sales growth (Goodman, 2009). The total global sales in 2002 reached $400.6 billion and in 2008 had risen to $808 billion (EFPIA, 2010). In 2019, the total revenue of the top 10 pharmaceutical companies was $456 billion

(FierceBiotech, 2020), and total worldwide sales for the industry reached $1.25 trillion (Statista, 2020). The largest single country market is the United States, reaching $484 billion in 2019, followed by China at $133 billion and Japan at $85 billion (Statista, 2019). In the United States, the cost of prescribed drugs accounts for some 14% of overall healthcare costs (PhARMA, 2019).

Profitability

For a drug to make a profit, sales revenue must exceed R&D, manufacture and marketing costs. Grabowski et al. (2002) found that only 34% of new drugs introduced between 1990 and 1994 brought in revenues that exceeded the average R&D cost. This quite surprising result needs to be interpreted with caution for various reasons. First, development costs vary widely, depending on the nature of the compound, the route of administration and the target indication, and so a drug may recoup its development cost even though its revenues fall below the average cost. Second, the development money is spent several years before any revenues come in, and sales predictions made at the time development decisions have to be taken are far from reliable. At any stage, the decision whether or not to proceed is based on a calculation of the drug's 'net present value' (NPV)—an amortized estimate of the future sales revenue minus the future development and marketing costs. If the NPV is positive, and sufficiently large to justify the allocation of development capacity, the project will generally go ahead, even if the money already spent cannot be fully recouped, as terminating it would mean that *none* of the costs would be recouped. At the beginning of a project, NPV estimates are extremely unreliable—little more than guesses—so most companies will not pay much attention to them for decision-making purposes until the project is close to launch, when sales revenues become more predictable. Furthermore, unprofitable drugs may make a real contribution to healthcare, and companies may choose to develop them for that reason.

Even though only 34% of registered drugs in the study of Grabowski et al. (2002) made a profit, the profits on those that did so more than compensated for the losses on the others, leaving the industry as a whole with a large overall profit during the review period in the early 1990s. Price control measures in healthcare now have to be considered (see Chapter 21), and R&D costs continue to rise. There will be continuing emphasis on the relative efficacy of drugs, and it will only be those new agents that have demonstrable superiority over generic competitors that will be able to command high prices (Eichler et al., 2010). A recent important study compares the profitability of the pharmaceutical industry with that of other major industries (Ledley et al., 2020) and concludes that profit margins are considerably higher even when increasing R&D costs are accounted for. The analyses used showed that there was considerable complexity underlying the differential profitability of pharmaceutical companies, and the profits were lower in the period 2014–18 than in earlier time points studied (Ledley et al., 2020). It is also worth noting that important sectors within the pharmaceutical industry take their 'profit' before a drug reaches the market. For many venture-capital funded companies, the target is to secure a lucrative buy-out from a large company that will then take the drug through full development and on to marketing. The drug may ultimately not be a large commercial success, but early investors have already taken their return.

Pattern of sales

The distribution of sales (2018 figures) by major pharmaceutical companies according to different therapeutic categories is shown in Table 22.1. Recent changes reflect a substantial increase in sales of anticancer drugs and a decrease in sales of drugs used to treat psychiatric disorders. The United States represents the largest market for pharmaceuticals. Together with Europe, China and Japan, these regions account for 88% of global sales. The rest of the established world market accounts for only 10%, with 3% in emerging markets (EFPIA, 2010; Statista, 2019).

One important area that has struggled to secure investment is antimicrobial therapy. For most new drugs, the target is to grow sales as quickly as possible during the patent-protected period. The strategy for a novel antimicrobial (especially for multiresistant organisms) needs to be different. Ideally, its use would be tightly controlled and limited to avoid promoting resistance. Current sales models do not support this approach, and investment and new financial models are required if we are to see a renaissance of R&D in this area.

Table 22.1 Top 10 therapeutic classes by estimated global sales in 2018

Therapeutic area	Sales ($US billions)
Oncology	99.5
Antidiabetics	78.7
Respiratory	60.5
Autoimmune disease	53.5
Antibiotics and vaccines	40.6
Anticoagulants	39.8
Pain	39.7
Mental health	35.5
Immunology	34.2
Hypertension	29.9

From Statista (2020). https://www.statista.com/ accessed 28 march 2021.

Blockbuster drugs

The analysis by Grabowski et al. (2002) showed that 70% of the industry's profits came from 20% of the drugs marketed, highlighting the commercial importance of finding 'blockbuster' drugs—defined as those achieving annual sales of $1 billion or more—as these are the ones that actually generate significant profits. An analysis of pharmaceutical company pipelines showed that 18 new blockbusters were registered in the period 2001–06, roughly four per year globally among the 30 or so new compounds that were being registered each year at that time. In 2000, a total of 44 marketed drugs achieved sales exceeding $1 billion, compared with 17 in 1995 and 35 in 1999. The contribution of blockbuster drugs to the overall global sales also increased from 18% in 1997 to 45% in 2001, reflecting the fact that sales growth in the blockbuster sector exceeded that in the market overall. The top 10 best-selling drugs in 2010 are shown in Table 22.2, and this should be compared with the top 10 best-selling drugs in 2019, shown in Table 22.3. In 2010, the best-selling drugs were mostly small molecules (seven) with three mAbs. By 2019, biologicals had dominated the list (seven) with only two small molecules and a vaccine completing the top 10. Munos (2009) analysed the peak sales achieved by 329 drugs and calculated that the probability of a new product achieving blockbuster status was only 21%, even though companies take a drug into clinical development only if they believe it has blockbuster potential.

The spate of pharmaceutical company mergers in the last 20 years has also been driven partly by the need for companies to remain in blockbuster territory despite the low rate of new drug introductions and the difficulty of predicting sales. By merging, companies are able to increase the number of compounds registered and thus

Table 22.2 Global sales of top 10 drugs in 2010

Rank	Drug	Trade name	Indication	Sales 2010 ($ billion)
1	Atorvastatin	Lipitor	Cholesterol lowering	12.7
2	Clopidogrel	Plavix	Antiplatelet anticoagulant	8.8
3	Fluticasone/salmeterol	Seretide	Asthma	8.5
4	Esomeprazole	Nexium	Gastric ulcer/reflux	8.3
5	Quetiapine	Seroquel	Schizophrenia	6.8
6	Cerivastatin	Crestor	Cholesterol lowering	6.7
7	Etanercept	Enbrel	Arthritis/psoriasis	6.2
8	Infliximab	Remicade	Arthritis/psoriasis	5.9
9	Adalimumab	Humira	Arthritis/psoriasis	5.9
10	Olanzepine	Zyprexa	Schizophrenia	5.7

From IMS. (2011). *The global use of medicines: outlook through 2015* (p. 27). IMS Institute for Healthcare Informatics.

Table 22.3 Global sales of top 10 drugs for 2018

Rank	Drug	Trade name	Indication	Sales ($ billions)
1	Adalimumab	Humira	Rheumatoid arthritis	19.2
2	Pembrolizumab	Keytruda	Oncology	11.1
3	Lenalidomide	Revlimid	Multiple myeloma	9.7
4	Apixaban	Eliquis	Anticoagulant	7.9
5	Nivolumab	Opdivo	Oncology	7.2
6	Bevacizumab	Avastin	Oncology	7.1
7	Rituximab	Rituxan	Oncology	6.5
8	Ustekinumab	Stelara	Immunology	6.4
9	Trastuzumab	Herceptin	Oncology	6.1
10	Pneumococcal conjugate vaccine	Prevnar	Infant protective vaccination	5.8

From Statista (2020). https://www.statista.com/ accessed 28 march 2021.

reduce the risk that the pipeline will contain no blockbusters. This may have had a negative effect on R&D performance and creativity, however (Kneller, 2010; LaMattina, 2011). Large companies have an ability to make a new treatment available rapidly across multiple jurisdictions, but the infrastructure required to support this is large and expensive. On this basis, a small but medically useful product will not be attractive to large companies but could be very attractive for a small company operating within a therapeutic niche. It is important that the ecosystem maintains a range of corporate models to ensure that the full range of novel therapeutics is available to patients, not just those of blockbuster potential.

Timelines

One important factor that determines profitability is the time taken to develop and launch a new drug, in particular, the time between patent approval and launch, which will determine the length of time during which competitors are barred from introducing cheap generic copies of the drug. A drug that is moderately successful by today's standards might achieve sales of about $400 million/year, so each week's delay in development, by reducing the competition-free sales window, will cost the company roughly $8 million.

Despite increasing expenditure on R&D costs and decreased output, the mean development time from first synthesis or isolation (i.e., excluding discovery research preceding synthesis of the development compound) to first launch was over 14 years in 1999, having increased somewhat over the preceding decade. Half of this time was taken up by discovery and preclinical development and half by clinical studies. A further 2 years was required for US Food & Drug Administration (FDA) review and approval. The long FDA review times during the 1980s have since come down substantially (Reichert, 2003), mainly because user fees and fast-track procedures for certain types of drug were introduced. Current estimates of time taken for R&D leading to a new marketed product are in the region of 10 years (EFPIA, 2019).

There are, of course, wide variations in development times between individual projects, although historically there has been little consistent difference between different therapeutic areas (with the exception of antiinfective drugs, for which development times are somewhat shorter, and anticancer drugs, for which they have been longer by about 2 years). Biopharmaceuticals have become more diverse, and many mAbs have been developed, and these have generally encountered more problems in development because their therapeutic and unwanted effects are sometimes unpredictable, and so clinical development times for biopharmaceuticals have tended to increase, although overall development timelines are shorter than for small-molecule therapeutics.

Information about the time taken for discovery—from the start of a project to the identification of a development compound—is sparse in the public literature. Management consultants McKinsey and Arthur Andersen estimate that in 1995, the time taken from the start of the discovery project to the start of clinical studies was extremely variable, ranging from 21 to 103 months. Both studies predicted a reduction in discovery time by the year 2000 to 46 months or less, owing to improved discovery technologies (Rang, 2006). It has taken until 2020 for this prediction to get close to reality.

Within the clinical development phase of development, the time taken to conduct phase I and phase III is relatively fixed. Much of the variation in time taken comes from the 'learning' phase II studies. Projects with a strong therapeutic strategy and clear targets for phase II tend to move rapidly, while those that test out several indications in phase II may be a lot slower. Human factors are also important; it is not unusual for a project to be led by different people in discovery, early clinical development and late clinical development. If a change in leader is accompanied by a change in strategy, there will usually be a time cost to this change.

Intensifying competition in the pharmaceutical marketplace also is demonstrated by the shrinking period of exclusivity during which the first drug in a therapeutic class is the sole drug in that class, thereby reducing the time a premium can be charged to recover the R&D expenditure. For example, cimetidine (Tagamet), an ulcer drug introduced in 1977, had an exclusivity period of 6 years before another drug in the same class, ranitidine (Zantac), was introduced. In contrast, celecoxib (Celebrex), the first selective cyclooxygenase-2 inhibitor (COX-2), which had a significant advantage over established nonsteroidal antiinflammatory drugs, was on the market only 3 months before a second, similar drug, rofecoxib (Vioxx), was approved. (Vioxx was withdrawn in 2004, because it was found to increase the risk of heart attacks: other COX-2 inhibitors were subsequently withdrawn or given restricted labels.)

Loss of patent protection opens up the competition to generic products (the same compound being manufactured and sold at a much lower price by companies that have not invested in the R&D underlying the original discovery), and the sales revenue from the branded compound generally falls sharply. A new facet to this is now the rise of biosimilars, as although it has taken some time to put the rules in place as to what constitutes a biosimilar, the earliest biological drugs have reached the end of their patent life and copies are arriving on the market. Over the period 2010–14 drugs generating combined revenues of $78 billion (Harrison, 2011) lost patent protection (Table 22.4). The current situation (Table 22.5) is less extreme, but a number of important drugs will shortly lose patent protection. These global figures vary from year to year as individual high-revenue drugs drop out of patent protection, and the revenue swings for an individual company are of course much more extreme than the global average, so maintaining a steady pipeline of new products and timing their introduction to compensate for losses as products become open to generic competition is a key part of a company's commercial strategy (FierceBiotech, 2020).

The situation is more complicated for biologicals, as they are made by recombinant DNA technology rather than chemical synthesis like small-molecule drugs. The molecules made are very much larger than conventional small molecules, the process more open to problems and the quality assurance of the finished product more difficult (see the comprehensive review by Kabir et al., 2019). This has meant that the system for evaluating and approving biosimilars has taken some time to put in place, and a significant number of biosimilars have only recently found their way to the market. They are subject to requirements for postlaunch pharmacovigilance not imposed on

Table 22.4 Selected drugs facing patent expiry in the United States 2010–12

Branded drug (INN drug name; company)	Indication	Worldwide 2009 sales (billion)*	Expected patent expiry
Aricept (donepezil; Eisai/Pfizer)	Alzheimer's-type dementia	¥303.8 (US$3.61)	Nov 2010
Lipitor (atorvastatin; Pfizer)	High cholesterol	US$11.43	2011
Zyprexa (olanzapine; Eli Lilly & Company)	Schizophrenia, bipolar 1 disorder	US$4.92	2011
Lexapro (escitalopram; Forest Laboratories/Lundbeck)	Depression and anxiety	DKK 7.77 (US$1.37)	2012
Actos (pioglitazone; Takeda)	Type 2 diabetes	¥334.5 (US$3.98)°	2012
Plavix (clopidogrel; Sanofi-Aventis/ Bristol-Myers Squibb)	Clot-related cardiovascular events	US$6.15	2012
Lovenox (enoxaparin; Sanofi-Aventis)	Acute deep vein thrombosis	€3.04($4.03)	2012
Seroquel (quetiapine; AstraZeneca)	Schizophrenia, bipolar disorder, major depressive disorder	US$4.87	2012

INN, International nonproprietary name.
From Harrison, C. (2011). The patent cliff steepens. *Nature Reviews. Drug Discovery, 10*, 12–13.
*Data from company annual reports.
°Europe and the Americas.

Table 22.5 Selected drugs facing patent expiry in 2020–22

Branded drug (INN, Company)	Indication	Worldwide 2019 sales (USD billions)	Expected patent expiry
Chantix (varenicline, Pfizer)	Smoking cessation	1.08	2020
Dexilant (dexlansoprazole, Takeda)	Gastric reflux	0.45	2020
Sprycel (dasatinib, BMS)	Chronic myeloid leukaemia	0.54	2020
Xarelto (rivaroxaban, Janssen)	Anticoagulant/stroke prevention	6.58	2020
Truvada (emtricitabine/tenofovir, Gilead)	HIV	2.64	2020
Afinitor (everolimus, Novartis)	Immunosuppressant/transplant rejection/Neuroendocrine tumours	1.0	2020
Forteo (teriparatide, Lilly)	Osteoporosis	0.64	2020
Januvia (sitagliptin, MSD)	Type II diabetes	3.68	2022
Vimpat (lacosamide, UCB)	Epilepsy	1.1	2022

INN, International nonproprietary name.
From Greyb. (2020). *Drug patents expiring 2020-2021-2022*. Retrieved from www.greyb.com. Accessed July, 20 and FiercePharma. (2020). *Special report: top 10 drugs losing US exclusivity 2020*. Retrieved from www.fiercepharma.com. Accessed July, 2020.

generic small molecules driven by concerns about differences in immunogenicity between the proprietary drug and its biosimilar (Kabir et al., 2019). Not surprisingly, the price differential between a biosimilar and the drug it is following may not be very large (estimated at 16%–40%) compared with the 80% or more price reduction seen with a generic small molecule (Kabir et al., 2019; PhARMA, 2019).

Pipelines and attrition rates

The number of new chemical entities (NCEs) registered as pharmaceuticals each year declined over the first decade of the century, or at best stayed flat, and various analyses (Drews, 2003a, 2003b; Kola & Landis, 2004; Munos, 2009) pointed to a serious 'innovation deficit'. According to these calculations, to sustain a revenue growth rate of 10%—considered to be a healthy level—the 10 largest pharmaceutical companies each needed to launch on average 3.1 new compounds each year, compared with 1.8 launches per company actually achieved in 2000—a rate insufficient to maintain even zero growth. A survey indicated that the top 10 pharmaceutical companies were producing 1.17 NCEs per year if based in the United States and 0.83 NCEs per year if based in Europe—a considerable shortfall (Pammolli et al., 2011). Goodman (2009) concluded that most pharmaceutical companies are not replacing the products they lose from patent expiry quickly enough and can only remain competitive by rigorous cost-cutting initiatives.

The number of potential products in development in each therapeutic area (Fig. 22.6) provides a measure of potential future launches. The figures shown may overestimate the numbers, because official notification of the start of clinical projects is obligatory, but projects may be terminated or put on hold without formal notification. Estimates of the number of active preclinical projects are even more unreliable, as companies are under no obligation to reveal this information, and the definition of what constitutes a project is variable. The number of clinical trials appears large in relation to the number of new compounds registered in each year, partly because each trial usually lasts for more than 1 year, and partly because many trials (i.e., different indications, different dosage forms) are generally performed with each compound, including previously registered compounds, as well as new ones.

The fact that in any year there are more phase II than phase I clinical projects in progress reflects the longer duration of phase II studies, which more than offsets the effect of attrition during phase I. The number of phase III projects is smaller, despite their longer duration, because of the attrition between phase II and phase III.

High attrition rates are a fact of life in pharmaceuticals and are the main reason why drug discovery and development is so expensive and why drug prices are so high in relation to manufacturing costs. The cumulative attrition based on projects in the mid-1990s predicted an overall success rate of 20% from the start of clinical development (phase I). An analysis quoted by the FDA (FDA Report, 2014) suggests a success rate of compounds entering phase I trials of only 8%, and this can be even lower for particular therapeutic areas (e.g., 5% for oncology) (Kola & Landis, 2004).

The main reasons currently for failure of compounds are summarized in Fig. 22.7 (Harrison, 2016). It can be seen that the situation has changed little since Kola and Landis (2004) showed that unsatisfactory pharmacokinetic properties and lack of therapeutic efficacy in patients were the commonest shortcomings in 1991, but that by 2000, the pharmacokinetic issues had largely been addressed. As discussed in Chapter 10, determined efforts have been made to control for pharmacokinetic properties in the discovery phase, and this appears to have reduced the failure rate during development. Accurate prediction of therapeutic efficacy in the discovery phase remains a problem, however, particularly in disease areas, such as psychiatric disorders, where animal models are unsatisfactory. In Fig. 22.7A, it can be seen that 52% of failures are due to lack of clinical efficacy regardless of therapeutic target and 24% due to inadequate safety (Harrison, 2016). The analysis in Fig. 22.7B (Harrison, 2016) shows that large numbers of drugs with novel mechanisms of action are failing in areas of high medical need such as cancer and CNS disorders. It has been estimated that in a typical research project, 20%–30% of the time is spent fine-tuning molecules to fit the available animal models of disease perfectly even though, in many cases, these models are not predictive of clinical efficacy (Bennani, 2011). It is especially concerning that drugs are still failing due to lack of efficacy in phase III clinical trials (Fig. 22.8) (Harrison, 2016), and that, although increasing numbers of compounds are reaching phase I and II clinical evaluation, the number of active phase III compounds has not increased. It has been suggested that the remedy is to make phase II trials more rigorous on the grounds that phase II failures are less disruptive and less costly than phase III failures (Arrowsmith, 2011; Harrison, 2016). Even having reached the registration phase, 23% of compounds subsequently fail to become marketed products (Kola & Landis, 2004). The problem of lack of predictability of long-term toxicity such that compounds need to be withdrawn after launch is still largely intractable.

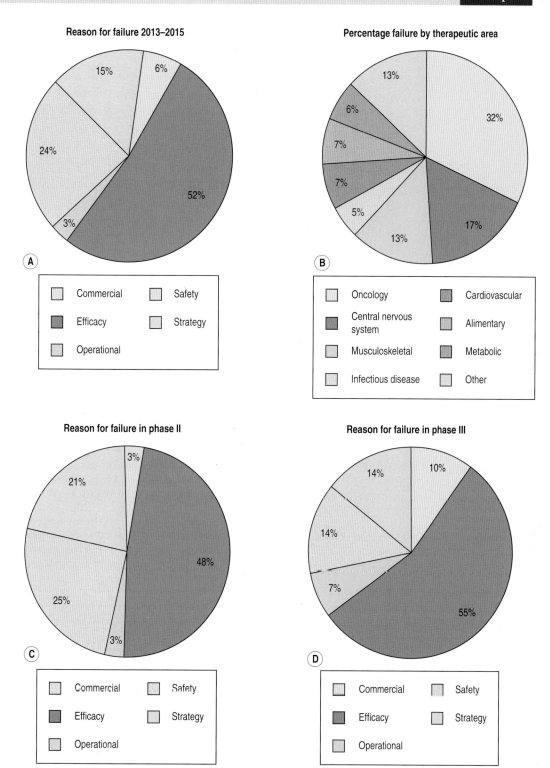

Fig. 22.7 Reasons for compound failure in development. (From Harrison, R. K. (2016). Phase II and phase III failures 2013–2016. *Nature Reviews. Drug Discovery, 15,* 817–818.)

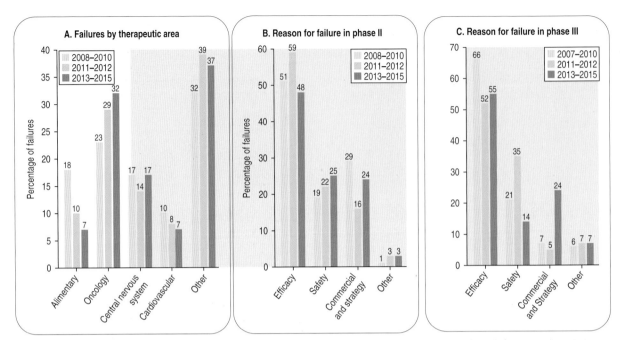

Fig. 22.8 Large numbers of drugs with novel mechanisms of action are failing in areas of high medical need. (From Harrison, R. K. (2016). Phase II and phase III failures 2013–2016. *Nature Reviews. Drug Discovery, 15*, 817–818.)

Biotechnology-derived medicines

An increasing share of research and development projects is devoted to the investigation of therapies using biotechnology-derived molecules (see Chapters 8, 9 and 13). The first such product was recombinant human insulin (Humulin), introduced by Lilly in 1982. From 1991 to 2003, 79 out of 469 (17%) new molecules registered were biopharmaceuticals. In 2002–08, the proportion was around 30%, and this rapidly increased to about 50% over the next few years. In 2002, an estimated 371 biopharmaceuticals were in clinical development (PhRMA Survey, 2002), with strong emphasis on new cancer therapies (178 preparations) and infectious diseases, including AIDS (68 preparations). At that time, the main growth area was mAbs. The first agent in this class, adalimumab, was approved by the FDA in 2002, but between then and 2010, an additional six were registered with three under review. In 2010, there were seven in phase III and 81 in phase I or II clinical trials (Nelson et al., 2010). Overall, biologicals have had a higher probability of success than small molecules, with 24% of agents entering phase I trials becoming marketed products (Kola & Landis, 2004).

Many biotechnology-based projects originate not in mainstream pharmaceutical companies but in specialized small biotechnology companies, which generally lack the money and experience to undertake development projects. This has resulted in increased in-licensing activities, whereby a large company licenses in and develops the substance, for which it pays fees, milestone payments and, eventually, royalties to the biotechnology company. A good example of this approach is the increase in the use of immunotherapy for cancer. In particular, this approach has been called the start of a new era in the treatment of small-cell lung cancer. Conventional chemotherapy with cytotoxic agents works initially, but survival rarely exceeds 10 months (Goetze, 2019). Combination of antibodies against the cell death receptor programmed death-ligand 1 (PD-L1) such as durvalumab or atezolizumab with chemotherapy has been found to improve overall survival and progression-free survival. This new class of antibody that also includes pembrolizumab (which targets PD-1) is characterized by usually only having a beneficial effect in combination with other drugs. This means that large companies have to collaborate with one another and with emerging biotech companies in order to access the most effective drug combination for treating a particular tumour (Mullard, 2019). Pembrolizumab has now been tested by Merck/MSD in over 1000 different trials, and the industry as a whole has conducted more than 2250 trials involving PD1/PD-L1 modulating agents (Mullard, 2019). This field of immune-oncology is about to become even more intensive with the emergence of small-molecule inhibitors targeting the PD-1/PD-L1 signalling pathway (Wu et al., 2020).

Recent introductions

An analysis of the 58 new substances approved by the FDA in the period 2001–02 showed that about half of the new synthetic compounds were directed at receptor targets (mostly G protein-coupled receptors [GPCRs] and some steroid receptors), all of which had been identified pharmacologically many years earlier, as had the transporter and enzyme targets. Only a minority of these compounds were 'first-in-class' drugs. In 2006, only about 30% of the drugs approved by the FDA were new chemical compounds, the rest being modified formulations or new uses for existing drugs (Austin, 2006). The 20% of compounds directed at infectious agents in 2002 were also mainly 'follow-up' compounds, directed at familiar targets, and so it is clear that during the 1990s, when these drugs were being discovered and developed, the industry was operating quite conservatively (DiMasi & Faden, 2011). Although, as described in Section 2, many new technologies are being applied in the hope of improving the speed and efficiency of drug discovery, drug targets and therapeutic approaches had not really changed. You are more likely to produce blockbusters, it was argued, by following the routes that produced blockbusters in the past than by trying new approaches with the aim of being 'first-in-class' (DiMasi & Faden, 2011). In a survey of 259 drugs registered by the FDA between 1999 and 2008 (Swinney & Anthony, 2011), it was found that only 75 of the 259 were first-in-class agents with novel mechanisms of action. Of the small-molecule drugs in the survey, target-based screening had produced 17 with 28 being discovered by using phenotypic disease model screening. Thus even though the industry was becoming more centred on molecular target-based screening, this was not the source of the majority of new drugs over that period. One worrying trend is the reduction in effort across the industry in the search for new drugs to treat psychiatric and neurological disorders, as, although this is the most difficult research area, the medical need for drugs has never been higher (Abbott, 2010; EFPIA, 2016; Kaitin & Milne, 2011).

Biopharmaceuticals registered between 1999 and 2008 include several protein mediators produced by recombinant methods and a number of mAbs. Vaccines were also strongly represented. Of the 75 first-in-class drugs registered by the FDA in this period, 50 (67%) were small molecules and 25 (33%) were biologicals. The trend towards biopharmaceuticals is set to continue, with cancer and inflammation/autoimmune diseases as the main therapeutic targets. A milestone was reached in 2012 when a biological became the world's top selling drug as a consequence of patent expiry for the previous top sellers (Hirschler, 2012).

Today, biologicals dominate the list of top selling drugs (Table 22.3), and there is no sign that this trend will end anytime soon. One change is in the emergence of alternative approaches to mAbs (as mentioned earlier) providing different ways to address the same target (see Chapter 9). Emerging therapies thus raise a number of issues around access to medicines and value for money (see Chapter 21 and later in this chapter).

Predicting the future?

Many models have been proposed as the ideal way to discover drugs, but there is now general cynicism and the intrinsic cyclical nature of drug discovery is likely to have been the real reason for swings from failure to success rather than the approach taken by the industry. Predicting the future, especially the facts and figures, is therefore a dangerous game! A number of factors have become apparent in the recent past that will change our world in ways that we probably could not have guessed at 10 years ago. The belief that small-molecule drug discovery could be industrialized was clearly a mistaken one, although mass screening using techniques such as phage display has been very successful in the biologicals field (see Chapter 8). Access to larger numbers of molecular targets, larger numbers of drug-like compounds and faster screening technology has not led to more registered drugs. Similarly, our knowledge of the human genome is only now having a major impact on drug discovery. We are learning more about disease processes day by day, but much of this knowledge is still difficult to translate into strategies for drug discovery. Senior figures in the pharmaceutical industry who said we needed to reinvent the industry (Bennani, 2011; Paul et al., 2010) have been vindicated, and this is now happening. The reduction in R&D spending of the industry, driven by a realization that spending more on R&D year on year did not work (Hirschler, 2011) has now been reversed and spending is again increasing year on year. The regulatory authorities accept that there is still more to be done in streamlining development (FDA, 2011) and developing strategies to kill drugs that are not clearly an improvement over what we already have as early as is feasible (Paul et al., 2010; Fig. 22.9). Some companies have seen the need to empower creative talent and admit that drug discovery is as much an art as a science (Bennani, 2011; Douglas et al., 2010; Paul et al., 2010). The crucial reorganization may already have happened, with much of the creative part of drug discovery moving over to the biotech sector or to academic centres for drug discovery (Kotz, 2011; Stephens et al., 2011). This in turn is leading to more partnerships between different pharmaceutical companies, and between pharmaceutical companies, biotech and academia. It is interesting to note that the academic contribution to drug discovery may have been underestimated in the past (Stephens et al., 2011). A recent study (Pammolli

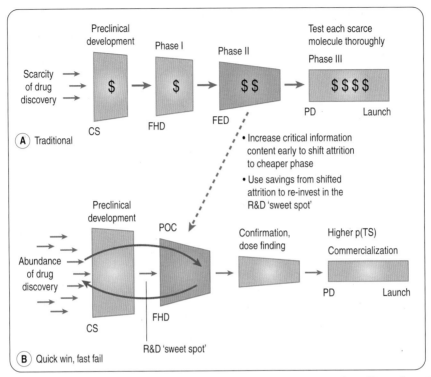

Fig. 22.9 The quick win/fast fail model for drug development. CS, candidate selection; FED, first efficacy dose; FHD, first human dose; PD, product decision. probability of success (p(TS)). (From Paul, S. M., Mytelka, D. S., Dunwiddie, C. T., Persinger, C. C., Munos, B. H., Lindborg, S. R., et al. (2010). How to improve R&D productivity: the pharmaceutical industry's grand challenge. *Nature Reviews. Drug Discovery, 9* 203–214.)

et al., 2020) analysed data from more than 50,000 projects between 1990 and 2017 and has concluded that attrition rates have been decreasing at all stages of clinical development. Most importantly, they found that R&D projects have become more targeted and novel both in terms of therapeutic indications and mechanism of action. A more cautionary note is sounded by Shih et al. (2018), who found in another industry-wide survey that companies were still playing catch up and often started projects in areas that others had already shown to be nonproductive. They also found that the tendency was to move to novel and unprecedented mechanisms for new projects, however.

The economics of our business have shifted geographically (IMS, 2011) with the US share of the global market declining from 41% in 2010 to 31% in 2015 but having recovered since then to 45% (Statista, 2019). The United States was still the largest market in 2018, but China has now risen to second place ahead of Japan and Western Europe. Increased spending on R&D in Asia, especially in China, does not seem to have justified the investment yet, and some companies have reduced their R&D efforts in China recently. The shift from proprietary medicines to generics has continued, and 90% of all prescriptions in

the United States are for generics (EFPIA, 2016; PhARMA, 2019). We are thus victims of our own success as the blockbusters of 2010 become the generics of 2020. Our world will look very different 5 years from now, with an increasingly complex social, legal, scientific and political environment. The pharmaceutical industry will continue to be important and governments will have to ensure that a fair reward for innovation (Aronson et al., 2012; Rajkumar, 2020) is still achievable, but how this will be done is at present unclear. There is clearly a problem already in making expensive medicines available to the patient (see Chapter 21), illustrated by the launch of cellular therapies where the financial cost is currently estimated to be in the region of $150,000–$475,000 per treatment, with no obvious fixed pricing structure provided by any one company (Walker & Johnson, 2016). Recently tafamidis (a stabilizer of the transthyretin [TTR] protein tetramer) was shown to reduce all-cause mortality and cardiovascular hospitalization and was approved for marketing by the FDA in May 2019 for treating TTR amyloid cardiomyopathy. It has been launched at a cost of $225,000 per annum, taking it out of the range that is affordable without co-payment assistance from the manufacturer (Masri et al., 2020).

This is the most exciting time there has ever been for drug discovery. Increasingly precise tools, such as cryo-electron microscopy allow us to define the structural biology of our targets, artificial intelligence aids in the design of novel molecules ranging from small molecules, through nucleotides and peptides to proteins such as mAbs. Preclinical development is still time-consuming, but advanced methods for clinical trial design allow earlier rejection of molecules that lack efficacy (see Chapter 17). Alternatives approaches are now being evaluated in parallel so that if a small-molecule drug is not found, then it may be possible to find a nucleotide-based medicine, a mAb or even a cell or gene therapy. The problem now is not whether we can discover a new treatment or not, and most of the previous technical barriers have been eliminated. In the last decade, treatments for a number of previously intractable diseases have been produced including the first effective treatment for cystic fibrosis caused by the *F508del* mutation (Heijerman et al., 2019), and the first oligonucleotide therapies have reached the market (see Chapter 9), with many more in the late-stage pipeline including potential genomic therapies for amyotrophic lateral sclerosis (ALS) (Hardiman & van den Berg, 2020) and Huntington's disease (Fishbeck & Wexler, 2019). FDA new drug approvals in 2019 show considerable novelty with the first approval of a nanobody, a number of antibody/drug conjugates and a gene therapy (Mullard, 2020). The issues now are whether we can use our novel treatment approach safely, and if so, is it affordable by the patient.

As this book was in its final stages of editing the world was rocked by the emergence of severe acute respiratory syndrome coronavirus 2 (SARS-Cov-2) and its worldwide spread. The application of modern sequencing technology meant that the genome of this virus was fully described in 2 weeks (compared with the 197 years to go from knowledge of the virus to a sequence for measles! [PhARMA, 2020]). This pandemic has led to more than 2000 clinical trials of new and repurposed drugs and the rapid development and clinical trial of 18 novel vaccines (PhARMA, 2020). In a little over a year we have seen the licensing of four novel and effective vaccines against SARS-Cov2 following large clinical trial programmes in multiple countries. This has re-set the paradigm for discovering and developing new vaccines. The use of other drugs for treating SARS Cov-2, in particular dexamethsone, remdesvir and tocilizumab has been validated by clinical trials. This has been as a result of an unprecedented level of integrated collaboration between governments, regulators, academics, healthcare systems and the pharmaceutical industry. It is likely that this pandemic experience will lead to long lasting changes in the way that novel therapies are discovered and developed.

References

Abbott, A. (2010). The drug deadlock. *Nature, 468,* 178–179.

Armitage, J., Holmes, M. V., & Preiss, D. (2019). Cholesterol ester transfer protein inhibition for preventing cardiovascular events. *Journal of the American College of Cardiology, 73,* 477–487.

Aronson, J. K., Ferner, R. E., & Hughes, D. A. (2012). Defining rewardable innovation in drug therapy. *Nature Reviews. Drug Discovery, 11,* 253–254.

Arrowsmith, J. (2011). Phase III and submission failures: 2007–10. *Nature Reviews. Drug Discovery, 10,* 1.

Austin, D. H. (2006). *Research and development in the pharmaceutical industry* (p. 55). Congress Budget Office.

Bennani, Y. L. (2011). Drug discovery in the next decade: innovation needed ASAP. *Drug Discovery Today, 16,* 779–792.

DiMasi, J. A., Hansen, R. W., & Grabowski, H. G. (2003). The price of innovation: new estimates of drug development costs. *Journal of Health Economics, 22,* 151–185.

DiMasi, J. A., & Faden, L. B. (2011). Competitiveness in follow-on drug R&D: A race or imitation? *Nature Reviews. Drug Discovery, 10,* 23–27.

DiMasi, J. A., Grabowski, H. G., & Hansen, R. W. (2016). Innovation in the pharmaceutical industry: new estimates of R&D costs. *Journal of Health Economics, 47,* 20–33.

Dorey, E. (2015). Cholesterol-busting PSK9 drugs. *The Pharmaceutical Journal, 294,* 7058.

Douglas, F. L., Narayanan, V. K., Mitchell, L., & Litan, R. E. (2010). The case for entrepreneurship in R&D in the pharmaceutical industry. *Nature Reviews. Drug Discovery, 9,* 683–689.

Drews, J. (2003a). Strategic trends in the drug industry. *Drug Discovery Today, 8,* 411–420.

Drews, J. (2003b). *In Quest of Tomorrow's Medicines* (4th ed.). New York: Springer-Verlag.

EFPIA. (2010). *The pharmaceutical industry in figures* (p. 40). Brussels: European Federation of Pharmaceutical Industry Associations.

EFPIA. (2016). *From innovation to outcomes, medicines costs in context.* 2016 slide set. see www.efpia.eu

EFPIA. (2019). *Pipeline review of innovative therapies.* 2019 slide set.

Eichler, H. G., Bioechl-Daum, B., Abadie, E., Barnett, D., König, F., & Pearson, S. (2010). Relative efficacy of drugs: An emerging issue between regulatory agencies and third-party payers. *Nature Reviews. Drug Discovery, 9,* 277–291.

EvaluatePharma. (2019). *World preview 2019, outlook to 2024* (12th ed.).

FDA Report. (2018). *Challenge and opportunity on the critical path to new medical products.* Retrieved from https://www.fda.gov/science-research/science-and-research-special-topics/critical-path-initiative.

FDA. (2021). *Advancing regulatory science at FDA: a strategic plan* (p. 34). FDA. https://www.fda.gov/science-research/science-and-research-special-topics/advancing-regulatory-science.

FierceBiotech. (2020). *Special report: The top 10 Pharma R&D budgets in 2019.* www.fiercebiotech.com/special-report/top-10-pharma-r-d-budgets-2019. Accessed July, 2020.

FiercePharma. (2020). *Special report: top 10 drugs losing US exclusivity 2020.* Retrieved from www.fiercepharma.com. Accessed July, 2020.

Fishbeck, K. H., & Wexler, N. S. (2019). Oligonucleotide treatment for Huntington's disease. *New England Journal of Medicine, 380*(24), 2373–2374.

Goetze, T. O. (2019). Immunotherapy: A new era in small-cell lung cancer. *The Lancet, 394,* 1884–1885.

Goodman, M. (2009). Pharmaceutical industry financial performance, *Nature Reviews. Drug Discovery, 8,* 927–928.

Grabowski, H., Vernon, J., & DiMasi, J. A. (2002). Returns on research and development for 1990s new drug introductions. *Pharmacoeconomics, 20,* 11–29.

Greyb. (2020). *Drug patents expiring 2020-2021-2022.* Retrieved from www.greyb.com. Accessed July, 20.

Hardiman, O., & van den Berg, L. H. (2020). The beginning of genomic therapies for ALS. *New England Journal of Medicine, 383,* 180–181.

Harrison, C. (2011). The patent cliff steepens. *Nature Reviews. Drug Discovery, 10,* 12–13.

Harrison, R. K. (2016). Phase II and phase III failures 2013—2015. *Nature Reviews. Drug Discovery, 15,* 817–818.

Heijerman, H. G. M., McKane, E. F., Downey, D. G., Van Braeckel, E., Rowe, S. M., Tullis, E. et al. (2019). Efficacy and safety of the elexacaftor plus tezacaftor plus ivacaftor combination regime in people with cystic fibrosis homozygous for the *F508del* mutation: a double blind randomized phase 3 trial. *The Lancet, 394,* 1940–1948.

Hirschler, B. (June 3, 2011). Drug R&D spending fell in 2010 and heading lower. *Reuters Business and Financial News.* Retrieved from www.reuters.com/assets/print?aid=USL6E7HO1BL20110626.

Hirschler, B. (April 11, 2012). Abbott drug tops sales as Lipitor, Plavix era ends, *Reuters Business and Financial News.* Retrieved from www.reuters.com/assets/print?aid=USL6E8FA3WO20120411.

IMS. (2011). *The global use of medicines: outlook through 2015* (p. 27). IMS Institute for Healthcare Informatics.

Kabir, E. R., Moreino, S. S., & Siam, M. K. S. (2019). The breakthrough of biosimilars: A twist in the narrative of biological therapy. *Biomolecules, 9,* 1–34.

Kaitin, K., & Milne, C. P. (2011). A dearth of new meds. *Scientific American, 305,* 16.

Kneller, R. (2010). The importance of new companies for drug discovery: Origins of a decade of new drugs. *Nature Reviews. Drug Discovery, 9,* 867–882.

Kola, I., & Landis, J. (2004). Can the pharmaceutical industry reduce attrition rates? *Nature Reviews. Drug Discovery, 3,* 711–716.

Kotz, J. (2011). Small (molecule) thinking in academia. *Science-Business eXchange, 4,* 617.

LaMattina, J. L. (2011). The impact of mergers on pharmaceutical R&D, *Nature Reviews. Drug Discovery, 10,* 559–560.

Ledley, F. D., McCoy, S. S., Vaughan, G., & Claery, E. G. (2020). Profitability of large pharmaceutical companies compared with other large public companies. *Journal of the American Medical Association, 323,* 834–843.

Masri, A., Chen, H., Wong, C., Fischer, K. L., Karam, M. D., Gellad, W. F., et al. (2020). Initial experience prescribing commercial tamfamidis the most expensive cardiac medication in history. *JAMA Cardiology, 5,* 1066–1067.

Mullard, A. (2011). Learning lessons from Pfizer's $800 million failure. *Nature Reviews. Drug Discovery, 10,* 163–164.

Mullard, A. (2017). R&D returns continue to fall. *Nature Reviews. Drug Discovery, 16,* 9.

Mullard, A. (2019). An audience with Roger Perlmutter. *Nature Reviews. Drug Discovery, 18,* 818–819.

Mullard, A. (2020). 2019 FDA drug approvals. *Nature Reviews. Drug Discovery, 19,* 79–84.

Munos, B. (2009). Lessons from 60 years of pharmaceutical innovation. *Nature Reviews. Drug Discovery, 8,* 959–968.

Nelson, A. L., Dhimolea, E., & Reichert, J. M. (2010). Development trends for human monoclonal antibody therapeutics. *Nature Reviews. Drug Discovery, 9,* 767–774.

Nishikido, T., & Ray, K. K. (2019). Non-antibody approaches to proprotein convertase subtilisin kexin 9 inhibition: antisense oligonucleotides, adnectins, vaccination and new attempts at small molecule inhibitors based on new discoveries. *Frontiers in Cardiovascular Medicine, 5,* 199.

Pammolli, F., Magazzini, L., & Riccaboni, M. (2011). The productivity crisis in pharmaceutical R&D. *Nature Reviews. Drug Discovery, 10,* 428–438.

Pammolli, F., Righetto, L., Abrignani, S., Pani, L., Pelicci, P. G., & Rabioso, E. (2020). The endless frontier? The recent increase of R&D productivity in pharmaceuticals. *Journal of Translational Medicine, 18,* 1–14.

Paul, S. M., Mytelka, D. S., Dunwiddie, C. T., Persinger, C. C., Munos, B. H., Lindborg, S. R., et al. (2010). How to improve R&D productivity: the pharmaceutical industry's grand challenge. *Nature Reviews. Drug Discovery, 9* 203–214.

PhRMA Survey. (2002). *Biotechnology medicines in development.* Retrieved from www.phrma.org/newmedicines/surveys.cfm.

PhARMA. (2019). *Biopharmaceuticals in perspective—slide set Summer.* Retrieved from www.phrma.com.

PhARMA. (2020). *PhRMA Covid-19 treatment progress.* Retrieved from www.phrma.com. Accessed July 12, 2020.

Rang, H. P. (2006). Drug discovery and development—facts and figures. *Drug discovery and development* (1st ed., pp. 311–327). Edinburgh: Churchill Livingston/Elsevier.

Rang, H. P., & Hill, R. G. (2013). Drug discovery and development—facts and figures. *Drug discovery and development* (2nd ed., pp. 321–334). Churchill Livingston/Elsevier, Edinburgh.

Rajkumar, S. V. (2020). The high cost of prescription drugs: causes and solutions. *Blood Cancer Journal, 10,* 71.

Reichert, J. M. (2003). Trends in development and approval times for new therapeutics in the United States. *Nature Reviews. Drug Discovery, 2,* 695–702.

Rosenson, R. S., Hegele, R. A., & Koenig, W. (2019). Cholesterol-lowering agents PSK9 inhibitors today and tomorrow. *Circulation Research, 124,* 364–385.

Shih, H. P., Zhang, X., & Aranov, A. M. (2018). Drug discovery effectiveness from the standpoint of therapeutic mechanisms and indications. *Nature Reviews. Drug Discovery, 17,* 19–33.

Stephens, A. J., Jensen, J. J., Wyller, K., Kilgore, P. C., Chatterjee, S., & Rohrbaugh, M. L. (2011). The role of public sector research in the discovery of drugs and vaccines. *New England Journal of Medicine, 364,* 535–541.

Swinney, D. C., & Anthony, J. (2011). How were new medicines discovered? *Nature Reviews. Drug Discovery, 10,* 507–519.

Tall, A. R., & Rader, D. J. (2018). Trials and tribulations of CETP inhibitors. *Circulation Research, 122,* 106–112.

Walker, A., & Johnson, R. (2016). Commercialization of cellular immunotherapies for cancer. *Biochemical Society Transactions, 44,* 329–332.

Wouters, O. J., McKee, M., & Luyten, J. (2020). Estimated research and development investment needed to bring a new medicine to market, 2009–2018. *Journal of the American Medical Association, 323,* 844–853.

Wu, Q., Jiang, L., Li, S. C., He, Q. J., Yang, B., & Cao, J. (2021). Small molecule inhibitors targeting the PD-1/PD-L1 signalling pathway. *Acta Pharmacologica Sinica, 42*(1), 1–9.

Index

Note: Page numbers followed by *b* indicates boxes, *f* indicates figures, and *t* indicates tables.

A

Abandonment, 286
Absorption
  assays and techniques, 139*t*
  cautions, 139–140
  first-pass hepatic clearance, 136
  oral drugs, 137
  passive permeability, 137–138
  prediction, 152–153
  proteolysis targeting chimeras (PROTACs), 136–137
  solubility measurements, 137
  tactics, 136–139
  troubleshooting decision tree, 138*f*
  Ussing chamber technique, 137–138
Absorption, distribution, metabolism, excretion (ADME)
  in-vitro screens, 99
  parameters, 99
ABvac40 (Araclon Biotech), 213
Accelerated stability tests, 235
Accelerated stress studies, antibody, 119
ACE inhibitors, 183
Acetazolamide, 8–9, 183
Aciclovir, 10 11
Acid secretion, 43
Actinomyces, 6
Actinomycin D, 6
Active metabolites identification, 149–150
  cautions, 150–151
  decision tree, 150*f*
  prodrugs, 150
  structure–activity relationship, 149–150
  tactics, 150–151
  time–response studies, 149–150
Active pharmaceutical ingredients (API), 234, 237
Actos, expiry, 341*t*
Acute myeloid leukaemia (AML), 131
Acyl glucuronides, 151
Adalimumab, 344
Adaptive cell therapy, 126–127
Adaptive pathways, 256–257
Addiction, therapeutic vaccines, 214–215, 215*f*
ADDvac1 (Axon Neuroscience SE), 213
Adenine deaminase severe combined immunodeficiency (ADA–SCID), 33–34
Adeno-associated virus (AAV)-based therapies, 129–131
Administrative rules, regulation, 308–309
Adoption pattern, new products, 316
Adrenaline, 6–7
  as trade name, 4–5
Advanced Therapy Medicinal Products (ATMPs), 301

Index

Adverse drug reactions (ADRs), 102
   documentation and review, 227
   mechanistic investigation, 228–229
   reproductive toxicity, 227
   serious, 227–228
   structured questionnaires, 227
Aequorin, 76–77
Aetiology, 20
AFFITOPE PD01A vaccine (AFFiRiS), 213
Afinitor, expiry, 341*t*
Aggregation, antibody, 118
Agonism, 159
Ahlquist, R., 65
Alkaloids, plant, 4
Allergen-specific immunotherapy (AIT), 211–212
Allergic disorders, therapeutic vaccines, 211–213
Alleviation, disease effects, 27
Allopurinol, 10–11
Allosteric pharmacology, 159
AlphaLISA, 76
AlphaScreen Technology, 76, 76*f*
Alzheimer's disease (AD), 213
   brain amyloid deposits, 270
   FDG-PET imaging, 270*f*
   functional MRI, 270–271
   magnetic resonance imaging (MRI), 269
   PD biomarkers, 269–270
American Medical Association (AMA), 312
Ames test, 181
Amiodarone, 175–176
Amphetamine, 12
Amphiphilic molecules, 239
Amyl nitrite, 3–4
Ancient Greeks, 1–2
Angiotensin antagonists, 183
Angiotensin I and II, 211
Animal disease models
   gene knock out, 168
   imaging approaches, 169
   species differences, 170
   structural methods, 169–170
   validity criteria, 170–171
Animal pharmacology, 162*t*
   profiling, 164–171
Antagonism, 159
Antiangiotensin II vaccine AngQb-Cyt006, 211
Antibodies
   discovery, 111–112
   monoclonal (mAbs), 344
   structure and properties, 109–110
   therapeutic *see* Therapeutic antibodies
Antibody-dependent cellular cytotoxicity, 39
Antidepressants, 175–176
Antidrug antibody (ADA) reaction, 112
Antimetabolite principle, 10–11
Antipyretics, 5
Antisense oligonucleotides (ASOs), 39, 44, 123–126
   chemical modification, 125
   drug targets, 123–125
   posthybridization mechanisms, 123–125
   RNA-like, 125
   toxic effects, 125
Anti-tumour necrosis factor (TNF), 12–13
Aphorisms, 223–224
Apixaban, 339*t*
Apothecaries' trade, 4–5
Aricept, expiry, 341*t*
Artemisinin, 6
Artificial intelligence (AI) technique, 50
Assay development
   miniaturization, 82

Assay development *(Continued)*
  readout/detection, 76–77
  validation, 68–71
Assay Guidance Website, 71
Astemizole, 175–176
Atezolizumab, 344–345
Atorvastatin, 339*t*
Atropine, 6
Attrition, drug, 101–104, 333*f*
Attrition rates, 342
Augmented toxicity, 102
Autologous ex vivo gene therapy, 129–131
Azathioprine, 10–11
AZT (zidovudine), 10–11

B

Bacillus subtilis, 190
Baclofen, 242–243
Bacterial/yeast-vectored cancer vaccines, 190, 202
Barbitone (barbital), 5
B cells screening, 112
Benefit, defines, 28
Benzene, 5
Beraprost, profiling, 169–170, 169*b*
Beta adrenoreceptor blocking drug, 225
Bevacizumab, 339*t*
Bile Salt Export Pump (BSEP), 103
Biliary clearance
  acidic and zwitterionic compounds, 148
  biliary transporter substrates, 148
  cautions, 149
  tactics, 149
Binders, 238
Binding assays, 163
Bioaxis, 25
Biochemical assays, 71–72, 71*f*
Biodistribution studies, PET imaging
  alternatively, labelled molecules, 266
  anticancer agents, 264–266
  blood–brain barrier penetration, species differences, 264*f*
  drug metabolism and pharmacokinetic (DMPK) radiotracer studies, 266
  monoclonal antibodies (mAbs), 266
  occupancy of a receptor (OR), 264
  passive distribution, 264
  principles, 263
  specific/nonspecific binding, 263–264
Bioelectronics, 42
Bioengineering, 14
Biological perspective
  function and dysfunction, 24–27
  organization levels, 25–26, 25*f*
Biological products, 37–40
Biology-oriented synthesis (BIOS), 97
Bioluminescence resonance energy transfer (BRET), 79
Biomarkers, 91
  classification, 154, 154*f*
Biomaterials, 35, 41–42
Biomedicine, developments, 2–3
Biomolecules, 65
Biopharmaceutical Classification System, 135–136
Biopharmaceuticals, 38*b*, 184–185, 345
  delivery and formulation, 241–242
  development, 8*t*, 15–16*t*
  efficacy, 302
  quality assessment, 301–302
  regulation, 300–303
  regulatory procedural considerations, 302–303
  research & development, 344
  safety, 302
Biopharmaceutics classification system (BCS), 235

Biophysical methods, high-throughput screening (HTS), 80
Biotechnology-derived medicines, 344–345
1,6-Bis(phosphocholine)-hexane, 94*f*
Black Box Warnings (FDA), 103
Black, James, 11–12
Blockbuster drugs, 5
    marketing, 312
    molecules, 328
    sales, 339–340
Blood CSF barrier (BCSFB), 144
Blood oxygenation level dependent (BOLD) contrast, 261
Boundary layer, dissolution process, 235
Breast cancer, 204
British Pharmacopoeia, 2
Buchheim, Rudolf, 3
Budget capping, 327–328*b*
Bulk phase, dissolution process, 235
Buprenorphine, 160
Burimamide, 11
Buserelin, 237

C

Caffeine, 183
Calcitonin, 237
Cancer
    immune-editing process, 198–199
    modified T cells, 40
Cancer testis antigens (CTAs), 198
Cancer vaccines
    bacterial/yeast-vectored cancer vaccines, 202
    cell-based, 199–201
    clinical trials
        breast cancer, 204
        colorectal cancer, 206
        lung cancer, 203–204
        melanoma, 203
        prostate cancer, 204–205
        renal cancer, 205–206
    combination immunotherapy, 202
    genetic cancer vaccines, 201
    immune evasion mechanisms, 198–199, 200*f*
    neoplastic changes, 197–198
    platforms, 199–202
    protein/peptide cancer vaccines, 201
    target antigens, 198
    tumorigenic process, 197–198
    viral vectors, 201–202
Candidate drug target profile (CDTP), 134, 136*t*
Cannabis, 183
Capsule formulations, 237, 238
Carbamazepine, 12
Carbonic anhydrase, 8–9
Carbutamide, 8–9
Carcinogenicity, 297
Carcinogenicity testing, 183–184
Cardiovascular system, toxicity, 102–103
CD19–CAR T-cell therapy, 128–129
Cell-based assays, 71–72
    advantages and disadvantages, 72*t*
    readouts, 76–77
    test systems, characteristics, 162*t*
    types, 72*f*
Cell-based Caco-2 permeability assay, 137–138
Cell-based cancer vaccines, 199–201
Cell line expression optimization, 119
Cell therapy, 2–3, 40, 127*t*, 185
    adaptive cell therapy, 126–127
    blood transfusion, 126–127
    chimeric antigen receptor (CAR) T-cell therapy, 126–128
    lymphocyte infusions, 126–127

Cellular models, 52
    lung epithelial barrier, 53*f*
Centers for Medicare and Medicaid Services (CMS), 323
Centralized procedure, 307
Central nervous system
    BBB properties, 145
    brain exposure, 144–145
    cautions, 145
    drug delivery systems, 242–243
    tactics, 144–145
    unbound concentration, 144
    in vitro efflux transporter assay, 144–145
Cereblon E3 Ligase Modulation Drugs (CELMoD), 37
Cerivastatin, 339*t*
Chantix, expiry, 341*t*
Charge heterogeneity, antibody, 118
Chemical Abstracts (CAs), 285
Chemical Genomics Center (NIH), 71
Chemical toxicity, 174
Chemistry
    20*th* century discoveries, 3
    developments, 3–4
    natural product, 6–7, 8*t*
    synthetic, 6, 8*t*
    see also Medicinal chemistry
Chemoreceptors, 65
Chemotherapy, 6, 7
Cheng–Prusoff equation, 163
'Cherry picking,' compounds, 66, 86
Children, special populations, 299
Chimeric antigen receptor (CAR) T-cell therapy, 40
    CAR T-cell manufacture, 128
    clinical trial outcomes, 128–129
    intracellular domain, 128
    principle, 127*f*
Chimpanzee adenovirus (ChAd), 189
Chinese hamster ovary (CHO) cell systems, 112
Chloramphenicol, 6
Chloroform, 3–4
Chlorothiazide, 8–9
Chlorpromazine, 12
Cholesterol ester transfer protein (CETP) inhibitor, 336–337
Choroideraemia, 41
Chromosomal abnormalities, 181–182
Chromosomal damage, 181–182
    mammalian cells, 181–182
    rodent haemopoietic cells, 182
Chronic hepatitis B (CHB) vaccine
    cellular immune responses, 192–193
    DNA HBsAg prime, 193
    immune tolerance, 193
    multicentre phase II GS-4774 trial, 193
    prophylactic vaccines, 193
Chronic toxicology studies, 178–181
    duration, 178–179, 180*t*
    experimental design, 179–180
    genotoxicity, 181
    immunotoxicity, 180
    long-term studies, 180–181
    mutagenicity test, 181–182
    recommended animals, 180*t*
    specific signs, 180
    specific testing, 181
Ciclosporin, 6
Ciliary clearance, 237
CIMAvax-EGF vaccine, 204
Cimetidine, 11, 340
Cinchona extract (quinine), 2, 4
Claims, patents, 282
Clearance
    active metabolites, 149–150

Clearance *(Continued)*
  biliary clearance, 148–149
  mechanisms, 145
  metabolic clearance, 145–148
  metabolite identification, 149
  optimization, 145
  prediction, 145
  renal clearance, 148
  in vitro and in vivo correlation (IVIVC) approach, 153
Clinical drug development
  adaptive pathways, 256–257
  discoveries, 12
  first in human (FIH) study, 248
  limitations, 245
  new medicine registration, 251–254
  paediatric drug development, 255
  pharmacokinetic/pharmacodynamic modelling, 251
  phase III studies, 251–254
  phase IV studies, 254–255
  phases, 247*t*
  phase 0 (microdose) studies, 255–256
  proof of concept study (POC), 250–251
  question-based drug development, 245–248
  safety measures, 249–250
  summary of product characteristics, 245, 246*f*
Clinical imaging, 259–280
  biodistribution, 263–266
  computed tomography, 261
  early phase development, 267–272
  human target validation, 262–263
  magnetic resonance imaging, 260–261
  oncology, 271–272
  optical imaging, 261–262
  patient stratification, 272–273
  pharmacodynamics, 267
  positron emission tomography, 259–260
  precision medicine, 273
  target interaction, 267
  ultrasound, 261–262
Clinical medicine, 14
Clinical studies, marketing, 315
Clinical tractability
  challenges and risks, 58
  disease prevention, 57
  early assessment, 57
  modality selection, 59
  on-target toxicity, 58
  patient selection, 57
Clinical trial application (CTA), 302
Clinical trials
  children, 299
  regulation, 304–305
Clopidogrel, 339*t*
Clozapine, 28
Clustered regularly interspaced short palindromic repeats [CRISPR]–CRISPR-associated
    protein [Cas] technology, 50–51, 131
Cocaine, 214–215
Colorectal cancer, 206
Colour quench effect, 73
Committee on the Safety of Drugs (UK), 14
Common Technical Document (CTD), 307–308
Comparability, 301–302
Compartment absorption and transit (CAT) model, 152–153
Complementarity-determining regions (CDRs), 112
Complement-dependent cytotoxicity, 39
Compound logistics, 85–86
Computed tomography (CT), 261
Concerned Member States (EU), 305
Confocal imaging, 79
Construct validity, 170–171
Continued Medical Education (CME), 312, 318

Controlled release, drugs, 241
Conus magus, 93–94
Conventional therapeutic drugs, 35–37
Copolymers, 239
Copyright, 289
Core battery, safety pharmacology test, 175, 176*t*
Corpora non agunt nisi fixata (Ehrlich), 7
Cosmeceuticals, 35
Cost-benefit analysis, 31
Cost-effectiveness, 30
Costs
    identification, 30
    research and development (R&D), 333–337
Cost-utility analysis, 30
CPHPC crosslinking agent, 94
CRISPR sequence, 41
Critical micelle concentration, 239
Critical path analysis, 222
Cryptate molecule, 75
Cure, permanent, 27
Cyclodextrins, 240
Cyclooxygenase-2 inhibitor (COX-2), 340
CYP
    induction, 142–143
    phenotyping, 142
    see also Cytochrome P450 (CYP450)
CYP inhibition
    competitive (reversible), 140, 141*f*
    cytochrome P450 (CYP450), 99, 142
    time-dependent (mechanism based) (TDI), 140–141, 142*f*
    uptake and efflux transporter inhibition, 141–142
CYT009-GhrQb vaccine (Cytos), 210
Cytochrome P450 (CYP450), 99
    inhibition, 99
Cytokine release, 185
Cytokine release syndrome (CRS), 39, 128–129
Cytotoxicity assays, 101

D

Darmstadt, 4–5
Data
    exclusivity, 308–309
    variability, 69*f*
Databases, 151
Decentralized procedure, 306
Delayed release, drugs, 241
DELFIA (dissociation-enhanced lanthanide fluoroimmuno assay), 71*f*, 75
Dementia, therapeutic vaccines, 213–214
Dendritic cell cancer vaccines, 199–201
Desferrioxamine (DFO), 266
Developability classification system (DCS), 235
Developmental toxicology studies, 297
Dexilant, expiry, 341*t*
Diabetes, 209–210
    type 1, 209–210
    type 2, 210
Diazoxide, 8–9
Dichloroisoprenaline, 11
Diethylene glycol, 13
Diethyl ether, 3–4
Digitalis, 2, 6
Diphenylhydantoin, 183
Direct to Consumer (DTC) advertising, 317
Disabilities, present, 22–23
Disease
    alleviation of effects, 27
    components, 22*f*
    concepts of, 19–22
    defined, 20
    nature of, 19–32, 25*f*

Disease (*Continued*)
  permanent cure, 27
  prevention, 23–24, 27, 57
Disease modification, 33–34
Disintegrating agents, 238
Disopyramide, 175–176
Displacement assay, 163
Dissociative fluorescence enhancement, 75
Dissolution process, 235
Dissolution rate, 235
Disvalue, 21–22
  components, 22–23
DNA vaccines, 201, 204
  hypertension, 211
  multiple sclerosis, 209
  type 2 diabetes, 210
  vector, 188–190
Documents, patents, 284
Dofetilide, 177
Domain of validity (DoV), 52
Dorzolamide, 8–9
Dose
  capping, 327–328*b*
  escalation protocol, 177–178
  prediction, 151–154
Dose range-finding (DRF) study, 177–178
Downstream antibody purification optimization, 119
Drapetomania, 21
Droperidol, 175–176
Drug delivery systems
  biopharmaceutical drug, 241–242
  central nervous system, 242–243
  liposomes, 240
  micelles, 239–240, 239*f*
  modified-release drug formulations, 241
  nanotechnology, 240, 241*t*
  polymers and surfactants, 238–239
  principles of, 238–243
Drug development
  attrition rates, 101–104, 333*f*, 342
  benefit/risk, 222
  clinical *see* Clinical drug development
  components, 219–222, 220*f*
  costs, 336–337
  costs associated, 219
  critical path analysis, 222
  data *vs.* question-based approach, 218*t*
  decision-making process, 223–224
  and discovery, 223
  efficacy assessment, 297–300
  environment, 303–304
  key decisions, 217, 218*f*
  leadership, 219
  model-based, 172–173
  nature of, 217–219
  orphan drugs, 303
  paediatric, 255
  patient safety, 222
  pipelines, 333*f*
  process, 293–304
  process-driven view, 217, 218*f*
  project management, 219
  project plan, 221*f*, 222
  project team and skills, 219
  quality assessment, 293–295
  quick win/fast fail model, 346*f*
  recent introductions, 345
  regulation, 293–304
  safety assessment, 295–297
  vasoactive amines, 222

Drug discovery
  assay development phase, 62–63
  clinical tractability, 57–58
  future trends, 345–347
  'golden' age, 43
  hit/lead identification, 63–64
  lead optimization, 64
  mechanism of action, 59–60
  modality selection, 59
  patents, 284
  pipelines, 333f, 342
  project planning, 62
  quick win/fast fail model, 346f
Drug-drug interactions (DDI)
  cautions, 144
  prediction, 143
  tactics, 140–143
Drug formulation, antibody, 119
Druggable target, 42
Drug-induced liver injury, 103
Drug-likeness, 95, 159–160
Drug-like small molecules, 176–177
Drug metabolism and pharmacokinetics (DMPK), 134–158
  human PK/dose prediction, 134
  optimization, 135
  proof of mechanisms, 134
  roles, drug discovery phases, 134, 135t
Drug Ordinance (1962) (Sweden), 291
Drugs
  adverse reactions, 102
  conventional, 35–37
  inhaled, 101
  intravenously administered, 101
Drug targets, 7–10, 8t
  candidate profile (CDTP), 134, 136t
  characteristics, 43–44
  distribution, 44, 44t
  modality selection, 59
  project selection criteria, 56–62
  receptors, 11–12
  selection challenges, 43
  vs therapeutic targets, 26–27
  unmet medical need, 56–57
Dubow, David, 311–312
Durvalumab, 344 345
Dyestuffs industry, 5
Dysfunction, 20
  function and, 24–27

E

Early adopters, 316
Early-stage drug discovery projects, 62
Ebers papyrus, 1
Effect, defined, 27, 28
Effectiveness, 27–28, 324
Efficacy, 27, 28
  consideration, 302
  doses, prediction, 154
Efflux transporter inhibition, 141–142
Efflux transporters, 141–142
EGFR receptor kinase inhibitors, 161f
Ehrlich, Paul, 3, 7, 65
Elderly, special populations, 299
Elion, Gertrude, 10–11
E-marketing, 317–318
Environment, drug development, 303–304
Enzyme-linked immunosorbent assay (ELISA), 76
  binding assay, 117
  receptor binding assay (RBA), 117

Enzymes, 65
Epilepsy models, 167–168*t*
Epileptogenesis models, 167–168*t*
Epinephrine, 4–5
Epstein–Barr virus (EBV) vaccines, 194
Equivalence, patents, 282
Ergot alkaloids, 6
Erythropoietin, 38
Esomeprazole, 339*t*
Estradiol, 237
Etanercept, 339*t*
Ethanol, 183
Ethnic differences, 299
E3 ubiquitin ligase complex, 37
Europe
    marketing, 305–307
    regulation, 304–305
European Commission, 307
European Economic Community (EEC), 291
European Medicines Agency (EMA), 293
European Patent Office, 285
Europium (Eu^{3+}) chelates, 75
Exon switching, 124*f*
Experimental medicine, 259
Exploratory toxicology studies, 177–178
External reference pricing (ERP), 321, 321*t*
Ex vivo autologous approach, 41

F

Face validity, 170
Fat mass and obesity (FTO) gene intron, 52
Fentanyl, 237
[^{18}F]-Fluorodeoxyglucose-positron emission tomography (FDG-PET) imaging
    Alzheimer's disease (AD), 270*f*
    oncology, 271
Financial-based agreements, 327–328*b*
First-in-class drug, 345
First in human (FIH) study, 248
    dose range, 248–249
    pharmacokinetic measures, 250
    single ascending dose (SAD), 248
    study design, 248
    study population, 249
FlashPlate, 73
Flow cytometry/FACS, 118
Fluorescence
    AlphaScreen, 76
    intensity, 74
    lifetime analysis, 76
    polarization (FP), 75
    quench assays, 74
    resonance energy transfer (FRET), 74, 74*f*
    technologies, 74–76
    time resolved, 74–75
Fluorescence correlation methods
    spectroscopy, 76
Fluorescence Imaging Plate Reader, 76–77
Fluorogenic assays, 74
Fluorometric assays, 76–77
Fluorophore, 74
Fluticasone/salmeterol, 339*t*
Focus groups, 315
Folic acid synthesis, 9*f*
Food and Drug Administration (FDA), 91
    Black Box Warnings, 103
    efficacy, 299
    IND approval, 301
    marketing, 305
    paediatric studies, 299
    patents, 287–288

Food and Drug Administration (*Continued*)
   recent introductions, 345
Food and Drugs Act (USA)
   1906, 13
   1937, 13
Food, Drug and Cosmetics Act, 273
Formal toxicology studies, 178
Formulation, 237–238
Forteo, expiry, 341*t*
Four humours, 1–2
Fragment-based screening, 80
France, health technology assessment (HTA), 312
Freedom to operate, 284
Frohlich, Bill, 311–312
Functional cell assay, 118
Functional MRI
   advantages, 276
   Alzheimer's disease (AD), 270–271
Function and dysfunction, 24–27
Furosemide, 8–9

G

Gene-editing technology, 41, 131, 132*f*
General pharmacology, 295
Gene silencing, 125, 125*f*
Gene therapy, 40–41
   adenine deaminase severe combined immunodeficiency (ADA–SCID),
      33–34
   autologous ex vivo gene therapy, 129–131, 130*f*
   gene-editing technology, 131
   objective, 129
   in vivo delivery, 129–131, 130*f*
Genetic cancer vaccines, 201
Genetic screens, 52
Genome, 26
Genome editing, 52
Genome-wide association studies (GWASs), 45–46, 47*f*
   databases, 46
   hearing loss, 48
   Mendelian randomization, 48
   obesity, 48
   principles, 46*f*
   single nucleotide polymorphisms, 45–46
   statistically significant, 45–46
Genomics, 43
Genotoxicity, 181, 182, 297
Germ theory of disease (Pasteur), 3
Ghrelin, 93–94, 94*f*
Glargine, 6–7
Glibenclamide, 8–9
Glutamic acid decarboxylase (GAD), 210
Glycogen synthase kinase-3 beta (GSK3β), 262
Glycosylation profile, antibody, 118
GOD-gels, 241
Good laboratory practice (GLP), 171
G-protein-coupled receptors (GPCRs), 37, 65, 93, 164–165
G-protein-coupled transmembrane receptors, 43
Guideline M3, 296
GVAX vaccines, 199, 206–207
GV1001 vaccine, 206

H

Halofantrine, 175–176
Haloperidol, 28
Harm, 21–22
Harris Interactive, 312
H_2 blockers, 43
Health, 20
   defined, 20

Health technology assessment (HTA)
    France, 312
    Germany, 322–323
    health authorities, 322
    United Kingdom, 322–323
    United States, 323
Hearing loss, genes involved, 48
Heat-killed *Mycobacterium vaccae*, 196
Hepatic metabolic clearance, 146
Hepatoxicity, 103
Herbal remedies, 1–2
hERG channel, 163
High content screening (HCS), 79–80
High Mobility Group Box1, 103
High-throughput electrophysiology assays, 78
High-throughput medicinal chemistry, 96
High-throughput screening (HTS), 65–90
    activity cascade, 68, 69*f*
    compound logistics, 85–86, 86*f*
    data analysis, 83–85
    future trends, 65–67
    historical perspective, 65–67
    lead discovery, 67–85
    profiling (HTP), 86–87
    robotics, 82–83
    screening libraries, 85–86
hIL1*b*Qb vaccine (Cytos), 210
Histone deacetylase (HDAC) inhibitor, 93*f*
Hitchings, George, 10–11
Holmes, Oliver Wendell, 2
Home-country patenting, 286
Homology-directed repair (HDR), 50–51
5HT receptor ligands, 163
HTRF (Homogeneous Time-Resolved Fluorescence), 75
HuMAb-Mouse, 112
Human antimouse antibody (HAMA) immune reactions, 112
Human genes, 43–44
Human immunodeficiency virus (HIV) vaccines
    CD8+ T-cell responses, 191
    chimpanzee adenovirus 63 (ChAd63) vector prime, 192
    'kick and kill' trials, 192
    nonhuman primate models, 191
    REDUC and BCN02 trials, 192
    RIVER trial, 192
    RV144 trial, 190
    STEP HVTN 502 and Phambili (HVTN503) trials, 190
    STEP trial, 190, 192
    Vacc-4X trial, 191
    VAX003 and 004 trials, 190
Human lifespan, 23*f*
Human papillomavirus (HPV) vaccines, 194–195
Human pharmacology studies, 297–298
Human target validation
    fMRI approaches, 262
    PET imaging, 263
Human telomerase reverse transcriptase (hTERT) protein, 204
Humoral immunity, 186
H56 (SSI) vaccine, 196
Hybridoma generation, 111–112
Hydralazine, 8–9
Hydroxypropyl methylcellulose (HPMC) capsule, 238
Hypertension, therapeutic vaccines, 210–211

I

Idiosyncratic toxicity, 102
Imaging studies, 259–280
    challenges to implementation, 274–276
    clinical drug development, 276
    as a surrogate marker, 273–274
    target occupancy studies, 276

Imaging studies *(Continued)*
   see also Clinical imaging
Imipramine, 183
Immune evasion mechanisms, 198–199, 200*f*
Immunization procedures, 41
Immunoglobulin G (IgG) isotype, 109, 110*f*
Immunotoxicity, 180, 184
IMS Health Inc, 312
Incremental cost-effectiveness ratios (ICERs), 322
Industrial applicability, invention, 284
Inert diluents/fillers, 238
Infection theory (Koch), 3
Inflammation, 33
Infliximab, 339*t*
Information sources, patents, 285
Inhaled drugs, 101
Innate gene silencing mechanism, 125*f*
Innovative Medicines Initiative (IMI), 328–329
Innovators, 316
In silico assessment, antibody, 118
Institute for quality and efficiency in Health Care (IQWiG), 322–323
Insulin, 6–7, 38
Insulin lispro, 6–7
Integrated Summaries of Efficacy (ISE), 308
Integrated Summaries of Safety (ISS), 308
 Intellectual property (IP), 281–289 *see also* Patents
Intelligent materials, 240
Intercontinental Marketing Services (IMS), 311–312
International Conference on Harmonization (ICH), 291–292
   classification, 298*t*
   clinical studies, 298*t*
   guideline E6, 304
   guideline M3, 296
   guideline Q5A-E, 300
   guideline Q6B, 300
   guideline S1A, 183
   guideline S7A, 175
   guideline S1B, 183
   guideline S1C, 183
   harmonization process, 292*f*
   terms of reference, 291
International Price Indexing (IPI), 323
Internet domain names, 289
Intranasal administration of drugs, 237
Intravenously administered drugs, 101
INVAC 1 vaccine, 204
Inventive step, 283–284
Investigational drug, 57–58
Investigational New Drug (IND)
   approval (FDA), 301
   regulation, 294*f*
Investigative skills, drug development, 219
In vitro and in vivo correlation (IVIVC) approach, 153
In vivo pharmacodynamic (PD) assays, 118
In vivo pharmacokinetic (PK) assays, 118
IonWorks Quattro, 78
Isotretinoin, 183
Ivermectin, 6

J

Januvia, expiry, 341*t*
Japan
   marketing, 307
   regulation, 305
Japanese Patent Office, 285

K

KefauverûHarris Drug Control Act, 312
Keratin 18 proteins, 103

Key opinion leaders (KOL), 318
Key stakeholder, 328
Kinetic determination, 117–118
Knockout databases, 50–51
Koch, Robert, 3

L

Label-free detection platforms, 79
Laggards/conservatives, 316
LANCE, 75
Law of Mass Action, 11
Lead discovery, high-throughput screening (HTS), 67–85
Lead-like property, 95
Lead optimization, 64
Lead optimization stage, 68
Lenalidomide, 339*t*
Levodopa, 242–243
Lidocaine, 295
Life-years saved per patient treated, 30
Ligand binding assays, 72–74
Ligand efficiency (LE), 96–97
Ligand-lipophilicity efficiency (LLE), 96–97
Lipitor, expiry, 341*t*
Lipophilic drug molecules, 239
Lipophilicity, 100
Liposomes, 240, 240*f*
Local tolerance studies, 297
Lovenox, expiry, 341*t*
Lowest observed adverse effect level (LOAEL), 248
Lubricants, 238
Lung cancer, vaccines, 203–204
Lung epithelial barrier, cellular models, 53*f*

M

'Magic' bullets, 7
Magnesium stearate, 238
Magnetic resonance imaging (MRI), 260–261
    Alzheimer's disease (AD), 269
    contrast-enhanced, 261
    functional, 261
    multiple sclerosis (MS), 268–269
    oncology, 271
    structural, 260
Major depressive disorder (MDD), 262
Major histocompatibility complex (MHC) molecules, 128–129
Managed entry agreements (MEA), 326–328, 327–328*b*
    taxonomy, 327*f*
Managerial skills, drug development, 219
Manhattan plot, 49*f*
Manufacturing classification system (MCS), 238
Market
    identification, 315
    research, 315
Market access (MA), 311, 318–319
Marketing, 311–331
    authorization, 305–307
    background, 311–312
    competition assessment, 316–317
    competitive differentiation, 328*b*
    e-marketing, 317–318
    environment, changing, 328–329
    Europe, 305–307
    future trends, 329–330
    health technology assessment (HTA), 321–323
    Japan, 307
    key stakeholder, 328
    managed entry agreements, 326–328
    market identification, 315

Marketing *(Continued)*
  new way, 330
  plans, 313
  R&D productivity, 328–329
  risk and uncertainty, 324–326
  traditional pharmaceutical, 315–318
  United States, 307
Mauvein, 4
Maximum tolerated dose (MTD), 177–178
McMaster Health Index, 30
Medicinal chemistry, 91–107
  attrition, 101–104
  lead identification/generation, 95–97
  lead optimization, 98–101
  New Chemical Entities (NCEs), 91
  target selection/validation, 92–94
Medicines Act (1968) (UK), 14, 291
Melanoma, vaccine, 203
Melphalan, 242–243
Mendelian inheritance, 45
Mendelian randomization, 48
6-Mercaptopurine, 10–11
Metabolic clearance optimization
  cautions, 147–148
  drug metabolizing enzymes, 145–146
  failure, 146
  hepatic metabolic clearance, 146
  nucleases, 146
  peptides, 146
  small molecules, 146
  tactics, 146–147
Metabolite identification, 149, 151
Methamphetamine, 214–215
Methylphenidate (Ritalin), 12
Mevastatin, 6
Micelles, 239–240, 239f, 241t
Microbeads, 73
Microfluidic encapsulation technologies, 112
Microplates, 73
Microtitre plates, 79
Miniaturization, 70t, 82
Minimal anticipated biological effect level (MABEL), 248
Minimal biologically active level (MABEL), 172
Mipomersen, 126
Modality agnostic approach, 61–62
Modified-release drug formulations, 241
Modified T cells, cancer, 40
Modified vaccinia ankara (MVA), 189
Molecular assays, 162t
Molecular profiling, 93
Monoclonal antibodies (mAbs), 38–39, 108, 266, 344
Monogenic inheritance, 45
Morbidity, 22–23
Morphine, 6
Multi-criteria decision analysis (MCDA), 229–230
Multiple sclerosis (MS), 208–209, 268–269
Multiwell plates, 82
Mutagenicity, 181
Mutual recognition, 306
Myelin-reactive T cells (MRTCs), 209

N

Nanoemulsions, 241t
Nanogels, 241t
Nanoprobes, 241t
Nanotechnology, 240, 241t
National Health Service (NHS), 322
National Institute for Health and Clinical Excellence (NICE),
  27–28, 319, 322

National Institutes of Health (NIH)
    Chemical Genomics Center, 71
National procedure, 305–306
Naturalist view, 21
Natural products, 6–7, 8*t*
Net present value (NPV), 338
NeuVax, 204
New Chemical Entities (NCEs), 91, 285, 342
New medicine registration, 253–254*t*
    data integrity, 252
    inclusion criteria, 252
    primary endpoint selection, 252
New Medicines Database, 316
Next-generation DNA sequencing (NGS), 119
Nicotine, 237
Nicotine addiction vaccines, 214
Nitroglycerin, 237
Nitrous oxide, 3–4
Nivolumab, 339*t*
Nonalcoholic steatohepatitis (NASH), 50
Nonclinical pharmacological studies, 174–185
    first-in-human studies, 174
    safety pharmacology, 175–177
    toxicology *see* Toxicology
Noncoding RNAs, 43–44
Nonhomologous end joining (NHEJ), 50–51
Noninsulin-dependent diabetes mellitus or adult-onset diabetes, 210
Nonlipophilic drugs, 240
Nonpatent regulatory exclusivity, 309
Nonspecific protein–protein interactions, antibody, 118
No observed adverse effect level (NOAEL), 172, 177–178
Normality, deviation from, 20–21
Normative view, 21–22
Nottingham Health Profile, 30
Novelty, 283, 300–303
Nucinersen, 124*f*
Nucleic acid-based vaccines, 188–190
Nucleotide therapy, 39–40
    antisense oligonucleotides, 123–126
    approved oligonucleotides, 126
    small interfering RNA, 123–126
    target organ, 125
Nusinersen treatment, 126
Nutriceuticals, 35

O

Obesity, genes associated, 48
Off-target binding, 118
Off-target pharmacology, 174
Olanzepine, 339*t*
Oligonucleotide therapy
    antisense oligonucleotides, 123–126
    approved oligonucleotides, 126
    small interfering RNA, 123–126
    target organ, 125
Oncostatin M (OSM), 48
OncoVAX, 206
On-target pharmacology, 174
Opioids, 237
Opioid vaccines, 214
Opportunity costs, 336
Optical imaging, 261–262
Oral bioavailability, 135–140
    prediction, 152–153
Organic Anion Transporter 3 (OAT3), 103
Organic anion transporters (OATs), 141, 148
Organic chemistry, 14
Oromucosal administration of drugs, 237
Orphan drugs, 303
Outcomes-based agreements, 327–328*b*

P

PABA (*p*-aminobenzoic acid), 9*f*
Paclitaxel, 6
Paediatric drug development, 255
Paediatric investigation plan (PIP), 255
Paediatric Regulation (2007) (EU), 299
Paediatric Research Enquiry Act (2007), 299
Paediatric use marketing authorization (PUMA), 299
p-aminobenzoic acid (PABA), 8, 9*f*
Parallel artificial membrane permeability assay (PAMPA), 137–138
Parallelization, 67
Paris Convention for the Protection of Industrial Property, 285–286
Passive distribution model, 264
Passive immunotherapy, 199
Passive targeting, 240
Pasteur, Louis, 3
Patent and Trademark Office (US), 285
Patent Cooperation Treaty, 287
Patents, 281–289
    bibliographic details, 282
    claims, 282
    defined, 281–282
    description, 282
    development compound protection, 285–289
    documents, 284
    drug discovery, 284
    expiry, 341*t*
    filing application, 285–289
    information sources, 285
    maintenance, 287
    New Chemical Entities (NCEs), 285
    offices, regional, 287
    pharmaceutical inventions, 283
    products and processes, 282
    professional evaluation, 284
    protection, 308
    requirements, 283–284
    rights enforcement, 288–289
    scientific evaluation, 284
    specification, 282
    state of the art (prior art), 284
    subject categories, 282
    Supplementary Protection Certificate, 308
    term extension, 287–288
Patients
    registry, 327–328*b*
    special populations, 299
    stratification, 259
Patisiran, 126
Payer's value system, 319
Pembrolizumab, 339*t*, 344–345
Penicillins, 6, 242–243
Peptide/protein-based vaccines, 188
Peptides, 38
Peptide transporter (PepT1), 138
Peptide vaccines, 212
Periodic safety update report (PSUR), 232
Perkin, William Henry, 4
Personalized medicine (PM), 303
Personalized peptide vaccine (PPV), 207
Personalized therapies, 303
P-glycoprotein (Pgp), 99–100, 141–142
Phage display, 39
Phage display technology, 113–114
Pharmaceutical Affairs Law (1943) (Japan), 291
Pharmaceutical Benefits Advisory Committee (Australia), 31
Pharmaceuticals, 1–18, 234–244
    19th century, 2
    administration routes, 236–237
    antecedents/origins, 1–2

Pharmaceuticals *(Continued)*
    dosage forms, 234, 236–237
    drug delivery systems, 238–243
    drug substance stability, 234
    emerging, 2–14
    formulation, 237–238, 243
    interventions, 35
    milestones, 14, 15–16*t*
    patents, 283
    preformulation studies, 234–236
    pricing, 309
    regulation *see* Regulation
    value proposition, 319
Pharmacodynamics (PD), 57–58, 259, 298
    clinical imaging, 267
Pharmacoeconomics, 28–31, 320
Pharmacoepidemiology, 28–31
Pharmacogenetic tests, 228*t*
Pharmacokinetic/pharmacodynamic (PK/PD) models, 172–173
Pharmacokinetics (PK), 151–154, 152*f*, 297 *see also* Drug metabolism and pharmacokinetics (DMPK)
Pharmacological hypothesis, 43
Pharmacological Institute, Dorpat, 3
Pharmacological tractability, 60–61
Pharmacology, 3, 159–173
    allosteric, 159
    binding assays, 163
    candidate drug, 162
    development phase, 171–172
    efficacy, 165–166
    evaluation, 159–163
    general, 295
    good laboratory practice (GLP), 171
    human, studies, 297–298
    nonclinical safety assessment, 174–185
    primary, 174, 295
    profiling, 164–171
    safety, 161, 175–177, 295–297
    secondary, 174–175
    selectivity screening, 162–163
    test systems, characteristics, 161, 162*t*
    in vitro, 165–166
    in vivo, 161, 166–167
Pharmacovigilance, 231–232
Phenobarbital, 6
Phenomenology, 20, 21
Phenome-wide association studies (PheWASs), 46, 47*f*
Phenotypic screening approach, 63
Phenytoin, 6
Phocomelia, 174, 291
Phosphothiorate single-stranded oligonucleotides, 125
Physiologically based pharmacokinetic (PBPK) model, 172–173
Pipelines, 333*f*, 342
Planar patch-clamp instruments, 78
Plasma cells screening, 112
Plasma concentration time profile, 154
Plavix, expiry, 341*t*
Pneumococcal conjugate vaccine, 339*t*
Polyclonality, 38–39
Polymers, 238–239
Population pharmacokinetic modelling (POPPK), 172–173
Positron emission tomography (PET), 259–260, 260*t*
    Alzheimer's disease (AD), 269, 270
    biodistribution, 263–266
    human target validation, 263
    transgenic models, 169
Postapproval safety studies (PASSs), 232
Postmarketing surveillance, 231–232
Poxviruses, 201–202
Precision medicine, 273

Precision medicine (PM), 259
Prediction, toxicity, 103–104
Predictive validity, 171
Preexposure prophylaxis (PrEP), 33–34
Preformulation studies
    components, 234
    dissolution rate, 235
    particle size and morphology, 236
    solubility, 235
    stability, 235–236
Pregabalin, 12
Prevention, disease, 23–24, 27
Price volume agreements, 327–328b
Pricing, 309, 319–324
    external reference, 321, 321t
    health technology assessorsÆ perspective, 321–323
    industry perspective, 323–324
    value-based pricing (VBP), 319–321
Primary pharmacodynamic studies, 160–161
Primary pharmacology, 174, 295
Prime vaccination using a recombinant replication-competent vaccinia virus (PROSTVAC-V), 201
Prior art (state of the art), patents, 284
Procaine, 5
Process-driven view, drug development, 217, 218f
Processes, patents, 282
Product characteristics, safety assessment, 230, 230–231t
Productivity (1970–2000), 17f
Product life-cycle
    decline phase, 314
    development phase, 313
    growth phase, 313
    introduction phase, 313
    maturity phase, 313–314
Products
    features/attributes/benefits/limitations (FABL), 316
    future, 329
    patents, 282
Profiling, 86–87
Profitability, 338
Prognosis, 22–23
Programmed death-ligand 1 (PD-L1), 344–345
Project evaluation and review technique (PERT) chart, 222
Promazine, 12
Promethazine, 12
Pronethalol, 11
Prontosil, 7–8
Proof of concept (POC) study
    designs, 251
    drug development, 92
Propranolol, 11
Proprotein convertase subtilisin–kexin type 9 (PCSK9), 48, 337
Prostate cancer vaccines, 204–205
PROSTVAC vaccine, 205
Protein/peptide cancer vaccines, 201
Proteins, 38, 44
Proteolysis targeting chimeras (PROTACs), 37, 136–137
Proteome, 26
Proteomics and metabolomics, 52
Provider
    therapeutic decision making, 319
    value system, 319
Public Health Service (USA), 31
Pulmonary administration of drugs, 237
Pyrimethamine, 10–11

Q

QT interval prolongation tests, 175–177
Quality-adjusted life years (QALYs), 30, 320

Quality assessment, 293–295
Quality by Design (QbD), 237
Quality chemical probe, 93
Quality module, 293
Quality-of-life estimate, 30
Quantitative systems pharmacology (QSP), 171–172
Question-based approach, 217, 218*t*
Question-based drug development, 245–248
Quetiapine, 339*t*
Quick win/fast fail model, 346*f*
Quinidine, 175–176
Quinine (*Cinchona* extract), 2, 4

R

Radioactive assays, homogeneous formats, 73
Reactive metabolites identification
  cautions, 151
  tactics, 151
Reactome, 50
Reagent production, 66
Receptors, 65
Receptor-targeted drugs, 11–12
Recombinant DNA technology, 8*t*
Recombinant human growth hormone, 38
Recombinant yeast-based vaccines, 190
Rectal administration of drugs, 237
Reference Member State (RMS), 306
Regulation, 290–310
  administrative rules, 308–309
  drug development process, 293–304
  Europe, 304–305
  historical perspective, 290–291
  international harmonization, 291–292
  Japan, 305
  procedures, 304–308
  process, 13–14
  roles/responsibilities, 292–293
  USA, 305
Relative biodistribution, 264
Renal cancer, 205–206
Renal clearance optimization, 148
  cautions, 148
  compounds, 148*f*
  tactics, 148
Renal toxicity, 103
Repeated-dose toxicity studies, 296*t*
Reporter gene assays, 77–78, 77*f*
Reproductive toxicology studies, 182–183, 227, 297
Research and development (R&D), 328–329, 333–337
  biotechnically derived medicines, 344
  compound attrition, 333*f*
  recent introductions, 345
  total global pharmaceutical, 334*f*
  US biopharmaceutical sector, 334*f*
Research Disclosure, 286
Reyes' syndrome, 28
Rheumatoid arthritis, 33
Risk, 324
Ritalin (methylphenidate), 12
Rituximab, 339*t*
RNA-based therapies, 126*t*
RNA-induced silencing complex (RISC), 39, 125
RNA interference, 125*f*
RNA vaccines, 189, 201
Robotics, high-throughput screening (HTS), 82–83
Rofecoxib, 340
Rosuvastatin, 103
Routine pharmacovigilance, 231–232

S

Safety
  biopharmaceuticals, 302
  clinical studies, 299–300
  pharmacology, 161, 295–297
  see also Chronic toxicology studies
Safety assessment, drug development
  benefit/risk assessment, 229–230
  in early clinical trials, 225–226
  identified risks management, 232
  missing/incomplete information, 232
  phase II clinical studies, 226–229
  phase III clinical studies, 229–230
  postmarketing surveillance, 231–232
  product characteristics, 230, 230–231*t*
  risk assessment, first-in-human studies, 226*t*
  routine pharmacovigilance, 231–232
  study design, 225–226
Safety pharmacology, 175–177
  core battery, 175
  follow-up studies, 175
  protocol-driven studies, 175
  QT interval prolongation tests, 175–177
  supplementary tests, 175
Sales
  pattern, 338, 338*t*
  revenues, 337–340
Salvarsan, 7–8, 65, 66*f*
Scaffolds
  privileged, 96
  'scaffold hunter' approach, 97
Scintillation proximity assays, 73, 73*f*
Scopolamine, 237
Screening process
  fragment-based, 80
  libraries, 85–86
Search tools, 151
Secondary pharmacodynamic studies, 160–161
Secondary pharmacology, 174–175
Selective local exposure, 236–237
Serious adverse events (SAE), 227–228
Seroquel, expiry, 341*t*
Sertürner, Friedrich, 4
Serum stability, antibody, 119
Severe acute respiratory syndrome coronavirus 2 (SARS-Cov-2), 347
Sickness Impact Profile, 30
Signal window, 69*f*
'Signatures,' biological, 4
Single ascending dose (SAD), 248
Single-dose studies, 296
Single-dose toxicity study protocol, 178*f*
Single nucleotide polymorphisms (SNPs), 45–46, 52
Small interfering RNAs (siRNAs), 39, 125
Small-molecule drugs, 35–37, 38*b*
Smoking, gene expression, 25
Solid gel formulations, 239
Solubility, 235
  antibody, 118–119
Solubilizing agent, 235
Special populations, 299
Spending, 333–337
Spinal muscular atrophy (SMA), 124*f*
Sprycel, expiry, 341*t*
Stakeholders
  key, 328
  values, 320*f*, 328
State of the art (prior art), patents, 284
Stem cell therapies, 185

Stokes shift, 74
Streptomycin, 6
Structural-based toxicity, 103
Structural classification of natural products (SCONP), 97
Structure-activity relationship (SAR), 67
Strychnine, 6
Subunit vaccines, 187–188
Sulfanilamides, 7–9, 290–291
Sulfonamides, 8, 183
    dynasty, 10*f*
Summary of product characteristics (SPC), 227, 230, 230–231*t*, 245
Supplementary Protection Certificate (SPC), 287–288
Surfactants, 238–239
Surgical shock, 12
Survival motor neuron (SMN) protein, 126
Suspected unexpected serious adverse reactions (SUSARs), 227–228
Sustained release, drugs, 241, 242*f*
Symptoms, 27
    present, 22–23
Synthetic chemistry, 6
Synthetic long peptides (SLPs), 188
Synucleinopathies, 213–214
Systemic exposure, 236–237

T

Tablets, formulation, 237
Tacrolimus, 6
Target
    biological studies, 64
    -directed drug discovery, 7–10
    engagement, 57–58
    interaction, 267
    interactions, 259
    pharmacological tractability, 60–61
    product profile, 62
    validation, 64, 259
    see also Drug targets
Target product profile (TTP), 62, 293
Target selection
    animal models, 45
    clinical context, 53, 53*t*
    CRISPR KO, 51*t*
    data expression, 48
    genetics, 45–48
    knockout databases, 50–51
    new targets validation, 51–52
    pathway analysis, 50
    public databases, 47*t*
    systematic literature searches, 50–51
    target mechanism of action, 52
    target modulation mechanisms, 44–45
    tractability assessment, 51
T-cell receptor (TCR)-T cells, 128–129
T cells, 211
Technical skills, drug development, 219
Temozolomide, 266
Teratogenicity, 181
Terfenadine, 175–176
Testosterone, 237
Tests
    characteristics, 161, 162*t*
    methods, hierarchy, 161
Tetracyclines, 6
TG4010, 203–204
TGN1412, 160
Thalidomide, 12, 291
Therapeutic antibodies
    alternative formats, 116*f*
    biological and biophysical assessment, 117–119
    chimerization and humanization, 112

Therapeutic antibodies *(Continued)*
  development project, 108–109
  disadvantages, 110
  discovery, 110–115
  examples, 109*t*
  Fc engineering, 115–117
  fragments, 115–117, 115*f*
  future perspective, 119–120
  manufacture, 117–119
  protein purity and fragmentation, 118
  serum half-life, 117
  structure and properties, 109–110, 110*f*
Therapeutics
  aims, 22–24
  bioelectronics, 42
  biological products, 37–40
  biomaterials, 41–42
  cell-based therapies, 40
  confirmatory, 299
  conventional therapeutic drugs, 35–37
  exploratory, 298
  gene editing, 41
  gene therapy, 40–41
  interventions, 19–20, 27, 33–35, 34*f*
  monoclonal antibodies, 38–39
  nucleotide-based therapies, 39–40
  outcomes, 27–28
  targets, 26–27
  therapeutic jungle, 312
  vaccines, 41
Therapeutic vaccines
  addiction, 215*f*
    cocaine and methamphetamine, 214–215
    nicotine addiction, 214
    opioid vaccines, 214
  allergic disorders, 211–213
  Alzheimer's disease, 213
  autoimmune diseases, 208–210
  biological feasibility, 186
  cancer vaccines, 197–208
  challenges, 186, 196–197, 197*f*
  chronic hepatitis B (CHB), 192–193
  dementia, 213–214
  diabetes, 209–210
  Epstein–Barr virus (EBV) vaccines, 194
  formulations and delivery systems, 187*f*
  HIV vaccines, 190–192
  human papillomavirus (HPV) vaccines, 194–195
  hypertension, 210–211
  immune exhaustion and dysfunction, 197
  for infectious diseases, 190–197
  live vectors, 189–190
  multiple sclerosis, 208–209
  nucleic acid-based vaccines, 188–190
  peptide/protein-based vaccines, 188
  subunit vaccines, 187–188
  synucleinopathies, 213–214
  tuberculosis vaccines, 195–196
  virus-like particles (VLPs), 188
  whole cell vaccines, 186–187
Thermal stability, antibody, 118
Thiazide diuretics, 175
Thioridazine, 175–176
Thought leaders, 318
Thyroxine, 6–7
Tight binders, 100–101
Tight capillary endothelium, 240
Time-dependent inhibition (TDI), 140–141, 142*f*
Timelines, 340–342
Time resolved fluorescence (TRF), 74–75
Tipapkinogen Sovacivec (TS) vaccine, 195

Tissue cross-reactivity studies, antibody, 119
Tissue plasminogen activator (tPA), 38
Tissues, measurement on isolated, 165–166
Tolbutamide, 8–9, 183
Tolerability, 297
Tolerance-inducing DC (tolDC)-based therapies, 209
Tool (reagent) production, 66
Torcetrapib, 336–337
Torsade de pointes, 175–176
Torsade des pointes syndrome, 102–103
Toxicity
    augmented, 102
    cardiovascular, 102–103
    idiosyncratic, 102
    on-target, 58
    prediction, 103–104
    renal, 103
    structural-based, 103
Toxicology
    acute, 179t
    ADME characteristics, 177
    in children, 184
    chronic studies, 178–181
    exploratory studies, 177–178
    formal studies, 178
    principle, 177
    regulatory, 296–297
    reproductive, 182–183
    reproductive/developmental, 297
    translational, 185
Tractability assessment, 51 see also Clinical tractability
Trademarks, 289
Transcriptome, 26
Transcriptomics, 52
Transcytosis, 243
Transdermal administration of drugs, 237
Transgenic mice, 112
Transgenic models
    gene knock out, 168
    imaging approaches, 169
    species differences, 170
    structural methods, 169–170
    validity criteria, 170–171
Translational toxicology, 185
Transplantation, 40
Transporters, 65
Trapping studies, 151
Trastuzumab, 339t
Trimethoprim, 10–11
Triptans, 237
TroVax vaccine, 205, 206
Truvada, expiry, 341t
Tuberculosis vaccines, 195–196
Tubocurarine, 6
Tumour-associated antigens (TAAs), 198
Tumour-associated peptides (TUMAPs), 205
Tumour-infiltrated lymphocytes (TILs), 198–199
Tumour-specific antigens (TSAs), 198

U

UK Biobank (UKBB), 46
UK Medicines Act 1968, 291
Uncertainty, 324
United States of America (USA)
    health technology assessment (HTA), 323
    marketing, 307
    regulation, 305
Uptake transporter inhibition, 141–142
Urokinase plasminogen-activator receptor (uPAR), 123–125
US Food and Drug Administration (FDA) Expedited Programs, 256–257t